Contemporary Issues in Cardiovascular Pathology

Cardiovascular Clinics Series

Brest	1/1	Hypertensive Cardiovascular Disease
Brest	1/2	Coronary Heart Disease
Brest	1/3	Cardiovascular Therapy
Downing	2/1	Congenital Heart Disease
White	2/3	International Cardiology
Gifford	3/1	Peripheral Vascular Disease
Engle	4/3	Pediatric Cardiology
Fowler	6/3	Diagnostic Methods in Cardiology
Vidt	7/1	Cleveland Clinic Cardiovascular Consultations
Brest et al.	7/2	Innovations in the Diagnosis and Management of Acute Myocardial Infarction
Spodick	7/3	Pericardial Diseases
Corday	8/1	Controversies in Cardiology
Rahimtoola	8/2	Coronary Bypass Surgery
Rios	8/3	Clinical Electrocardiographic Correlations
Onesti, Brest	9/1	Hypertension
Kotler, Segal	9/2	Clinical Echocardiography
Brandenburg	10/3	Office Cardiology
Castellanos	11/1	Cardiac Arrhythmias: Mechanisms and Management
Engle	11/2	Pediatric Cardiovascular Disease
Rackley	11/3	Critical Care Cardiology
Noble, Rothbaum	12/1	Geriatric Cardiology
Vidt	12/2	Cardiovascular Therapy
Rahimtoola	13/1	Controversies in Coronary Artery Disease
Spittell	13/2	Clinical Vascular Disease
Fowler	13/3	Noninvasive Diagnostic Methods in Cardiology
Goldberg	14/1	Coronary Artery Spasm and Thrombosis
Dreifus	14/2	Pacemaker Therapy
Conti	14/3	Cardiac Drug Therapy
Schroeder	15/1	Invasive Cardiology
Wenger	15/2	Exercise and the Heart
Josephson	15/3	Sudden Cardiac Death
Dreifus	16/1	Cardiac Arrhythmias: Electrophysiologic Techniques and Management
Frankl, Brest	16/2	Valvular Heart Disease: Comprehensive Evaluation and Management
Rackley	16/3	Advances in Critical Care Cardiology
Kotler, Steiner	17/1	Cardiac Imaging: New Technologies and Clinical Applications
Fisk	17/2	The Right Heart
McGoon	17/3	Cardiac Surgery, ed. 2
Mehta	18/1	Thrombosis and Platelets in Myocardial Ischemia

Contemporary Issues in Cardiovascular Pathology

Bruce F. Waller, M.D. | Editor

Professor of Pathology and Medicine
Director, Section of Cardiovascular Pathology
Indiana University School of Medicine
Research Associate
Krannert Institute of Cardiology
Indianapolis, Indiana

Cardiovascular Clinics

Albert N. Brest, M.D. | Editor-in-Chief

James C. Wilson Professor of Medicine
Director, Division of Cardiology
Jefferson Medical College
Philadelphia, Pennsylvania

F.A. DAVIS COMPANY, PHILADELPHIA

Printed in the United States of America

NOTE: As new scientific information becomes available through basic and clinical research, recommended treatments and drug therapies undergo changes. The author(s) and publisher have done everything possible to make this book accurate, up-to-date, and in accord with accepted standards at the time of publication. However, the reader is advised always to check product information (package inserts) for changes and new information regarding dose and contraindications before administering any drug. Caution is especially urged when using new or infrequently ordered drugs.

Library of Congress Cataloging in Publication Data

Cardiovascular clinics. 18/2

Philadelphia, F. A. Davis, 1969-
v. ill. 27 cm.
Editor: v. 1- A. N. Brest.
Key title: Cardiovascular clinics, ISSN 0069-0384.
1. Cardiovascular system—Diseases—Collected works. I. Brest, Albert N., ed.
[DNLM: W1 CA77N]
RC681.A1C27 616.1 70-6558
ISBN 0-8036-9031-2 MARC-S

Preface

In 1972 and 1973, Jesse E. Edwards, M.D., edited two outstanding issues of the CARDIOVASCULAR CLINICS, devoted to topics in cardiovascular pathology. During the subsequent 14 years, a broad range of new areas of investigation has emerged in cardiac pathology, resulting primarily from technical and therapeutic advances in clinical cardiology and cardiovascular surgery. Echocardiography, computed tomography, transluminal balloon angioplasty, laser radiation, and cardiac transplantation are some of the new clinical areas that have prompted intense interest in clinicopathologic correlations. This "renaissance" period of cardiovascular pathology was the stimulus to prepare another volume of CARDIOVASCULAR CLINICS devoted to cardiac pathology.

We have assembled a group of authors who have played major roles in contributing to our understanding in these new areas of cardiac pathology. Each chapter has been written with the general aim of providing subject material that will aid in the understanding and diagnosis of disease processes or shed light on the mechanism(s) of new therapeutic interventions. I hope that this volume will be valuable to cardiologists, surgeons, radiologists, and pathologists.

I express my appreciation to all of the contributors for their state-of-the-art presentations. I also thank Dr. Albert Brest for the opportunity to serve as Guest Editor for this issue, and Dr. Brest's secretary, Annette Foluch, for her assistance in assembling the manuscripts. A very special thanks goes to Sylvia K. Fields, Ed.D., Senior Medical Editor of F. A. Davis Company, for her dedication to making this issue a reality and her reassurance during times of frustration.

Bruce F. Waller, M.D.
Guest Editor

Editor's Commentary

Two early issues of the CARDIOVASCULAR CLINICS were devoted to clinicopathologic correlations. These two issues dealt with a wide variety of cardiac conditions, and most of that material is still as timely and informative as it was originally. No attempt is made in the current book either to duplicate or to update the earlier material. Instead, the present volume concentrates on those contemporary issues that currently occupy center stage in the practice of cardiovascular medicine. The subjects covered range from atherogenesis, thrombosis, thrombolytic therapy, balloon angioplasty, laser radiation, and coronary bypass grafts to myocarditis, cardiomyopathy, endomyocardial biopsy, and cardiac transplantation, and from bioprosthetic heart valve failure and pathology of cardiovascular prostheses to the floppy heart valve syndrome and the very elderly heart. Each of these contemporary subjects is examined in detail by distinguished investigators with broad experience. I am extremely grateful to Bruce Waller for his guidance in the development of this material, and we, in turn, are deeply indebted to the contributing authors for their exemplary contributions.

Albert N. Brest, M.D.
Editor-in-Chief

Contributors

James B. Atkinson, M.D., Ph.D.
Assistant Professor of Pathology
Vanderbilt University
Nashville, Tennessee

Margaret E. Billingham, M.D.
Associate Professor of Pathology
Director, Cardiac Pathology
Department of Pathology
Stanford University Medical Center
Stanford, California

J. Butany, M.B.B.S., F.R.C.P.C.
Assistant Professor, Department of Pathology
University of Toronto
Director, Autopsy Service
Department of Pathology
Toronto General Hospital
Toronto, Ontario, Canada

Randal S. Cassling, M.D.
Fellow, Division of Adult Cardiology
University of Texas Health Sciences
Center at San Antonio
San Antonio, Texas

Ming C. Chan, M.D.
Vice Chairman of Medicine
The Third Teaching Hospital
Beijing Medical University
Beijing, People's Republic of China

Paul J. Corso, M.D.
Associate Clinical Professor of Surgery
The George Washington University
Senior Attending Cardiac Surgeon
Washington Hospital Center
Washington, D.C.

Jesse E. Edwards, M.D.
Professor of Pathology
University of Minnesota
Minneapolis, Minnesota
Senior Consultant, Anatomic Pathology
United Hospital
St. Paul, Minnesota

William D. Edwards, M.D.
Associate Professor of Pathology
Mayo Medical School
Consultant, Department of Pathology
Mayo Clinic and Mayo Foundation
Rochester, Minnesota

John T. Fallon, M.D., Ph.D.
Associate Professor of Pathology
Harvard Medical School
Associate Pathologist
Massachusetts General Hospital
Chief of Pathology
Shriners Burns Institute
Boston, Massachusetts

John J. Fenoglio, Jr., M.D.
Department of Pathology
Columbia University College of Physicians and Surgeons
New York, New York

Mervyn B. Forman, M.D.
Assistant Professor of Medicine and Cardiology
Vanderbilt University
Nashville, Tennessee

Jorge M. Garcia, M.D.
Associate Clinical Professor of Surgery
The George Washington University
Director, Division of Cardiovascular Surgery
Washington Hospital Center
Washington, D.C.

Charles J. Gauntt, Ph.D.
Professor, Department of Microbiology
University of Texas Health Sciences Center at San Antonio
San Antonio, Texas

Avrum I. Gotlieb, M.D.
Associate Professor of Pathology
Director, Vascular Research Laboratory
Department of Pathology
Banting and Best Diabetes Centre
Toronto General Hospital
Staff Pathologist
St. Michael's Hospital
Toronto General Hospital
Toronto, Ontario, Canada

Hamner Hannah III, M.D.
Chairman, Section of Cardiothoracic Surgery
University of Missouri
Menorah Medical Center
Kansas City, Missouri

Jody L. Kujovich
Medical Student
Harvard/MIT Program in Health Sciences and Technology
Boston, Massachusetts

Garrett Lee, M.D.
Director of Research
Northern California Heart and Lung Institute
Mt. Diablo Hospital Medical Center
Concord, California

Robert J. Levy, M.D.
Associate Professor of Pediatrics, Communicable Diseases, and Pharmaceutics
University of Michigan Medical School
Ann Arbor, Michigan

J. T. Lie, M.D.
Professor of Pathology
Mayo Medical School and Mayo Graduate School of Medicine
Consultant in Pathology, Cardiovascular Diseases, and Internal Medicine
Mayo Clinic and Mayo Foundation
Rochester, Minnesota

Charles C. Marboe, M.D.
Department of Pathology
Columbia University College of Physicians and Surgeons
New York, New York

Dean T. Mason, M.D.
Chairman, Department of Cardiovascular Medicine
St. Mary's Hospital and Medical Center
Physician-in-Chief
Western Heart Institute
San Francisco, California

Bruce M. McManus, M.D., Ph.D.
Professor, Department of Pathology and Microbiology
Director, Cardiovascular Registry
University of Nebraska Medical Center
Omaha, Nebraska

Randy Morgan, B.S.
Supervisor, Necropsy Assistants
Supervisor, Cardiovascular Pathology Registry
Department of Pathology
Indiana University School of Medicine
Indianapolis, Indiana

Augusto D. Pichard, M.D.
Professor of Medicine
The George Washington University
Director, Cardiac Catheterization Laboratory
Washington Hospital Center
Washington, D.C.

Robert L. Reis, M.D.
Chief, Cardiovascular Surgery
Cedars Medical Center
Miami, Florida

Frederick J. Schoen, M.D., Ph.D.
Director, Cardiac Pathology
Brigham and Women's Hospital
Associate Professor of Pathology
Harvard Medical School
Boston, Massachusetts

Malcolm D. Silver, M.D., Ph.D., F.R.C.P.C., F.R.C.P.A.
Professor and Chairman
Department of Pathology
University of Toronto
Chief of Pathology
Toronto General Hospital
Toronto, Ontario, Canada

Martin St. John Sutton, M.D.
Associate Professor of Medicine
Harvard Medical School
Director, Non-Invasive Cardiac Laboratories
Brigham and Women's Hospital
Boston, Massachusetts

Renu Virmani, M.D.
Professor of Pathology
Georgetown University
Washington, D.C.
Associate Professor of Pathology
Vanderbilt University
Nashville, Tennessee
Chairperson, Department of Cardiovascular Pathology
The Armed Forces Institute of Pathology
Washington, D.C.

Bruce F. Waller, M.D.
Professor of Pathology and Medicine
Director, Section of Cardiovascular Pathology
Indiana University School of Medicine
Research Associate
Krannert Institute of Cardiology
Indianapolis, Indiana

Michael K. K. Wong, Ph.D.
Medical Student
Faculty of Medicine
University of Toronto
Medical Scientist
Canadian Heart Foundation
Toronto, Ontario, Canada

Contents

PART 1

Pathology of Atherosclerotic Coronary Heart Disease

CHAPTER 1

Atherosclerosis: Activation of the Injured Vessel Wall*

Avrum I. Gotlieb, M.D.
Michael K. K. Wong, Ph.D.

Effective prevention and management of atherosclerosis requires an understanding of the sequence of events leading to the initiation and growth of the fibrofatty plaque.[1] An area of intense investigation into understanding the pathogenesis of atherosclerosis is the cell biology of the vessel wall. Since the advent of tissue culture methods to study pure populations of large vessel endothelial[2–5] and smooth muscle cells,[6] the role of these vascular wall cells in the development and the subsequent growth of the fibrofatty plaque has been extensively investigated to give new insight into human atherogenesis. The major contribution of cell biology has been to show that the vascular endothelial cells are very active metabolically and are able to interact with other important physiologic processes that occur at the blood–vascular wall interface, including coagulation,[7–10] fibrinolysis,[11] platelet aggregation,[12,13] leukocyte adherence, and migration.[14–17] Smooth muscle cells have been shown to be very active metabolically, synthesizing the matrix components of the atherosclerotic plaque.[6,18–20] It has also been shown that endothelial cells have the potential to modulate smooth muscle cell function within the vessel wall and vice versa by the release of locally acting polypeptides and glycoproteins and by direct intercellular communications.[21] The studies to be reviewed in this chapter support two concepts. The first is that the endothelial and smooth muscle cells maintain the physiologic homeostasis of the vessel wall. The second is that new stable states are achieved by these cells when normal homeostasis is lost following injury. In these new stable states, the vessel continues to function as a conduit for blood flow but is more likely to form the pathobiologic fibrofatty plaque (Fig. 1–1).

---

* This work was supported by grant T-435 from the Heart and Stroke Foundation of Ontario and grant MT-6485 from the Medical Research Council of Canada. Dr. Wong holds a Medical Scientist Award from the Canadian Heart Foundation.

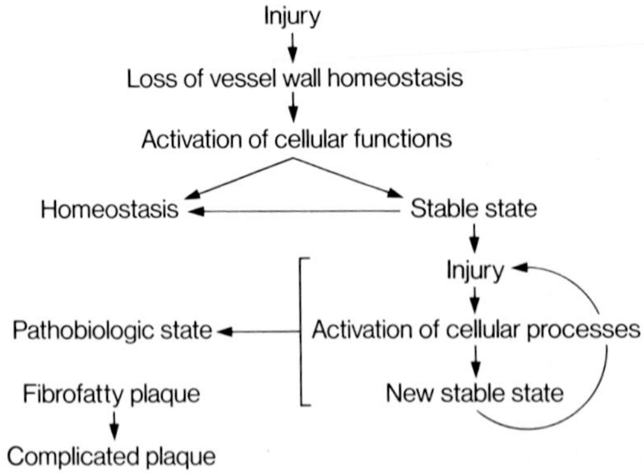

Figure 1–1. Hypothesis for the pathogenesis of atherosclerosis. Atherogenesis is a multistep process in which the endothelial cell and smooth muscle cell of the vessel actively mediate three states: homeostasis, stable, and pathobiologic. The response of these cells to injury can return the vessel wall to homeostasis or result in the establishment of a new stable state. Further injury results in the progression of the vessel wall through a series of stable states that eventually lead to the pathobiologic fibrofatty plaque. Although much evidence to date is consistent with this concept, further experimentation is required to test the hypothesis directly.

ENDOTHELIAL INJURY

Injury to the endothelium is important in the initiation of plaque formation.[22–27] The endothelial cell plays a central role in the physiologic homeostasis of the vessel wall via its ability to function as a thromboresistant surface, a macromolecular barrier, and an active metabolic unit. Although severe injury to the endothelial cell can often lead to cell death and endothelial denudation,[28] less severe injury may result in a change in endothelial cell function[29] such that the cell, although present, is no longer capable of carrying out one or several of its regulatory functions in the vessel wall.

Denuding Injury

A variety of factors have been shown to induce severe endothelial cell injury. It is likely that the cells of the wall interact with these factors over a period of several years to predispose a specific area of the vessel wall to the development of an atherosclerotic plaque. Some factors may act synergistically over time, whereas others are transient and act in sequence to promote development of the plaque. Because there is a predisposition to the development of atherosclerotic plaques in areas of abnormal hemodynamic stress, such as at bifurcations and branch points, this factor is probably important[30] in endothelial injury. Numerous studies support this concept. In many of these areas the endothelium shows increased permeability, and there is an increased turnover of endothelial cells indicating cell loss.[31] Inasmuch as extensive endothelial denudation is not found, it is possible that the injury is very small, perhaps even a few cells wide, and is repaired rapidly. Persistent abnormal chronic flow, as can occur in stenotic atherosclerotic vessels, can induce endothelial trauma leading to cell death, which is then rapidly repaired.[32] How then does the hemodynamic stress cause injury?

There has been considerable debate as to whether low or high shear forces[33] are responsible for the injury. Although the question is not settled, there is evidence that suggests that both types may be important. Studies of the human carotid bifurcation using scale models of pressure-fixed postmortem human arteries suggest that areas of low shear predispose to the development of atherosclerotic plaques[34] inasmuch as intimal thickening was shown to be inversely correlated to the magnitude of shear stress. These authors suggest that increased heart rate should increase the oscillatory flow fields at the outer and side walls of the carotid sinus and thus should enhance the progression of the atherosclerosis. Postulated mechanisms include an increased fluid residence time, which may interfere with endothelial metabolism,[33,34] and disturbance of the stability of intercellular junctions in the endothelial monolayer. It is of interest that in hypertension the increased endothelial permeability observed was thought to be due to opened intercellular junctions.[35]

Hemodynamic stresses and flow are also capable of affecting endothelial cells in subtle ways by regulating endothelial cell structure and function. Very prominent changes in endothelial shape and orientation can be regulated by local blood flow.[36] Flow also affects the metabolic function of the endothelial cell. A change in shear, whether it be an increase or a decrease, results in increased pinocytotic activity of the endothelial cells.[37] In addition, flow stimulates PGI_2[38,39] and histamine[40] release from endothelial cells.

There is evidence that high levels of serum cholesterol may cause endothelial denudation,[41] whereas moderate hypercholesterolemia causes functional endothelial injury by increasing permeability.[42] The frank denudation appears to occur after numerous lipid-laden macrophages appear in the subendothelial space. Thus, in this case, endothelial denudation seems to be a secondary response to the presence of the foam cells in the subendothelial space.[43] Certain metabolic diseases such as homocystinuria result in endothelial denudation.[44] In endotoxemia, increased endothelial turnover is thought to be due to focal endothelial denudation and rapid repair.[45] The replication rate of aortic endothelium is also increased in hypertension,[46,47] indicating cell loss. Immunologic injury has also been shown to induce experimental atherosclerosis[48,49] and may also be associated with the accelerated atherosclerosis seen in human organ transplants.[50,51]

Dysfunctional Injury

The endothelial cell may be considered an important homeostatic regulator of the vessel wall. As already noted, it regulates procoagulation-anticoagulation, fibrinolysis, platelet aggregation-antiaggregation, leukocyte adhesion-nonadhesion, and cell growth promotion-inhibition—all processes whose disruption is considered important in the pathogenesis of the plaque. Thus, any primary change in endothelial cell function that promotes atherogenic processes could be thought of as an endothelial dysfunctional injury resulting in loss of physiologic homeostasis. Although studies in this area of endothelial cell dysfunction are at an early stage of development, several lines of research are being actively considered. For example, because endothelial cells contain factors that are mitogenic and inhibitory for smooth muscle cell growth, dysfunction could be regarded as a disequilibrium in growth factors favoring mitogenesis.[52] Although this interaction of growth factors appears to be important in plaque formation, to date there are no data to support actual growth factor dysfunction or disequilibrium. What has been shown is that injury induced by endotoxin or tumor promoter results in the release by endothelial cells of a platelet-derived growth factor–like molecule that is known to stimulate smooth muscle cell growth.[53] Another example of dysfunction is that hypercholesterolemia may alter endothelial cells in a way that promotes adhesion of monocytes.[14,16,17] One study has shown that the effect of lipid-rich LDL particles is mediated by a direct effect on the endothelial cells and not on the monocytes.[54] This adhesion is very important inasmuch as numerous studies have implicated the monocyte as a participant in the early stages of the formation of fatty streak–type lesions.[14–17] The monocyte accumulation may also be due to the release of chemotactic factors from hypercholesterolemic medial smooth muscle cells that act specifically on hypercholesterolemic monocytes.[55] Endothelial cell participation in the inflammatory process can be induced by several stimuli including interleukin-1[56] and leukotrienes C_4 and D_4.[57] Leukotrienes C_4 and D_4 stimulate endothelial cells to synthesize platelet-activating factor, which induces adherence of polymorphonuclear leukocytes.[57] With respect to coagulation, Stern and coworkers[10] have shown that endothelial cells alone can participate in procoagulant reactions leading to the formation of a cell-associated fibrin thrombus. Endotoxin-injured endothelial cells demonstrate induced tissue factor activity, which promotes fibrin formation via this endothelial cell–dependent pathway of coagulation.[10] As already noted, hemodynamic stress also causes functional changes in the cell. Thus, injured or activated endothelial cells may carry out responses that can lead to further vascular injury or to reestablishment of homeostasis. Although this area of research is in its infancy at present, it promises to be one of the most fascinating areas of endothelial cell pathobiology.

RESPONSE OF THE ENDOTHELIAL CELL TO INJURY

Endothelial injury may be of a denuding nature or of a functional nature. The mechanisms involved in the responses of these forms of injury are likely to be different, and it is via these responses that homeostasis or new stable states are achieved.

Denuding Injury Repair

The endothelial cell has internal systems to regulate wound repair, which can be modulated by a variety of factors. We have recently reported on several experiments showing that following denudation, the cytoskeleton of the endothelial cell is activated in a precise temporal sequence to mediate rapid reendothelialization.

The endothelial cell cytoskeleton is made up of three major fibrous protein systems:[58] microfilaments,[59–63] microtubules,[64] and intermediate filaments.[65,66] Microfilaments are organized within endothelial cells as peripheral and central bundles (Fig. 1–2). Endothelial cells also contain centrosomes, which consist of the paracentral paired centrioles and the amorphous material around them. The centrosome is an organizer of microtubule structure and function.[67] These cytoskeletal systems have been studied in vivo[59–62,71] (Fig. 1–2) and in vitro (Fig. 1–3).[58,63–70,72–75] These systems are dynamic in nature and are important in regulating the shape of the endothelial cell. Small wounds created by the removal of a single cell from a confluent monolayer are rapidly reendothelialized by the simple spreading of the endothelial cells adjacent to the denuded area.[68] Cell migration and cell proliferation are not required for single cell wound closure. Larger wounds, however, require cell spreading followed by endothelial cell migration in order to close the wound.[63] We have found that the microtubules and their associated centrosome,[64,69–71] and the F-actin microfilaments,[63,68,72] play a central role in regulating cell spreading and migration. We have shown that the initial response to the loss of a single endothelial cell is the extrusion of thin, broad cellular processes called

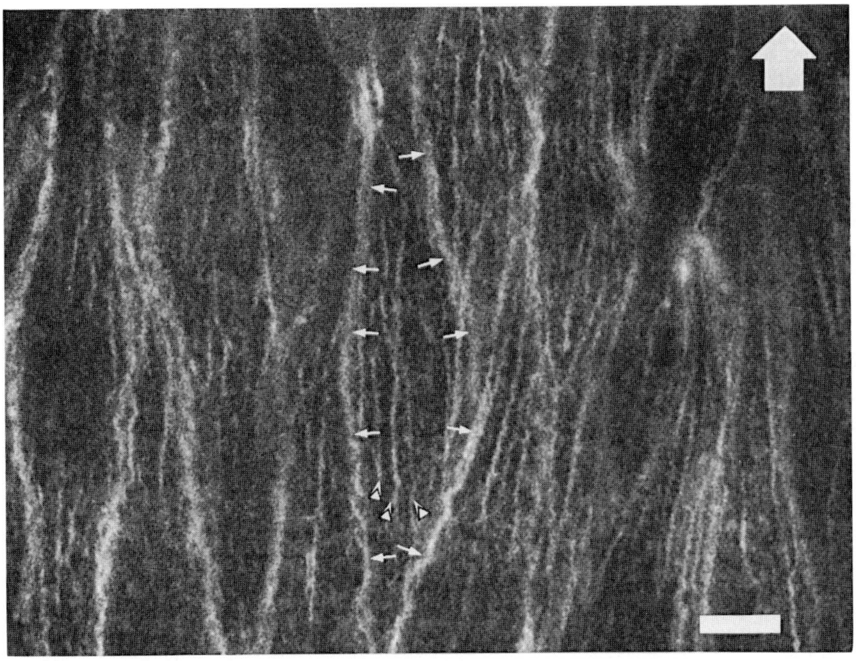

Figure 1 – 2. Photomicrograph of the abdominal aorta of a rabbit stained with rhodamine-phalloidin to localize endothelial cell F-actin microfilaments. *Small arrows* outline the prominent peripheral microfilament bundle of one endothelial cell, while *arrowheads* point out three individual central microfilament bundles (stress fibers) of the same cell. The *large arrow* denotes the direction of blood flow. Bar = 10 μm.

lamellipodia from all of the cells around the wound (Fig. 1 – 3*C*). These lamellipodia are closely associated with peripheral actin microfilaments that we have termed "the dense peripheral band" (DPB)[63,73] (Fig. 1 – 3*C*). If this DPB is disrupted, then rapid reendothelialization cannot occur. We have also shown that if the repair process cannot be carried out rapidly, within about an hour, by the spreading of lamellipodia from neighboring endothelial cells, then these cells undergo a specific rearrangement of their cytoskeleton that allows them to migrate into the area and close the wound.[74] The cells begin to elongate, and there is a redistribution of the centrosome by microtubules from a random location within the cell toward the side of the cell nucleus that faces the direction of cell movement. The DPB becomes markedly reduced in these migrating cells, and prominent central microfilament bundles oriented parallel to the direction of cell migration appear as the cells move into the area of the wound[63] (Fig. 1 – 3*D*). Adjacent cells behind it spread somewhat to fill in the gap. The centrosomal redistribution occurs rapidly; it depends on the presence of intact mictrotubules and can be regulated by external agents such as platelet-derived growth factor and insulin.[75] Although the mechanism for the loss of the DPB is not known at present, it is likely that actin-associated proteins may be involved in enhancing the depolymerization of the peripheral actin.[76]

Our studies suggest a key role for the DPB in normal endothelial cell function. The DPB is a structure unique to the confluent cell monolayer in that it is not present in subconfluent cultures and begins to form just as confluency is reached (Fig. 1 – 3*A*). We have shown that the DPB contains many other cytoskeletal proteins besides actin.[73] Hence, the DPB may be contractile and can potentially stabilize the cell

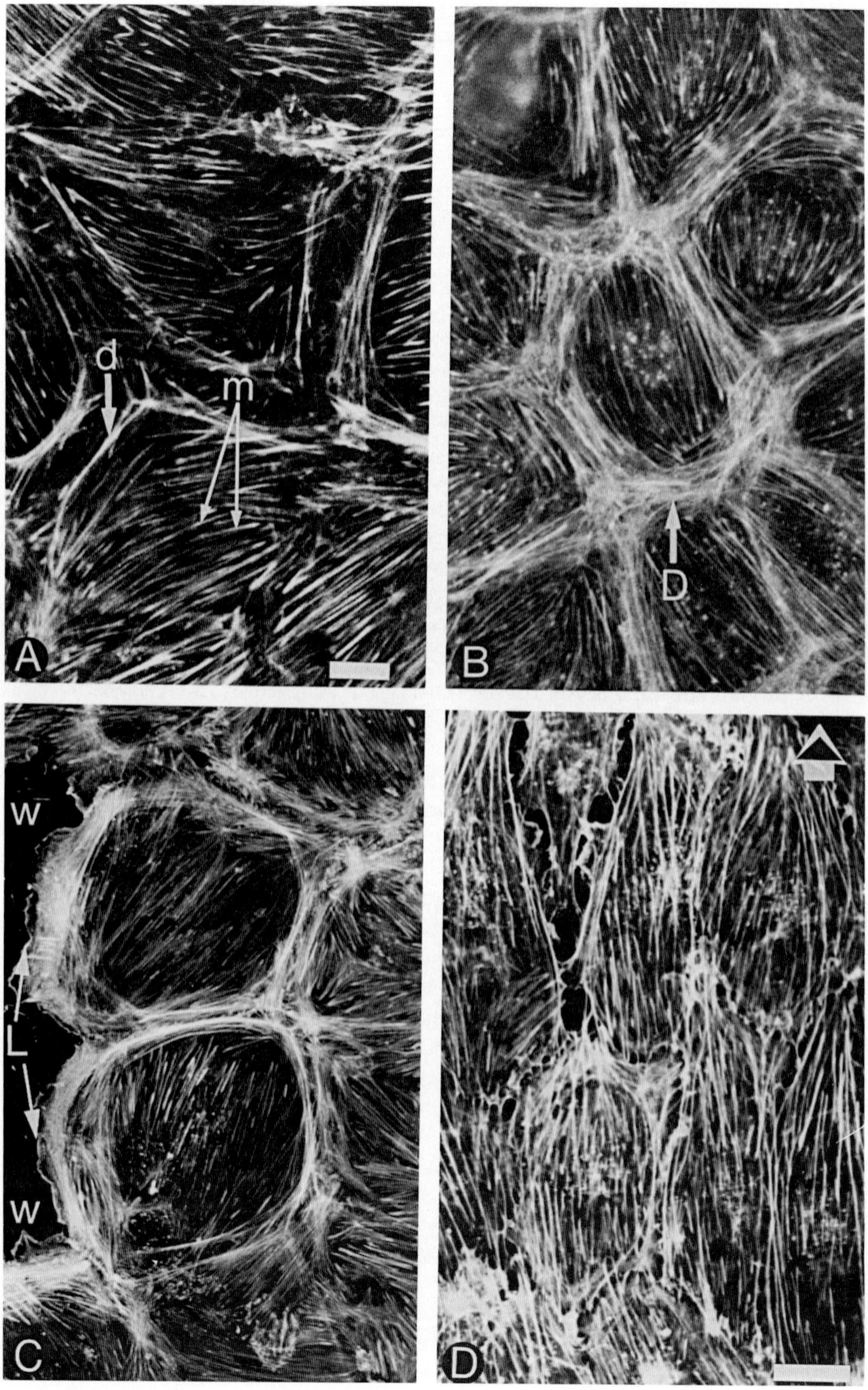

Figure 1–3. See legend on facing page.

against forces that will pull cells apart and alter cell shape. We have suggested that this property is mediated through the association of the DPB with adherens-type junctions containing vinculin,[73] which maintain endothelial cells adherent to one another. Thus, disruption of the DPB will lead to disruption of endothelial integrity. This idea is supported by the observations that reversible pulmonary edema caused by ethchlorvynol may be related to the loss of the endothelial DPB[77] and that thrombin-induced shape changes are mediated by changes in the DPB[78] (Fig. 1–4).

Thus, the cytoskeleton of the endothelial cell provides the cell with the internal machinery to carry out very precise cell shape changes. Following loss of vessel-wall homeostasis, as occurs in denudation, the cytoskeletal systems are one of the important cellular processes to be activated in order to promote cell spreading and migration to repair the denudation rapidly. We propose that these cytoskeletal activities are cellular processes activated after all denuding injuries. These processes can be regulated by external agents, by the subendothelial matrix,[79] and by flow. We have shown that endothelial cell spreading is enhanced by platelet releasate.[80] Langille and associates[32] have shown that different flow conditions either enhance or retard the migration of endothelial cells during the repair of a small endothelial denudation.

Although the monolayer is physically reestablished, dysfunction may still exist. The regenerated endothelium following reestablishment of the monolayer shows changes in gap and tight junction morphology associated with increased permeability.[81] Monocytes are more adherent to the regenerated endothelium.[82] In addition, the media beneath the regenerated endothelium in large wounds show enhanced accumulation of glycosaminoglycans[83] and lipids.[84]

Although the rapid response to repair following denudation is mediated by cytoskeletal factors, cell turnover occurs as well.[85] Endothelial cell proliferation occurs after cell migration at sites that are close to the wound and at a distance from the wound.[86] The normal intact endothelium is very quiescent, with a thymidine index rate of 0.04 percent. Although the stimulus for proliferation is not known, a loss of contact inhibition appears to be important. In addition, the regulation of cell surface proteins that have been identified in quiescent monolayers may be associated with senescence.[87,88] Recently, it has been shown that smooth muscle cells produce an inhibitor of endothelial cell growth.[89] At the site of proliferation, there may be some disruption of the normal alignment of endothelial cells, which subsequently realign under the influence of flow.

Interestingly, the few experiments in which the effect of risk factors on rate of repair was studied showed that neither hypertension nor hyperlipidemia altered the rate of endothelial repair.[81,90,91]

Figure 1–3. Photomicrograph of cultured endothelial cells stained with rhodamine-phalloidin demonstrating the presence or absence of the dense peripheral band of microfilaments under different conditions. *A*, EC culture just as confluency is reached. Note the presence of central microfilaments (m) and the commencement of DPB formation (d). *B*, EC culture 2 to 3 days postconfluent. Note the well-developed DPBs (D) present about the circumference of each cell. *C*, ECs in confluent cultures responding to a very small circular denuding wound (w) by the extrusion of lamellipodia (L). Note the splaying of the DPB on the side of the cell participating in lamellipodia extrusion and the continuing presence of the DPB around the remaining circumference of the cell. *D*, EC in confluent culture undergoing cell migration in response to a large scrape wound inflicted 36 hours previously. The *large arrow* is located on the cells at the wound edge, and its direction points out the direction of cell migration. Note the loss of the DPB within these migrating cells. Bar in $A = 10\ \mu m$ for *A*, *B*, and *C*. Bar in $D = 20\ \mu m$.

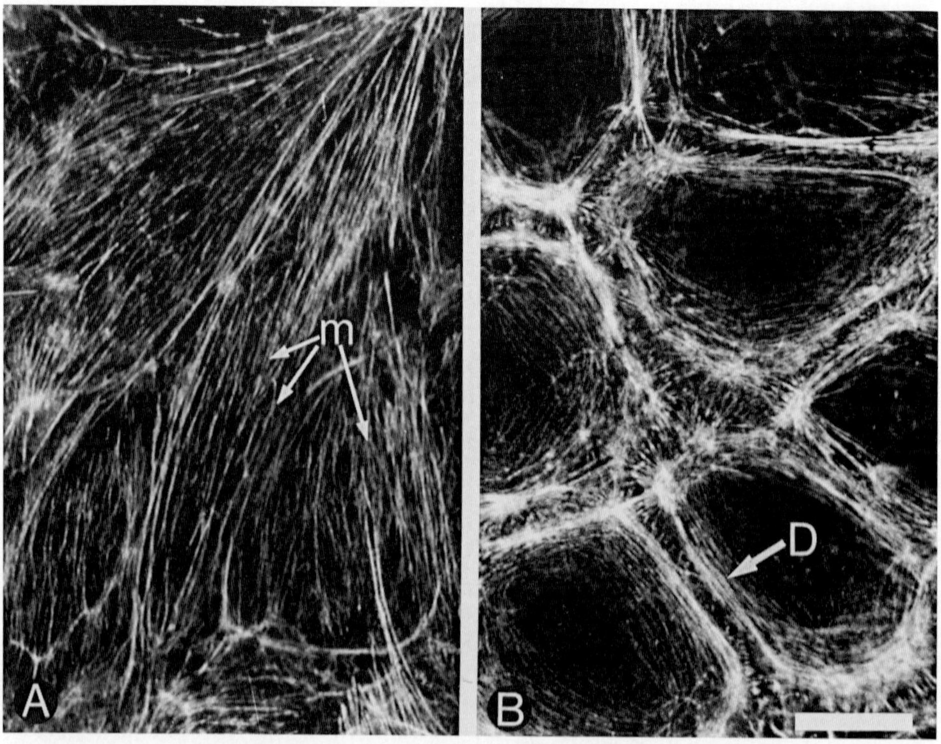

Figure 1-4. Photomicrograph of a confluent culture of endothelial cells incubated with 4 units/ml of human thrombin and subsequently fixed and stained with rhodamine-phalloidin at various time points. *A*, Cells after 2 hours incubation with thrombin. Note loss of the DPB, the prominence of central microfilament (m) bundles and the elongated shape of the cells. *B*, ECs 1 hour after the washout of thrombin. Note the reappearance of the DPB (D) and the reestablishment of the characteristic cobblestone monolayer. Bar = 20 μm.

Dysfunctional Injury Repair

A change in a function may be considered either to be an "injury" or a response to a physiologic perturbation. Thus, dysfunction must be considered with respect to the microenvironment.

In dysfunctional injury, one can only speculate at this time as to how the cell may respond in order to reestablish homeostasis. One possible response is for the vessel wall to use other systems available to achieve the same end. Thus, if secretion of one growth factor is faulty, then another growth factor might be synthesized and secreted, or a decrease in growth inhibitors might occur. Similarly, the endothelial cell has been shown to possess at least three mechanisms by which it can respond to increase its antithrombotic potential. These include the synthesis and secretion of prostacyclin,[92] plasminogen activators,[11] and protein S[93,94]—a regulatory vitamin K-dependent plasma protein that is required for the function of the anticoagulant-activated protein C. Thus, dysfunction in one mechanism may lead to compensation by the others. Although these types of regulatory interactions have not yet been studied in any detail, the therapeutic potential of enhancing one system when another is dysfunctional should be considered.

RESPONSE OF THE SMOOTH MUSCLE CELL TO INJURY

The smooth muscle cell is the principal cell in the fibrofatty plaque.[95] The smooth muscle cell may form part of the plaque, as a cell that has migrated from the media into the intima, as an intimal smooth muscle cell present in the intima,[96] or as part of diffuse intimal thickening that occurs with increasing age.[97–99] Factors such as the platelet-derived growth factor are chemotactic to smooth muscle cells.[100] Injury to the endothelium also promotes smooth muscle cell proliferation. The size and extent of the injury is important. Small denuding injuries to the normal endothelium do not result in smooth muscle cell proliferation.[101,102] Larger injuries, often accompanied by some smooth muscle cell damage, result in smooth muscle cell hyperplasia.[103–105] It is likely then that small injuries to neointima or the atherosclerotic plaque will invoke further proliferation.

About 85 percent of the volume of the medial smooth muscle cell is made up of numerous myofilaments, dense bodies, and intermediate filaments. The cellular organelles including the smooth and rough endoplasmic reticulum, the mitochondria, and the Golgi complex are sparse (Fig. 1–5). These organelles synthesize and secrete the small amounts of collagen, matrix proteins, elastin, and glycosaminoglycans necessary for maintaining the homeostasis of the vessel wall. In the elastic arteries, the smooth muscle cells are neatly arranged in lamellar units made up of subgroups of musculoelastic fascicles.[106] Once a response to injury is initiated by as yet unknown factors, the smooth muscle cells undergo modulation from a "contract-

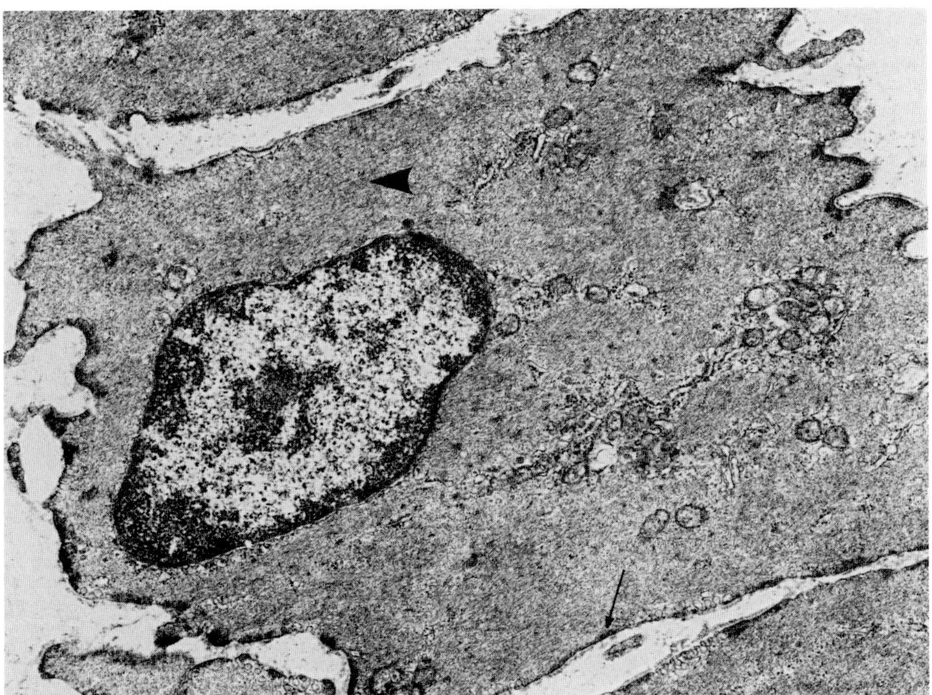

Figure 1–5. An electron micrograph of a normal aortic medial smooth muscle cell. Note the sparse organelles, dense bodies *(arrow),* and myofilaments *(arrowhead).* (Original magnification ×19,500; reduced 7 percent.)

ile" to a "synthetic" state.[107] These terms have been used to describe the two phenotypic states.[107] In the synthetic state, the intracellular organelles including the smooth and rough endoplasmic reticulum and the Golgi complex become very prominent, whereas the myofilaments and dense bodies markedly decrease in volume (Fig. 1-6). The smooth muscle cell, although it has lost much of its contractile apparatus, still has many features of a contractile cell including the presence of alpha-adrenergic receptors[108] and smooth-muscle myosin isoforms.[109] Not only does the "synthetic" smooth muscle secrete more, but also the pattern of secretion appears to be different. The normal medium contains predominantly type III collagen with little type I, whereas the atherosclerotic plaque contains much more type I than type III.[110] Glycosaminoglycan patterns also change.[111-113] Comparing the plaque with the normal vessel wall, the former contains more dermatan sulfate relative to chondroitin sulfate and heparan sulfate. However, others have reported that the plaque has an increase in chondroitin sulfates A and C as well.[113] These changes may promote trapping of lipid in the matrix of the plaque.[114] The synthetic cells also appear to metabolize lipids differently than the contractile cell, which may give rise to intracellular lipid accumulation.[115]

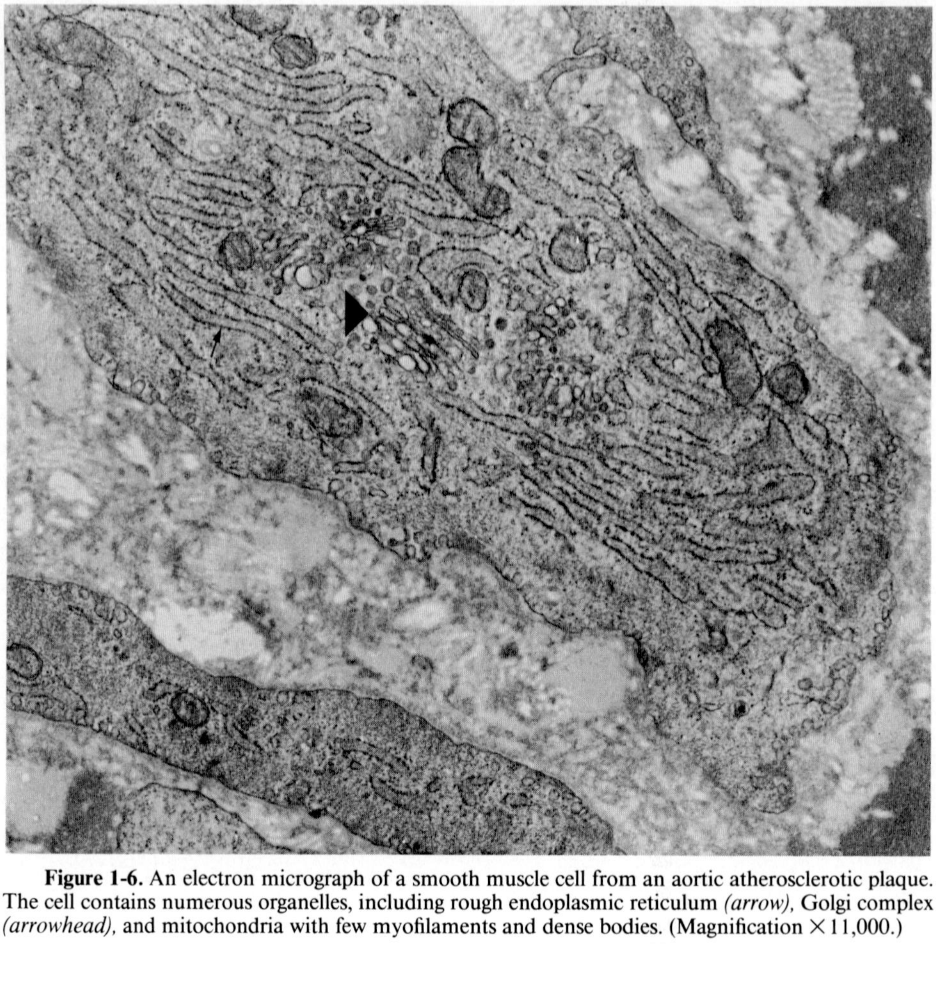

Figure 1-6. An electron micrograph of a smooth muscle cell from an aortic atherosclerotic plaque. The cell contains numerous organelles, including rough endoplasmic reticulum *(arrow)*, Golgi complex *(arrowhead)*, and mitochondria with few myofilaments and dense bodies. (Magnification ×11,000.)

Smooth muscle cells are capable of very active proliferation. In the last few years, it has become apparent that there are numerous substances that are capable of regulating smooth muscle cell proliferation. Although the precise regulation of smooth muscle cells in vivo are not yet known, several reasonable ideas have been entertained. When endothelial denudation occurs, platelets adhere and release platelet-derived growth factor, which is a very potent mitogen for smooth muscle cells.[116] In addition, lipoproteins have been shown to enhance smooth muscle cell proliferation.[117] In the hypercholesterolemic lesions, the numerous monocyte/macrophage–derived foam cells are also capable of releasing macrophage-derived growth factor, which is mitogenic for smooth muscle cells.[118] Even if an intact endothelium is present, there are still mechanisms by which smooth muscle cell proliferation could occur. Endothelial cells contain both endothelial cell–derived growth factor and a platelet-derived growth factor.[119,120] Thus, any condition that promotes secretion of these factors may stimulate smooth muscle cell proliferation. Endotoxin and tumor promoters have been shown to release mitogens from the in vitro endothelium.[53] Smooth muscle cells in neonatal media,[121] in primary culture,[122] and derived from the neointima[123] secrete platelet-derived growth factor, which can stimulate their own growth in an autocrine fashion. In addition, vasoactive substances such as serotonin[124] and catecholamines[125] stimulate smooth muscle cell growth. Growth of the smooth muscle cell is regulated by inhibitors as well. It has been shown that smooth muscle cell proliferation stops when the overlying endothelial layer is reestablished.[126] Heparin and heparin-like factors released from endothelial cells inhibit or reduce smooth muscle cell proliferation.[127–129] The smooth muscles themselves contain heparan sulfate molecules on the cell surface, which reduces smooth muscle cell growth.[130] Enhancement of these inhibitory pathways may be important in the future in reducing the smooth muscle cell proliferation that occurs following wall injury in such procedures as angioplasty[131–133] and aortocoronary saphenous vein bypass.[134,135]

It is interesting that the neointima once formed by smooth muscle cell proliferation becomes thromboresistant.[136,137] A few platelets may adhere to the wall, but no platelet pavementing occurs as is the case immediately following denudation of the normal intact endothelium.

It is also of interest that the smooth muscle cells respond dramatically to injury within the first 2 weeks, but the rate of proliferation following this becomes reduced.[138] Smooth muscle cell proliferation does not persist indefinitely, and the lumen will not close off in large vessels. Wall tension or pressure may be important in regulating this process. Langille and O'Donnell have shown that changes in vessel wall diameter following injury are modulated by the presence of endothelium.[139]

GROWTH OF ATHEROSCLEROTIC PLAQUE

The steps involved in the final development of the clinically important stenotic fibrofatty plaque are not well known. Fatty streak lesions[140–142] or other types of precursor lesions[143,144] have been postulated to predispose the vessel wall to become the pathologic atheroma. It appears that the fibrofatty plaque becomes established following chronic injury. Organization of mural thrombi is important in growth as well. The steps in the development of focal areas of calcification and the role of the well-developed areas of focal nonspecific chronic inflammation also are not known. An important feature is neovascularization of the plaque. Thin-walled vessels derived from the vasa vasorum appear in the intima and media.[145] These vessels are thought to be fragile and can cause spontaneous intramural hemorrhage, which may result in acute increases in the plaque size.[146,147] If the fibrous capsule is thin, it may rupture and luminal thrombosis will occur. The plaque also increases in size by the organization of mural thrombi on the surface of the plaque. The narrowed lumen predisposes to both abnormal flow and subsequent endothelial denudation on the surface of plaques, each of which promote thrombosis.

STABLE AND PATHOBIOLOGIC STATES

The new information derived from cell biology has shown that a bewildering array of biologic processes is likely to occur both at the surface and within the vessel wall. These processes interact with each other, subserving similar or diametrically opposed functions, and act to maintain physiologic homeostasis in the face of physiologic perturbations and injury.

We have proposed that it is now more meaningful to consider atherosclerosis as a condition in which there is a loss of the very precise homeostasis maintained on the surface and within the vessel wall. The strategy in this approach is first to define those processes that are important in maintaining the physiologic hemostasis of the wall and to characterize the regulation of these processes. The next step is to understand how the endothelial and smooth muscle cells of the wall become activated either to restore homeostasis or to maintain new stable states. The development of the atherosclerotic plaque from stable states appears to be a complex process in which the cells of the wall are no longer able to maintain their present state and are unable as well to establish a new stable state.

For example, if injury to the vessel is mild and acute, the endothelium repairs itself by activating the cytoskeletal systems and cell proliferation, if necessary, to restore the integrity of the endothelium that serves the function of regulating physiologic homeostasis. If reendothelialization is delayed, then the smooth muscle cells attempt to reestablish physiologic homeostasis. Instead, a new stable state is achieved that may, however, act as a nidus for subsequent development of the fibrofatty plaque.

We suggest that the neointima is an example of a new stable state. Clowes and associates[148] have characterized a model of neointimal formation in a chronically denuded artery in which intimal thickness does not change after the initial intense proliferation. They showed that the artery existed for a year in a stable state without endothelium, owing to a balance between loss and low-grade chronic proliferation of the smooth muscle cells. Inasmuch as there was some evidence of platelet aggregation, this proliferation may be regulated by platelet-derived growth factor or even by platelet serotonin, which is also mitogenic to smooth muscle cells and may in fact act synergistically with platelet-derived growth factor.[124] Studies have shown that the smooth muscle cells of the neointima form a relatively thromboresistant internal lining.[136,137] Why this occurs is not known, but smooth muscle cells are able to synthesize prostaglandin I_2 (prostacyclin), the potent inhibitor of platelet aggregation.[149] This neointima, when reinjured, invokes a more dramatic thrombotic response by activating both the coagulation system and platelets. In contrast, following injury to the normal endothelium, only platelets adhere, and only for a short time. Thus, the neointima, which we are suggesting is a stable state, may progress more rapidly to an atherosclerotic plaque following further injury. From a therapeutic viewpoint, it has been shown that prostacyclin and heparin in combination greatly suppress platelet and fibrin deposition following neointimal injury.[150] This finding has direct application to the prevention of restenosis following angioplasty.

The progression of fibrofatty plaque growth and development can be considered as a series of steps in which the cells of the wall attempt to reestablish homeostasis. If this cannot be accomplished, then a new stable state is achieved, which may temporize for the moment but which in turn becomes the fertile environment for the development of future fibrofatty plaques. Both fatty streak lesions and focal or diffuse intimal thickening[98,99] may indeed be stable states that require further definable steps to lead eventually to the development of the fibrofatty plaque and the complicated lesion. The concept of a multistep process in the pathogenesis of atherosclerosis is consistent with the findings of human population studies which showed that fatty streak-type lesions and intimal thickening characterized by smooth muscle cell proliferation did not differ greatly among populations with or without significant atherosclerosis.[151] Hence it is likely that therapeutic agents will have to be targeted to the physiologic, stable, or pathobiologic states because in a multistep pathogenesis, different biologic and pathobiologic processes may be active at each state.

ACKNOWLEDGMENT

We thank Ms. Sue Sarju for secretarial support.

REFERENCES

1. Gotlieb, AI: Smooth muscle and endothelial cell function in the pathogenesis of atherosclerosis. CMAJ 126:903, 1982.
2. Jaffe, EA, Nachman, RL, Becker, CG, et al: Culture of human endothelial cells derived from umbilical veins. Identification by morphologic and immunologic criteria. J Clin Invest 52:2745, 1973.
3. Gimbrone, MA, Jr, Cotran, RS, and Folkman, J: Human vascular endothelial cells in culture: Growth and DNA synthesis. J Cell Biol 60:673, 1974.
4. Booyse, FM, Sedlak, BJ, and Rafelson, ME: Culture of arterial endothelial cells: Characterization and growth of bovine aortic cells. Thromb Diath Haemorrh 34:825, 1975.
5. Ryan, US, Clements, E, Habliston, D, et al: Isolation and culture of pulmonary artery endothelial cells. Tissue Cell 10:535, 1978.
6. Ross, R: The smooth muscle cell. II. Growth of smooth muscle in culture and formation of elastic fibres. J Cell Biol 50:172, 1971.
7. Jaffe, EA, Hoyer, LW, and Nachman, RL: Synthesis of antihemophilic factor antigen by cultured human endothelial cells. J Clin Invest 52:2757, 1973.
8. Engelberg, H: Heparin, heparin fractions, and the atherosclerotic process. Sem Thromb Hemost 11:48, 1985.
9. de Groot, PG, Gonsalves, MP, C. Loesberg, M, et al: Thrombin-induced release of von Willebrand factor from endothelial cells is mediated by phospholipid methylation. J Biol Chem 259:13329, 1984.
10. Stern, D, Nawroth, P, Handley, D, et al: An endothelial cell-dependent pathway of coagulation. Proc Natl Acad Sci USA 82:2523, 1985.
11. Loskutoff, DJ and Edgington, TS: Synthesis of fibrinolytic activator and inhibitor by endothelial cells. Proc Natl Acad Sci USA 74:3903, 1977.

12. Groves, HM, Kinlough-Rathbone, RL, Richardson, M, et al: Platelet interaction with damaged rabbit aorta. Lab Invest 40:194, 1979.
13. Kinlough-Rathbone, RL, Packham, MA, and Mustard, JF: Vessel injury: Platelet adherence and platelet survival. Arteriosclerosis 3:529, 1983.
14. Gerrity, RG: The role of the monocyte in atherogenesis. I. Transition of blood-borne monocytes into foam cells in fatty lesions. Am J Pathol 103:181, 1981.
15. Gerrity, RG: The role of the monocyte in atherogenesis. II. Migration of foam cells from atherosclerotic lesions. Am J Pathol 103:191, 1981.
16. Joris, I, Zand, T, Nannari, JJ, et al: Studies on the pathogenesis of atherosclerosis. I. Adhesion and emigration of mononuclear cells in the aorta of hypercholesterolemic rats. Am J Pathol 113:341, 1983.
17. Faggiotto, A, Ross, R, and Harker, L: Studies of hypercholesterolemia in the nonhuman primate. I. Changes that lead to fatty streak formation. Arteriosclerosis 4:323, 1984.
18. McCullagh, KG, Duance, VC, and Bishop, KA: The distribution of collagen types I, II, III and V (AB) in normal and atherosclerotic human aorta. J Pathol 130:45, 1980.
19. Vijayagopal, P, Radhakrishnamurthyu, B, Srinivasan, SR, et al: Studies of biological properties of proteoglycans from bovine aorta. Lab Invest 42:190, 1980.
20. Wight, TN and Hascall, VC: Proteoglycans in primate arteries. III. Characterization of the proteoglycans synthesized by arterial smooth muscle cells in culture. J Cell Biol 96:167, 1983.
21. Davies, PF, Ganz, P, and Diehl, PS: Methods in laboratory investigation. Reversible microcarrier-mediated junctional communication between endothelial and smooth muscle cell monolayers: An in vitro model of vascular cell interactions. Lab Invest 85:710, 1985.
22. Ross, R, Glomset, J, and Harker, L: Response to injury and atherogenesis. Am J Pathol 86:675, 1977.
23. Ross, R: The pathogenesis of atherosclerosis—an update. N Engl J Med 314:488, 1986.
24. Fishman, JA, Ryan, GB, and Karnovsky, MJ: Endothelial regeneration in the rat carotid artery and the significance of endothelial denudation in the pathogenesis of myointimal thickening. Lab Invest 32:339, 1975.
25. Stemerman, MB, Spaet, TH, Pitlick, F, et al: Intimal healing: The pattern of reendothelialization and intimal thickening. Am J Pathol 87:125, 1977.
26. Hirsch, EZ and Robertson, AL, Jr: Selective acute arterial injury and repair. I. Methodology and surface characteristics. Atherosclerosis 28:271, 1977.
27. Schwartz, SM, Haudenschild, CC, and Eddy, EM: Endothelial regeneration. I. Quantitative analysis of initial stages of endothelial regeneration in rat aortic intima. Lab Invest 38:568, 1978.
28. Thorgeirsson, G and Robertson, AL: The vascular endothelium—pathobiological significance. Am J Pathol 93:801, 1978.
29. Hansson, GK and Schwartz, SM: Endothelial cell dysfunction without cell loss. In Cryer, A: Biomedical Interactions at the Endothelium. Elsevier Science and Publishers, New York, 1983, p 343.
30. Nerem, RM and Cornhill, JF: Hemodynamics and atherogenesis. Atherosclerosis 36:151, 1980.
31. Caplan, BA, Gerrity, RG, and Schwartz, CJ: Endothelial cell morphology in focal areas of in vivo Evans Blue uptake in the young pig aorta. I. Quantitative light microscopic findings. Exp Mol Pathol 21:102, 1974.
32. Langille, BL, Reidy, MA, and Kline, RL: Injury and repair of endothelium at sites of flow disturbances near abdominal aortic coarctations in rabbits. Arteriosclerosis 6:146, 1986.
33. Bell FP, Somer, JB, Craig, IH, et al: Patterns of aortic Evans Blue uptake in vivo and in vitro. Atherosclerosis 16:369, 1972.
34. Ku, DN, Giddens, DP, Zarins, CK, et al: Pulsatile flow and atherosclerosis in the human carotid bifurcation. Arteriosclerosis 5:293, 1985.
35. Gabbiani, G, Badonnel, MC, and Rona, G: Cytoplasmic contractile apparatus in aortic endothelial cells of hypertensive rats. Lab Invest 32:227, 1975.
36. Langille, BL and Adamson, SL: Relationship between blood flow direction and endothelial cell orientation at arterial branch sites in rabbits and mice. Circ Res 48:481, 1981.
37. Davies, PF, Dewey, CF, Bussolàri, SR, et al: Influence of hemodynamic forces on vascular endothelial function. In vitro studies of shear stress and pinocytosis in bovine aortic cells. J Clin Invest 73:1121, 1984.
38. Grabowski, EF, Jaffe, EA, and Weksler, BB: Prostacyclin production by cultured endothelial cell monolayers exposed to step increases in shear stress. J Lab Clin Med 105:36, 1985.
39. Frangos, JA, Eskin, SG, McIntyre, LV, et al: Flow effects on prostacyclin production by cultured human endothelial cells. Science 227:1477, 1985.

40. DeForrest, JM and Hollis, TM: Shear stress and aortic histamine synthesis. Am J Physiol 234:H701, 1978.
41. Ross, R and Harker, L: Hyperlipidemia and atherosclerosis: Chronic hyperlipidemia initiates and maintains lesions by endothelial cell desquamation and lipid accumulation. Science 193:1094, 1976.
42. Gerrity, RG and Schwartz, CJ: Endothelial cell injury in early mild hypercholesterolemia. Prog Biochem Pharmacol 14:213, 1977.
43. Faggiotto, A and Ross, R: Studies of hypercholesterolemia in the nonhuman primate. II. Fatty streak conversion to fibrous plaque. Arteriosclerosis 4:341, 1984.
44. Harker, L, Ross, R, Slichter, S, et al: Homocystine-induced arteriosclerosis: The role of endothelial cell injury and platelet response in its genesis. J Clin Invest 58:731, 1976.
45. Reidy, MA and Schwartz, SM: Endothelial injury and regeneration. IV. Endotoxin: A nondenuding injury to aortic endothelium. Lab Invest 48:25 1983.
46. Gabbiani, G, Elemer, G, Guelpha, CH, et al: Morphologic and functional changes of the aortic intima during experimental hypertension. Am J Pathol 96:399, 1979.
47. Schwartz, SM and Benditt, EP: Aortic endothelial cell replication. I. Effects of age and hypertension in the rat. Circ Res 41:248, 1977.
48. Minick, CR, Murphy, GE, and Campbell, WG: Experimental induction of athero-arteriosclerosis by the synergy of allergic injury to arteries and lipid-rich diet. I. Effect of repeated injections of horse serum in rabbits fed a dietary cholesterol supplement. J Exp Med 124:635, 1966.
49. Minick, CR, Alonso, DR, and Rankin, L: Role of immunologic arterial injury in atherogenesis. Thromb Haemostasis 39:304, 1978.
50. Gotlieb, AI, Crosby, D, Lemire, GC, et al: A study of human cardiac allograft in a patient with four year survival. CMAJ 19:154, 1974.
51. Alonso, DR, Starek, P, and Minick, CR: Studies on the pathogenesis of athero-arteriosclerosis induced in rabbit cardiac allografts by the synergy of graft rejection and hypercholesterolemia. Am J Pathol 87:415, 1977.
52. Schwartz, SM, Gajdusek, CM, and Selden, SC, III: Vascular growth control: The role of the endothelium. Arteriosclerosis 1:107, 1981.
53. Fox, PL and DiCorleto, PE: Regeneration of the production of a platelet derived growth factor-like protein by cultured bovine aortic endothelial cells. J Cell Physiol 121:298, 1984.
54. Alderson, LM, Endemann, G, Lindsey, S, et al: LDL enhances monocytes adhesion to endothelial cells in vitro. Am J Pathol 123:334, 1986.
55. Gerrity, RG, Goss, JA, and Soby, L: Control of monocyte recruitment by chemotactic factor(s) in lesion-prone areas of swine aorta. Arteriosclerosis 5:55, 1985.
56. Bevilacqua, MP, Pober, JS, Cotran, RS, et al: Interleukin 1 (IL-1) acts upon vascular endothelium to stimulate procoagulant activity and leukocyte adhesion. J Cell Biochem (Suppl) 9A:148, 1985.
57. McIntyre, TM, Zimmerman, GA, and Prescott, SM: Leukotrienes C and D stimulate human endothelial cells to synthesize platelet activating factor and bind neutrophils. Proc Natl Acad Sci USA 83:2204, 1986.
58. Kalnins, VI, Subrahmanyan, L, and Gotlieb, AI: The reorganization of cytoskeletal fibre systems in spreading porcine endothelial cells in culture. Eur J Cell Biol 24:36, 1981.
59. Yohro, T and Burnstock, G: Filament bundles and contractility of endothelial cells in coronary arteries. Z Zellforsch Mikrosk Anat 138:85, 1973.
60. Wong, AJ, Pollard, TD, and Herman, IM: Actin filament stress fibres in vascular endothelial cells in vivo. Science 219:867, 1983.
61. White, GE, Gimbrone, MA, and Fujiwara, K: Factors influencing the expression of stress fibres in vascular endothelial cells in situ. J Cell Biol 97:416, 1983.
62. Rogers, KA and Kalnins, VI: A method for examining the endothelial cytoskeleton in situ using immunofluorescence. J Histochem Cytochem 31:1317, 1983.
63. Gotlieb AI, Spector, W, Wong, MKK, et al: In vitro reendothelialization: Microfilament bundle reorganization in migrating porcine endothelial cells. Arteriosclerosis 4:91, 1984.
64. Gotlieb, AI, McBurnie-May, L, Subrahmanyan, L, et al: Distribution of microtubule organizing centers in migrating sheets of endothelial cells. J Cell Biol 91:589, 1981.
65. Franke, WW, Schmid, E, Osborn, M, et al: Intermediate-sized filaments of human endothelial cells. J Cell Biol 81:570, 1979.
66. Bose, SH and Meltzer, DI: Visualization of the 10-nm filament vimentin rings in vascular endothelial cells in situ: Close resemblance to vimentin cytoskeletons found in monolayers in vitro. Exp Cell Res 135:299, 1981.

67. Brinkley, BR: Microtubule organizing centers. Ann Rev Cell Biol 1:145, 1985.
68. Wong, MKK and Gotlieb, AI: In vitro reendothelialization of a single-cell wound. Role of microfilament bundles in rapid lamellipodia mediated wound closure. Lab Invest 51:75, 1984.
69. Gotlieb, AI, Subrahmanyan, L, and Kalnins, VI: Microtubule-organizing centers and cell migration. Effect of inhibition of migration and microtubule disruption in endothelial cells. J Cell Biol 96:1266, 1983.
70. Rogers, KA, Boden, P, Kalnins, VI, et al: The distribution of centrosomes in endothelial cells of non-wounded and wounded aortic organ cultures. Cell Tissue Res 1985.
71. Rogers, KA, McGee, N, and Kalnins, VI: The preferential orientation of centrioles towards the heart in endothelial cells of major blood vessels is reestablished following reversal of a segment. Proc Natl Acad Sci USA 82:3272, 1985.
72. Gotlieb, AI and Spector, W: Migration into an experimental wound: A comparison of porcine aortic endothelial and smooth muscle cells and the effect of culture irradiation. Am J Pathol 103:271, 1981.
73. Wong, MKK and Gotlieb, AI: Endothelial cell monolayer integrity. 1. Characterization of dense peripheral band of microfilaments. Arteriosclerosis 6:212, 1986.
74. Wong, MKK and Gotlieb, AI: Small endothelial wound repair—a two step process. Fed Proc 44:1662, 1985.
75. Mascardo, RN and Sherline, P: Insulin and multiplication-stimulating activity induce a very rapid centrosomal orientation response to wounding in endothelial cell monolayers. Diabetes 33:1099, 1984.
76. Chaponnier, R, Borgia, R, Rungger-Brandel, E, et al: An actin-destabilizing factor is present in human plasma. Experientia 35:1039, 1979.
77. Wysolmerski, R and Lagunoff, D: The effect of ethchlorvynol on cultured endothelial cells. A model for the study of the mechanism of increased vascular permeability. Am J Pathol 119:550, 1985.
78. Wong, MKK and Gotlieb, AI: The dense peripheral band: A dynamic microfilament structure present in confluent endothelial cell monolayers. J Cell Biol 99:198a, 1984.
79. Pratt, BM, Harris, AS, Morrow, JS, et al: Mechanisms of cytoskeletal regulation. Modulation of aortic endothelial cell spectrin by the extracellular matrix. Am J Pathol 117:349, 1984.
80. Gotlieb, AI, and Wong, MKK: The effects of platelet poor plasma serum on endothelial cell spreading. Artery 9:59, 1981.
81. Stemerman, MB: Effects of moderate hypercholesterolemia on rabbit endothelium. Arteriosclerosis 1:25, 1981.
82. DiCorleto, PE and de la Motte, CA: Characterization of the adhesion of the human monocyte cell line U-937 to cultured endothelial cells. J Clin Invest 75:1153, 1985.
83. Alavi, M, Dunnet, CW, and Moore, S: Lipid composition of rabbit aortic wall following removal of endothelium by balloon catheter. Arteriosclerosis 3:413, 1983.
84. Richardson, M, Ihnatowycz, IO, and Moore, S: Glycosaminoglycan distribution in rabbit aortic wall following balloon catheter deendothelialization: An ultrastructural study. Lab Invest 43:509, 1980.
85. Schwartz, SM, Gajdusek, CM, Reidy, MA, et al: Maintenance of integrity in aortic endothelium. Fed Proc 39: 2618, 1980.
86. Haudenschild, CC and Schwartz, SM: Endothelial regeneration. II. Restitution of endothelial continuity. Lab Invest 41:407, 1979.
87. Vlodavsky, I, Johnson, LK, and Gospodarowicz, D: Appearance in confluent vascular endothelial cell monolayers of a specific cell surface protein (CSP-60) not detected in actively growing endothelial cells or in cell types growing in multiple layers. Proc Acad Sci USA 76:2306, 1979.
88. Heimark, RL and Schwartz, SM: The role of membrane-membrane interactions in the regulation of endothelial cell growth. J Cell Biol 100:1934, 1985.
89. Schumacher, BL, Grant, D, and Eisenstein, R: Smooth muscle cells produce an inhibitor of endothelial cell growth. Arteriosclerosis 5:110, 1985.
90. Ramsay, MM, Walker, LN, and Bowyer, DE: Narrow superficial injury to rabbit aortic endothelium. Atherosclerosis 43:233, 1982.
91. Prescott, MF and Muller, KP: Endothelial regeneration in hypertensive and genetically hypercholesterolemic rats. Arteriosclerosis 3:306, 1983.
92. Weksler, V, Marcus, A, and Jaffe, E: Synthesis of prostaglandin I_2 (prostacyclin) by cultured human and bovine endothelial cells. Proc Natl Acad Sci USA 74:3903, 1977.
93. Walker, F: Protein S and the regulation of activated protein C. Semin Thromb Hemostasis 10:131, 1984.
94. Stern, D, Brett, J, Harris, K, et al: Participation of endothelial cells in the Protein C–Protein S anticoagulant pathway: The synthesis and release of protein S. J Cell Biol 102:1971, 1986.

95. Thomas, WA and Kim, DN: Biology of disease: Atherosclerosis as a hyperplastic and/or neoplastic process. Lab. Invest 48:245, 1983.
96. Scott, RF, Thomas, WA, Lee, WM, et al: Distribution of intimal smooth muscle cell masses and their relationship to early atherosclerosis in the abdominal aortas of young swine. Atherosclerosis 34:291, 1979.
97. French, JE, Jennings, MA, and Florey, HW: Morphological studies on atherosclerosis in swine. Ann NY Acad Sci 127:780, 1965.
98. Scott, RF, Thomas, WA, Lee, WM, et al. Distribution of intimal smooth muscle cell masses and their relationship to early atherosclerosis in the abdominal aortas of young swine. Atherosclerosis 34:291, 1979.
99. Stout, LC, Whorton, EB, and Vaghela, M: Pathogenesis of diffuse intimal thickening (DIT) in non-human primate thoracic aortas. Atherosclerosis 47:1, 1983.
100. Grotendorst, GR, Chang, T, Seppa, HEJ, et al: Platelet-derived growth factor is a chemoattractant for vascular smooth muscle cells. J Cell Physiol 112:161, 1982.
101. Walker, LN, Ramsay, MM, Bowyer, DE: Endothelial healing following defined injury to rabbit aorta. Depth of injury and mode of repair. Atherosclerosis 47:123, 1983.
102. Reidy, MA and Silver, M: Endothelial regeneration. VII. Lack of intimal proliferation after defined injury to rat aorta. Am J Pathol 118:173, 1985.
103. Poole, JCF, Cromwell, SB, and Benditt, EP: Behaviour of smooth muscle cells and formation of extracellular structures in the reaction of arterial wall to injury. Am J Pathol 62:391, 1971.
104. Webster, WS, Bishop, SP, and Geer, JC: Experimental aortic intimal thickening. I. Morphology and source of intimal cells. Am J Pathol 76:245, 1974.
105. Spaet, TH, Stemerman, MB, Veith, FJ, et al: Intimal injury and regrowth in the rabbit aorta: Medial smooth muscle cells as a source of neointima. Cir Res 36:58, 1975.
106. Clark, JM and Glagov, S: Transmural organization of the arterial media. The lamellar unit revisited. Arteriosclerosis 5:519, 1985.
107. Campbell, GR and Campbell, JH: Smooth muscle phenotypic changes in arterial wall homeostasis: Implications for the pathogenesis of atherosclerosis. Exp Mol Pathol 42:139, 1985.
108. Colucci, WS, Black, TA, Gimbrone, MA, et al: Regulation of alpha-adrenergic receptor coupled calcium flux in cultured vascular smooth muscle cells. Hypertension 6:119, 1984.
109. Owens, GK, Loeb, A, Gordon, D, et al: Expression of smooth muscle specific isoactin in cultured vascular smooth muscle cells: Relationship between growth and cytodifferentiation. J Cell Biol 102:343, 1986.
110. McCullagh, KG, Duance, VC, and Bishop, KA: The distribution of collagen types I, III, and V (AB) in normal and atherosclerotic human aorta. J Pathol 130:45, 1980.
111. Stevens, RL, Colombo, M, Gonzales, JJ, et al: The glycosaminoglycans of the human artery and their changes in atherosclerosis. J Clin Invest 58:470, 1976.
112. Srinivasan, SR, Dolan, P, Radhakrishnamurthy, B, et al: Isolation of lipoprotein-acid mucopolysaccharide complexes from fatty streaks of human aortas. Atherosclerosis 16:95, 1972.
113. Yla-Herttuala, S, Sumuvuori, H, Karkola, K, et al: Glycosaminoglycans in normal and atherosclerotic human coronary arteries. Lab Invest 54:402, 1986.
114. Iverius, PH: The interaction between plasma lipoproteins and connective tissue glycosaminoglycans. J Biol Chem 247:2607, 1972.
115. Campbell, JH, Reardon, MF, Campbell, GR, et al: Metabolism of atherogenic lipoproteins by smooth muscle cells of different phenotype in culture. Arteriosclerosis 5:318, 1985.
116. Ross, R, Glomset, J, Kariya, B, et al: A platelet dependent serum factor that stimulates the proliferation of arterial smooth muscle cells in vitro. Proc Nat Acad Sci USA 71:1207, 1974.
117. Fischer-Dzoga, K, Fraser, R, and Wissler, RW: Stimulation of proliferation in stationary primary cultures of monkey and rabbit aortic smooth muscle cells. I. Effects of lipoprotein fractions of hyperlipemic serum and lymph. Exp Mol Pathol 24:346, 1976.
118. Martin, BM, Gimbrone, MA, Unanue, ER, et al: Stimulation of nonlymphoid mesenchymal cell proliferation by a macrophage-derived growth factor. J Immunol 126:1510, 1981.
119. Gajdusek, CM, DiCorleto, P, Ross, R, et al: An endothelial cell-derived growth factor. J Cell Biol 85:467, 1980.
120. DiCorleto, PE and Bowen-Pope, DF: Cultured endothelial cells produced a platelet-derived growth factor-like protein. Proc Natl Acad Sci USA 80:1919, 1983.
121. Seifert, RA, Schwartz, SM, and Bowen-Pope, DF: Developmentally regulated production of platelet derived growth factor–like molecules. Nature 311:669, 1984.

122. Nilsson, J, Sjlund, M, Palmberg, L, et al: Arterial smooth muscle cells in primary culture produce a platelet derived growth factor-like protein. Proc Natl. Acad Sci 82:4418, 1985.
123. Walker, LN, Bowen-Pope, DF, and Reidy, MA: Secreting of platelet derived growth factor (PDGF)-like activity in arterial smooth muscle cell is induced as a response to injury (abstr). J Cell Biol 99:416a, 1984.
124. Nemecek, GM, Coughlin, SR, Handley, DA, et al: Stimulation of aortic smooth muscle cell mitogenesis by serotonin. Proc Natl. Acad Sci USA 83:674, 1986.
125. Blaes, N and Boissel, JP: Growth stimulating effect of catecholamines on rat aortic smooth muscle cells in culture. J Cell Physiol 116:167, 1983.
126. Fishman, JA, Ryan, GB, and Karnovsky, MJ: Endothelial regeneration in the rat carotid artery and the significance of endothelial denudation in the pathogenesis of myointimal thickening. Lab Invest 32:339, 1975.
127. Guyton, JR, Rosenberg, RD, Clowes, AW, et al: Inhibition of rat arterial smooth muscle cell proliferation by heparin. Circ Res 46:625, 1980.
128. Castellot, JJ, Beeler, SL, Rosenberg, RD, et al: Structural determinants of the capacity of heparin to inhibit the proliferation of vascular smooth muscle cells. J Cell Physiol 120:315, 1984.
129. Castellot, JJ, Choay, J, Lormeau, JC, et al: Structural determinants of the capacity of heparin to inhibit the proliferation of vascular smooth muscle cells. II. Evidence for a pentasaccharide sequence that contains a 3-0-sulfate group. J Cell Biol 102:1979, 1986.
130. Fritze, LMS, Reilly, CF, and Rosenberg, RD: An antiproliferative heparin sulfate species produced by postconfluent smooth muscle cells. J Cell Biol 100:1041, 1985.
131. Waller, BF, McManus, BM, Gorfinkel, HJ, et al: Status of the major epicardial coronary arteries 80 to 150 days after percutaneous transluminal coronary angioplasty. Am J Cardiol 51:81, 1983.
132. Faxon, DP, Samborn, TA, Weber, VJ, et al: Restenosis following transluminal angioplasty in experimental atherosclerosis. Arteriosclerosis 4:189, 1984.
133. Austin, GE, Ratliff, NB, Hollman, J, et al: Intimal proliferation of smooth muscle cells as an explanation for recurrent coronary artery stenosis after percutaneous transluminal coronary angioplasty. JACC 6:369, 1985.
134. Campeau, L, Enjalbert, M, Lesperance, J, et al: Arteriosclerosis and late closure of aorto-coronary saphenous vein grafts: Sequential angiographic studies at 2 weeks, 1 year, 5-7 years, and 10-12 years after surgery. Circulation 68 (Suppl II): II-1. 1983.
135. Fuster, V and Chesebro, JJ: Aorto-coronary vein-graft disease: Experimental and clinical approach for the understanding of the role of platelets and platelet inhibitors. Circulation 72(Suppl V): V-65, 1985.
136. Groves, HM, Kinlough-Rathbone, RL, Richardson, M, et al: Thrombin generation and fibrin formation following injury to rabbit neointima: Studies of vessel wall reactivity and platelet survival. Lab Invest 64:605, 1982.
137. Mustard JF: The role of platelets and thrombosis in the development of atherosclerosis and its complications. Ann R Coll Phys Surg Can 14:22, 1981.
138. Clowes, AW, Reidy, MA, and Clowes, MM: Kinetics of cellular proliferation after arterial injury. I. Smooth muscle growth in the absence of endothelium. Lab Invest 49:327, 1983.
139. Langille, BL and O'Donnell, F: Reduction in arterial diameter produced by chronic decreases in blood flow are endothelium dependent. Science 231:405, 1986.
140. Geer, JC, McGill, HC, and Strong, JP: The fine structure of human atherosclerotic lesions. Am J Pathol 38:263, 1961.
141. Balis, JR, Haust, MD, and More, RH: Electron microscopic studies in human atherosclerosis: Cellular elements in aortic fatty streaks. Exp Mol Pathol 3:511, 1964.
142. McGill, HC: Persistent problems in the pathogenesis of atherosclerosis. Arteriosclerosis 4:443, 1984.
143. Smith, EB, Evans, PH, and Pownham, MD: Lipid in the aortic intima: The correlation of morphological and chemical characteristics. J Atherosclerosis Res 7:171, 1967.
144. Bocan, RMA, Schifani, TA, and Guyton, JR: Ultrastructure of the human aortic fibrolipid lesion. Formation of the atherosclerotic lipid rich core. Am J Pathol 123:413, 1986.
145. Heistad, DD and Armstrong, ML: Blood flow through vasa vasorum of coronary arteries in atherosclerotic monkeys. Arteriosclerosis 6:326, 1986.
146. Paterson, JC: Capillary rupture with intimal hemorrhage as a causative factor in coronary thrombosis. Arch Pathol 25:474, 1938.
147. Barger, AC, Beeuwkes, R, Lainey, LL, et al: Hypothesis: Vasa vasorum and neovascularization of human coronary arteries. N Engl J Med 310:175, 1984.

148. Clowes, AW, Clowes, MM, and Reidy, MA: Kinetics of cellular proliferation after arterial injury. III. Endothelial and smooth muscle cell growth in chronically denuded vessels. Lab Invest 54:295, 1986.
149. Moncada, S, Herman, AG, Higgs, EA, et al: Differential formation of prostacyclin (PGX or PGI_2) by layers of the arterial wall: An explanation for the anti-thrombotic properties of vascular endothelium. Thromb Res 11:323, 1977.
150. Adelman, B, Stemerman, MB, and Handin, RI: Interaction of platelets and fibrin with injured rabbit aortic neointima. Effect of prostaglandin I_2 and heparin. Arteriosclerosis 3:141, 1983.
151. Tracy, RE, Kissling, GE, Lopez, CR, et al: Histometric component of aortic atherosclerosis which vary or remain constant among eight populations. Lab Invest 54:34, 1986.

CHAPTER 2

Coronary Thrombosis and Acute Myocardial Infarction

J. T. Lie, M.D.

A HISTORIC PERSPECTIVE

The role of coronary thrombosis in the genesis of acute myocardial infarction remains controversial.[1–5] The evolution of the traditional concept of ischemic heart disease, from recognition of the existence of coronary circulation by William Harvey (1578–1657) in 1649 to the first bedside diagnosis of coronary thrombosis by Adam Hammer (1818–1878) in 1878, was a languid 229-year process.[6,7] Hammer's report[7] appeared more than 100 years after William Heberden's lecture on angina pectoris,[8] and preceded Carl Weigert's description of the pathology of acute myocardial infarction.[9] Hammer's report was followed, in this country, in 1896, by George Dock's report[10] of a 36-year-old man in whom the clinical diagnosis of occlusion of the right coronary artery was confirmed at autopsy. Then came similar reports by the Russian physicians Obrastzow and Straschesko in 1910,[11] and by our own James Bryan Herrick in 1912.[12]

Compared with any of the preceding reports, Herrick's classic article[12] attracted more widespread interest and exerted greater influence in bringing the concept of acute coronary artery occlusion causing myocardial infarction to the attention of the entire medical profession. The terms "coronary thrombosis" and "coronary occlusion" became virtually synonymous with myocardial infarction. This view was held for many years, until Blumgart and colleagues[13,14] demonstrated pathologic specimens in which coronary occlusion was found in the absence of myocardial infarction. The presence of a functional collateral circulation in hearts with coronary artery disease seemed to have protected the myocardium. Blumgart recognized that patients with acute myocardial infarction might not exhibit coronary thrombosis at autopsy. He did not, however, speculate on the pathogenesis of myocardial infarction without total occlusion. The prevailing view then became that myocardial infarction was the consequence of progressive coronary atherosclerosis or increased flow demand over a fixed coronary reserve. More recently, there has been a steady stream of reports of myocardial infarction in the presence of "normal" coronary arteries (or more correctly, in the absence of critical or significant coronary artery disease), for which there are many possible explanations but none that is completely satisfactory.[15] Finally, the relationship between fixed (atherosclerotic) and dynamic (vasospastic) obstruction of the coronary artery in the genesis of acute myocardial infarction remains unsettled, as the two opposing mechanisms of coronary artery occlusion are not mutually exclusive.[16-20]

PATHOPHYSIOLOGY AND ANATOMIC BASIS OF CORONARY HEART DISEASE

The traditional view of the pathophysiology of myocardial ischemia and myocardial infarction is an unfavorable balance between coronary blood flow and the metabolic needs of the myocardium. The supply and demand imbalance has usually been attributed to the inability of the coronary circulation to supply the increased amount of oxygen required by augmented myocardial demands. However, myocardial ischemia may not necessarily be preceded by an increase in oxygen demand; decreased oxygen delivery from reduction in coronary blood flow may be a more important pathophysiologic mechanism of myocardial ischemia in many clinical settings. We now know that coronary stenoses frequently behave as though the obstruction to flow is variable and not as rigidly fixed as previously believed. The conditions that reduce coronary blood flow, which are transient and dynamic in nature, may modify the threshold for ischemia, especially in patients with fixed obstructive disease of the coronary arteries.[20-22]

The clinical spectrum of ischemic heart disease encompasses asymptomatic coronary artery disease, the various angina syndromes, myocardial infarction, and sudden death (Fig. 2–1). In an autopsy population, in which a qualitative and quantitative assessment of myocardial and coronary artery pathology is possible, about two thirds of all fatalities from ischemic heart disease had two or more coronary arteries with critical stenoses (Table 2–1). The prevalence of double- or triple-

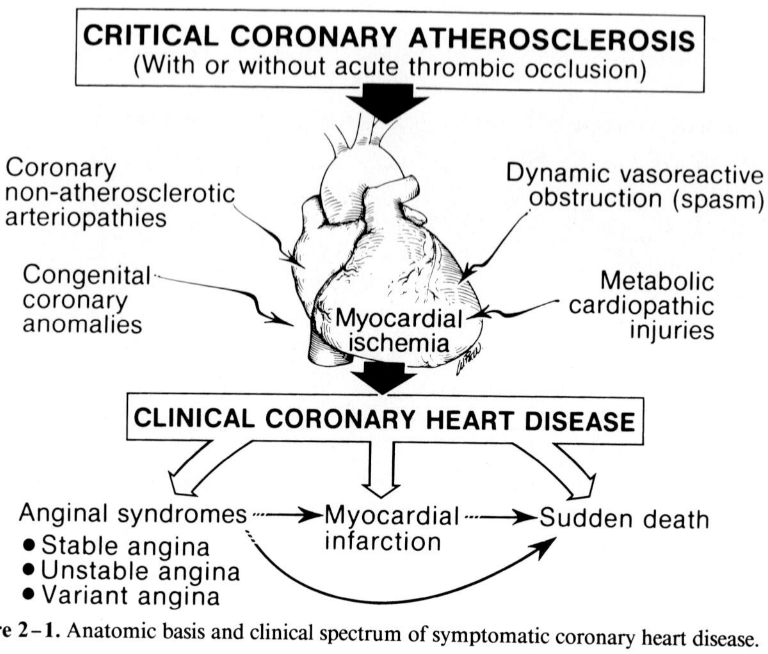

Figure 2–1. Anatomic basis and clinical spectrum of symptomatic coronary heart disease.

Table 2–1. Anatomic Findings in Fatal Ischemic Heart Disease: A Cumulative Autopsy Series of 824 Cases

Clinicopathologic Subgroup	Stable Angina	Unstable Angina	Variant Angina	Myocardial Infarction: *Transmural*	Myocardial Infarction: *Nontransmural*	Sudden Death*
Number of patients	58	76	32	247	209	202
Critical coronary stenosis†						
Single-vessel disease	15 (26%)	14 (18%)	9 (28%)	47 (19%)	27 (13%)	36 (18%)
Double-vessel disease	17 (29%)	19 (35%)	9 (28%)	52 (21%)	63 (30%)	47 (23%)
Triple-vessel disease	21 (37%)	31 (41%)	12 (38%)	94 (38%)	90 (43%)	93 (46%)
Left main artery disease	5 (8%)	12 (16%)	2 (6%)	54 (22%)	29 (14%)	26 (13%)
Acute coronary thrombosis	4 (7%)	7 (9%)	7 (22%)	151 (61%)	25 (12%)	36 (18%)
Myocardial infarction						
Recent (<4 wk)	3 (6%)	27 (36%)	13 (41%)	247 (100%)	209 (100%)	63 (31%)
Healed (>4 wk)	24 (42%)	36 (47%)	12 (38%)	84 (34%)	98 (47%)	71 (35%)
Cardiac hypertrophy (Heart weight >400 g)	27 (47%)	41 (54%)	15 (46%)	160 (65%)	119 (57%)	123 (61%)
Average heart weight	415 g	430 g	420 g	465 g	480 g	435 g

* Death occurring within 1 hour of onset of acute terminal event.

† Coronary artery with >75% reduction in cross-sectional luminal area. Left main artery disease is not counted in the single-vessel disease group, and in all instances is seen in the double- or triple-vessel disease group.

vessel, fixed coronary artery disease of this magnitude was independent of the clinical subsets of fatal ischemic heart disease. The incidence of histologically documented acute coronary thrombosis varied greatly, from 7 percent in patients with stable angina to 61 percent in patients with transmural myocardial infarction (Fig. 2–2). This trend is in general agreement with that reported by other investigators,[23–30] although the number of vessels with critical stenosis may vary according to the source and the selection criteria of the case material. Critical stenosis is defined as 75 percent or greater reduction in cross-sectional area of the artery.

Fixed Atherosclerotic Disease and Coronary Spasm

Although atherosclerotic disease of the coronary arteries, with or without thrombosis, is the most common and most important cause of myocardial ischemia, transient and dynamic obstructions are the alternative mechanisms that have become better understood in the past two decades.[20–22,31–33] These mechanisms can be classified into two broad categories: those that cause a dynamic coronary stenosis and those that reduce the coronary vasodilatory reserve capacity (Table 2–2).

Atherosclerosis is often considered to produce rigid, fixed arterial segments incapable of vasospastic response, but such is not the case. The majority of diseased coronary arteries have an eccentric lumen (Fig. 2–3); that is, an arch of the vessel wall remains uninvolved, or only minimally involved, and is capable of contraction. MacAlpin[34] has calculated that normal coronary vasomotion in this setting might be sufficient to occlude the lumen, and he has further shown that most cases of angiographically documented coronary artery spasm involved a vessel with fixed atherosclerotic disease.[35] Tests on pharmacologic reactivity of human epicardial coronary arteries revealed that morphologic characteristics of the atherosclerotic plaques within the vessel lumen and the degree of myocardial dysfunction did not qualita-

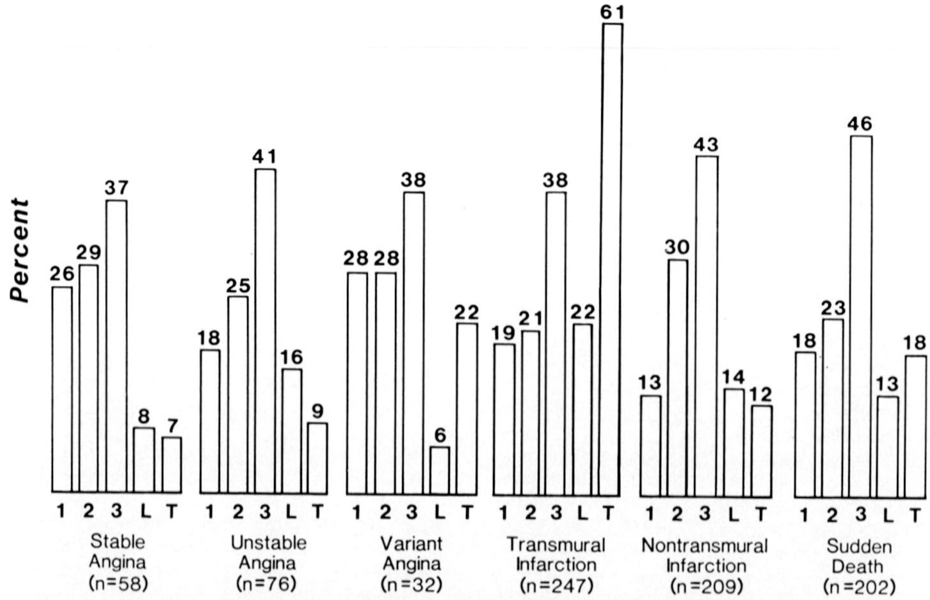

Figure 2-2. Frequency distribution of number of coronary arteries with critical stenosis (≥ 75 percent reduction in luminal area) and of acute thrombosis in various clinical subsets of fatal cases of coronary heart disease. 1 = single-vessel disease; 2 = double-vessel disease; 3 = triple-vessel disease; L = left main coronary artery disease; T = acute coronary thrombosis.

Table 2-2. Vascular Factors in Myocardial Ischemia

- I. Obstructive coronary artery disease
  - A. Fixed lesions, with or without thrombosis
    - 1. Atherosclerosis
    - 2. Nonatherosclerotic disease (e.g., arteritis, aneurysms, dysplasia, and dissection)
  - B. Transient obstruction
    - 1. Systolic arterial compression
      - a. Myocardial bridging
      - b. Left ventricular-aortic pressure gradient
    - 2. Arterial constriction
      - a. Vasospasm
      - b. Hypertonus
- II. Inadequate coronary vascular reserve flow capacity
  - A. Structural
    - 1. Hypertrophy
    - 2. Other mechanisms
  - B. Functional
    - 1. Hemodynamic
      - a. Diastolic transmural compression
      - b. Coronary "steal"
    - 2. Arteriolar unresponsiveness or deregulation
      - a. Idiopathic
      - b. Smoking
      - c. Drug-induced

Modified from Gorlin.[22]

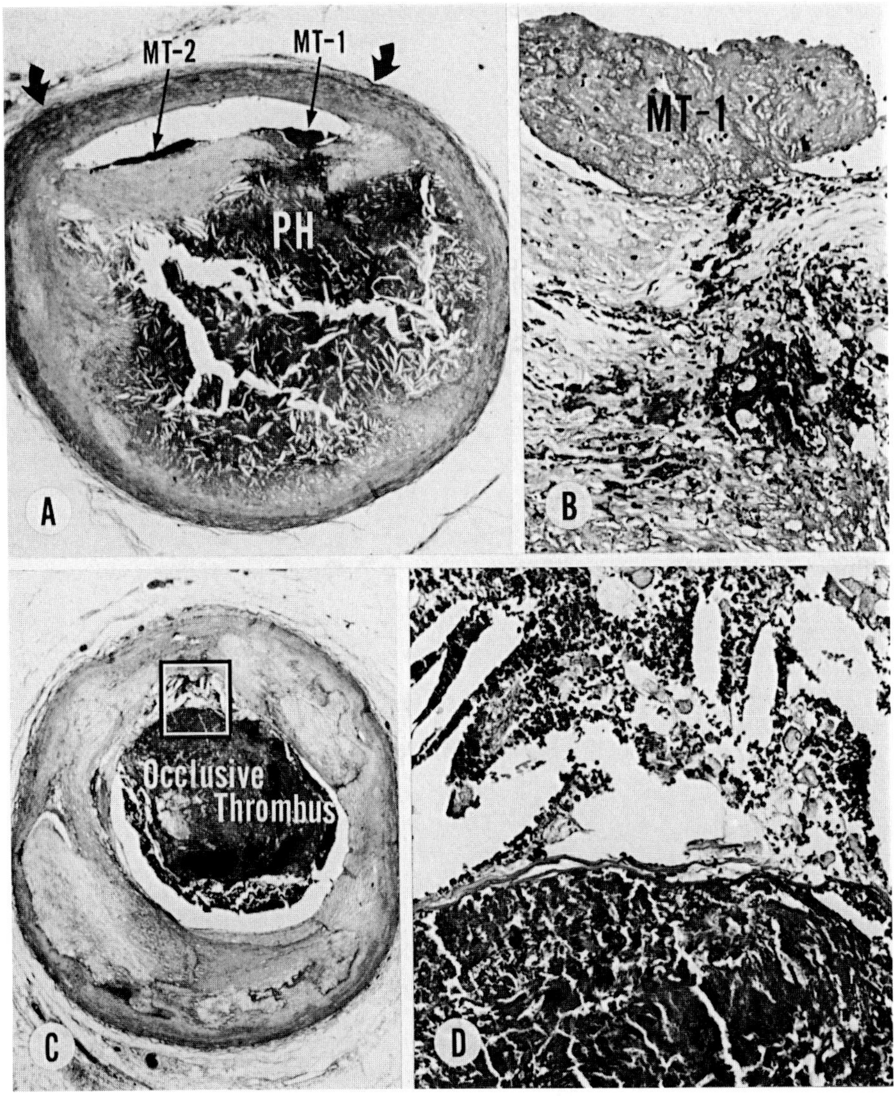

Figure 2-3. *A,* Coronary atherosclerosis with a large fatty plaque and an eccentric, slit-like lumen bound by an arch of normal muscular media *(curved arrows)* and two mural thrombi, MT-1 and MT-2 *(straight arrows). B,* Mural thrombus MT-1 seen at higher magnification. *C,* Coronary atherosclerosis with a concentric lumen and an occlusive thrombus attached to eroded intimal surface, seen at higher magnification in *D.* (Hematoxylin and eosin; magnification *A* and *C,* ×16; *B* and *D,* ×160.)

tively alter the contractile responses of the coronary arteries to various vasoactive agents.[36]

Coronary artery spasm cannot be and has not been convincingly demonstrated anatomically at postmortem.[37] However, some evidence of coronary artery spasm has been reported in 0.26 to 3.4 percent of all patients undergoing selective coronary arteriography.[35] According to a study reported by Bertrand and associates,[38] the overall frequency of drug-provoked coronary artery spasm in 1089 consecutive patients undergoing coronary arteriography was 12.3 percent. Among the various clinical subsets (Table 2-3), the frequency was highest in patients with angina at rest (38

Table 2–3. Frequency of Provoked Spasm in 1089 Consecutive Patients Undergoing Coronary Arteriography

Patient Subgroup	Number of Patients	Coronary Artery with Fixed Lesion				Spasm	
		0	*1*	*2*	*3*	*n*	%
Atypical chest pain	248	221	22	5	0	3	1.2
Exertional angina pectoris	117	23	38	26	30	5	4.3
Angina on effort and at rest	138	58	22	34	24	19	13.8
Angina pectoris at rest	203	93	55	29	26	77	38.0
Recent myocardial infarction	116	7	54	31	24	23	20.0
Old myocardial infarction	64	3	26	20	15	4	6.2
Valvular heart disease	154	132	16	5	1	3	2.0
Cardiomyopathy	49	44	4	1	0	0	0.0
Total	1089	581	237	151	120	134	12.3

Based on the data of Bertrand et al.[38]

percent) and lowest in those with atypical chest pain (1.2 percent) and exertional angina (4.3 percent), which did not differ significantly from the control groups (valvular disease 2 percent, and cardiomyopathy 0 percent). Vasoconstriction of small intramyocardial arteries and inadequate coronary flow reserve capacity have also been implicated in the genesis of myocardial ischemia.[22,23]

ACUTE CORONARY THROMBOSIS

Among patients who died of ischemic heart disease, the prevalence of critical coronary artery disease is similar in all clinical categories, but the incidence of acute coronary artery thrombosis is highly variable (see Fig. 2–2). Despite numerous pathologic studies, there is still disagreement on the cause-and-effect relationship of acute coronary thrombosis and myocardial infarction.[1–5,39–41] Discrepancies and variation in definition, methodology, and patient selection have prolonged the controversy. The recognition that the frequency of acute coronary artery thrombosis varies with different types of myocardial infarction and sudden death has been a major step toward clarification of this important issue (Table 2–4).

The salient pathologic features of coronary artery thrombosis may be summarized as follows:

1. Less than 20 percent of sudden coronary death patients have coronary thrombosis, whereas coronary thrombi are found in more than 50 percent of patients who survived a myocardial infarction for 24 hours or longer. Among patients who survived more than 24 hours, the incidence of coronary thrombosis is about three to four times higher in those with transmural infarction (60 to 90 percent) than in those with subendocardial infarction (20 to 30 percent). Coronary thrombosis is also three to four times more common in patients with cardiogenic shock than in those without.[39–47]

2. Acute coronary thrombi may be nonocclusive (mural) or occlusive (Fig. 2–4). The majority of occlusive thrombi are single and short (less than 2 cm) and are found almost exclusively in the major extramural coronary arteries. Thrombosis rarely occurs in a normal or near-normal coronary artery (see Figs. 2–3 and 2–4).[51] Rapid, spontaneous resolution of thromboemboli has been documented as a proba-

Table 2–4. Frequency of Coronary Artery Thrombosis in Acute Myocardial Infarction and Sudden Coronary Death

Category of Fatal Event (First Author and Year)	Number of Cases	Frequency of Coronary Thrombosis (%)
Transmural infarction		
Miller, 1951[42]	93	90
Chapman, 1968[43]	292	91
Sinapius, 1972[44]	170	96
Davies, 1976[45]	469	95
Bulkley, 1977[46]	102	95
Horie, 1978[47]	185	92
Subendocardial infarction		
Miller, 1951[42]	50	20
Davies, 1976[45]	31	13
Sudden coronary death (survival time)		
Spain, 1960 (<1 hr)[48]	363	16
Lie, 1975 (<6 hr)[49]	120	17
Baroldi, 1979 (<10 min)[50]	151	12

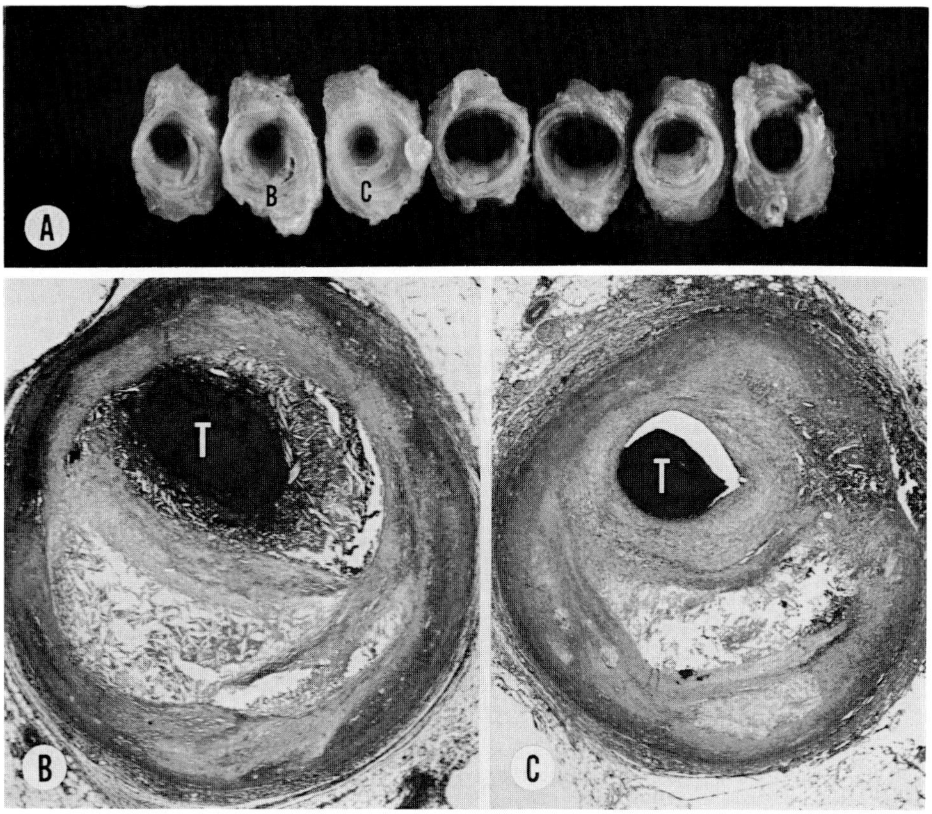

Figure 2–4. *A,* Serial, 5 mm, cross sections of right coronary artery with a long (3.5 cm) occlusive thrombus, occurring at proximal segment *(left-hand side)* and propagating distally *(right-hand side).* Note that thrombus occurs in artery with severe atherosclerosis and critical stenosis. Two selected cross sections are shown as photomicrographs in *B* and *C.* Note that thrombus (T) in *B* is admixed with extruded atheromatous material after plaque ulceration and rupture. (Hematoxylin and eosin; *B* and *C,* original magnification ×16; reduced 5 percent.)

ble cause of myocardial infarction occurring in patients with angiographically normal coronary arteries,[52-55] but this is by no means proven in all cases.

According to the angiographic studies by DeWood and coworkers,[56] in the first 4 hours of the onset of symptoms, the coronary artery supplying the infarcted area is occluded in more than 87 percent of patients. The occlusion rates drop to 32 percent within 12 hours[56] and to about 50 percent at 2 to 3 weeks.[57] In pathologic specimens, an acute occlusive coronary thrombus seldom undergoes complete spontaneous lysis in less than 2 to 3 days (Fig. 2–5).

3. Irrespective of whether the histologic study was carried out on random samples or serial sections, the majority (60 to 100 percent) of acute coronary thrombi have been shown to be initiated by ulceration or fissuring, hemorrhage, and rupture of the underlying atherosclerotic plaques.[58-65] The histologic appearance of the thrombosis-associated plaque rupture often indicates that the disruption is from within the plaque with extrusion of atheromatous debris into the lumen and tell-tale admixture of plaque contents with the thrombus (Fig. 2–6).

However, not all plaque hemorrhage and ulceration are associated with thrombosis, nor are all coronary thrombi occlusive (see Fig. 2–4). All occlusive lesions of the coronary arteries, presumed to be thrombi on gross appearance, should be verified histologically. Plaque hemorrhage and luminal occlusion by atheromatous material (Fig. 2–7) or old organized thrombi (Fig. 2–8) can be deceiving to the naked eye and are often mistaken as acute thrombosis when not examined histologically.

A Unifying Concept

Coronary artery spasm and coronary thrombosis are not two independent and mutually exclusive mechanisms of vascular occlusion in the genesis of myocardial

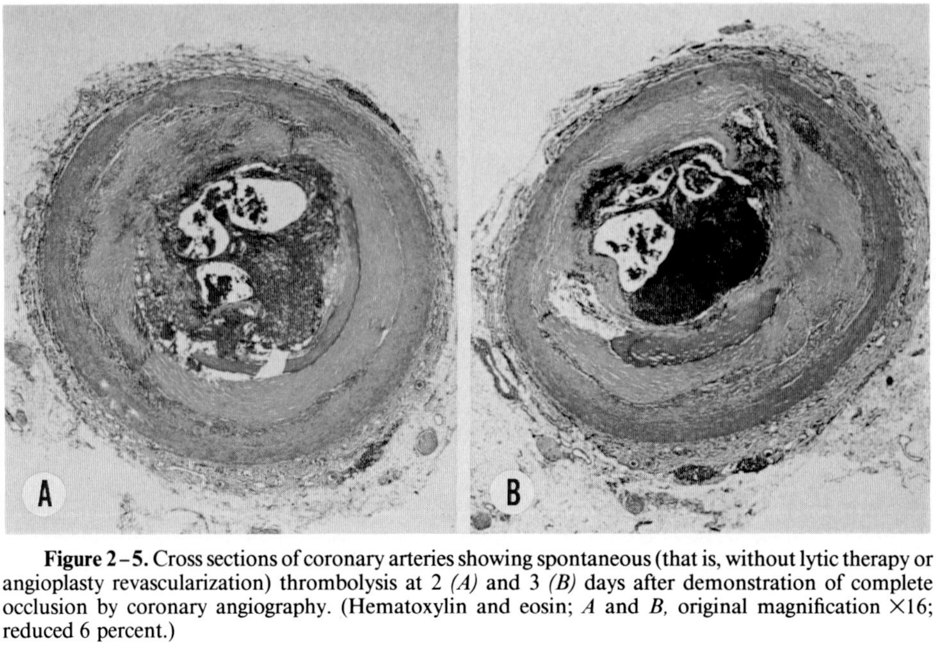

Figure 2–5. Cross sections of coronary arteries showing spontaneous (that is, without lytic therapy or angioplasty revascularization) thrombolysis at 2 *(A)* and 3 *(B)* days after demonstration of complete occlusion by coronary angiography. (Hematoxylin and eosin; *A* and *B*, original magnification ×16; reduced 6 percent.)

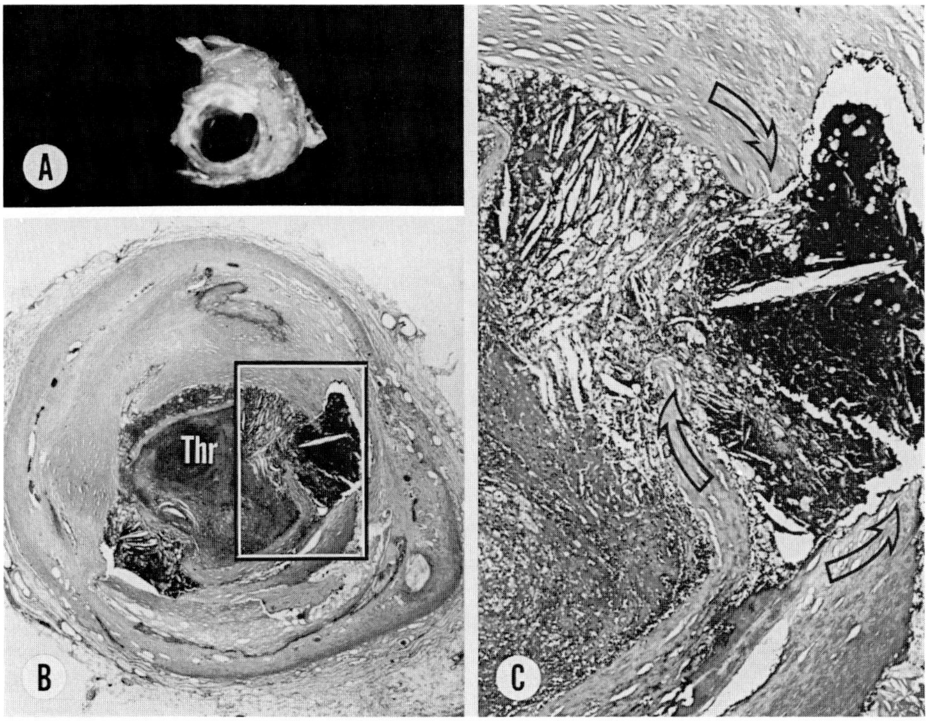

Figure 2–6. *A,* Cross section of coronary artery with occlusive thrombus. *B,* Photomicrograph of same coronary artery revealing that thrombus (Thr) is initiated by plaque hemorrhage and rupture. *C,* Close-up view of boxed area in *B,* to show rupture site *(arrows)* and extrusion of plaque contents into lumen. (Hematoxylin and eosin; original magnifications *B,* ×16; *C,* ×64; reduced 5 percent.)

ischemia and infarction. Coronary spasm may cause intimal tear and plaque rupture. Platelet aggregation, the precursor of thrombosis, may be induced by exposed intimal collagen following endothelial injury and plaque rupture. Endothelial injury may impair the synthesis of prostacycline, a powerful coronary vasodilator, whereas platelet aggregation is associated with the release of thromboxane A_2, a potent coronary vasoconstrictor. An imbalance of prostacycline-thromboxane A_2 production may initiate or perpetuate coronary spasm, and thus it forms common links among vascular injury, coronary spasm, and thrombosis.[5,66,67]

Coronary Embolism and Intramyocardial Platelet Aggregates

The first fatal case of coronary thrombosis that was correctly diagnosed before death by Adam Hammer, in1878, was probably embolic in origin.[7] However, coronary embolism as the cause of death or myocardial infarction is uncommon; its reported autopsy incidence ranges from 0.06 to 1.1 percent.[68–70] The most frequent sources of coronary emboli are bland or septic thrombi from cardiac valves or mural thrombi from the cardiac chambers.[69–71] Thromboemboli do not necessarily occur in diseased (atherosclerotic) arteries; they are usually lodged at branch points or in the smaller-caliber distal segments of the coronary arteries, as well as in their intramural

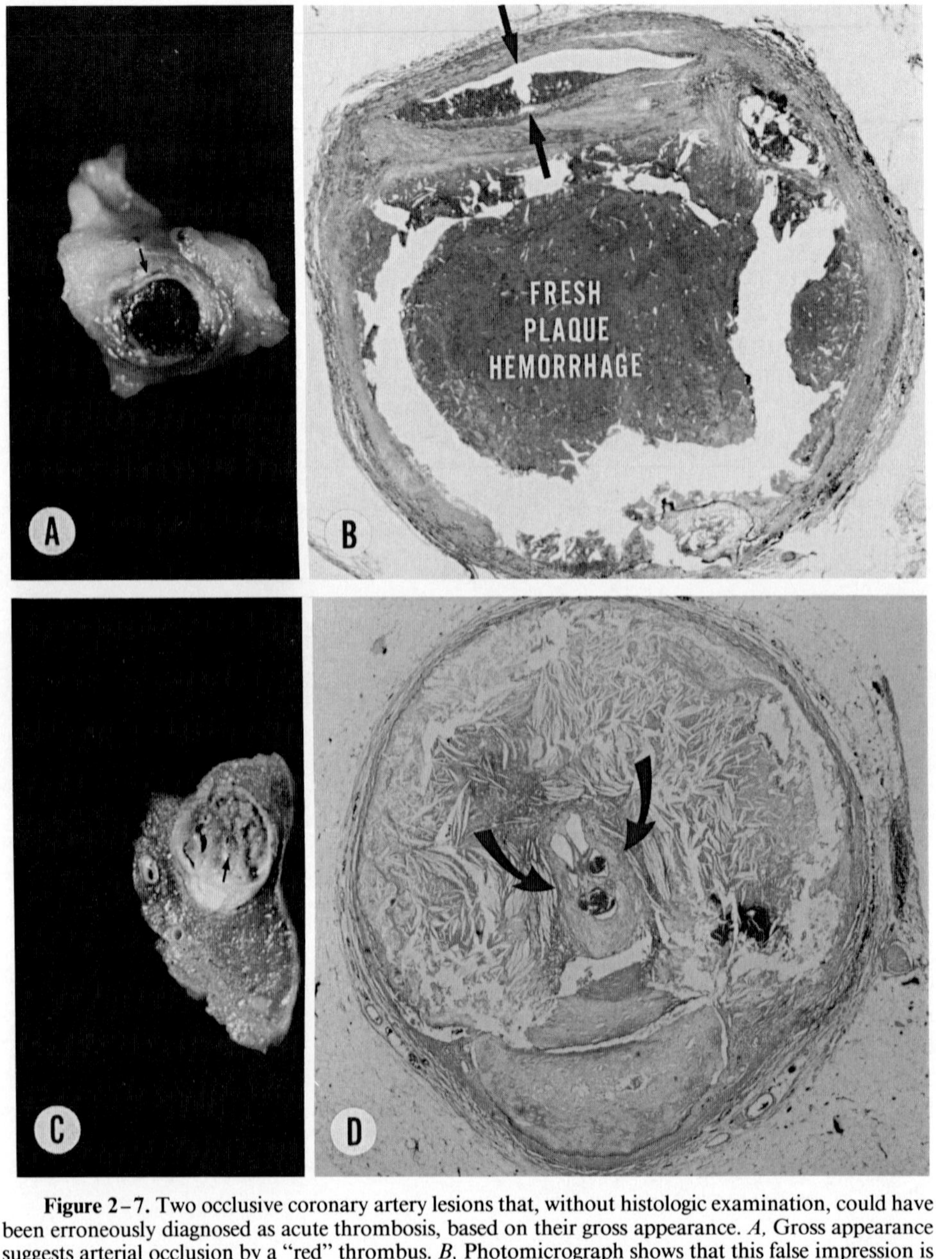

Figure 2–7. Two occlusive coronary artery lesions that, without histologic examination, could have been erroneously diagnosed as acute thrombosis, based on their gross appearance. *A,* Gross appearance suggests arterial occlusion by a "red" thrombus. *B,* Photomicrograph shows that this false impression is created by plaque hemorrhage and inconspicuous slit-like lumen *(arrows). C,* Gross appearance mimicks arterial occlusion by a pale fibrin-platelet "white" thrombus. *D,* Photomicrograph shows that this false impression is created by fatty atheromatous material surrounding a central minuscule lumen *(arrows).* (Hematoxylin and eosin; *B* and *D,* magnification ×16.)

branches (Fig. 2–9). In studies of autopsy populations, emboli were found in the distribution of the left coronary artery in more than 70 percent of cases, and multiple emboli were found in 15 to 25 percent of patients.[69,70] More than two thirds of cases were unrecognized clinically, according to one study.[70]

Previous autopsy studies[49,72–74] have reported intramyocardial platelet aggregates in up to 54 percent of victims of sudden coronary death. These findings may have been interpreted as indicative of hyperactive platelets undergoing spontaneous intravascular agglutination. Recent additional studies[75,76] support the view that platelet aggregates in the myocardium represent an embolic occlusion of the microcirculation and are a potential cause of unstable angina, ischemia-induced ventricular fibrillation, and sudden death. Likewise, platelet hyperaggregability may be the underlying cause of chest pain in patients with angiographically normal coronary arteries.[77]

Small Vessel Disease

There is considerable renewed interest in the role of small vessel disease of the heart in the genesis of myocardial ischemia.[22,33] The intramyocardial small arteries and arterioles are unaffected by atherosclerosis, but they may exhibit significant proliferative changes, with wall thickening and luminal narrowing in a variety of conditions (Fig. 2–10), including hypertension, diabetes mellitus, collagen-vascular diseases, amyloidosis, and cardiomyopathies.[78,79] However, there is still uncertainty

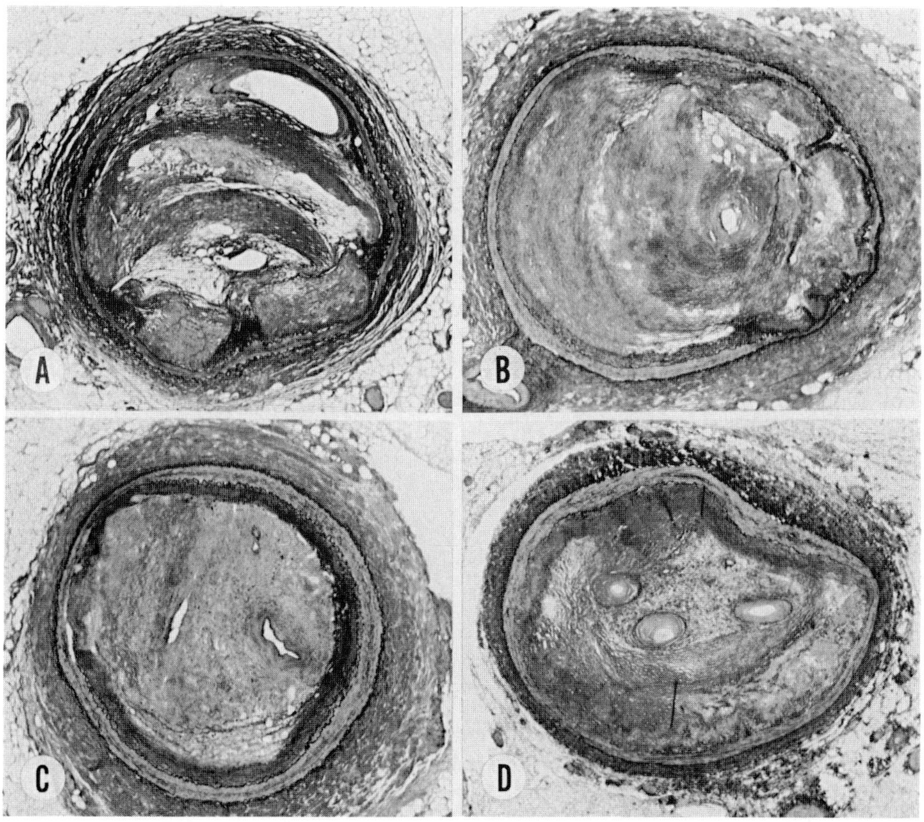

Figure 2–8. Old occlusive disease of coronary arteries that, without histologic examination, could have been erroneously diagnosed as acute thrombosis, based on their gross appearance. *A* and *B*, Examples of occlusion by build-up of atherosclerotic plaques. *C* and *D*, Examples of old, organized thrombi with minute recanalized channels that would escape detection by naked-eye inspection. (Hematoxylin and eosin; original magnification ×16; reduced 5 percent.)

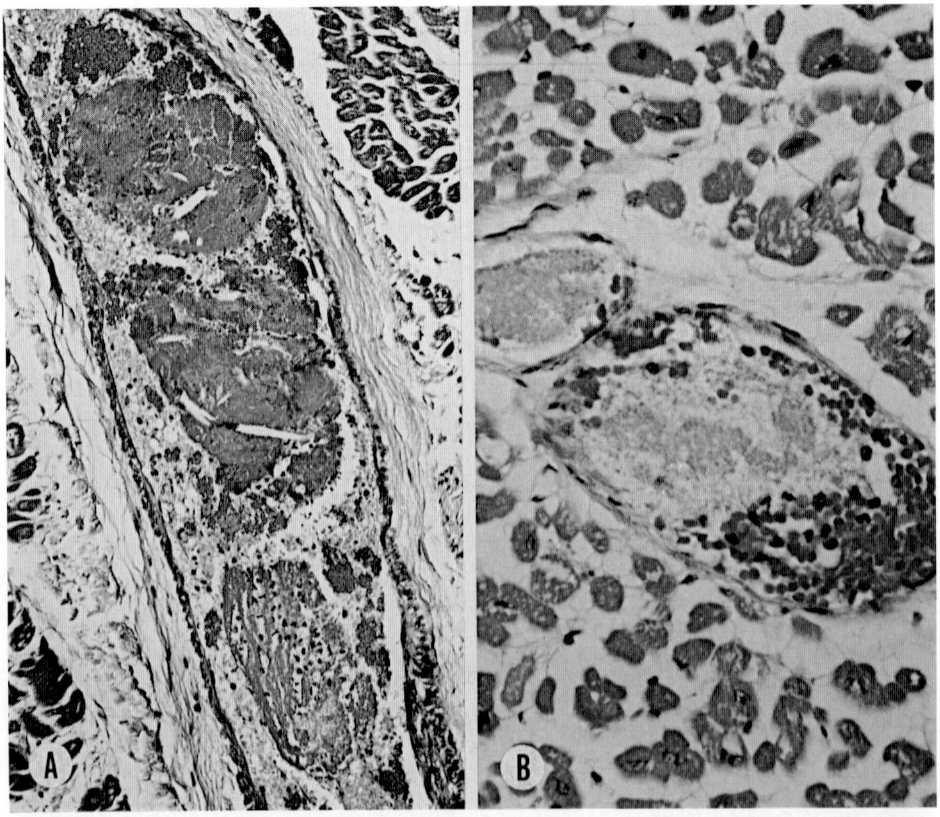

Figure 2–9. Two types of occlusive disease of coronary microcirculation. *A,* Embolic material from ruptured atherosclerotic plaque upstream in a diseased epicardial coronary artery. *B,* Platelet aggregates in microcirculation in a patient with unstable angina and sudden cardiac death. (Hematoxylin and eosin; *A* and *B,* original magnification ×160; reduced 6 percent.)

regarding the functional significance of "small vessel disease," because it may also be found in asymptomatic patients. In ischemic heart disease, subendocardial myocardial infarction was frequently associated with narrowing of the small arteries, even in the absence of major coronary artery stenosis. However, transmural myocardial infarction occurred almost always with large (extramural) coronary artery disease, either alone or in combination with narrowing of the small arteries.[80]

MYOCARDIAL INFARCTION

Transmural, Subendocardial, and Mixed Varieties

Myocardial infarctions are traditionally classified as *transmural* (extending beyond one half to two thirds of the ventricular wall thickness) or *subendocardial* (confined to the inner half or one third of the ventricular wall-thickness).[42] The majority of transmural infarcts have an occlusive thrombus in the vessel subtending the infarcted zone, whereas subendocardial infarcts are seldom associated with acute coronary thrombosis.[81] A *mixed* infarct, with combined topographic features of both transmural and subendocardial infarctions (Fig. 2–11), occurs perhaps more commonly than is generally recognized.

The existence of a "border zone" in myocardial infarction has been inferred from biochemical, electrocardiographic, and histochemical studies.[82,83] If it exists, salvage of the border zone is potentially beneficial in limiting the infarct size and reduction of mortality. A morphologic study[82] showed that in most infarcts, an irregular but sharp boundary demarcated normal and infarcted myocardium with no intermediate zone. Three-dimensional analysis of the infarcts revealed no true islands but instead demonstrated a region composed of highly complex interdigitating peninsulas (Fig. 2–12).

Myocardial Vulnerability

The number of normal, ischemic, and necrotic myocytes differs in different areas of the region at risk during the early critical hours of myocardial infarction. In the canine heart, virtually all myocytes are necrotic after 6 hours of ischemia.[84] The

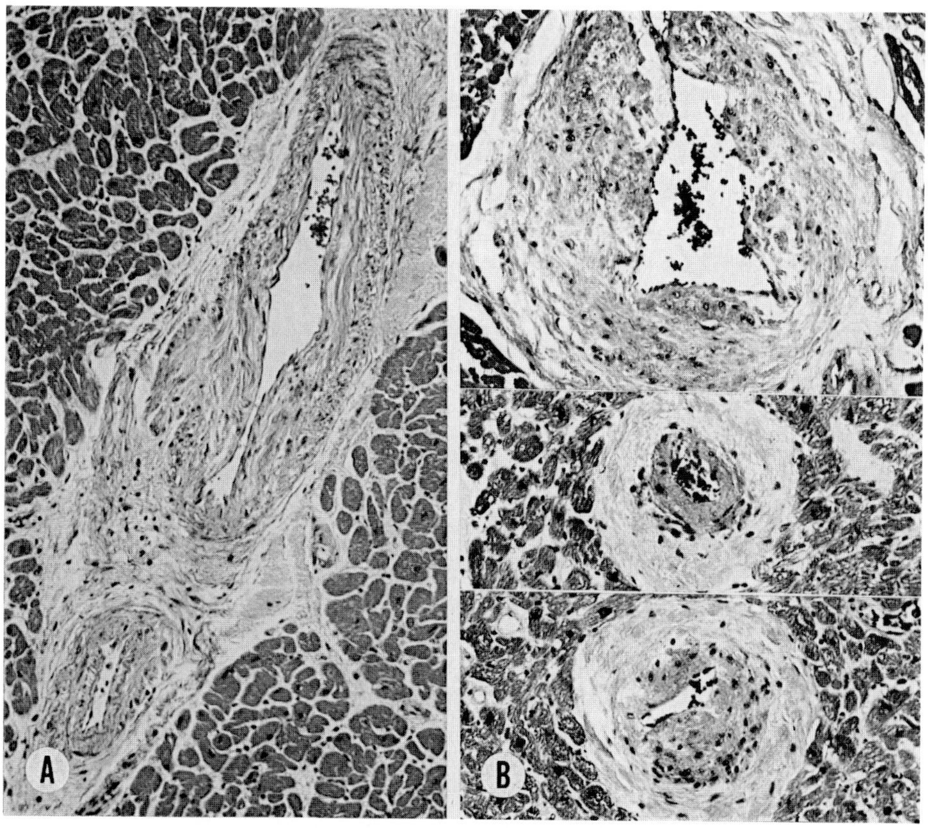

Figure 2–10. Small-vessel disease of intramyocardial branches of coronary arteries in hypertensive heart disease *(A)* and diabetes mellitus *(B)*. (Hematoxylin and eosin; *A* and *B*, original magnification ×160; reduced 5 percent.)

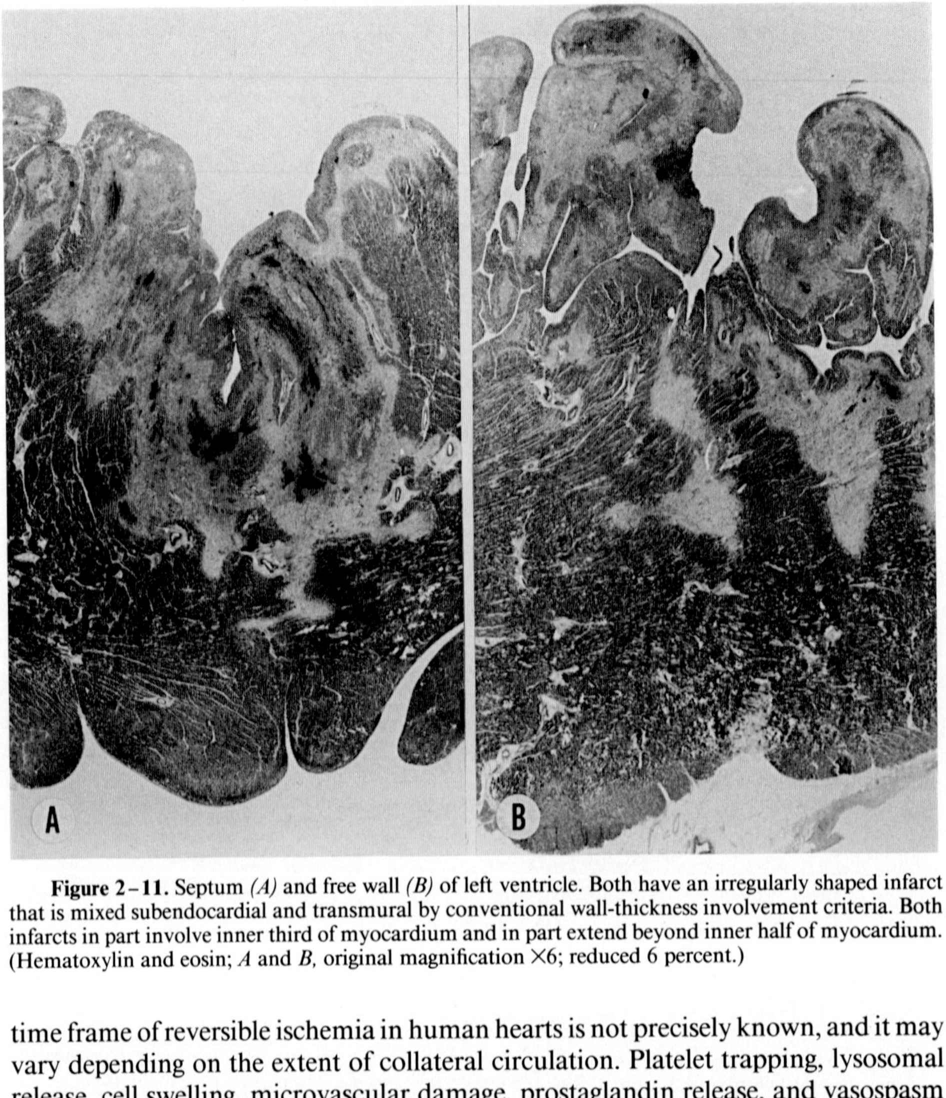

Figure 2–11. Septum *(A)* and free wall *(B)* of left ventricle. Both have an irregularly shaped infarct that is mixed subendocardial and transmural by conventional wall-thickness involvement criteria. Both infarcts in part involve inner third of myocardium and in part extend beyond inner half of myocardium. (Hematoxylin and eosin; *A* and *B*, original magnification ×6; reduced 6 percent.)

time frame of reversible ischemia in human hearts is not precisely known, and it may vary depending on the extent of collateral circulation. Platelet trapping, lysosomal release, cell swelling, microvascular damage, prostaglandin release, and vasospasm are some of the factors influencing the viability of ischemic myocardium.[5]

Hypertrophied myocardium is more susceptible to ischemic injury than nonhypertrophied myocardium. Diminished subendocardial adenosine triphosphate stores appear to be an intrinsic property of severely hypertrophied myocardium and probably contribute to its enhanced sensitivity to ischemia.[85]

CONCLUSION

Coronary thrombosis is an important cause but not a prerequisite of acute myocardial infarction. Coronary thrombosis seldom occurs without pre-existing atherosclerotic obstructive arterial disease and is virtually always initiated by plaque ulceration and rupture. Fixed (atherosclerotic-thrombotic) and dynamic (vasospastic) obstructions of the coronary arteries are not mutually exclusive mechanisms in the genesis of acute myocardial infarction.

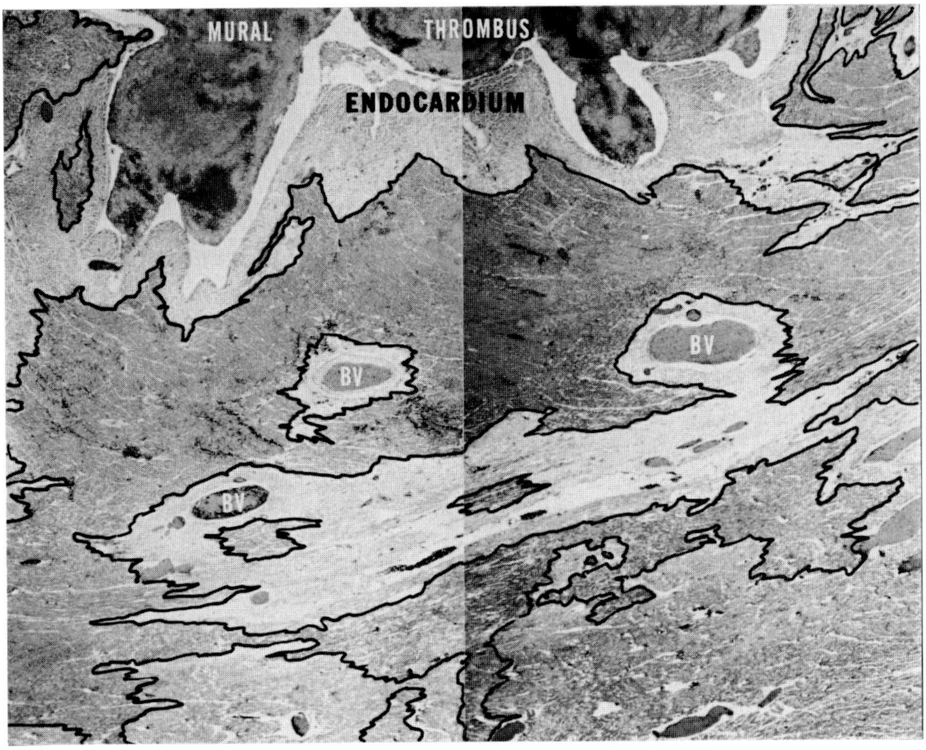

Figure 2-12. Montage of photomicrograph of an infarct composed of complex interdigitating "peninsulas." There is an irregular but sharp boundary demarcating normal and infarcted myocardium with no intermediate zone. BV = blood vessel. (Hematoxylin and eosin; magnification ×16.)

REFERENCES

1. Chandler, AB, Chapman, I, Erhardt, LR, et al: Coronary thrombosis in myocardial infarction. Am J Cardiol 34:823, 1974.
2. Baroldi, G: Coronary thrombosis: Facts and beliefs. Am Heart J 91:683, 1976.
3. Silver, MD, Baroldi, G, and Mariani, F: The relationship between acute occlusive coronary thrombi and myocardial infarction studied in 100 consecutive patients. Circulation 61:219, 1980.
4. Buja, LM and Willerson, JT: Clinicopathologic correlates of acute ischemic heart disease syndromes. Am J Med 47:343, 1981.
5. Oliva, PB: The role of coronary artery spasm in acute myocardial infarction. Cardiovasc Clin 14(1):45, 1983.
6. Lie, JT: Recognizing coronary heart disease: Selected historical vignettes from the period of William Harvey (1578–1657) to Adam Hammer (1818–1878). Mayo Clin Proc 53:811, 1978.
7. Lie, JT: Centenary of the first correct antemortem diagnosis of coronary thrombosis by Adam Hammer (1818–1878): English translation of the original report. Am J Cardiol 42:849, 1978.
8. Heberden, W: Some account of a disorder of the breast. Medical Transactions of the Royal College of Physicians (London) 2:59, 1772.
9. Weigert, C: Meber die pathologischen Gerinnungsvorgänge. Virchows Arch [Pathol Anat] 79:87, 1880.
10. Dock, G: Some notes on the coronary arteries. Med Surg Rep 75:1, 1896.
11. Obrastzow, WP and Straschesko, ND: Zur Kenntnis der Thrombose der Koronarterien des Herzens. Z Klin Med 71:116, 1910.
12. Herrick, JB: Clinical features of sudden obstruction of the coronary arteries. JAMA 59:2015, 1912.
13. Blumgart, HL, Schlesinger, MJ, and Davis, D: Studies on the relation of the clinical manifestations of

angina pectoris, coronary thrombosis, and myocardial infarction to the pathologic findings, with particular reference to significance of collateral circulation. Am Heart J 19:1, 1941.
14. Blumgart, HL, Schlesinger, MJ, and Zoll, PM: Angina pectoris, coronary failure, and acute myocardial infarction: Role of coronary occlusion and collateral circulation. JAMA 16:91, 1941.
15. Erlebacher, JA: Transmural myocardial infarction with "normal" coronary arteries. Am Heart J 98:421, 1979.
16. Hellstrom, HR: Vasospasm in ischemic heart disease—a hypothesis. Prospect Biol Med 16:427, 1973.
17. Hillis, LD and Braunwald, E: Coronary artery spasm. N Engl J Med 299:695, 1978.
18. Conti, CR: Myocardial infarction: Thoughts about pathogenesis and the role of coronary artery spasm. Am Heart J 110:187, 1985.
19. Chahine, RA: Coronary artery spasm: The pendulum continues swinging. J Am Coll Cardiol 7:446, 1986.
20. Maseri, A, Chierchia, S, and Davies, G: Pathophysiology of coronary occlusion in acute infarction. Circulation 73:233, 1986.
21. Brown, BG, Bolson, EL and Dodge, HT: Dynamic mechanisms in human coronary stenosis. Circulation 70:917, 1984.
22. Gorlin, R: Dynamic vascular basis in the genesis of myocardial ischemia. J Am Coll Cardiol 1:897, 1983.
23. Hamby, RI: Clinical-Anatomical Correlates in Coronary Artery Disease. Futura Publishing, Mount Kisco, NY, 1979, pp 79–171.
24. Fuster, V, Frye, RL, Connolly, DC, et al: Arteriographic patterns early in the onset of the coronary syndromes. Br Heart J 37:1250, 1975.
25. Ehrlich, JC and Shinohara, Y: Low incidence of coronary thrombosis in myocardial infarction. A restudy of serial block technique. Arch Pathol 78:432, 1964.
26. Roberts, WC and Buja, LM: The frequency and significance of coronary artery thrombi and other observations in fatal acute myocardial infarction. A study of 107 necropsy studies. Am J Med 52:425, 1972.
27. Roberts, WC: The coronary arteries and left ventricle in clinically isolated angina pectoris. A necropsy analysis. Circulation 54:388, 1976.
28. Roberts, WC and Jones, AA: Quantitation of coronary arterial narrowing at autopsy in sudden coronary death: Analysis of 31 patients and comparison with 25 control subjects. Am J Cardiol 44:39, 1979.
29. Roberts, WC and Virmani, R: Quantitation of coronary arterial narrowing in clinically isolated unstable angina pectoris: An analysis of 22 necropsy patients. Am J Med 67:792, 1979.
30. Roberts, WC and Jones, AA: Quantitation of coronary arterial narrowing at necropsy in acute transmural myocardial infarction: Analysis and comparison of findings in 27 patients and 22 controls. Circulation 61:786, 1980.
31. Maseri, A and Chierchia, S: Coronary artery spasm: Demonstration, definition, diagnosis, and consequences. Prog Cardiovasc Dis 25:169, 1982.
32. Oliva, PB: Coronary arterial spasm and vasomotion: Current concepts regarding their role in ischemic heart disease. Chest 81:740; 82:105, 1982.
33. Pepine, CJ and Feldman, RL: Dynamic coronary blood flow reduction: Supply side considerations. Int J Cardiol 3:3, 1983.
34. MacAlpin, RN: Contribution of dynamic vascular wall thickening to luminal narrowing during coronary arterial constriction. Circulation 61:296, 1980.
35. MacAlpin, RN: Relation of coronary arterial spasm to sites of organic stenosis. Am J Cardiol 46:143, 1980.
36. Ginsburg, R, Bristow, MR, Davis, K, et al: Quantitative pharmacologic responses of normal and atherosclerotic isolated human epicardial coronary arteries. Circulation 69:430, 1984.
37. El-Maraghi, NRH and Sealey, BJ: Recurrent myocardial infarction in a young man due to coronary artery spasm demonstrated at autopsy. Circulation 61:199, 1980.
38. Bertrand, ME, LaBlanche, JM, Tilmant, PY, et al: Frequency of provoked coronary arterial spasm in 1089 consecutive patients undergoing coronary arteriography. Circulation 65:1299, 1982.
39. Chapman, I: The cause-effect relationship between recent coronary artery occlusion and acute myocardial infarction. Am Heart J 87:267, 1974.
40. Roberts, WC: Coronary thrombosis and fatal myocardial ischemia. Circulation 49:1, 1974.
41. Chandler, AB: Mechanism and frequency of thrombosis in the coronary circulation. Thromb Res 4(Suppl I):3, 1974.

42. Miller, RD, Burchell, HD, and Edwards, JE: Myocardial infarction with and without acute coronary occlusion: A pathologic study. Arch Intern Med 88:597, 1951.
43. Chapman, I: Relationships of recent coronary artery occlusion and acute myocardial infarction. J Mt Sinai Hosp 35:149, 1968.
44. Sinapius, D: Beziehungen zwischen koronarthrombosen and myokardinfarkten. Stsh Med Wochenschr 97:443, 1972.
45. Davies, MJ, Woolf, N, and Robertson, WB: Pathology of acute myocardial infarction with particular reference to occlusive coronary thrombi. Br Heart J 38:659, 1976.
46. Bulkley, BH and Hutchins, GM: Coronary thrombosis: The major cause of acute myocardial infarction in atherosclerotic coronary artery disease. Circulation 55, 56(Suppl 3):64, 1977.
47. Horie, T, Sekiguchi, M, and Hirosawa, K: Coronary thrombosis in pathogenesis of acute myocardial infarction: Histopathological study of coronary arteries in 108 necropsied cases using serial section. Br Heart J 40:153, 1978.
48. Spain, DM and Bradess, VA: The relationship of coronary thrombosis to coronary atherosclerosis and ischemic heart disease. Am J Med Sci 240:701, 1960.
49. Lie, JT and Titus, JL: Pathology of the myocardium and the conduction system in sudden coronary death. Circulation 52(Suppl 3):41, 1975.
50. Baroldi, G, Falzi, G, and Mariani, F: Sudden coronary death: A postmortem study in 208 selected cases compared to 97 control subjects. Am Heart J 98:20, 1979.
51. Schuster, E, Achaff, S, Bell, W, et al: Multiple coronary thromboses in previously normal coronary arteries: A rare cause of acute myocardial infarction. Am Heart J 99:506, 1980.
52. O'Reilly, RJ and Spellberg, RD: Rapid resolution of coronary arterial emboli: Myocardial infarction and subsequent normal coronary arteriograms. Ann Intern Med 81:348, 1974.
53. Bertrand, ME, Lefebvre, JM, Laisne, CL, et al: Coronary arteriography in acute transmural myocardial infarction. Am Heart J 97:61, 1979.
54. Sanborn, TA, Faxon, DP, Kellett, MA, et al: Serial angiographic evidence of rapid resolution of coronary artery stenosis. Chest 84:302, 1983.
55. Ong, L, Reiser, P. Coromilas, J, et al: Left ventricular function and rapid release of creatine kinase MB in acute myocardial infarction: Evidence for spontaneous reperfusion. N Engl J Med 309:1, 1983.
56. DeWood, MA, Spores, J, Notske, RN, et al: Prevalence of total coronary occlusion during the early hours of transmural myocardial infarction. N Engl J Med 303:897, 1980.
57. Bertrain, ME, Lefebvre, JM, Laisne, CL, et al: Coronary arteriography in acute transmural myocardial infarction. Am Heart J 97:61, 1979.
58. Constantinides, P: Plaque fissures in human coronary thrombosis. Atherosclerosis 6:1, 1966.
59. Freidman, M and Van den Bovenkamp, GJ: The pathogenesis of coronary thrombus. Am J Pathol 48:19, 1966.
60. Chapman, I: Morphogenesis of occluding coronary artery thrombosis. Arch Pathol 80:256, 1965.
61. Bouch, DC and Montgomery, GL: Cardiac lesions in fatal cases of recent myocardial ischemia from a coronary care unit. Br Heart J 32:795, 1970.
62. Freidman, M: The coronary thrombus: Its origin and fate. Hum Pathol 2:81, 1971.
63. Jorgensen, L, Chandler, AB, and Borchgrevink, CF: Acute lesions of coronary arteries in anticoagulant-treated and in untreated patients. Atherosclerosis 13:21, 1971.
64. Falk, E: Plaque rupture with severe pre-existing stenosis precipitating coronary thrombosis: Characteristics of coronary atherosclerotic plaques underlying fatal occlusive thrombi. Br Heart J 50:127, 1983.
65. Davies, MJ and Thomas, AC: Plaque fissuring—the cause of acute myocardial infarction, sudden ischemic death, and crescendo angina. Br Heart J 53:363, 1985.
66. Hellstrom, HR: Evidence in favor of the vasospastic cause of coronary artery thrombosis. Am Heart J 97:449, 1979.
67. Buja, LM, Hillis, LD, Petty, CS, et al: The role of coronary arterial spasm in ischemic heart disease. Arch Pathol Lab Med 105:221, 1981.
68. Levy, RL, Gruenn, HG, and Kurtz, D: Facts on disease of coronary arteries, based on survey of clinical and pathologic records of 762 cases. Am J Med Sci 187:376, 1934.
69. Wenger, NK and Bauer, S: Coronary embolism: Review of the literature and presentation of fifteen cases. Am J Med 25:549, 1958.
70. Prizel, KR, Hutchins, GM, and Bulkley, BH: Coronary artery embolism and myocardial infarction: A clinicopathologic study of 55 patients. Ann Intern Med 88:155, 1978.
71. Roberts, WC: Coronary embolism: A review of causes, consequences and diagnostic considerations. Cardiovasc Med 3:699, 1978.

72. Haerem, JW: Platelet aggregates in intramyocardial vessels of patients dying suddenly and unexpectedly of coronary artery disease. Atherosclerosis 15:199, 1972.
73. Haerem, JW: Mural platelet microthrombi and major acute lesions of main epicardial arteries in sudden cardiac death. Atherosclerosis 19:529, 1974.
74. El-Maraghi, N and Genton, E: The relevance of platelet and fibrin thromboembolism of the coronary microcirculation with special reference to sudden cardiac death. Circulation 62:936, 1980.
75. Falk, E: Unstable angina with fatal outcome: Dynamic coronary thrombosis leading to infarction and/or sudden death. Circulation 71:699, 1985.
76. Davis, MJ, Thomas, AC, Knapman, PA, et al: Intramyocardial platelet aggregation in patients with unstable angina suffering from sudden cardiac death. Circulation 73:418, 1986.
77. Rubenfire, M, Blevin, RD, Barnhart, M, et al: Platelet hyperaggregability in patients with chest pain and angiographically normal coronary arteries. Am J Cardiol 57:657, 1986.
78. James, TN: Small arteries of the heart. Circulation 56:2, 1977.
79. Geer, JC, Bishop, SP, and James, TN: Pathology of small intramural coronary arteries. Pathol Annu 14(2):125, 1979.
80. Parl, F, Gutstein, WH, and Glasser, M: Relationship of small and large coronary artery disease to myocardial ischemia. Arch Pathol Lab Med 104:70, 1980.
81. Geer, JC, Crago, CA, Little, WC, et al: Subendocardial ischemic myocardial lesions associated with severe coronary atherosclerosis. Am J Pathol 98:663, 1980.
82. Factor, SM, Sonnenblick, EH, and Kirk, ES: The histologic border zone of acute myocardial infarction—islands or peninsulas. Am J Pathol 92:111, 1978.
83. Hearse, DJ and Yellon, DM: The "border zone" in evolving myocardial infarction: Controversy or confusion? Am J Cardiol 47:1321, 1981.
84. Reimer, KA, Lowe, JE, Rusmussen, MM, et al: The wavefront phenomenon of ischemic cell death. Circulation 56:786, 1977.
85. Peyton, RB, Jones, RN, Atlarian, D, et al: Depressed high-energy phosphate content in hypertrophied ventricles of animal and man. Ann Surg 196:278, 1982.

CHAPTER 3

Aortocoronary Saphenous Vein Bypass Grafts*

Renu Virmani, M.D.
James B. Atkinson, M.D., Ph.D.
Mervyn B. Forman, M.D.

Approximately 700,000 Americans die yearly from coronary atherosclerosis.[1] Coronary bypass grafting for obstructive coronary artery disease, which was developed in the 1960s and refined in the 1970s, has dramatically changed the management of patients with ischemic heart disease. Its true role remains controversial, despite numerous randomized and nonrandomized studies. However, there is little doubt that surgery alleviates anginal symptoms and substantially prolongs life of patients with left main coronary artery disease and three-vessel disease.[2]

RANDOMIZED TRIALS IN CORONARY BYPASS SURGERY

The overall goals of both medical and surgical treatment remain the same, that is, improvement in the quality of life by reducing angina, improvement in left ventricular function, elimination of resistant ventricular tachyarrhythmias, reduction in the incidence of myocardial infarction, and an increased and productive lifespan.[3] Both medical and surgical advances for ischemic heart disease have progressed rapidly in the last 5 years, with the introduction of effective thrombolytic agents, balloon angioplasty, and calcium channel blockers, and with the decrease in perioperative mortality.[4] Also, an increasing number of patients are being treated with both coronary artery bypass grafts and nonsurgical treatments simultaneously, to reduce cost and complications. Therefore, comparisons between surgical and medical management are difficult today because of the heterogeneity of coronary artery disease.

---

*The opinions or assertions contained herein are the private views of the authors and are not to be construed as official or as reflecting the views of the Department of the Army or the Department of Defense.

The Veterans Administration Coronary Bypass Surgery Cooperative Study in 1972 to 1974,[5,6] the European Coronary Surgery Study (ECSS) in 1973 to 1976,[7] and the Coronary Artery Surgery Study (CASS) in 1974 to 1979[8,9] were randomized trials aimed at determining whether assignment to medical or surgical therapy offers a significant advantage for long-term survival. Despite obvious differences in study populations, the time frame of the investigation, the number of grafts anastomosed, differences in medical and surgical mortality, and differences in medical management, certain conclusions can be drawn as stated by Killip and Ryan:[10]

1. Bypass surgery improves survival in patients with significant left main coronary artery disease.
2. Bypass surgery improves survival in patients with three-vessel disease and reduced ventricular function.
3. Bypass surgery does not protect patients from the risk of subsequent myocardial infarction.
4. Graft patency deteriorates with time.
5. Accelerated changes of atherosclerosis develop in the bypassed vessels.

NATURAL HISTORY OF SAPHENOUS VEIN BYPASS GRAFTS

At the time of introduction of coronary artery bypass grafting, the long-term patency of grafted veins was not well known. In the first 5 years after surgery, graft patency rates appeared to be high, and atherosclerosis within grafts was a relatively minor problem.[11] Attrition rates between 7 and 12 percent occur less than 1 month after surgery. An additional 10 percent failure rate occurs between 1 month and 1 year after surgery. Beyond the first year and up to 6 years, the attrition rate of vein grafts is approximately 2.5 percent per year.[12] Similar patency rates have been reported by several groups.[13-15] Currently, patency rates of approximately 70 percent can be expected at 10 years.[16]

CAUSES OF EARLY GRAFT CLOSURE

Early graft closure can result from mechanical problems, including faulty surgical technique, inadequate size of the coronary vessels, and poor run-off.[16] A fine deposit of platelet, fibrin, erythrocytes, and polymorphonuclear leukocytes in the intima of the vein graft is consistently seen in patients who die shortly after operation (Fig. 3-1). Also, various blood elements can be seen within intima of some patients, suggesting insudation of blood elements secondary to increased permeability of the endothelium, probably from high arterial pressure within the lumen.[17] In an experimental model of saphenous vein grafts,[18] it has been shown that the endothelium sloughs and microthrombi with platelets form, and this development may be related to vessel wall injury caused by high flow or "jet" lesions. In humans, thrombus is probably a response to the endothelial injury that is probably an unavoidable consequence of manipulation and preparation of the graft.[20] The incidence of a fine layer of fibrin thrombus on the intima of saphenous vein grafts has been reported to be as high as 73 percent in patients who die within 24 hours of surgery.[21] Whereas occlusive thrombi rarely form within 24 hours of implantation, they are one of the major

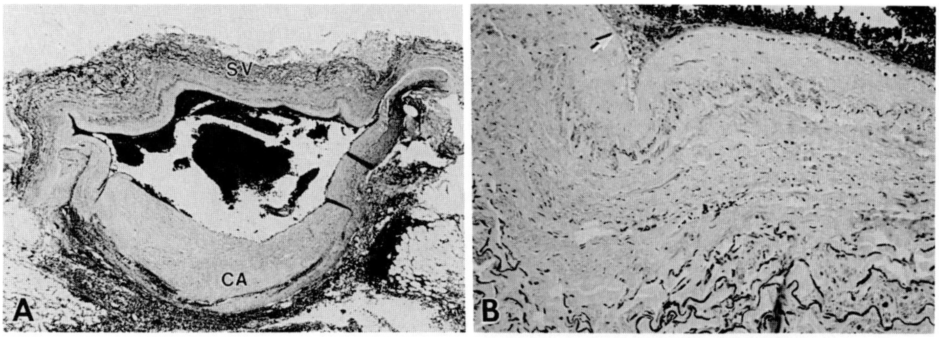

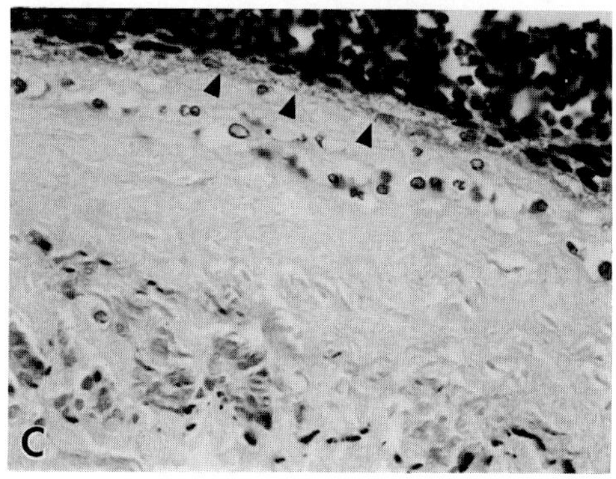

Figure 3-1. A 60-year-old man underwent saphenous vein bypass surgery for unstable angina and died 6 hours after surgery with postoperative difficulty in maintaining systemic pressures. At autopsy the heart weighed 540 g. The bypass grafts were intact, but all vein grafts proximal and at site of anastomosis showed a thin layer of platelet deposition on the endothelial surface. *A,* Anastomotic site of vein graft (SV) to left obtuse marginal coronary artery (CA). *B,* Platelet fibrin deposit close to the anastomotic site in the vein graft *(arrow). C,* Vein graft with a fine layer of platelet deposition *(arrowheads).* (Movat stain; original magnification *A* ×15, *B* ×160, *C* ×600; reduced 44 percent.)

causes (33 percent) of occlusion within 30 days of operation.[22] The incidence of thrombus reached 75 percent in patients who died more than 1 month after operation.[22] Patients treated with warfarin or dipyridamole and aspirin have a higher patency rate after coronary bypass surgery.[23,24]

Another cause of early graft closure is compression; that is, loss of circumference of coronary artery occurs when part of the intrinsic coronary wall is everted or compressed by suturing during construction of graft artery anastomosis.[22] Griffith and associates[22] have calculated the percent reduction in luminal area for coronary arteries with internal diameter of 2 mm or 1 mm. In a 2 mm artery, suture bites that are 0.5 mm or 1.0 mm back from the edge of the arteriotomy result in reduction of the cross-sectional area of the coronary lumen by 29 and 54 percent, respectively. In a 1 mm artery, on the other hand, the same two sutures will reduce the area by 52 and 89 percent, respectively. This obviously occurs only in the case of eversion of the wall.

Another important factor is the presence of severe atherosclerotic plaque in the distal segment of the coronary artery. Plaque results in reduced internal circumference of the arterial wall available for anastomosis; if plaque is present distal to the anastomosis, this will cause decreased coronary artery lumen, reduced flow, and thereby a predisposition to thrombosis.[22] If atherosclerotic plaque is present at the site of anastomosis, it can cause the plaque to detach from the coronary wall where anastomosis is being created. This detachment can result in coronary artery dissection at the level of the vein graft, as well as distal to the anastomosis (Fig. 3-2). The length of the dissection, however, is usually short. Spray and Roberts[19] report a 17 percent incidence, whereas Griffith and coworkers[22] report an 8 percent incidence. Although the incidence of dissection is low, it is another cause of lumen compression.

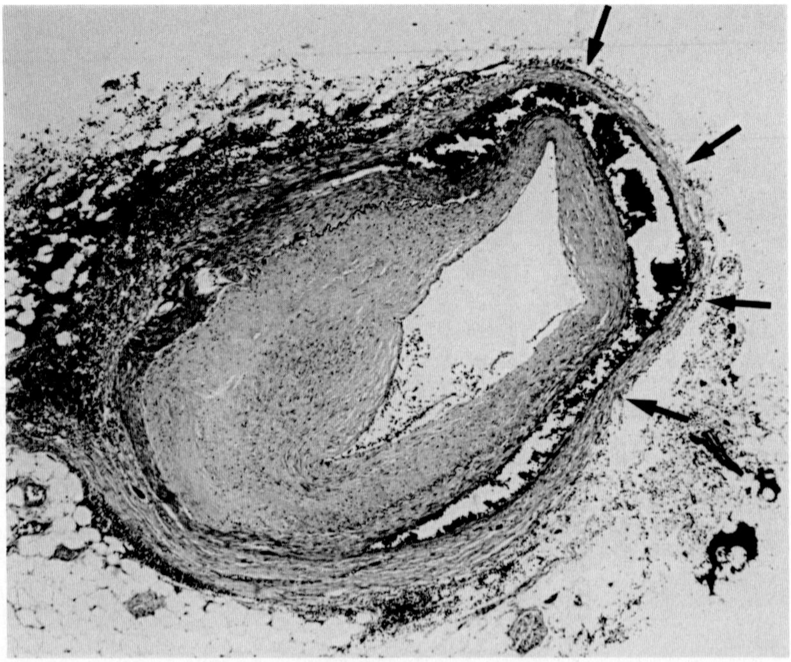

Figure 3–2. Histologic section of coronary artery taken distal to the anastomotic site. Note presence of dissection *(arrows)* involving 50 percent of the circumference of the artery. The media of the coronary artery is dissected; however, the dissection extended less than 1 cm in length. (Movat stain; magnification ×40.)

MORPHOLOGIC CHANGES IN LONG-TERM SAPHENOUS VEIN BYPASS GRAFTS

Graft Changes Between One Month and One Year After Surgery

Grafts that are in place for up to 1 year uniformly demonstrate intimal fibrous proliferation, characterized by intimal thickening with a vascular, highly cellular connective tissue comprising proliferating smooth muscle cells in a loose matrix of acid mucopolysaccharide and collagen (Fig. 3–3). Electron microscopic studies have shown that the cellular component is a smooth muscle cell, with myofibrils, dense bodies, and basement membranes.[17] However, Kern and coworkers[25] considered the cell with rough endoplasmic reticulum to be a fibroblast. The pathogenesis of fibrointimal proliferation is speculative; it may represent reparative responses to ischemia or hemodynamic stresses (such as systemic hypertension), resulting in endothelial damage with platelet aggregation, smooth muscle proliferation, and intimal thickening.[26] Brody and colleagues,[18] employing the canine model of vein-to-vein and artery-vein-artery anastomosis, concluded that the initial necrosis and inflammatory changes in the media are ischemic in origin and that the disruption of vasa vasorum may be responsible for the resultant intimal thickening. Inasmuch as the degree of fibrointimal proliferation may vary along the length of a vein graft or even among different grafts in the same patient,[27–29] ischemia alone cannot entirely account for these changes. Flow rate may modify the extent of fibrointimal proliferation, inasmuch as increased flow may produce recurrent endothelial damage, result-

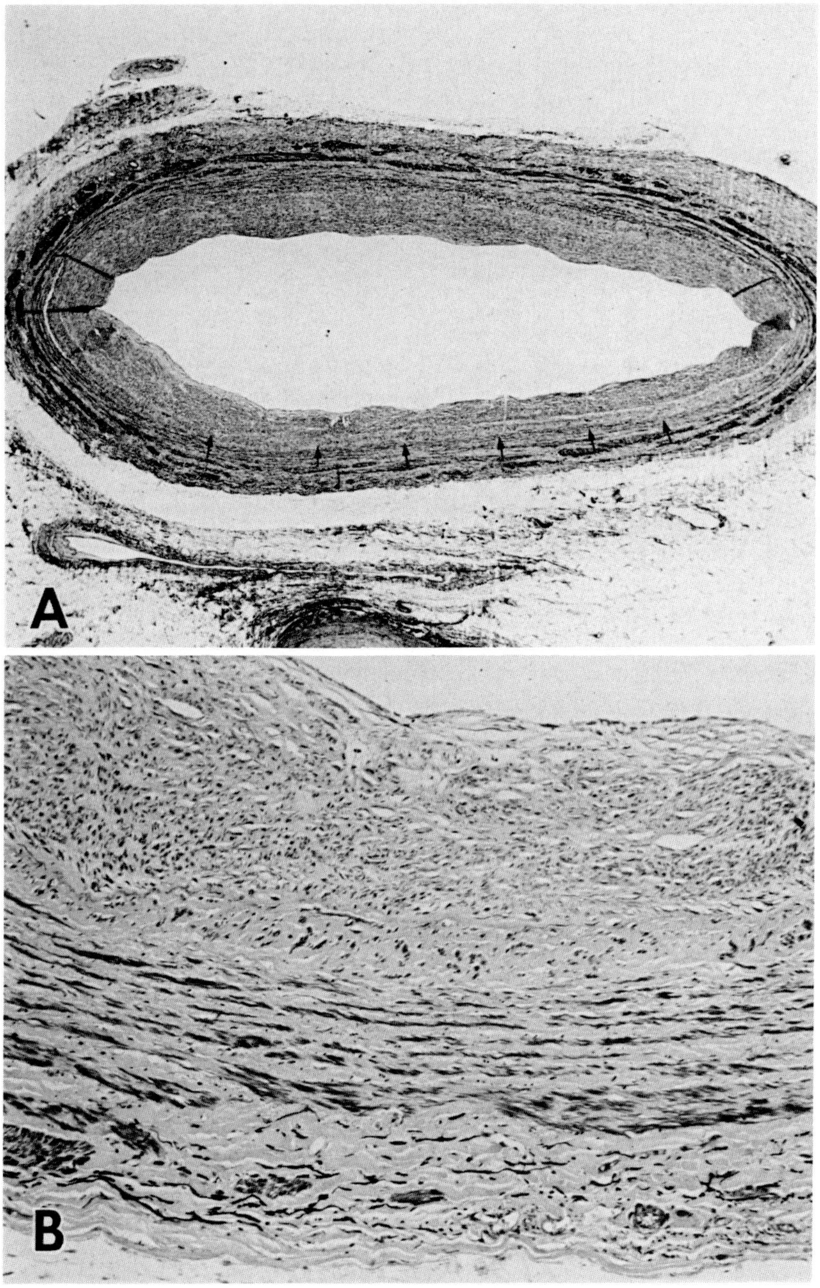

Figure 3-3. *A,* Section of a saphenous vein graft in place for 8 months. There is uniform concentric circumferential intimal proliferation *(arrows). B,* Higher magnification of wall of vein graft shown in *A.* Note elastic fibers in adventitia *(black)* but not in the media; the intima shows presence of smooth muscle cells *(dark gray)* and collagen in a background of acid mucopolysaccharide. (Movat pentachrome stain; magnification *A* ×15, *B* ×100.)

ing in fibrin-platelet deposition, thrombosis, and repair.[19] However, we and others[30,31] have not observed mural thrombus (fibrin, erythrocytes, iron) in vein grafts manifesting fibrointimal proliferation.

Fibrointimal proliferation in humans and in experimental animals shows progression in intimal proliferation and fibrosis at varying rates and locations. During the early phase of graft implantation, the fibrointimal proliferation is uneven and patchy in distribution but with time becomes circumferential and diffuse.[32] The presence of fibrointimal proliferation may be beneficial, because it induces moderate reduction of the internal diameter of the vein graft and reduces it to the approximate size of the recipient artery, thereby promoting a greater velocity of flow.[32]

Graft Changes After One Year of Surgery

We have recently reported our findings[30] involving 117 saphenous vein grafts that had been in place 12 to 168 months prior to death (mean 62.7 ± 37.5 months) in 56 patients (50 males, 6 females), mean age 59.6 ± 9.1 years. Cause of death was sudden in 21, acute myocardial infarction in 11, and congestive heart failure in 5. Six patients died during or shortly after reoperation for coronary artery bypass. Other causes of death included malignant neoplasms in 4 patients, pulmonary embolism in 2, rupture of an aortic aneurysm in 1, sepsis in 2, cerebrovascular accident in 1, and poisoning in 1.

All patients had one or more risk factors for accelerated coronary atherosclerosis (Table 3–1). Thirty-two patients (57 percent) had systemic hypertension, 15 patients (27 percent) had diabetes mellitus, 17 patients (30 percent) had a documented history of hyperlipidemia, and 19 (34 percent) had a family history of premature coronary

Table 3–1. Cardiovascular History in 56 Patients With Saphenous Vein Aortocoronary Bypass Grafts, at Necropsy

Risk Factors for Accelerated Coronary Artery Disease*	No. Patients
Systemic hypertension	32
Diabetes mellitus	15
Hyperlipidemia	
Hypercholesterolemia	13
Hypercholesterolemia + hypertriglyceridemia	4
Smoking	33
Family history of premature coronary heart disease	19
Cardiovascular history	
Angina pectoris	44
Acute myocardial infarction	37
Congestive heart failure	21

* Risk factors had been clearly documented in these patients subsequent to placement of aortocoronary bypass grafts. Systemic hypertension was defined as blood pressure greater than 140/90 mmHg; diabetes mellitus was assessed by determining whether patients were being treated at the time of death or a serum glucose level greater than 130 mg/dl. Hypercholesterolemia was defined as a serum cholesterol level greater than 240 mg/dl, and hypertriglyceridemia was a serum triglyceride level greater than 200 mg/dl.

From Atkinson et al.,[30] with permission.

heart disease. The vast majority of patients had angina pectoris (44 patients), and 37 had suffered acute myocardial infarction as documented by electrocardiographic and/or enzyme changes. Twenty-one patients (38 percent) were symptomatic from congestive heart failure.

Morphologic Findings

A total of 117 saphenous vein grafts had been in place 12 to 168 months prior to death (mean 62.7 months). Three characteristic types of morphologic changes were found (Table 3–2). Atherosclerosis, as defined by the World Health Organization,[33] was present in 25 vein grafts (Fig. 3–4). Ten of the atherosclerotic grafts were occluded by recent thrombus, and the others had various degrees of luminal narrowing secondary to atherosclerosis. One atherosclerotic vein graft had aneurysmal dilatation. Sixty-six vein grafts had various degrees of fibrointimal proliferation in the absence of atherosclerotic change, with prominent internal elastic laminae and smooth muscle proliferation, collagen, and acid mucopolysaccharide ground substance (Fig. 3–5). Twenty-six saphenous vein grafts were totally occluded with fibrous tissue (Fig. 3–6). Atherosclerotic vein grafts had been in place longer than those with fibrointimal proliferation (Table 3–2).

Fibrointimal proliferation occurred exclusively in 25 patients, atherosclerotic change alone in 9, and fibrosis alone occurred in 6. The majority of patients had a single type of lesion in their grafts, although 16 patients had more than one morphologic lesion (Table 3–2). Some degree of fibrointimal proliferation was found in all the atherosclerotic grafts, but significant fibrointimal proliferation (greater than 25 percent cross-sectional area narrowing) was never noted in atherosclerotic grafts.

The various degrees of cross-sectional area luminal narrowing of saphenous vein grafts determined at autopsy is shown in Table 3–2. Nearly one fourth of grafts with atherosclerosis and fibrointimal proliferation had significant narrowing at necropsy (greater than 75 percent cross-sectional area luminal narrowing). Total occlusion was secondary to fibrointimal proliferation in two vein grafts and to atherosclerosis in eight.

There was no statistical difference when comparing mean heart weight with the type of morphologic change (Table 3–3). The mean number of four major coronary arteries (left main, left anterior descending, left circumflex, and right) with greater than 75 percent cross-sectional area luminal narrowing is shown in Table 3–3 and was also similar among the three groups. Histologic evidence of acute and/or healed myocardial infarction at necropsy was found in 12 of 15 patients with atherosclerotic vein grafts, 33 of 39 patients with fibrointimal proliferation in their grafts, and 18 of 19 patients with fibrotic vein grafts. Ten patients had no evidence of infarction, either healed or acute.

Correlation of Vein Graft Morphology with Cardiovascular Risk Factors

Cardiovascular risk factors were correlated with the specific type of vein graft morphology (atherosclerosis or fibrointimal proliferation) (Table 3–4). Systemic hypertension was present in 76 percent of saphenous vein grafts with fibrointimal proliferation, as compared with 24 percent of atherosclerotic grafts. Forty percent of atherosclerotic vein grafts occurred in patients with diabetes mellitus, as compared with 18 percent of grafts with fibrointimal proliferation. Sixty-eight percent of atherosclerotic vein grafts were found in patients with hypercholesterolemia in contrast to only 15 percent with fibrointimal proliferation. The differences between the

Table 3–2. Morphology of 117 Saphenous Vein Grafts Implanted Longer Than 12 Months in 56 Patients, at Necropsy

Morphology of Graft Implants				**No. Grafts**
Atherosclerosis				25
Recent thrombus				10
Aneurysm				1
Fibrointimal proliferation				66
Fibrosis with total occlusion				26
Distribution of Vein Grafts				**No. Patients**
Fibrointimal proliferation				25
Atherosclerosis				9
Fibrosis				6
Fibrointimal proliferation + atherosclerosis				3
Fibrointimal proliferation + fibrosis				10
Atherosclerosis + fibrosis				2
Atherosclerosis + fibrointimal proliferation + fibrosis				1
Number of Grafts with Various Degrees of Cross-sectional Area Luminal Narrowing				
	0–25%	*26–50%*	*51–75%*	*>75%*
Atherosclerosis	0	4(16%)	5(20%)	16(64%)
Fibrointimal proliferation	17(26%)	29(44%)	14(21%)	6(9%)
Total	17(18%)	33(36%)	19(21%)	22(24%)

From Atkinson et al.,[30] with permission.

atherosclerotic grafts and those with fibrointimal proliferation for the two risk factors (systemic hypertension, hypercholesterolemia) were statistically significant (Table 3–4). The majority of grafts (17 of 22) from hypertensive patients that did not demonstrate fibrointimal proliferation were fibrotic. No statistically significant differences were noted among the two morphologic groups with regard to history of smoking, family history of premature coronary heart disease, acute myocardial infarction, or congestive heart failure.

In 8 of our 56 patients, accurate documentation of cardiovascular risk factors and/or values for total serum cholesterol, serum glucose, and blood pressure were not available. We therefore excluded these patients from statistical analysis. Grafts with less than 25 percent cross-sectional area luminal narrowing by fibrointimal proliferation in four patients were also excluded, because mild degrees of fibrointimal proliferation can be seen in saphenous veins at the time of implantation. Of the remaining 74 grafts in 44 patients, statistically significant differences were seen in the atherosclerotic and fibrointimal proliferation groups with regard to elevated cholesterol and systemic hypertension, but no statistically significant differences were noted for diabetes mellitus. The mean total serum cholesterol levels obtained after surgery were significantly greater in patients with atherosclerotic grafts, compared with those with fibrointimal proliferation ($p < 0.001$)(Fig. 3–7). Although the mean serum glucose level was also higher in patients with atherosclerotic grafts (163 ± 38 mg/dl) than in patients with fibrointimal proliferation (127 ± 10 mg/dl), the differences were not statistically significant. Patients with fibrointimal proliferation had higher systolic and diastolic blood pressures than did patients with atherosclerotic grafts, but these differences reached statistical significance only for systolic blood pressure ($p < 0.05$)(Fig. 3–8). The number of separate measurements made for cholesterol, glucose, and blood pressure were 5.4 ± 0.7, 5.0 ± 0.7, and 4.1 ± 0.6 per patient, respectively, subsequent to coronary artery bypass graft placement.

Role of Risk Factors in the Development of Atherosclerosis Versus Diffuse Intimal Change (Table 3–5)

The role of hyperlipidemia in the development of atherosclerosis in grafts is controversial. In hypercholesterolemic animals, there is a greater propensity for the development of atherosclerosis in vein grafts,[38–42] compared with native coronary arteries or grafted internal mammary arteries.[42] In vitro, canine venous grafts incorporate lipids at accelerated rates compared with normal arteries and veins.[43] The role of hyperlipidemia in the pathogenesis of atherosclerosis in human grafts is less clear, although some studies have confirmed the animal data. Lie and associates[34] found atherosclerosis in 78 percent of grafts implanted longer than 12 months in hyperlipidemic patients, as compared with 11.5 percent in patients with normal lipids. This has been confirmed by Barboriak and colleagues;[44] however, in other morphologic[37] and angiographic[45] studies, no correlation between hyperlipidemia and atherosclerosis was present, suggesting that other etiologic factors may also be involved. Campeau

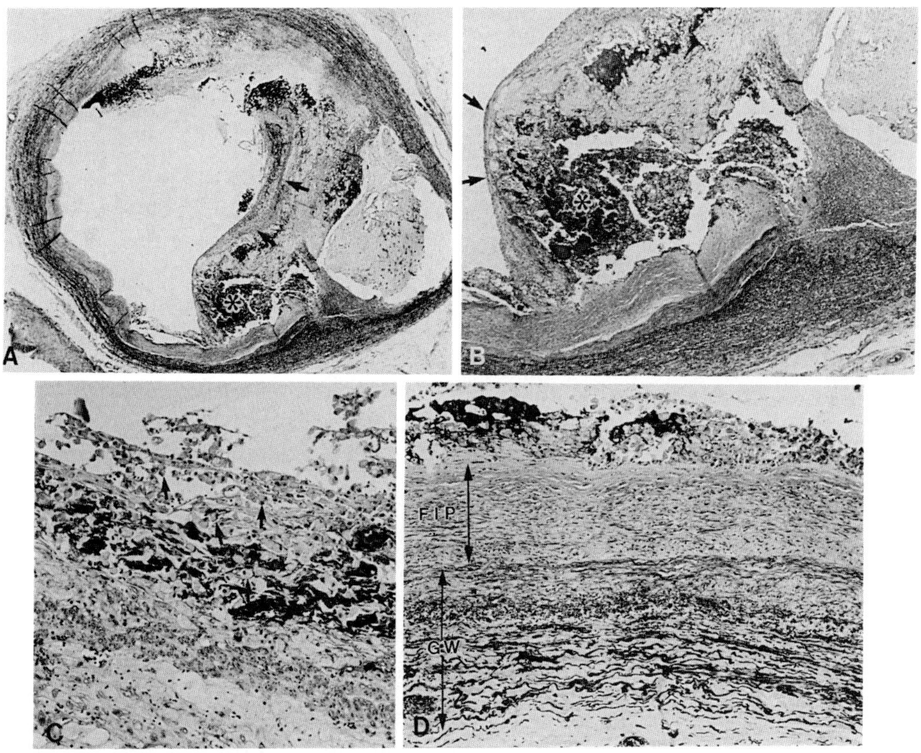

Figure 3–4. Atherosclerotic saphenous vein graft from a 62-year-old man who had undergone saphenous vein-graft placement 56 months before death. His risk factors included diabetes mellitus and systemic hypertension. *A,* Photomicrograph showing eccentric atherosclerotic plaque with a fibrous cap *(arrows)* and hemorrhage within a plaque (*). *B,* Higher magnification of hemorrhage (*) into a plaque covered by a thin layer of fibrous cap *(arrows)*. *C,* Extensive foam cell deposition *(arrows)* in the subintimal region with fibrin interspersed *(black)*. *D,* Saphenous vein graft wall (GW) and superimposed fibrointimal proliferation (FIP) with foam cells in the superficial layers of the intima interspersed with fibrin deposits *(black)*. (Movat stain; magnification A ×15, B ×40, C ×160, D ×100; reduced 45 percent.)

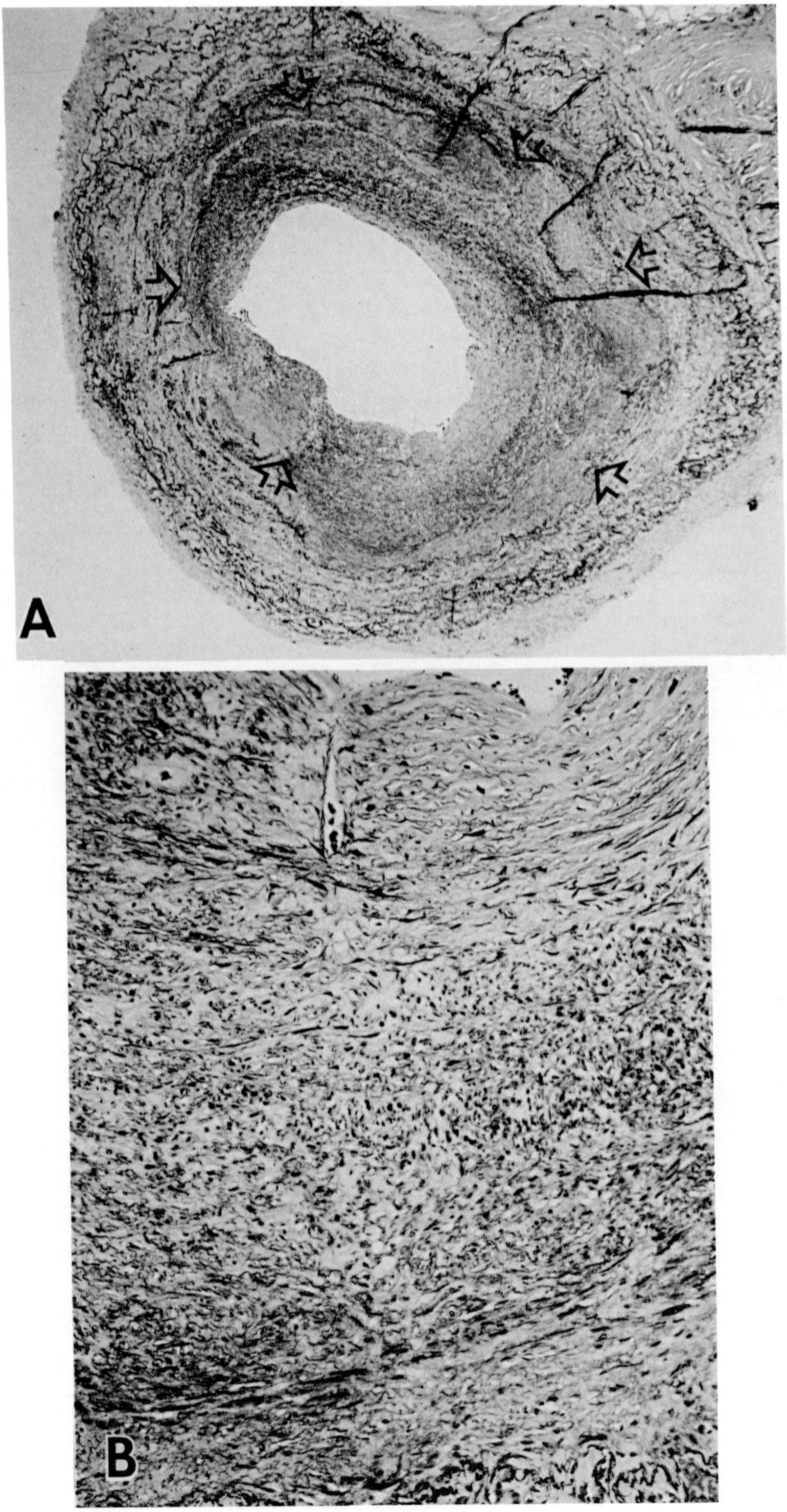

Figure 3-5. See facing page for legend.

Table 3–3. Morphologic Features in Hearts from 56 Patients with Saphenous Vein Graft Implants

	Atherosclerotic Grafts (15 pts)*	**Fibrointimal Proliferation Grafts (39 pts)***	**Fibrotic Grafts (19 pts)***	**Total**
Duration of vein graft†	75.9 ± 42.7	57.4 ± 33.4	56.5 ± 41.2	62.7 ± 37.5
Heart weight (g)	520 ± 96	609 ± 168	640 ± 172	598 ± 150
Graft implantation‡				
Right coronary artery	10	25	9	44
Left anterior descending coronary artery§	7	28	9	44
Left circumflex coronary artery‖	8	13	8	29
Mean number of coronary arteries > 75% narrowed	2.7 ± 1.0	2.4 ± 1.1	2.8 ± 0.9	2.6 ± 1.1
Myocardial infarction				
Acute myocardial infarction	1(7%)	0	1(5%)	2(4%)
Healed myocardial infarction	4(27%)	24(62%	11(58%)	39(70%)
Acute and healed myocardial infarction	7(47%)	9(23%)	6(32%)	22(41%)

* Patients with more than one type of lesion in vein grafts were counted twice according to the type of morphologic change.

† $p < 0.05$ for atherosclerotic versus fibrointimal proliferation grafts.

‡ Includes posterior descending branch in hearts with dominant right coronary artery.

§ Includes left diagonal branches.

‖ Includes left obtuse marginal branch.

From Atkinson et al.,[30] with permission.

Table 3–4. Correlation of Saphenous Vein Graft Morphology with Cardiovascular Risk Factors in 56 Patients

Risk Factors	**Atherosclerosis (Total Grafts 25) No. (%) of Grafts**	**Fibrointimal Proliferation (Total Grafts 66) No. (%) of Grafts**
Systemic hypertension	6(24)	50(76)
Diabetes mellitus	10(40)	12(18)
Hypercholesterolemia	17(68)	10(15)
Smoking	15(60)	40(61)
Family history of premature coronary heart disease	9(36)	17(26)
Past history of		
Acute myocardial infarction	17(68)	44(67)
Angina pectoris	23(92)	48(73)
Congestive heart failure	9(36)	23(35)

From Atkinson et al.,[30] with permission.

Figure 3–5. Fibrointimal proliferation in a saphenous vein graft in place for 12 months. The patient had a history of systemic hypertension and was a smoker. *A,* Note presence of extensive fibrointimal tissue within the vein wall *(open arrows). B,* Higher magnification showing smooth muscle cells (dark gray) in a background of acid mucopolysaccharide. There was almost total absence of collagen. (Movat stain; magnification *A* ×25, *B* ×160.)

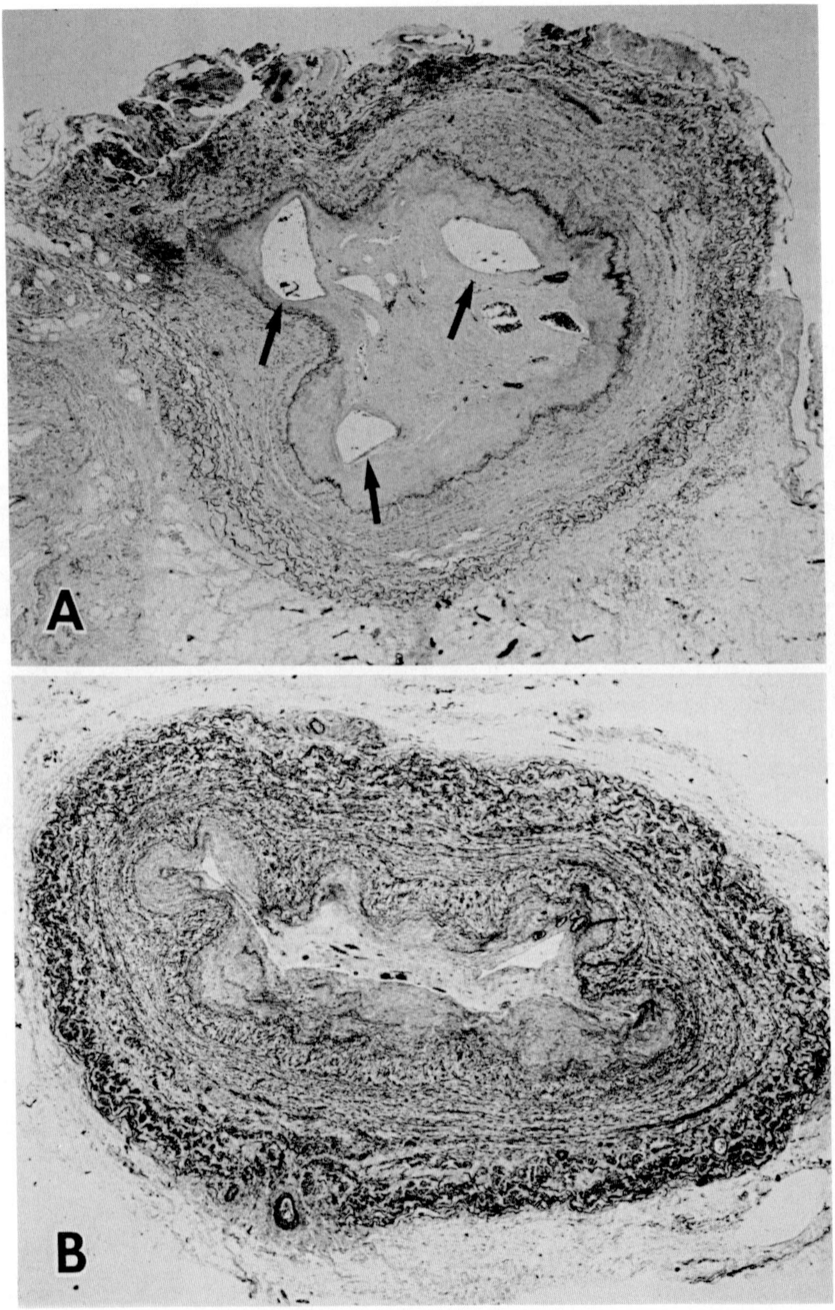

Figure 3–6. *A,* Fibrotic saphenous vein grafts. Note total occlusion of the vein graft by fibrous tissue with multiluminal channels interspersed *(arrows),* representing recanalized thrombus. *B,* Collapsed fibrotic vein graft with the lumen occupied by fibrous tissue. The compression of vein graft could be secondary to fibrous tissue retraction. Only a few multiluminal channels are seen. (Movat stain; magnification ×25.)

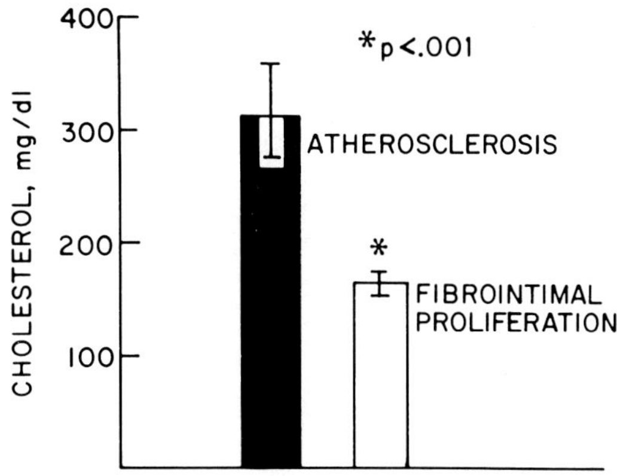

Figure 3-7. Total serum cholesterol levels in patients with atherosclerotic grafts, as compared with those in patients with fibrointimal proliferation. Values were obtained from 44 patients, representing a total of 74 grafts (25 with atherosclerosis and 49 with fibrointimal proliferation). (From Atkinson et al.,[30] with permission.)

and associates[16] recently reported progression of new lesions in saphenous vein grafts after 1 year of implantation in patients who had high levels of very low-density and low-density lipoproteins and low levels of high-density lipoproteins. Total plasma cholesterol and triglyceride levels were also higher in patients with new lesions. All lesions that appeared after 1 year were designated "atherosclerotic," based on patterns of irregularity by angiography.[46] Our study, which was based on histologic confirmation of atherosclerosis, demonstrates that "atherosclerosis" is not the predominant change in vein grafts that have been in place for greater than 1 year; in fact, fibrointimal proliferation is encountered more frequently. However, the natural progression of fibrointimal proliferation may be interrupted by the presence of risk factors, with hypercholesterolemia producing atherosclerotic change and systemic hypertension leading to greater luminal narrowing by unrelenting proliferation of fibrointimal tissue.

Although there are inherent problems in a retrospective study of a selected patient population such as ours, this is the first study to our knowledge to show a relationship between the presence of systemic hypertension and the development of significant (greater than 25 percent cross-sectional area luminal narrowing) fibrointimal proliferation. Hypertension may lead to hemodynamic and/or ischemic endothelial damage with resultant repair and intimal hyperplasia. Although a relationship

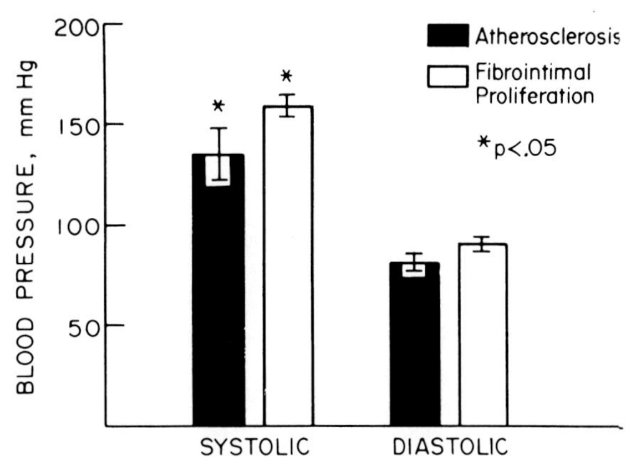

Figure 3-8. Graph showing systolic and diastolic blood pressures in patients with atherosclerotic vein grafts, compared with those with fibrointimal proliferation. Values were obtained from 44 patients, representing a total of 74 grafts (25 with atherosclerosis and 49 with fibrointimal proliferation). (From Atkinson et al.,[30] with permission.)

Table 3–5. Reports of Morphologic Changes in Long-Term Saphenous Vein Bypass Grafts

Author	Year	No. Pts	Duration of SVBG (mo)	DIT	Atherosclerosis	Th
Barboriak[32]	1976	11*	23.7 ± 3.1	11	1	4
Lie[34]	1977	23	13–75	14	9†	0
Bulkley[26]	1977	9	1–54	8	4	6
Batayias[35]	1977	12	6 mo to >36	12	3	2
Walts[36]	1982	5	5 to 8 yr	—	5	5
Bourassa[1]	1983	19	>24 mo	—	8	—
Smith[37]	1983	24	7–116 mo	21	11	3
Atkinson[30]	1985	56	62.7 ± 37.5	39	15‡	9

* Eight patients had hyperlipidemia, one had systemic hypertension.
† Only 11.5% of grafts of normolipemic patients manifested histologic changes of atherosclerosis compared with 78.6% of those from hyperlipemic patients.
‡ Elevated cholesterol was present in 67% compared with 16% in patients with DIT.
DIT = diffuse intimal thickening; SVBG = saphenous vein bypass graft; Th = thrombus, recent.

between hyperlipidemia and development of atherosclerosis in vein grafts has been demonstrated by others, our study is among the few in which atherosclerosis in vein grafts has been confirmed morphologically. Inasmuch as morphologic lesions vary from graft to graft in the same patient, it is likely that other risk factors may also be important etiologically. Technical, hemodynamic, or pre-existing changes in vein grafts may all contribute to the development of either fibrointimal proliferation or atherosclerosis. Because known cardiac risk factors play at least a contributory role in the development of different morphologic lesions, continued reduction in risk factors in patients who have undergone bypass surgery may help to prolong the patency of these grafts.

CORRELATION OF SAPHENOUS-VEIN-BYPASS GRAFT ANGIOGRAMS WITH HISTOLOGIC CHANGES AT NECROPSY

Previous studies of saphenous vein (SV) bypass grafts have either been angiographic or morphologic, and few have correlated angiograms with histology. Nine necropsy patients who had received 21 saphenous vein implants 12 to 120 (mean 67 ± 42) months before death were studied (Table 3–6).[47] All patients had severe coronary artery disease. Three types of histologic changes were found: atherosclerosis in nine grafts, fibrointimal proliferation in eight grafts, and total occlusion with fibrosis in four (Table 3–7). All patients had premortem angiograms 0 to 3 (mean 0.8 ± 0.1) months before death.

Premortem Angiography (Tables 3–6 and 3–7)

Two patterns were found at angiography. Five SV grafts demonstrated generalized irregularity with or without localized stenotic lesions and were interpreted as having atheromatous change (Fig. 3–9). Eight grafts had smooth walls with areas of tubular narrowing of a variable length, believed to represent fibrointimal hyperplasia (Fig. 3–10). Eight grafts were totally occluded at their origin.

Table 3-6. Clinical Findings in 9 Patients With Long-Term Saphenous Vein Bypass Grafts

No.	Age (Yr)	Sex	DM	TC	SH	FH	CS	AP	AMI	CHF	Duration SVBG (mo)	Interval Between Angio and Death (days)
1	65	M	0	0	+	0	+	+	0	0	12	30
2	69	M	0	+	+	0	+	+	+	0	39	2
3	58	M	0	0	+	+	+	+	0	+	45	30
4	64	M	0	0	+	+	0	+	0	0	120	2
5	62	F	+	0	+	+	0	+	+	+	14	90
6	64	M	0	0	0	+	0	+	+	0	64	5
7	67	M	0	0	+	0	+	+	+	0	105	4
8	49	M	+	+	+	0	0	+	+	0	96	60
9	52	M	0	0	0	0	+	+	+	+	111	3

Angio = angiography; AMI = acute myocardial infarction; AP = angina pectoris; CHF = congestive heart failure; CS = cigarette smoking; DM = diabetes mellitus; F = female; FH = family history of coronary disease; M = male; SH = systemic hypertension; SVBG = saphenous vein bypass graft; and TC = total serum cholesterol > 250 mg/dl.

From Atkinson et al.,[47] with permission.

Table 3-7. Correlation of Angiographic Findings and Morphologic Changes in Long-Term Saphenous Vein Bypass Grafts

No.	Angiographic Narrowing of SVBG (% diameter)	Anatomic Narrowing of SVBG (% XSA)	No CAs > 75% Narrowing in XSA	AMI	HMI	Postmortem Angiography
1	OM—100	100 (F)	4	+	0	+
	R—100	100 (F)				
	LAD—Normal	72 (FIP)*				
2	LD—Normal	25 (FIP)	3	0	0	+
	LAD—50	19 (FIP)†				
	OM—Normal	25 (FIP)				
	R—100	100 (F)				
3	LAD—50	53 (FIP)†	4	0	0	+
	R—Normal	54 (FIP)*				
4	R—100	100 (A)	3	0	0	+
	LAD—95	39 (FIP)†				
	OM—Normal	25 (A)				
5	LAD—100	100 (A)	4	0	0	+
	PD—50	38 (A)†				
6	R—50	75 (A)	4	0	+	+
	LAD—100	100 (F)				
7	R—100	100 (A)	3	+	0	+
	LAD—90	100 (A)				
	OM—Normal	50 (A)				
8	LAD—Normal	63 (FIP)*	4	+	+	0
9	OM—75	80 (A)	4	+	+	0

AMI = acute myocardial infarction; A = atherosclerosis; CAs = coronary arteries; F = fibrosis; FIP = fibrointimal proliferation; HMI = healed myocardial infarction; LAD = left anterior descending coronary artery; LC-left circumflex coronary artery; LD-left diagonal branch of left anterior descending coronary artery; OM-obtuse marginal coronary artery; PD-posterior descending branch of right coronary artery; R-right coronary artery; SVBG-saphenous vein bypass graft; XSA = cross-sectional area.

Values for anatomic narrowing at necropsy were obtained by computer-linked planimetry.

* Underestimation by premortem angiography.

† Overestimation by premortem angiography.

From Atkinson et al.,[47] with permission.

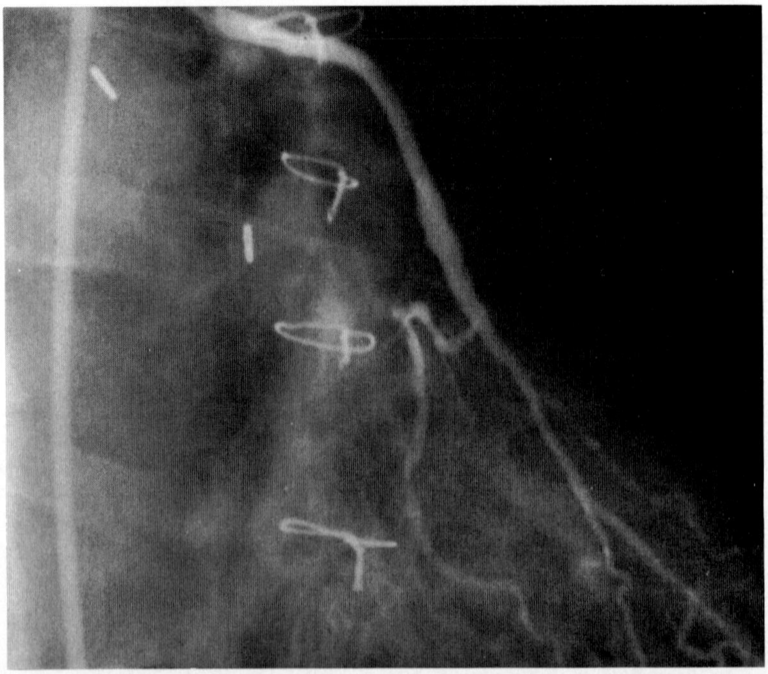

Figure 3-9. Cineangiogram in the left anterior oblique projection showing generalized irregularity of the obtuse marginal graft, believed to represent atherosclerotic change that was confirmed at autopsy. Selective angiography was performed 4 days before death. (From Atkinson et al.,[47] with permission.)

Morphologic Evaluation

Three characteristic lesions were found: fibrointimal proliferation in eight, total fibrotic occlusion in four, and atherosclerosis in nine. Planimetry confirmed the extent of luminal narrowing estimated by visual inspection in all cases. Three grafts were greater than 50 percent narrowed in diameter by atherosclerosis, whereas five were totally occluded with hemorrhage into plaques and superimposed thrombosis.

Correlation of Premortem Angiograms and Necropsy Findings

In seven grafts, premortem angiograms incorrectly assessed the extent of luminal narrowing—three underestimations (Fig. 3-10) and four overestimations of luminal narrowing (Fig. 3-11). Six incorrectly assessed grafts had fibrointimal proliferation, and one had atherosclerosis with 26 to 50 percent cross-sectional narrowing at necropsy. Postmortem angiograms in seven hearts confirmed the correlations between the premortem angiographic and histologic findings.

Causes of Underestimation and Overestimation of Degrees of Luminal Narrowing By Angiography Versus Histology

Angiography underestimates the degree of coronary narrowing compared with histology,[48] varying from 5 to 33 percent. The possible causes for this discrepancy have been listed as nonperfusion of coronary arteries at necropsy, diffuse atherosclerosis, eccentric slit-like lumens, and postmortem shrinkage and fixation artifacts.

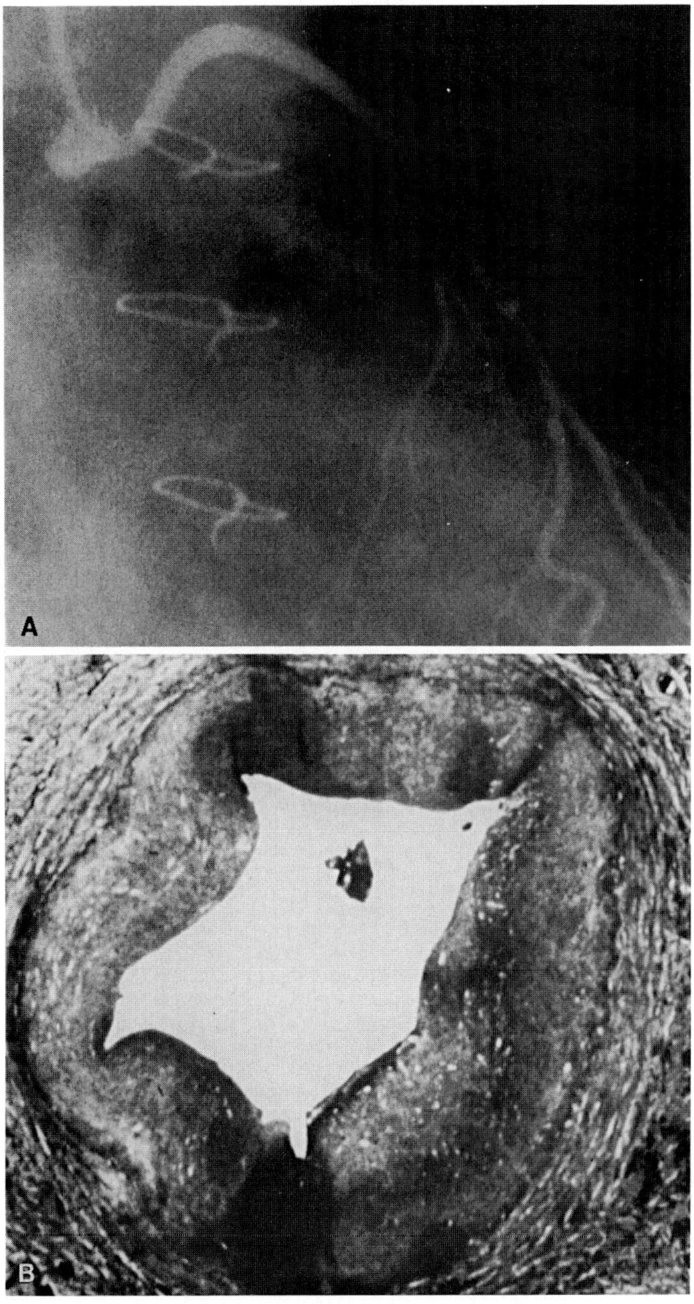

Figure 3-10. Patient 1 (Tables 3-6, 3-7) underwent catheterization 3 weeks before death. *A*, Angiogram of the anterior descending coronary graft in the left anterior oblique projection shows tubular narrowing with no focal stenotic lesions, and the graft was estimated to have less than 25 percent diameter reduction. *B*, At autopsy, there was up to 75 percent cross-sectional area narrowing by fibrointimal proliferation. The angiogram underestimated the extent of narrowing in this graft. (Movat stain; magnification ×30.) (From Atkinson et al.,[47] with permission.)

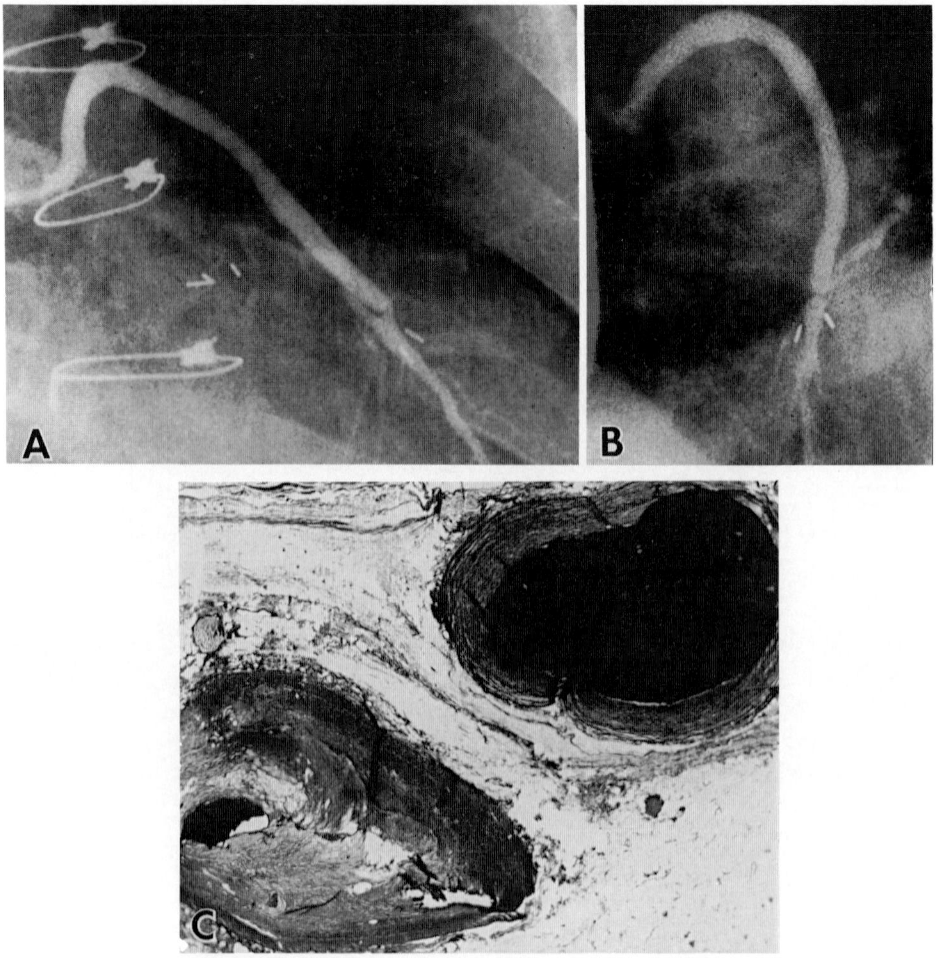

Figure 3-11. Patient 2 (Tables 3-6 and 3-7) underwent angiography 2 days before death. The right *(A)* and left *(B)* anterior oblique projections revealed generalized tubular narrowing of the anterior descending graft with focal stenotic lesion of up to 50 percent diameter reduction *(arrows)*. The histologic section at autopsy through the site of maximal narrowing of the vein graft showed less than 25 percent cross-sectional area reduction by fibrointimal proliferation, but a 90 percent cross-sectional luminal narrowing of the native left anterior descending coronary artery just proximal to the anastomotic site *(C)*. The angiogram therefore had overestimated the extent of narrowing in the vein graft. (Movat pentachrome stain; original magnification ×18; reduced 28 percent.) (From Atkinson et al.,[47] with permission.)

Atherosclerosis in vein grafts is usually diffuse and could result in underestimation, but only one of the seven vein grafts that were incorrectly assessed in this study had atherosclerosis. Postmortem shrinkage artifacts have also been incriminated and may result in reduction of tissue size of up to 20 percent. Smooth muscle and elastic fibers in grafts with fibrointimal proliferation may accentuate these changes. Shrinkage artifacts have been minimized by performance of postmortem angiography in seven of eight of our patients. Angiography also has its limitations, because it permits only a two-dimensional view of a three-dimensional structure.

In six of eight grafts with fibrointimal proliferation in our study,[47] angiograms tended to overestimate or underestimate luminal narrowing. Smooth muscle, a prominent component of the intima of saphenous veins that develop fibrointimal proliferation, may undergo transient spasm or dilatation, resulting in incorrect assessment of the grafts at angiography. Focal spasm in saphenous vein (SV) grafts has been reported in two patients,[49,50] and both had recurrent Prinzmetal's angina following coronary bypass surgery. The increased smooth muscle cells that are present in the intima of many of these grafts may have a hyper-reactive response to either endogenous vasoconstrictors or dilators.[51–53]

Our results[47] indicate that selective angiography of SV grafts is a precise and reliable means of assessing graft patency in the majority of patients. However, grafts with narrowing by fibrointimal proliferation are prone to erroneous assessment by angiography, perhaps owing to spasm or dilatation. Spasm had not been recognized in any of our patients clinically, and other factors may certainly be responsible for the angiographic findings.

INTERNAL MAMMARY ARTERY VERSUS SAPHENOUS VEIN AS A BYPASS GRAFT

The use of internal mammary artery as a graft has had a checkered existence. The Vineberg operation—implantation of the left internal mammary artery into a tunnel of left ventricular muscle, first described around 1950—demonstrated that the mammary artery could remain patent over a long time.[54] At the Cleveland Clinic from 1960 to 1965, the Vineberg procedure was increasingly used, because Sones confirmed patency by angiography.[55] In 1968 Spencer and associates[56] demonstrated in animals that the internal mammary artery could be directly anastomosed to left anterior descending coronary artery, and that year the first internal mammary anastomosis was performed in a human being.[56] However, its routine use was inhibited because of concerns about adequacy of flow rates. Finally, in 1984, reports from Montreal of 10-year angiographic studies comparing vein graft patency with mammary artery patency showed that 30 percent of vein grafts became occluded and that another 30 percent developed atherosclerosis, whereas 95 percent of internal mammary artery grafts remained open.[57] This has led to an increased use of internal mammary artery anastomoses, including sequential anastomoses and bilateral mammary anastomoses.[54] Also, it has been shown that the internal mammary artery can enlarge, probably in response to increased peripheral resistance to blood flow as atherosclerosis further occludes native vessels.[54] In a recent report, Loop and coworkers[58] compared retrospectively 2306 mammary artery anastomoses with 3625 saphenous vein grafts to the left anterior descending coronary artery over 7 years, representing the largest data currently available. The 10-year actuarial survival rate among the group receiving the internal mammary artery graft as compared with that of the group receiving vein grafts was 93.4 percent versus 88 percent ($p = 0.05$) for one-vessel; 90 percent versus 79.5 percent ($p < 0.0001$) for two-vessel; and 82.6 percent versus 71 percent ($p < 0.0001$) for those with three-vessel disease. The frequency of infarction was also decreased, but not the frequency of recurrence of angina or arrhythmias. This study shows that most patients undergoing bypass surgery who have severe stenosis of the anterior descending artery should receive an internal-mammary-artery graft to that artery, along with other vein grafts to other vessels as indicated.

REFERENCES

1. Eisenberg, MS: The problem of sudden cardiac death. In Eisenberg, MS and Hallstrom, AP (eds): Sudden Cardiac Death in the Community. Praeger, New York, 1984, p 2.
2. Carr, KW, Engler, RL, and Ross, J, Jr: Do coronary artery bypass operations prolong life? (Medical Progress). West J Med 136:295, 1982.
3. Rahimtoola, SH: Coronary bypass surgery—a perspective. In Rahimtoola, SH and Brest, AN (eds): Coronary Bypass Surgery. FA Davis, Philadelphia, 1977, p 11.
4. Christian, CB, Mack, JW, and Wetstein, L: Current status of coronary artery bypass grafting for coronary artery atherosclerosis. In Symposium on the Latest Advances in Cardiac Surgery. Surg Clin North Am 65(3):509, 1985.
5. Murphy, ML, Hultgren, HN, Detre, K, et al: Treatment of chronic stable angina: A preliminary report of survival data of the randomized Veterans Administration cooperative study. N Engl J Med 297:621, 1977.
6. Detre, KM, Peduzzi, P, Takaro, T, et al: Eleven-year survival in the Veterans Administration randomized trial of coronary bypass surgery for stable angina. N Engl J Med 311:1333, 1984.
7. European Coronary Surgery Study Group: Long-term results of a prospective randomized study of coronary artery bypass surgery in stable angina pectoris. Lancet 2:1173, 1982.
8. CASS Principal Investigators: Coronary Artery Surgery Study (CASS): A randomized trial of coronary artery bypass surgery: Survival data. Circulation 68:939, 1983.
9. CASS Principal Investigators: Comparison of coronary bypass surgery and medical therapy in patients 65 years of age or older. A nonrandomized study from the Coronary Artery Surgery Study (CASS) Registry. N Engl J Med 313:217, 1985.
10. Killip, T and Ryan, TJ: Randomized trials in coronary bypass surgery. Circulation 71:418, 1985.
11. Campeau, L, Lesperance, J, Corbara, J, et al: Aortocoronary saphenous vein bypass graft changes 5 to 7 years after surgery. Circulation 58 (Suppl I):I-170, 1978.
12. Bourassa, MG, Campeau, L, Lesperance, J, et al: Changes in grafts and in coronary arteries after saphenous vein aortocoronary bypass surgery. In Hammermeister, KE (ed): Coronary Bypass Surgery. The Late Results. Praeger Scientific, New York, 1983, p 293.
13. Seides, SF, Borer, JS, Kent, KM, et al: Long-term anatomic fate of coronary-artery bypass grafts and functional status of patients five years after operation. N Engl J Med 298:1213, 1978.
14. Lawrie, GM, Morris, GC, Howell, JF, et al: Results of coronary bypass more than 5 years after operation in 434 patients. Clinical, treadmill exercise and angiographic correlations. Am J Cardiol 40:665, 1977.
15. Hamby, RI, Aintablian, A, Handler, M, et al: Aortocoronary saphenous vein bypass grafts. Long-term patency, morphology and blood flow in patients with patent grafts early after surgery. Circulation 60:901, 1979.
16. Campeau, L, Enjalbert, M, Lesperance, J, et al: The relation of risk factors to the development of atherosclerosis in saphenous-vein bypass grafts and the progression of disease in the native circulation. A study 10 years after aortocoronary bypass surgery. N Engl J Med 311:1329, 1984.
17. Unni, KK, Kottke, BA, Titus, JL, et al: Pathologic changes in aortocoronary saphenous vein grafts. Am J Cardiol 34:526, 1974.
18. Brody, WR, Angell, WW and Kosek, JC: Histologic fate of the venous coronary artery bypass in dogs. Am J Pathol 66:111, 1972.
19. Spray, TL and Roberts, WC: Status of the grafts and the native coronary arteries proximal and distal to coronary anastomotic sites of aortocoronary bypass grafts. Circulation 55:741, 1977.
20. Bulkley, BH: Pathology of coronary artery bypass graft surgery. Am Heart J 98:539, 1979.
21. Bulkley, BH and Hutchins, GM: Pathology of coronary artery bypass graft surgery. Arch Pathol Lab Med 102:273, 1978.
22. Griffith, LSC, Bulkley, BH, Hutchins, GM, et al: Occlusive changes at the coronary artery bypass graft anastomosis. Morphologic study of 95 grafts. J Thorac Cardiovasc Surg 73:668, 1977.
23. McEnany, MT, DeSanctis, RW, Harthorne, JW, et al: Effect of antithrombolytic therapy on aortocoronary vein graft patency rates. Circulation 54(Suppl II):124, 1976.
24. Chesebro, JH, Fuster, V, Elveback, LR, et al: Effect of dipyridamole and aspirin on late vein-graft patency after coronary bypass operations. N Engl J Med 310:209, 1984.
25. Kern, WH, Dermer, GB, and Lindesmith, GG: The intimal proliferation in aortic-coronary saphenous vein grafts. Light and electron microscopic studies. Am Heart J 84:771, 1972.
26. Bulkley, BH and Hutchins, GM: Accelerated "atherosclerosis": A morphologic study of 97 saphenous vein coronary artery bypass grafts. Circulation 55:163, 1977.

27. Brody, WR, Kosek, JC, and Angell, WW: Changes in vein grafts following aorto-coronary bypass induced by pressure and ischemia. J Thorac Cardiovasc Surg 68:847, 1972.
28. Marti, MC, Bouchardy, B, and Cox, JN: Aortocoronary bypass with autogenous saphenous vein grafts: Histopathologic aspects. Virchows Arch [Pathol Anat] 352, 255, 1971.
29. McNamara, JJ, Darling, RC, and Linton, RR: Segmental stenosis of saphenous vein autografts. N Engl J Med 277:290, 1967.
30. Atkinson, JB, Forman, MB, Vaughn, WK, et al: Morphologic changes in long-term saphenous vein bypass grafts. Chest 88:341, 1985.
31. Smith, SH and Geer, JC: Morphology of saphenous vein-coronary artery bypass grafts seven to 116 months after surgery. Arch Pathol Lab Med 107:13, 1983.
32. Barboriak, JJ, Batayias, GE, Pintar, K, et al: Pathological changes in surgically removed aortocoronary vein grafts. Ann Thorac Surg 21:524, 1976.
33. World Health Organization: Classification of atherosclerotic lesions report of a study group. Technical Report Series. Publication 143, World Health Organization, Geneva, 1958, pp 3–20.
34. Lie, JT, Lawrie, GM, and Morris, GC: Aortocoronary bypass saphenous vein graft atherosclerosis. Anatomic study of 99 vein grafts from normal and hyperlipoproteinemic patients up to 75 months postoperatively. Am J Cardiol 40:906, 1977.
35. Batayias, GE, Barboriak, JJ, Korns, ME, et al: The spectrum of pathologic changes in aortocoronary saphenous vein grafts. Circulation 56:11, 1977.
36. Walts, AE, Fishbein, MC Sustaita, H, et al: Ruptured atheromatous plaques in saphenous vein coronary artery bypass: A mechanism of acute, thrombotic, late graft occlusion. Circulation 65:197, 1982.
37. Smith, SH and Geer, JC: Morphology of saphenous vein-artery bypass grafts. Seven to 116 months after surgery. Arch Pathol Lab Med 107:13, 1983.
38. Sako, Y: Susceptibility of autologous vein grafts to atheromatous degeneration. Surg Forum 12:247, 1961.
39. Friedman, M: Spontaneous atherosclerosis and experimental thromboatherosclerosis. Arch Pathol 76:571, 1963.
40. Scott, HW, Jr, Morgan, CV, Bolasny, BL, et al: Experimental atherosclerosis in autogenous venous grafts. Arch Surg 101:677, 1970.
41. King, P, Royle, JP: Autogenous vein grafting in atheromatous rabbits. Cardiovasc Res 6:627, 1972.
42. Rossiter, SJ, Brody, WR, Kosek, JC, et al: Internal mammary artery versus autogenous vein for coronary artery bypass graft. Circulation 50:1236, 1974.
43. Larson, RM, Hagen, PO, and Fuchs, JCA: Lipid biosynthesis in arteries, veins and venous grafts. Circulation 50(Suppl 3):139, 1974.
44. Barboriak, JJ, Pintar, K, and Korns, ME: Atherosclerosis in aortocoronary vein grafts. Lancet 2:621, 1974.
45. Grondin, CM, Campeau, L, Lesperance, J, et al: Atherosclerotic changes in coronary vein grafts six years after operation: Angiographic aspect in 110 patients. J Thorac Cardiovasc Surg 77:24, 1979.
46. Campeau, L, Enjalbert, M, Lesperance, J, et al: Atherosclerosis and late closure of aortocoronary saphenous vein grafts: Sequential angiographic studies at 2 weeks, 1 year, 5 to 7 years and 10 to 12 years after surgery. Circulation 68 (Suppl II):1, 1983.
47. Atkinson, JB, Forman, MB, Perry, JM, et al: Correlation of saphenous vein bypass graft angiograms with histologic changes at necropsy. Am J Cardiol 55:952, 1985.
48. Isner, JM, Kishel, J, Kent, KM, et al: Accuracy of angiographic determination of left main coronary arterial narrowing. Angiographic-histologic correlative analysis in 28 patients. Circulation 63:1056, 1981.
49. Victor, MF, Kimbiris, D, Iskandrian, AS, et al: Spasm of a saphenous vein bypass graft. A possible mechanism for occlusion of the venous graft. Chest 80:413, 1981.
50. Walinsky, P: Angiographic documentation of spontaneous spasm of saphenous vein coronary artery bypass graft. Am Heart, J 103:290, 1982.
51. Kalsner, S and Richards, R: Coronary arteries of cardiac patients are hyperreactive and contain stores of amines: A mechanism for coronary spasm. Science 223:1435, 1981.
52. Ellis, EF, Oelz, O, Roberts, LJ, II, et al: Coronary arterial smooth muscle contraction by a substance released from platelets: Evidence that it is thromboxane A_2. Science 193:1135, 1976.
53. Roy, L, Knapp, HR, Robertson, RM, et al: Endogenous prostacyclin (PGI_2) biosynthesis is stimulated by cardiac catherization and angiography in man. Circulation 68(Suppl III):104, 1983.
54. Spencer, FC: The internal mammary artery: The ideal coronary bypass graft? N Engl J Med 314:50, 1986.

55. Effler, DB, Groves, LK, Sones, FM, Jr, et al: Increased myocardial perfusion by internal mammary artery implant: Vineberg's operation. Am Surg 158:526, 1963.
56. Spencer, FC, Green, GE, Tice, DA, et al: Surgical therapy for coronary artery disease. Curr Probl Surg, September 1970.
57. Grondin, CM, Campeau, L, Lesperance, J, et al: Comparison of late changes in internal mammary artery and saphenous vein grafts in two consecutive series of patients 10 years after operation. Circulation 70:I-208, 1984.
58. Loop, FD, Lytle, BW, Cosgrove, DM, et al: Influence of the internal-mammary-artery graft on 10-year survival and other cardiac events. N Engl J Med 314:1, 1986.

CHAPTER 4

Pathology of New Interventional Procedures in Coronary Disease

Bruce F. Waller, M.D.

During the last decade we have witnessed the development and continuing evolution of several important procedures used for the treatment of patients with symptomatic coronary atherosclerosis. Experimental and clinical results of these therapeutic interventions predictably have stimulated interest in the pathologic changes produced by these procedures. This chapter summarizes certain morphologic-histologic changes resulting from the experimental or clinical use of five new therapeutic interventions: (1) coronary artery and aortocoronary saphenous vein bypass graft *balloon angioplasty;* (2) *thrombolysis therapy* for evolving acute myocardial infarction; (3) *laser irradiation;* (4) ventricular *endocardial resection,* and *catheter ablation* of sites causing chronic life-threatening ventricular arrhythmias; and (5) temporary left and right *ventricular assist devices.*

PERCUTANEOUS TRANSLUMINAL BALLOON ANGIOPLASTY

Several reports of percutaneous transluminal balloon angioplasty (TBA) have demonstrated its clinical usefulness as a nonoperative treatment of atherosclerotic coronary artery disease[1-6] and obstructed aortocoronary saphenous vein bypass grafts.[7-11] Despite the therapeutic successes of TBA in the treatment of patients with obstructed vessels, the exact mechanism by which TBA improves vessel patency remains unclear. The purpose of this section of this chapter is to review morphologic and histologic changes observed in coronary arteries and aortocoronary saphenous vein bypass grafts previously subjected to TBA procedures.

Atherosclerotic Coronary Arteries

Morphologic observations in coronary arteries of patients undergoing TBA are limited.[12-20] This section reviews certain clinical and morphologic findings in 11 patients receiving coronary artery TBA: six patients examined personally[13-16] and five examined by others.[12,18-20]

Personal Series

Six men had percutaneous transluminal coronary angioplasty with subsequent morphologic coronary artery examination: three had TBA 4 hours to 7 days *(early)* before coronary bypass surgery and either coronary endarterectomy (two patients) or death (one patient) (Figures 4-1 through 4-4), and three had TBA 80 to 150 days *(late)* before sudden death (Figures 4-4 through 4-9).

Clinical Observations

Early. Each of three patients, aged 43, 52, and 54 years, had exertional angina pectoris ranging from 1 to 18 months before TBA. Coronary angiography and TBA performed 4 hours before death (one patient) or 4 hours to 7 days before coronary artery endarterectomy at the time of aortocoronary artery bypass surgery (two patients) disclosed severe (80 to 99 percent diameter reduction) luminal narrowing of the left anterior descending (LAD) or right (R) coronary arteries. At TBA, one patient had the LAD coronary artery dilated, with reduction in mean intracoronary gradient of 45 mmHg, before the onset of chest pain, hypotension, ventricular fibrillation, and subsequent death at bypass operation. The dilation procedure was angiographically successful. The two remaining patients also developed chest pain during or shortly after the TBA procedure and underwent coronary endarterectomy and aortocoronary bypass grafting. The dilation procedure in the latter two patients was complicated by difficulties crossing the severely obstructed lesion.[13,14]

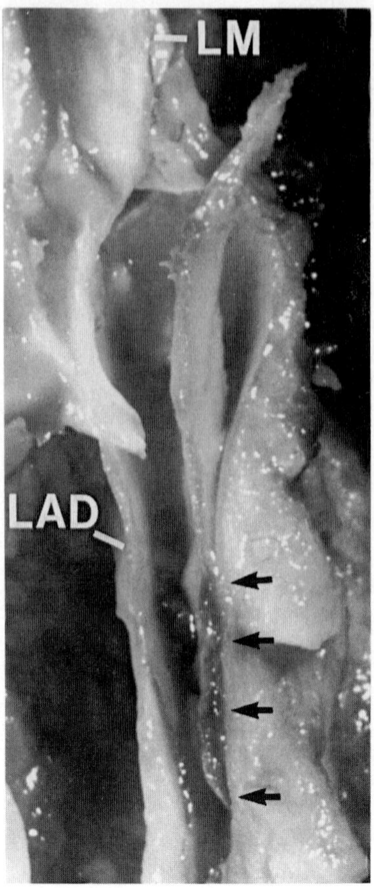

Figure 4-1. Coronary dissection *(arrows)* is present at site of TBA in the left anterior descending (LAD) coronary artery. LM = left main coronary artery. (From Waller,[13] reprinted with permission of Clinical Cardiology Publishing Co., Inc., and the Foundation for Advances in Clinical Medicine, the JBI Building, Box 521, Mahwah, NJ.)

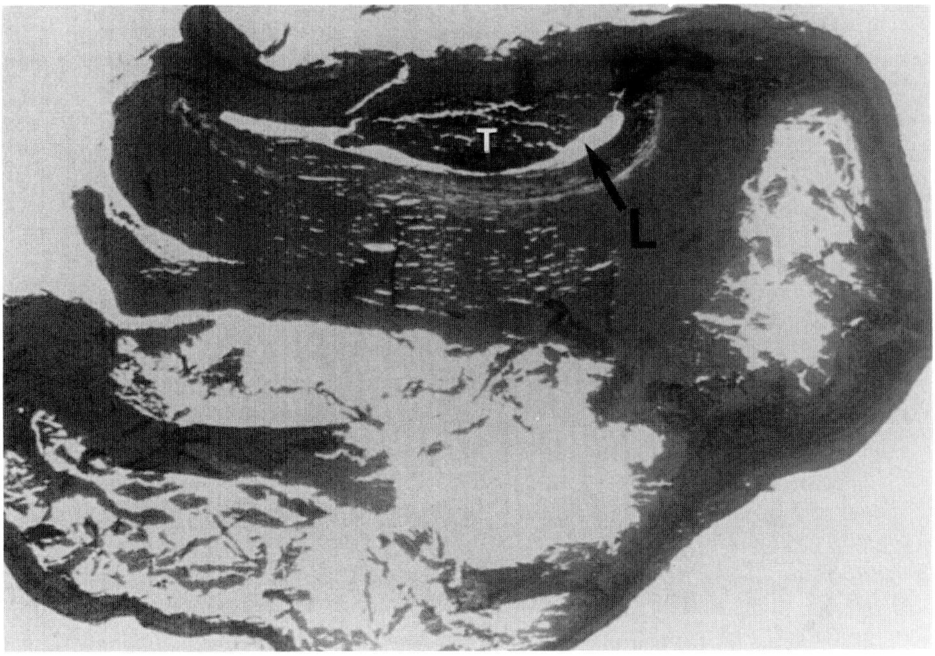

Figure 4-2. Histologic section of right endarterectomy specimen in the area of attempted transluminal balloon angioplasty showing severe plaque hemorrhage and thrombus (T) in an already severely narrowed lumen (L). (van Gieson stain; original magnification ×28; reduced 21 percent.) (From Waller,[13] reprinted with permission of Clinical Cardiology Publishing Co., Inc., and the Foundation for Advances in Clinical Medicine, the JBI Building, Box 521, Mahwah, NJ.)

Late. Each of the three patients had exertional angina pectoris for 1 to 2 months before TBA. Coronary angiography and TBA performed 80, 90, and 150 days, respectively, before death disclosed severe (76 to 95 percent diameter reduction) luminal narrowing of the LAD coronary artery. At TBA, the LAD was dilated 55, 50, and 65 percent, respectively, and the corresponding mean intracoronary pressure gradient fell 17, 38, and 43 mmHg, respectively (see Figs. 4-4, 4-6, 4-8). Each patient had angina pectoris with marked ST segment depression during exercise testing before TBA and no angina and only J point depression (two patients) or no electrocardiographic changes (one patient) during exercise testing 1 to 11 days after TBA. Thus, these three men had clinically, hemodynamically, and angiographically successful TBA procedures. Two of the three patients remained angina-free following TBA, but the third patient developed recurrent angina pectoris 45 days before death. Of the two clinically asymptomatic patients, one died suddenly at home (sudden coronary death) and the other was killed in an automobile accident while intoxicated (alcohol) (noncardiac cause of death). The symptomatic patient died suddenly (without apparent preceding chest pain) at work (sudden coronary death).

Morphologic Observations

Early. At necropsy, in the single patient dying 4 hours after angiographically successful TBA, dissection of the LAD coronary artery at the site of TBA was observed (see Fig. 4-1). Histologic assessment of atherosclerotic plaques from endarterectomy specimens obtained 4 hours to 7 days after TBA disclosed extensive plaque hemorrhage or plaque hemorrhage with localized dissection in the areas of attempted angioplasty.[13] The sites of TBA in the LAD coronary artery and in two R coronary

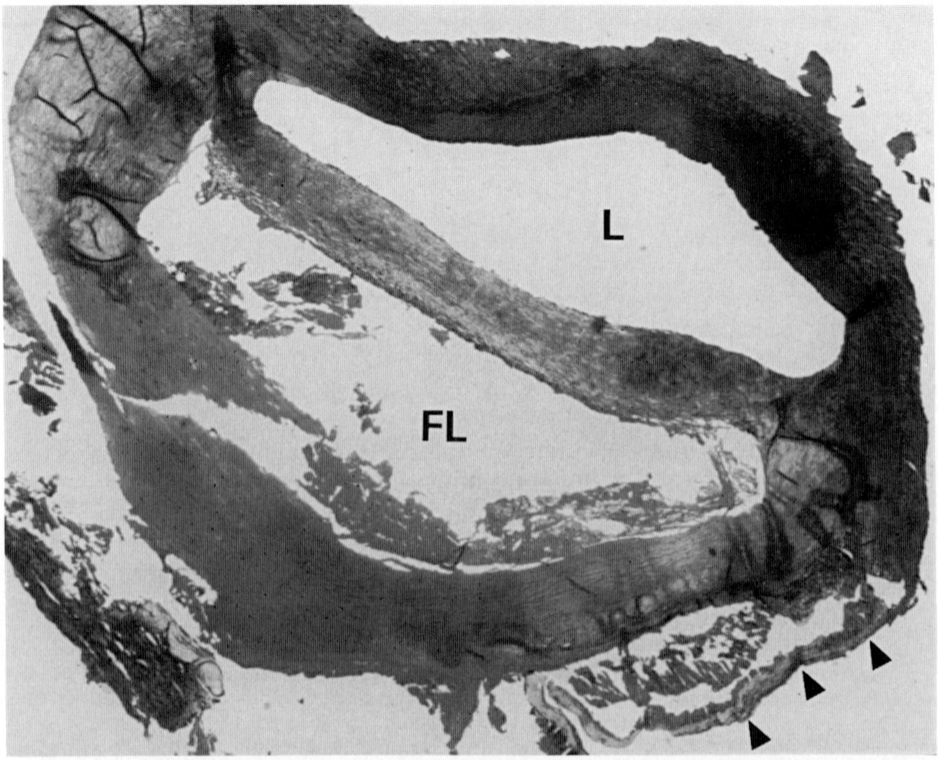

Figure 4-3. Histologic section of the right coronary endarterectomy specimen at the site of attempted transluminal balloon angioplasty showing coronary dissection with an intimal flap separating true lumen (L) and false lumen (FL). Extensive hemorrhage is present in the outer wall of the FL and in the adventitial layer of the coronary artery *(arrowheads).* (van Gieson stain, original magnification ×28; reduced 10 percent.) (From Waller,[13] reprinted with permission of Clinical Cardiology Publishing Co., Inc., and the Foundation for Advances in Clinical Medicine, the JBI Building, Box 521, Mahwah, NJ.)

artery endarterectomy specimens were narrowed 76 to 95 percent in cross-sectional area by atherosclerotic plaques (see Figs. 4-2, 4-3).

Late. At necropsy, in the three patients dying 80, 90, and 150 days after clinically successful TBA, no foci of myocardial necrosis or fibrosis were present.[16] The site of TBA on the LAD coronary artery in each patient was narrowed 76 to 95 percent in cross-sectional area by atherosclerotic plaques (see Figs. 4-5, 4-7, 4-9). A 5 mm long segment of LAD containing the site of TBA in each patient was serially sectioned at 10 μ intervals. A total of 72 histologic sections in the areas of TBA were examined. Histologic assessment of atherosclerotic plaques in the areas of the TBA compared with other areas of atherosclerotic plaque in the same artery or other coronary arteries in the same patient disclosed no distinctive morphologic differences.[14,16] While "splits," "tears," and "breaks" have been described histologically in coronary arteries of humans and experimental animals immediately after the TBA procedure,[21-26] these distinctive acute morphologic lesions or healed modifications of these lesions were not recognized late in these three patients.[16]

Other Investigators

Morphologic analysis at necropsy of coronary arteries from five additional patients undergoing TBA have been reported to date: four patients dying *early*[12,19,20]

(Figs. 4–10 through 4–13) and one patient dying *late*[18] (Fig. 4–14) after the procedure.

Early Observations. At necropsy, four patients (three women, one man) have been reported in whom the LAD coronary artery had been successfully dilated a few (approximately 4 to 90) hours before death. Block and colleagues[12] reported atherosclerotic plaque "splitting" with extension into the media in two patients (see Fig. 4–10). In one patient the medial dissection was more extensive, with involvement of the "outer media" by dissecting hematoma. Mizuno and colleagues[19] serially sectioned the TBA site in one patient and observed intimal-splitting and medial-splitting leading to coronary artery dissection (see Fig. 4–11). Soward and associates[20] recently reported plaque splitting, medial dissection and lifting of the plaque from the media at the site of previous TBA (see Figs. 4–12, 4–13).

Late Observations. A report by Essed and associates[18] describes morphologic changes at the site of TBA that occurred 5 months before death. To date, this patient represents the latest necropsy followup of previously dilated coronary arteries. Cross sections of the LAD showed extensive disruption of the media with extensive proximal and distal dissection and partial absence of the pre-existent muscular layer (see Fig. 4–14). A large intimal "crack" with partial "flap" formation created a "false channel," which after 5 months had filled with fibrocellular material. The fibrocellular proliferation covered surrounding portions of atherosclerotic plaque in addition to the area of previous plaque fracture, producing a severely narrowed coronary

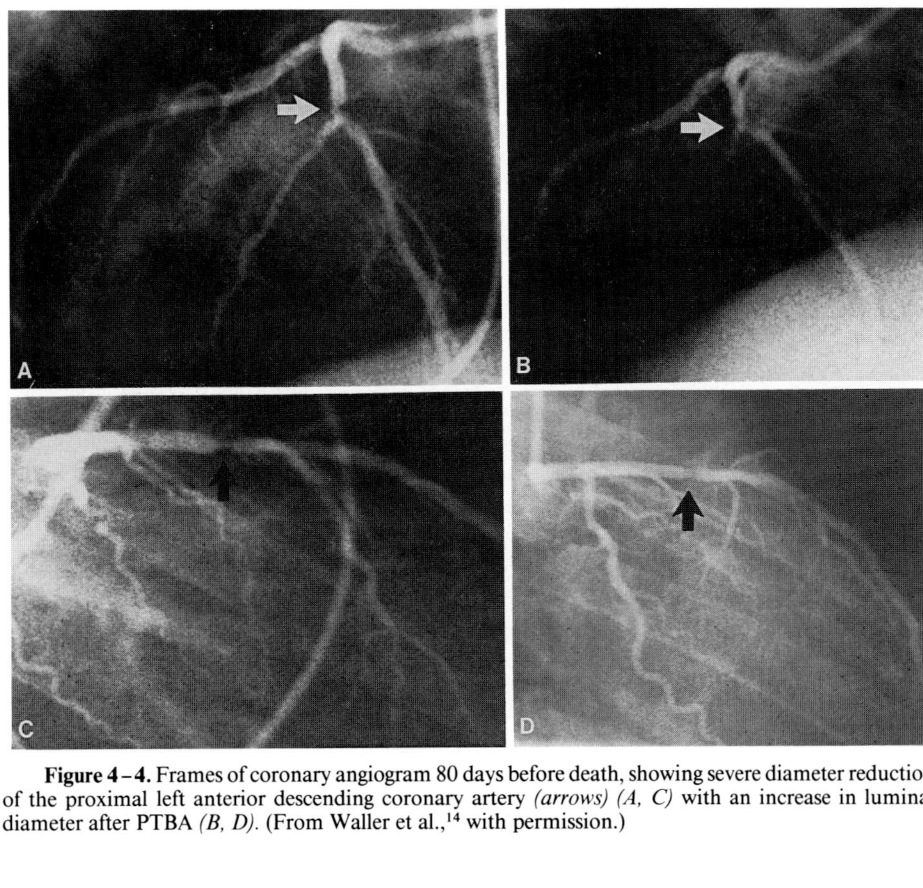

Figure 4–4. Frames of coronary angiogram 80 days before death, showing severe diameter reduction of the proximal left anterior descending coronary artery *(arrows) (A, C)* with an increase in luminal diameter after PTBA *(B, D)*. (From Waller et al.,[14] with permission.)

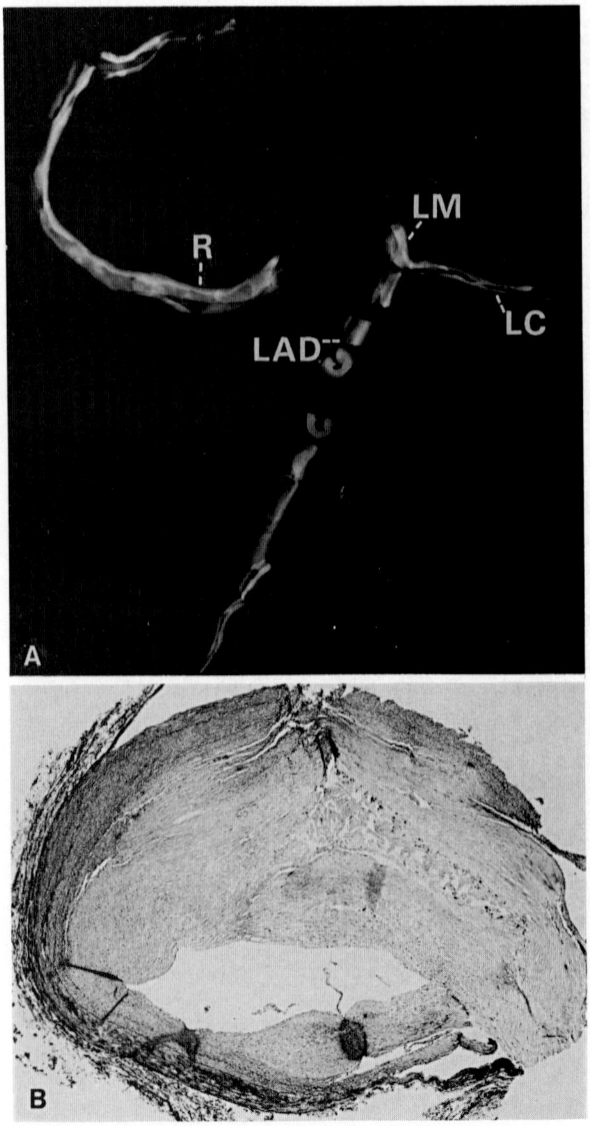

Figure 4-5. *A,* Postmortem radiograph of excised coronary tree showing no calcific deposits. *B,* Histologic section of the left anterior descending (LAD) coronary artery at the site of previous PTBA showing severe luminal narrowing by atherosclerotic plaque. (Movat stain; magnification ×26, reduced 7 percent.) LC = left circumflex, LM = left main, R = right. (From Waller et al.,[14] with permission.)

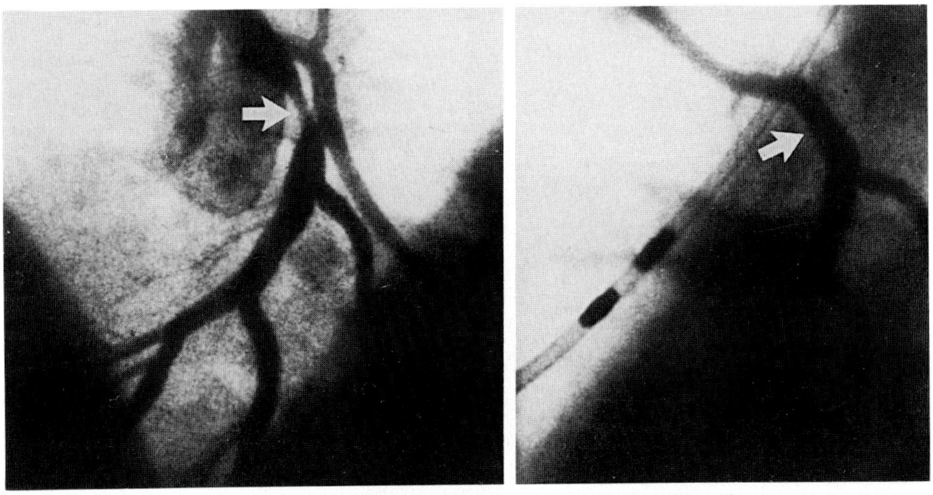

Figure 4–6. Frames of coronary angiogram 90 days before death, showing an increase in diameter of the left anterior descending coronary artery after transluminal balloon angioplasty *(arrows)* (See Fig. 4–7). (From Waller et al.,[14] with permission.)

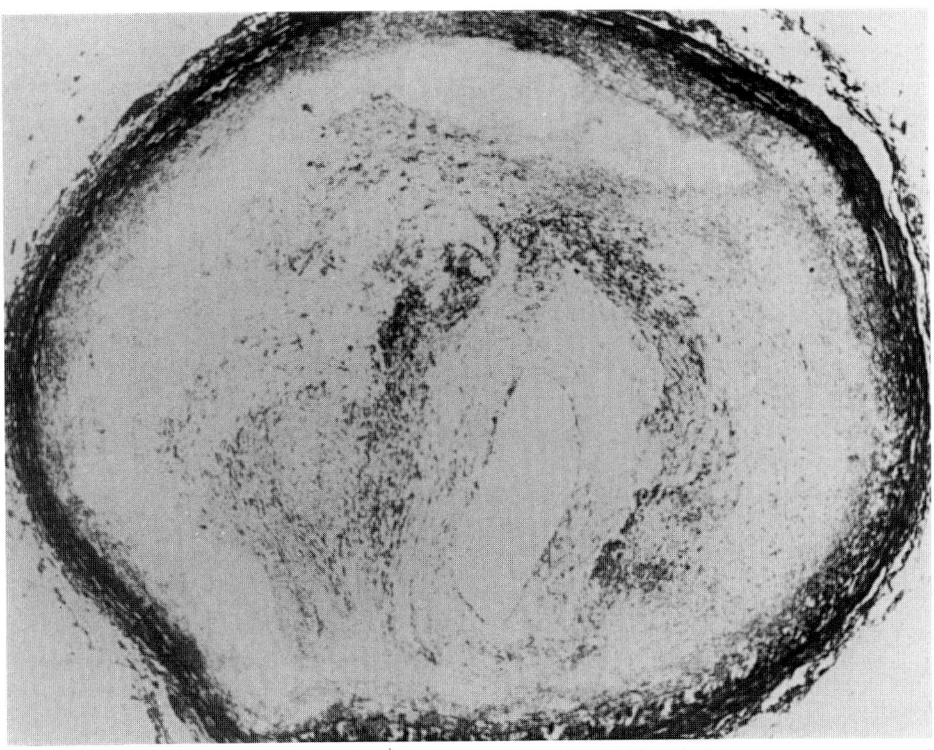

Figure 4–7. Histologic section of the left anterior descending coronary artery at the site of previous transluminal balloon angioplasty procedure, showing severe luminal narrowing by atherosclerotic plaque (see Fig. 4–6). (Movat stain; original magnification ×22; reduced 9 percent.) (From Waller et al.,[14] with permission.)

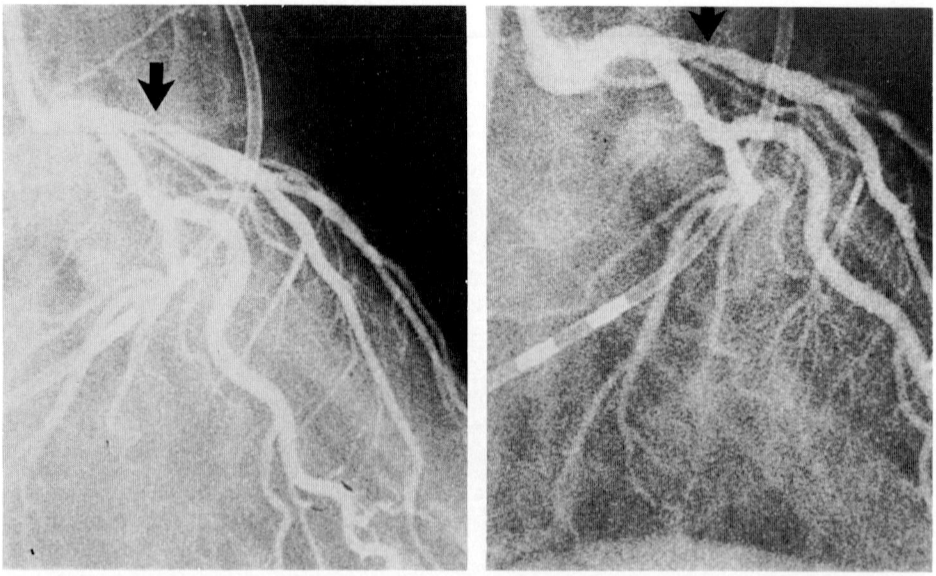

Figure 4–8. Frames of coronary angiogram 150 days before death, showing an increase in diameter of the left anterior descending coronary artery after transluminal balloon angioplasty *(arrows)* (see Fig. 4–9). (From Waller et al.,[14] with permission.)

artery. Essed and colleagues[18] speculate that the wall laceration with exposure of smooth muscle cells to blood products may have initiated the excessive fibrocellular response.

Mechanism(s) of Coronary Artery Balloon Angioplasty (Fig. 4–15)

Plaque Compression. Dotter and Judkins[1] in their original description of the angioplasty procedure (as well as Gruntzig[2] 12 years later) initially attributed the mechanism of TBA to *redistribution* and *compression* of intimal atherosclerotic plaque (Fig. 4–15*A*). Inflation of the angioplasty balloon within an arterial stenosis was believed to "compress" atherosclerotic plaque components against the arterial wall, thereby resulting in a larger vessel lumen. However, the vast majority of atherosclerotic plaques in human coronary arteries are composed of dense fibrocollagenous tissue with varying amounts of calcific deposits and far lesser amounts of intracellular and extracellular lipid (that is, "hard plaques"). Thus, it appears unlikely that plaque "compression" plays a major role in human coronary artery TBA dilation. In experimental animal models, vessel-induced injury plus high-cholesterol diets are used to create atherosclerotic lesions. The atherosclerotic lesions induced in these models are composed almost entirely of lipid-laden foam cells without dense collagen and calcific deposits (that is, "soft plaques").[23,25] Thus, in contrast to the mechanism(s) of TBA in human arteries, "compression" or "redistribution" of plaque may contribute to luminal expansion in the experimental model.

Plaque Fracture. Data from angioplasty results in experimental models,[22,23,25] from angioplasty results in human necropsy coronary arteries,[21,24,26] and from results in human vessels examined following successful or complicated

TBA procedures[12,19,20] suggest the major mechanism of human coronary angioplasty is by atherosclerotic plaque *"breaking," "cracking," "splitting,"* or *"fracture"* (Fig. 4–15*B*). Plaque "fractures," "breaks" (also called dissection clefts), and "cracks" extending from the lumen for variable lengths into the plaque and occasionally separation of intimal plaque from the medial layer provide a means of improving vessel patency by creating additional channels or avenues for coronary blood flow. Healing and repair changes at the angioplasty site eventually may remodel the acute pathologic lesion(s) to alter or eliminate the aforementioned distinctive features. The healing process at the TBA site per se also may increase luminal size (as has been noted angiographically[27]) or decrease luminal size (restenosis).

PLAQUE FRACTURE, INTIMAL FLAPS, AND LOCALIZED MEDIAL DISSECTION. Waller and colleagues[15] reported plaque fracture, "intimal atherosclerotic flaps," and localized medial dissection as the major mechanism of TBA in human coronary arteries examined from patients undergoing TBA during life (Fig. 4–15*E*). Initial and persistent luminal cross-sectional area expansion appears to require deep *intimal* fractures (occasionally creating intimal "flaps") with localized tears or dissection of the underlying *media.*[15] Failure to obtain localized and limited medial

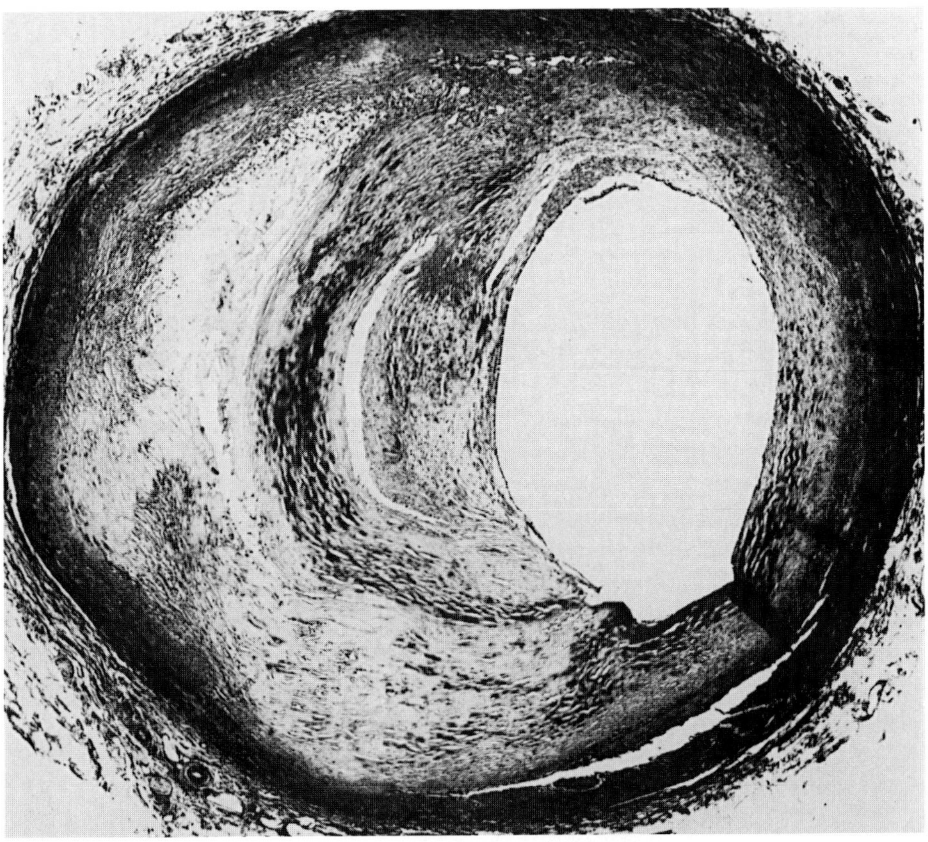

Figure 4–9. Histologic section of the left anterior descending coronary artery at the site of a previous transluminal balloon angioplasty procedure showing severe luminal narrowing by atherosclerotic plaque (see Fig. 4–8). (Movat stain; original magnification ×22; reduced 19 percent.) (From Waller et al.,[14] with permission.)

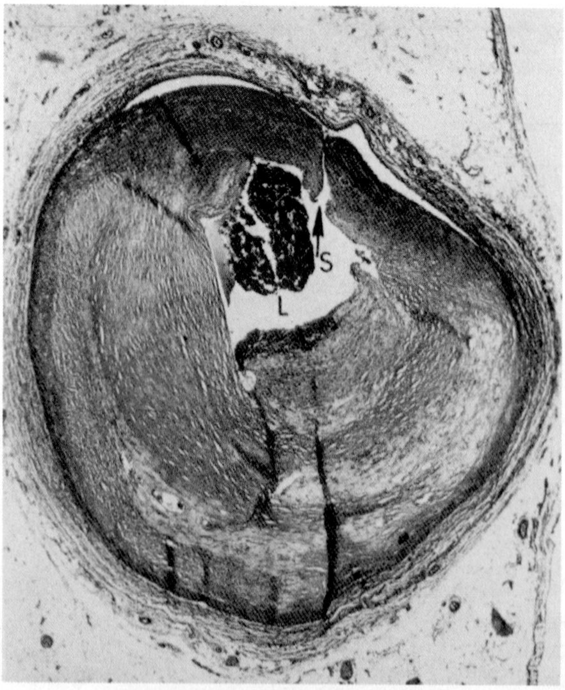

Figure 4-10. Section of left anterior descending artery at site of angioplasty showing a split (S) *(arrow)* in the thinnest portion of a fibrous atherosclerotic plaque. The split extends into the media with circumferential extension. The lumen (L) is partly occluded by a small thrombus. (From Block et al.,[12] with permission.)

involvement in addition to the intimal damage may be a cause of early "restenosis" following initially successful TBA.

Stretching of Plaque-Free Wall Segment. An additional mechanism of coronary artery dilation appears to be "stretching" of plaque-free wall segments of eccentric atherosclerotic lesions (Fig. 4-15*C*).[13,28,29] Inflation of angioplasty balloons across eccentric plaque lesions may distend or "stretch" the normal wall segment and produce little or no damage to the plaque on the remaining portions of the arterial wall. Stretching of the plaque-free wall segment may result initially in coronary luminal (diameter and cross-sectional area) increase, but several weeks later gradual "relaxation" of this overstretched segment ("restitution of tone") decreases the coronary lumen toward the predilation state. The decrease in coronary luminal area toward the predilation state may provide another explanation for early "restenosis

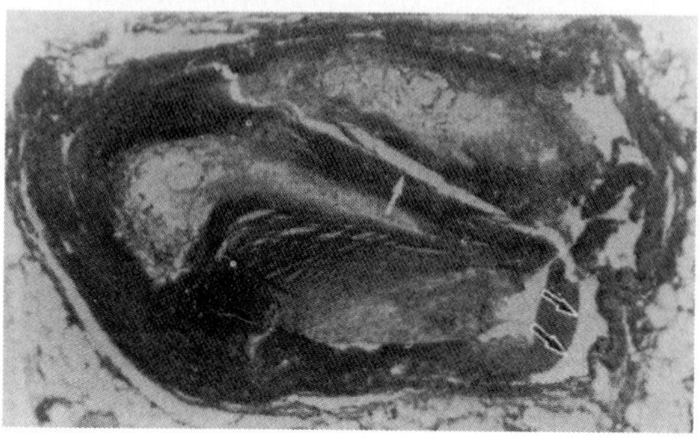

Figure 4-11. Histologic appearance of the dilated left anterior descending artery showing intimal and medial splitting, which have led to medial dissection *(black arrows)* and plaque fracture *(white arrow)*. (From Mizuno et al.,[19] with permission.)

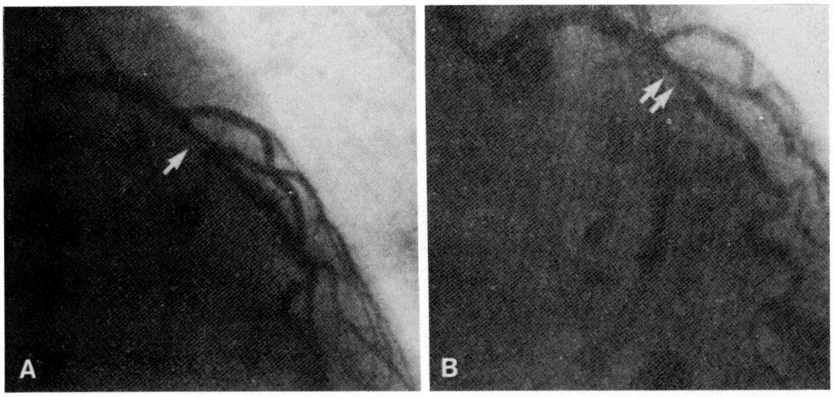

Figure 4–12. Frames from coronary angiogram showing severe left anterior descending artery stenosis *(arrows)* before *(A)* and after *(B)* PTBA (see Fig. 4–13). (From Soward et al.,[20] with permission.)

after an initially angiographically successful dilation.[18] The high frequency of eccentric-type coronary lumen in severely diseased vessels[30,31] suggests that stretching of the plaque-free wall segment may be a more frequent mechanism of clinically successful coronary angioplasty than previously thought. On the basis of examination of 200 atherosclerotic coronary artery sections, Vlodaver and Edwards[30] found *eccentric* coronary lumen (eccentric polymorphous and eccentric slit-like) in 70 percent of cross sections examined and *concentric* lumen in the remaining 30 percent of sections. Baroldi[31] examined 1069 sites of severe (greater than 70 percent) diameter reduction and found that 46 percent of the coronary luminal shapes were concentric,

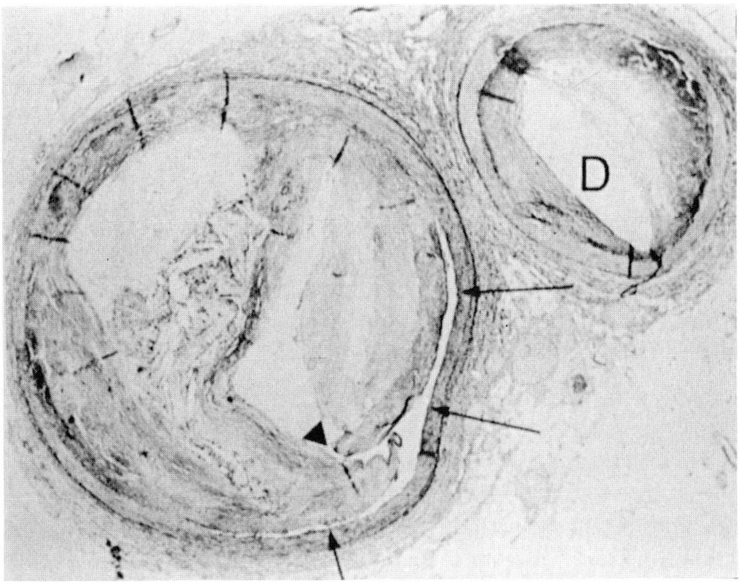

Figure 4–13. Histologic section of proximal left anterior descending artery and adjacent diagonal branch (D). Atherosclerotic plaque narrows the lumen. The plaque shows disruption and splitting *(arrowhead)* and is dissected and lifted from the media. (From Soward et al.,[20] with permission.)

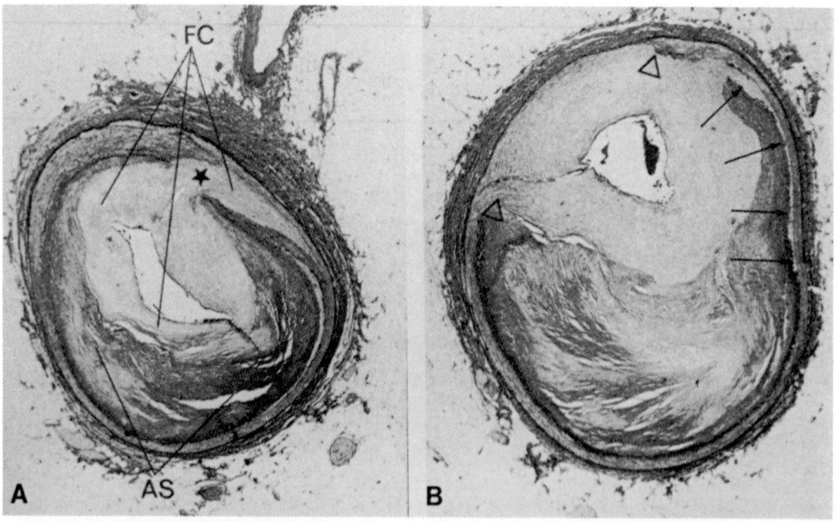

Figure 4–14. Cross section of left anterior descending artery showing *(A)* disruption of the medial layer (*) and medial dissection. The false channel and the major part of the lumen are filled with fibrocellular tissue (FC). The preexistent atherosclerotic plaque (AS) is easily distinguished. *B*, More distal segment of the same artery shows dehiscence of the sclerotic plaque from the underlying media *(closed arrows)*. The media shows a localized interruption *(open arrowheads)*. (From Essed et al.,[28] with permission.)

24 percent eccentric (lateral lumen position but still encircled by plaque), and 30 percent "semilunar" (a variable arc of disease-free wall). Recently, Saner and colleagues[29] studied 100 coronary artery segments narrowed 50 to 90 percent in cross-sectional area by atherosclerotic plaque. Of these 100 segments, 17 to 23 percent (average 20 percent) of the vessel circumference was disease-free. The percent of disease-free wall arc length did not differ significantly with increasing severity of luminal obstruction, proximal or distal location of the lesion, or the location of the lesion among the various coronary arteries.[29]

Stretching and Compression. A fifth, although less likely, mechanism for TBA of coronary arteries is the combination of vessel stretching with minimal or mild plaque compression (Fig. 4–15*D*). In this situation, an oversized angioplasty balloon may stretch a localized coronary segment that is concentrically narrowed by fibrocollagenous plaque.

Clinical-Pathologic Correlations

Isner and Fortin[32] reported morphologic observations in coronary arteries that had *not* been subjected to previous TBA procedures. In 49 percent of 70 patients examined, plaque fractures and dissection clefts (cracks) similar to those described in TBA arteries were observed. These findings emphasize two points: (1) the need for *precise* angiographic-morphologic correlations in the histologic evaluation of arteries subjected to TBA[16] and (2) the presence of similar plaque "cracks" and "breaks" in non–TBA–treated arteries, which suggests that such lesions may not be the sole basis for successful angioplasty and that vessel dilation and stretching (and perhaps plaque compression) are additional important mechanisms.

Aortocoronary Saphenous Vein Bypass Grafts

Morphologic changes in obstructed aortocoronary saphenous vein bypass grafts following TBA have recently been reported.[7,8] This section summarizes clinical and morphologic observations in two patients undergoing TBA of obstructed saphenous vein bypass grafts—operatively excised segments of bypass graft *early* (less than or equal to 1 year) (Figs. 4–16 through 4–19) and *late* (greater than 1 year) (Figs. 4–20 through 4–23) after aortocoronary bypass graft surgery—and reviews possible mechanisms of graft dilation.

Angioplasty of Saphenous Vein Graft *Early* After Bypass Surgery

Clinical Features. A 63-year-old man with angina pectoris underwent unsuccessful TBA of the LAD coronary artery and had an aortocoronary saphenous

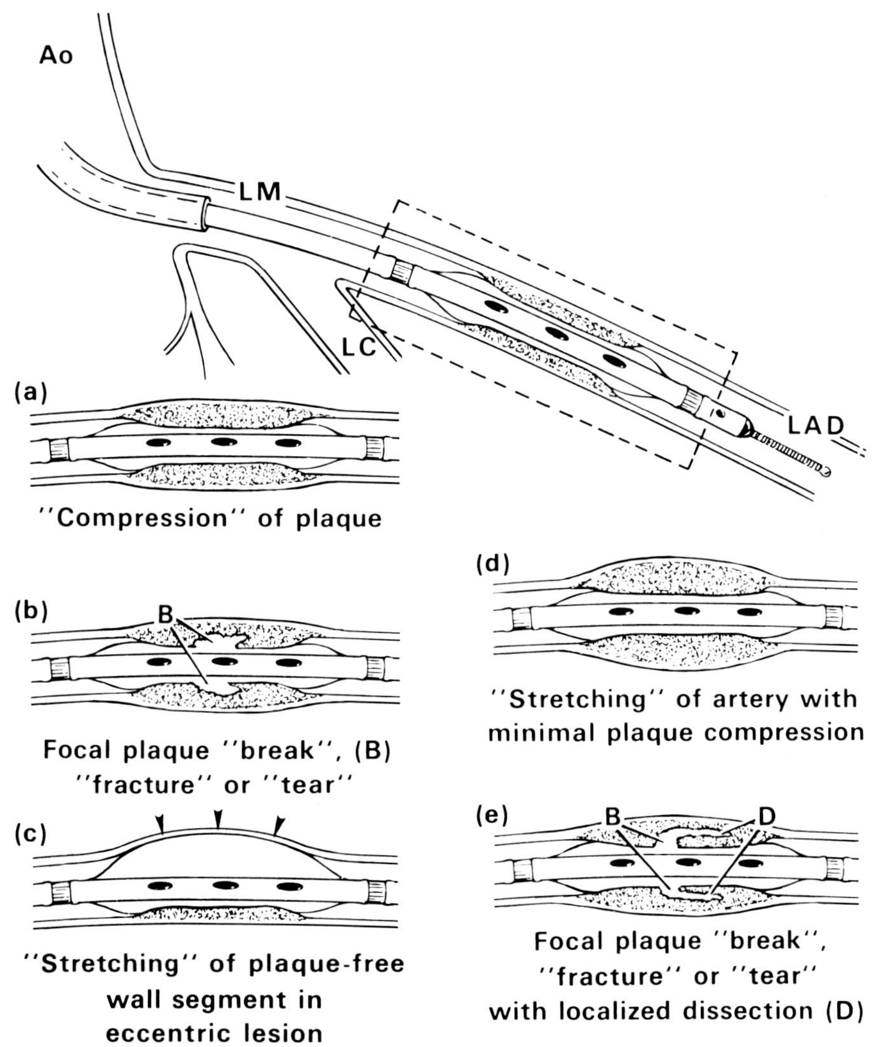

Figure 4–15. Diagram showing possible mechanisms of coronary artery balloon angioplasty (Ao = aorta; LAD = left anterior descending coronary artery; LC = left circumflex coronary artery; LM = left main coronary artery). (From Waller,[28] with permission.)

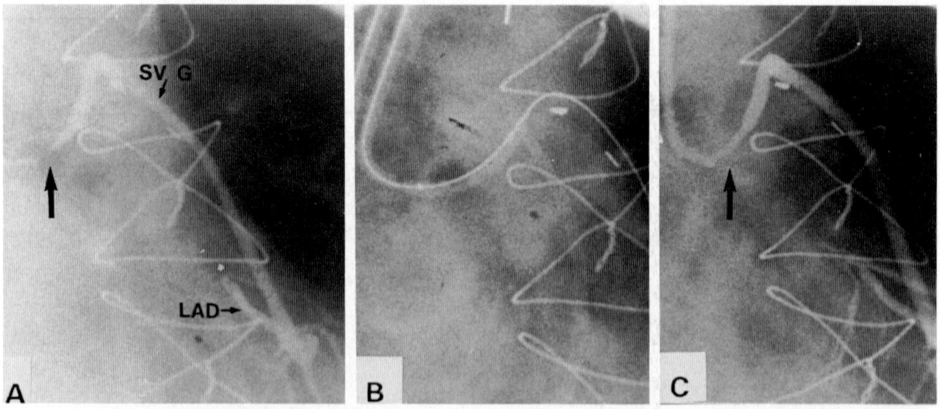

Figure 4–16. Angiographic frames of a saphenous vein bypass graft (SV G) before and after transluminal balloon angioplasty 1 month before graft excision and 2 months after graft insertion. *A,* Severe luminal narrowing of the bypass graft near the aortic anastomotic site *(arrow). B,* Inflated angioplasty balloon located within the proximal saphenous vein graft. *C,* Marked increase in luminal diameter of saphenous vein graft following angioplasty *(arrow).* LAD = left anterior descending coronary artery. (From Waller et al.,[8] with permission.)

vein bypass graft inserted into the LAD. Seven weeks after bypass surgery, the patient had recurrent angina and angiography disclosed 95 percent symmetric diameter reduction of the bypass graft near its proximal (aortic) anastomotic site. The stenotic area was dilated, with multiple balloon inflations resulting in a marked increase in graft luminal diameter (see Fig. 4–16). Four weeks after successful graft TBA, the patient had recurrent angina. Repeat angiography disclosed severe graft narrowing

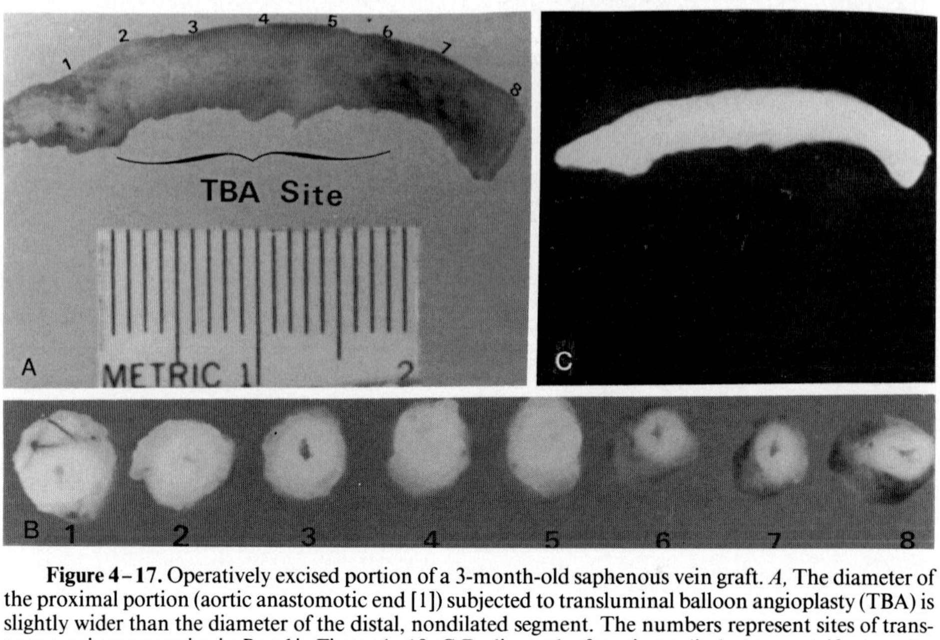

Figure 4–17. Operatively excised portion of a 3-month-old saphenous vein graft. *A,* The diameter of the proximal portion (aortic anastomotic end [1]) subjected to transluminal balloon angioplasty (TBA) is slightly wider than the diameter of the distal, nondilated segment. The numbers represent sites of transverse sections appearing in *B* and in Figure 4–18. *C,* Radiograph of specimen discloses no calcific deposits. (From Waller et al.,[8] with permission.)

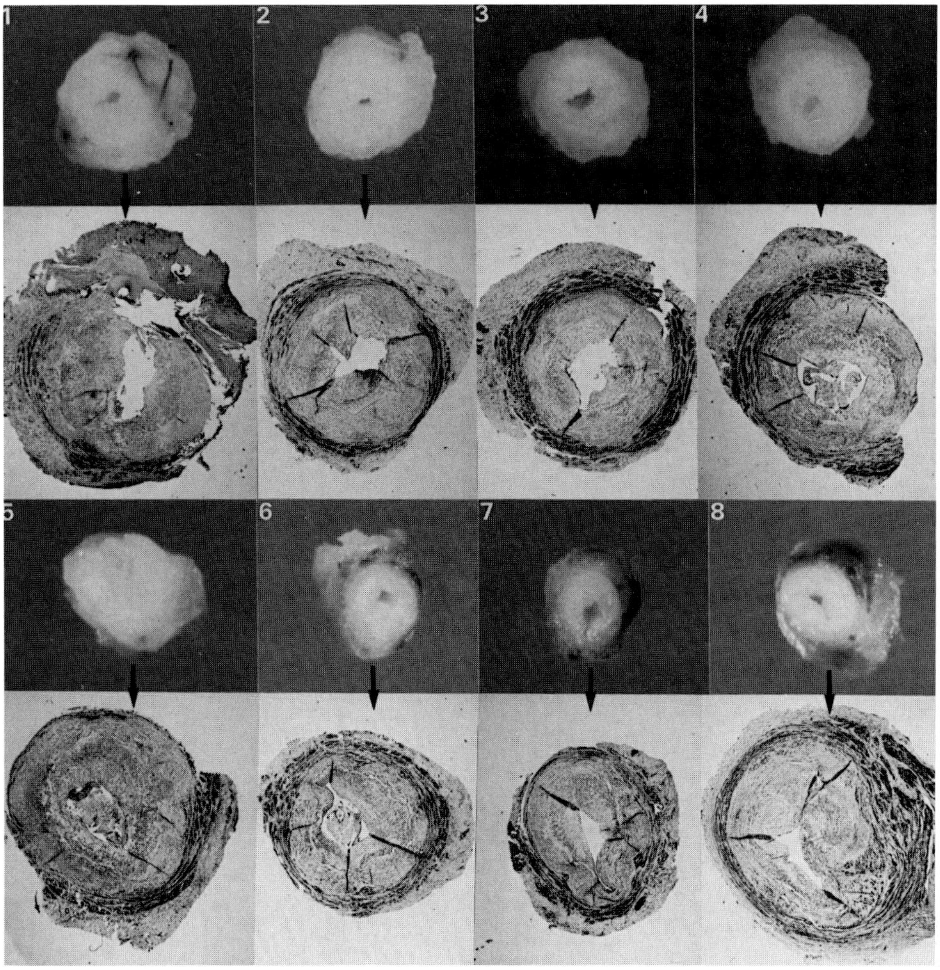

Figure 4–18. Morphologic and histologic photographs of the eight segments of saphenous vein graft, corresponding to the sites labeled in Figure 4–17. Segments 1 through 6 are from the area of balloon inflation and dilation, and segments 7 and 8 are from nondilated portions of the graft (that is, "controls"). Each of the eight segments had diffuse and severe cross-sectional area luminal narrowing by intimal thickening consisting of fibrocollagenous tissue. No segments contained atherosclerotic plaque or calcium deposits. No distinctive histologic changes were observed in the segments subjected to transluminal balloon angioplasty, compared with control segments. (Elastic stains; original magnification ×6; reduced 32 percent.) (From Waller et al.,[8] with permission.)

(restenosis) at the previous dilation site. This time, however, the stenotic segment was not smooth and symmetric but appeared irregular and asymmetric. The proximal portion of the graft was excised at repeat coronary bypass surgery.

Morphologic Features. The operatively excised portion of saphenous vein (Fig. 4–17) contained the proximal site of maximal balloon inflation and a short distal portion in which the catheter and guide wire had passed but in which balloon inflation had not occurred. The excised graft was free of calcific deposits. The lumen of the bypass graft was diffusely and severely (more than 75 percent cross-sectional area) narrowed by cellular fibrocollagenous tissue without foam cells or cholesterol clefts ("intimal fibrous hyperplasia, fibrous proliferation") (see Fig. 4–18). Areas of

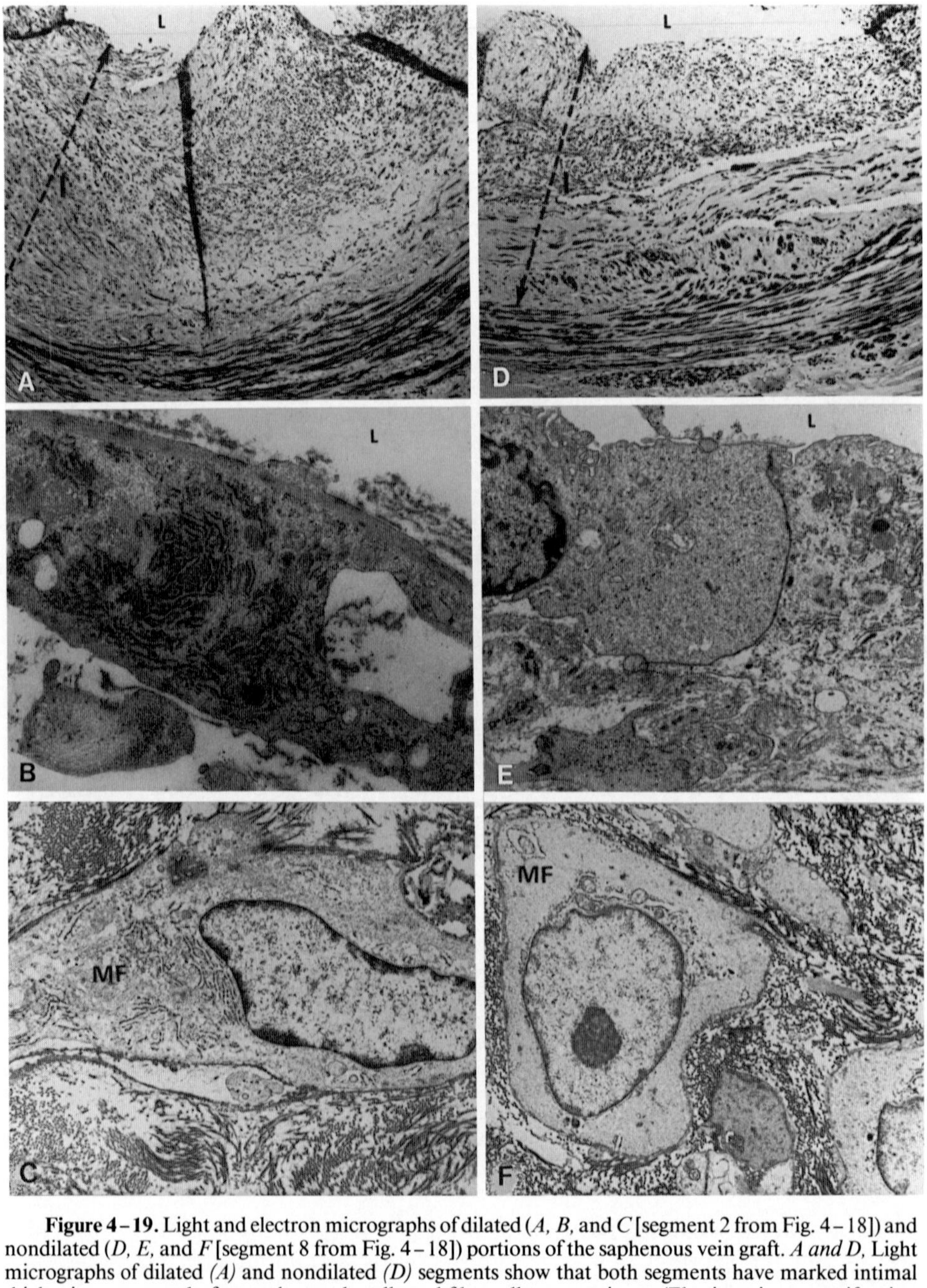

Figure 4–19. Light and electron micrographs of dilated (*A, B,* and *C* [segment 2 from Fig. 4–18]) and nondilated (*D, E,* and *F* [segment 8 from Fig. 4–18]) portions of the saphenous vein graft. *A and D,* Light micrographs of dilated *(A)* and nondilated *(D)* segments show that both segments have marked intimal thickening composed of smooth muscle cells and fibrocollagenous tissue. (Elastic stains; magnification ×40, reduced 30 percent.) *B and E,* Electron micrographs at the luminal border of dilated *(B)* and nondilated *(E)* segments show a loss of endothelial cells, with micropinocytotic vesicles bordering the lumen in *E.* A short segment of basement membrane is visible at the lower right. (Magnification ×8300, reduced 30 percent.) *C and F,* Electron micrographs from deeper portions of the intimal thickening of the dilated *(C),* and nondilated *(F)* segments show similar types of myofibroblastic cells (MF) and dense bundles of collagen fibrils. (Magnification ×8300, reduced 30 percent.) (From Waller et al.,[8] with permission.)

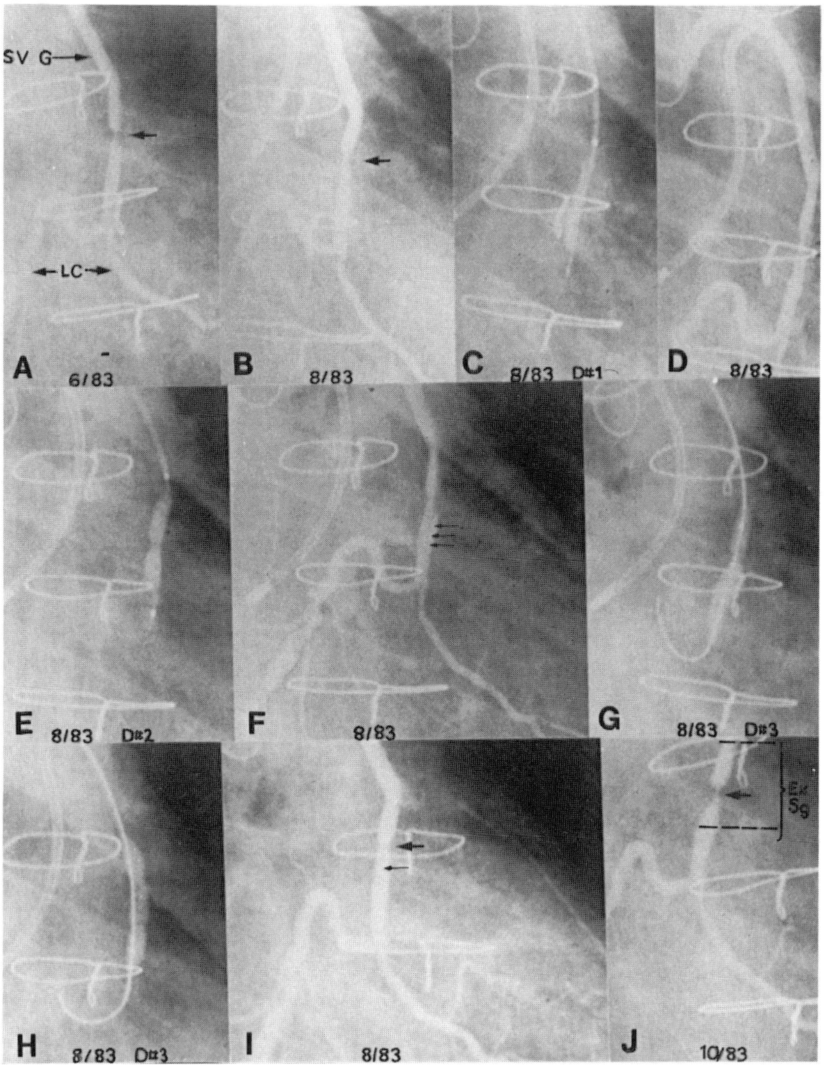

Figure 4-20. Serial angiographic frames of a saphenous vein (SV) bypass graft (G) before and after two transluminal balloon angioplasty (TBA) procedures. *A,* Severe luminal narrowing in the mid-portion of the SV G *(arrow)* 52 months after insertion. TBA (not shown) resulted in decreased luminal narrowing (from 95 percent to 20 percent) (LC = left circumflex coronary artery). *B,* Restenosis at graft 2 months later at previous TBA site *(arrow). C through I,* Second TBA (54 months after insertion) showing serial dilations (D#1 to D#3) using progressively larger balloons, variable inflation pressures, and inflation durations. *F and I* show a localized "break," "fracture," or "dissection" line at the site of TBA *(small arrows).* The second TBA resulted in decreased luminal narrowing (from 95 percent to 10 percent). *J,* Restenosis of the graft 2 months later (56 months after insertion) at the previous TBA sites. The boxed area indicates the operatively excised segment (Ex Sg) of the saphenous vein graft. Numbers in each frame indicate month and year. (From Waller et al.,[9] with permission.)

dilated and nondilated graft contained similar amounts of intimal thickening. Serial 10 μ sections of the angioplastic site did not disclose morphologic evidence ("cracks," "tears," "breaks") of previous TBA (see Figs. 4-18, 4-19). Furthermore, histologic assessment did not disclose any significant or distinctive morphologic lesion(s) in the intimal, medial, or adventitial layers of dilated or nondilated portions of the saphenous vein graft.

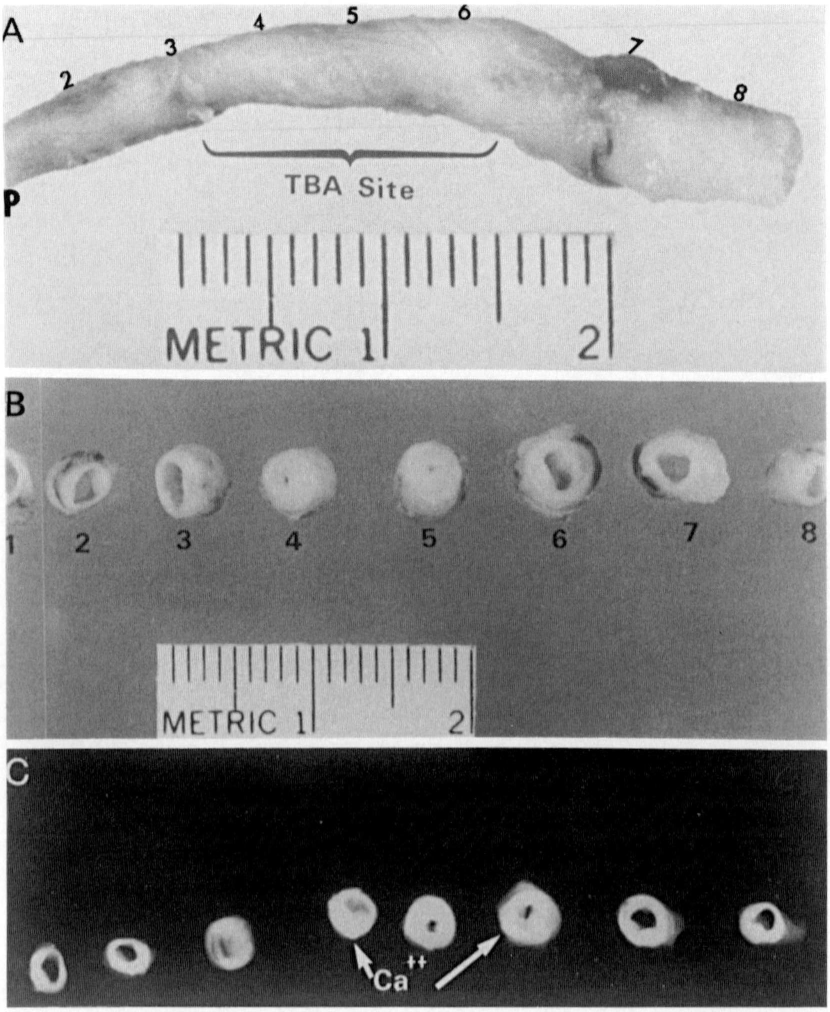

Figure 4–21. Operatively excised portion of a 56-month-old saphenous vein graft. *A*, The brackets indicate the site of two TBA procedures located in the mid-portion of the graft (P = proximal end). The numbers represent sites of transverse sections appearing in *B* and in Figure 4–22. *C*, Radiograph of transverse section discloses foci of calcific (Ca^{++}) deposits. (From Waller et al.,[8] with permission.)

Angioplasty of Saphenous Vein Graft *Late* After Bypass Surgery

Clinical Features. A 42-year-old man underwent aortocoronary bypass grafting for persistent pain following acute myocardial infarction. Fifty-two months after graft insertion (and an intervening second bypass operation), the patient had recurrent angina. Angiography disclosed a left circumflex (LC) saphenous vein bypass graft narrowed 95 percent in diameter on its midportion (body). TBA of the LC graft resulted in increased luminal diameter (see Fig. 4–20). Two months later (54 months after graft insertion), a second TBA was performed for restenosis of the LC graft at the previous TBA site. Multiple dilations again greatly improved the graft luminal diameter (95 percent diameter reduction to 10 percent diameter reduction) (see Fig. 4–20). During this TBA, a localized dissection and "crack" or "fracture" was apparent at the angioplasty site (see Fig. 4–23). Two months later (56 months

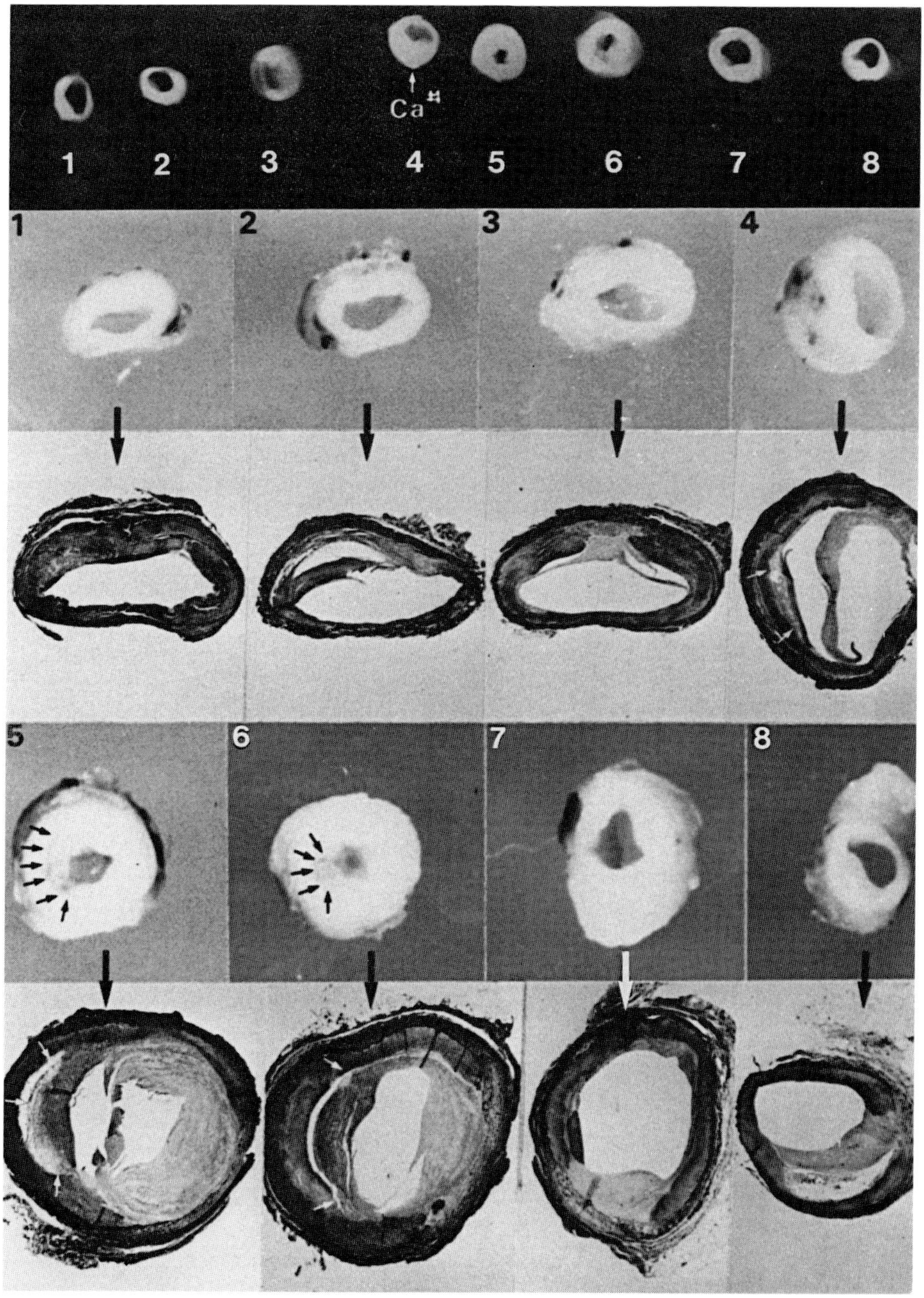

Figure 4-22. Photographs of morphologic and histologic segments of saphenous vein graft corresponding to the sites labeled in Figure 4-21. Each of the segments shows diffuse but variable degrees of intimal thickening composed of atherosclerotic plaque. The segment with the most severe luminal narrowing (5) corresponds to the area of previous transluminal balloon angioplasty procedures *(small arrows)*. (From Waller et al.,[8] with permission.)

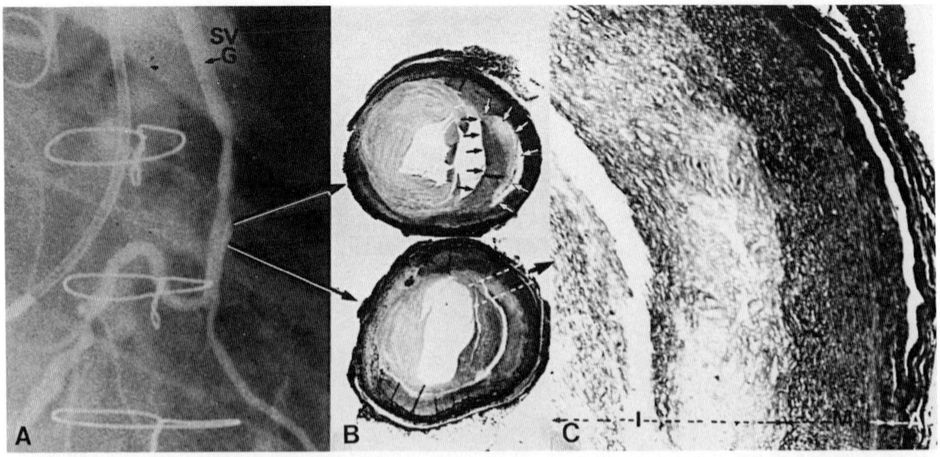

Figure 4–23. Angiographic morphologic-histologic correlation at the site of angioplasty dissection 2 months before graft excision. *A,* Angiographic frame of saphenous vein bypass graft (SV G) following transluminal balloon angioplasty showing a line of dissection. *B,* Corresponding morphologic segments *(large arrows)* of SV G in area of angiographic dissection showing severe luminal cross-sectional area narrowing with an "intimal flap" *(small arrows)* and a partially healed intimal "fracture." *C,* Higher magnification (×80, reduced 35 percent) of boxed area in *B* showing the intimal (I) fracture site. The intimal thickening is composed of fibrocollagenous tissue, foam cells, and cholesterol clefts. (M = media; A = adventitia.) (Elastic stains.) (From Waller et al.,[8] with permission.)

after insertion and two previous TBA procedures), the graft was again severely stenotic at the TBA site. The midportion of the LC graft was excised at repeat bypass operation.

Morphologic Features. The operatively excised portion of graft had foci of calcific deposits in the area of previous TBA (see Fig. 4–21). The lumen of the graft was diffusely narrowed but variable in degrees of intimal thickening. The maximal narrowing (in the area of TBA) consisted of foam cells, cholesterol clefts, fibrocollagenous tissue, foci of myofibroblasts, and calcific deposits characteristic of atherosclerotic plaque (see Fig. 4–22). Other areas of the graft were narrowed by predominantly fibrocollagenous tissue. The site of angioplasty dissection (see Fig. 4–23) had partial separation of the intima from the media. This "intimal flap" had begun to reattach to the wall of the graft (healing of localized plaque "tear").

Clinical-Morphologic Correlations in Saphenous Vein Graft Angioplasty

Each of the aforementioned patients had one or more clinically successful percutaneous transluminal angioplasty dilations of a stenotic saphenous vein bypass graft early (2 months) or late (52 to 54 months) after graft insertion. *Angiographic similarities* between the early and late saphenous vein grafts included an increase in luminal diameter associated with a decrease in mean trans-stenotic gradient following angioplasty, and restenosis of the graft at the site of previous dilation 1 or 2 months later. *Angiographic differences* between the grafts included the absence of "cracks," "breaks," or "splits" following the second angioplasty procedure in the early graft. An additional angiographic difference between the grafts was the stenosis location. The site of stenosis in the early graft was at the proximal end of the graft (aortic anastomosis), whereas the site of stenosis in the late graft was in the graft body (midportion). *Morphologic similarities* between the grafts included diffuse intimal thickening by fibrocollagenous tissue with fibrotic medial and adventitial layers. *Morphologic differences* between the grafts were distinctive: the early graft had thickened intima without atherosclerotic plaque changes or calcific deposits and no morphologic evidence of previous dilations, whereas the late graft had thickened intima typical of atherosclerotic plaque with focal calcific deposits and morphologic evidence of TBA injury.

Therapeutic Implications for Saphenous Vein Angioplasty Derived From Morphologic Observations (Figs. 4–24, 4–25)

The fate of an aortocoronary saphenous vein bypass graft appears dependent on several factors relevant to the time interval from bypass grafting to graft obstruction. Graft occlusion developing *within 1 month of bypass graft insertion* is almost invariably secondary to graft thrombosis related to technical factors such as stenosis at aortic or coronary anastomotic sites, intraoperative vein trauma, or poor distal run-off secondary to severe atherosclerosis or reduced caliber of the distal native vessel.[33–35] These technical factors may limit the role of TBA in successfully relieving saphenous vein graft obstruction occurring within 1 month of bypass operation.

Functionally significant graft stenoses developing *between 1 month and 1 year following graft insertion* nearly always are characterized by intimal thickening histologically composed of cellular or acellular fibrocollagenous tissue. The venous medial and adventitial layers become fibrotic and the graft resembles a thick, fibrous tube. Focally stenotic lesions produced by this intimal thickening appear amenable to dilation by TBA, as illustrated in the first patient described previously. However, in view of the histologic composition of the intima, the dilating mechanism is probably not "intimal compression" or intimal "fracture"[36] but rather graft "stretching" (see Fig. 4–24*a′*). Depending on the degree of graft stretching, the dilating procedure may have limited therapeutic success (weeks or months), with graft "restenosis" representing gradual "restitution of tone" of an overstretched graft segment.

Saphenous vein graft stenoses occurring *beyond 1 year and generally after 3 years following graft insertion* usually consists of atherosclerotic plaque in addition to intimal fibrous thickening.[33,34,37,39] The atherosclerotic plaque in saphenous vein grafts appears histologically similar to that observed in native coronary arteries: foam cells, cholesterol clefts, blood product debris, fibrocollagenous tissue and calcific deposits.[38,39] Focal stenoses produced by this type of lesion also appear amenable to dilation by TBA, as illustrated in the second patient described earlier. The mechanism(s) of graft dilation in this setting appear(s) similar to that proposed for coronary artery angioplasty: plaque "splitting," "cracking," or "breaking" with or without localized intimal-medial dissection (see Fig. 4–24*a* to *c*). Therapeutic limitations in dilating saphenous vein grafts narrowed by atherosclerotic plaque should be similar to that observed in atherosclerotic coronary arteries subjected to TBA.

In addition to age of the bypass graft, at least two other anatomic factors appear to influence the therapeutic success of TBA of saphenous vein grafts: *length of stenosis* and *location of stenosis*. Long stenotic segments (greater than 15 to 20 mm) of saphenous vein are frequently technically more difficult to dilate and are associated with a lower primary therapeutic success compared with short stenotic segments (less than or equal to 5 mm).[36,40] Graft stenoses may be located at the anastomotic sites (aorta-graft or coronary-graft) or within the body of the graft (see Fig. 4–11). Angiographic studies[7,9,36,40] have suggested that saphenous vein graft stenoses at the coronary graft anastomotic site have the best therapeutic results, followed by

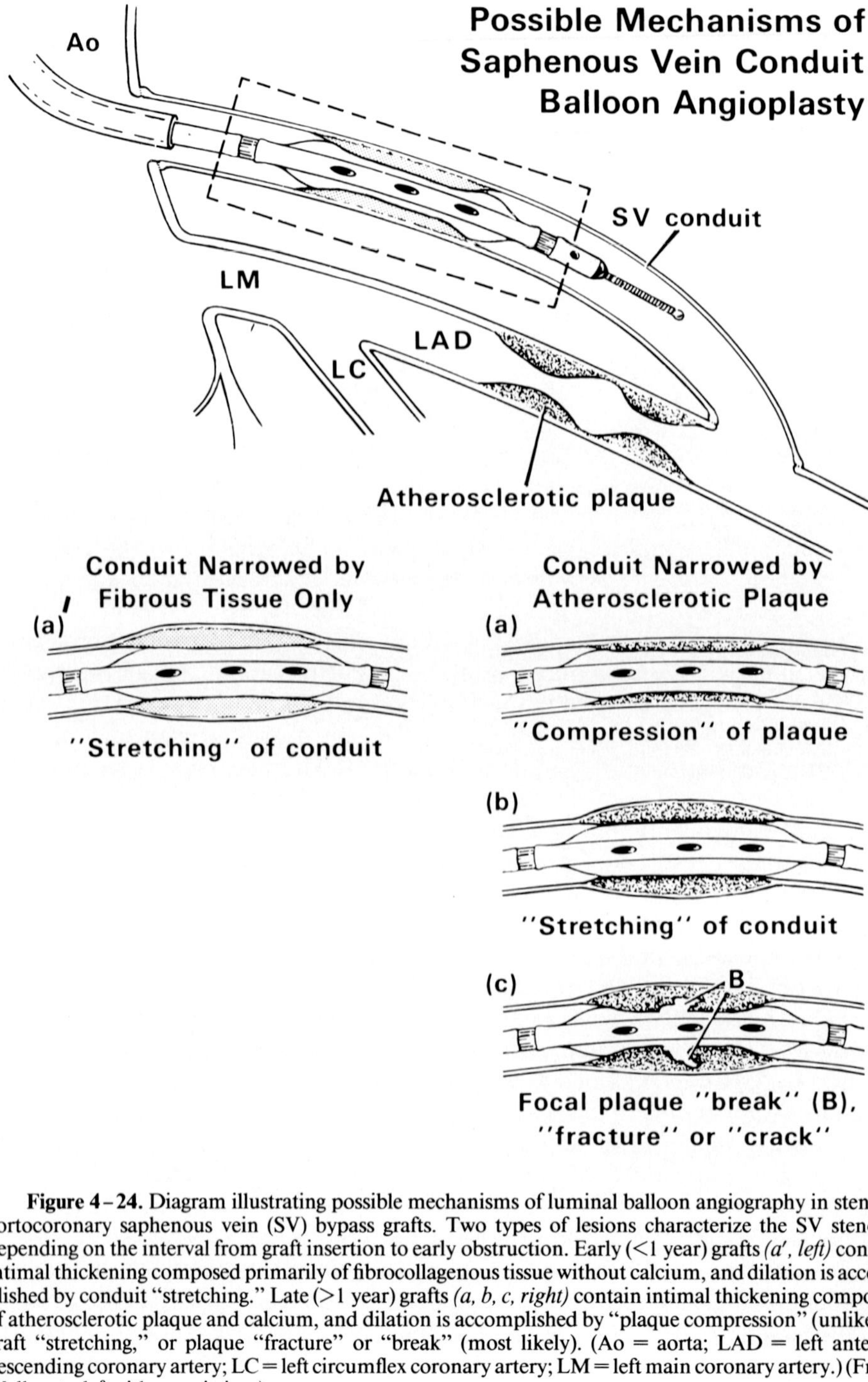

Figure 4-24. Diagram illustrating possible mechanisms of luminal balloon angiography in stenotic aortocoronary saphenous vein (SV) bypass grafts. Two types of lesions characterize the SV stenoses depending on the interval from graft insertion to early obstruction. Early (<1 year) grafts *(a', left)* contain intimal thickening composed primarily of fibrocollagenous tissue without calcium, and dilation is accomplished by conduit "stretching." Late (>1 year) grafts *(a, b, c, right)* contain intimal thickening composed of atherosclerotic plaque and calcium, and dilation is accomplished by "plaque compression" (unlikely), graft "stretching," or plaque "fracture" or "break" (most likely). (Ao = aorta; LAD = left anterior descending coronary artery; LC = left circumflex coronary artery; LM = left main coronary artery.) (From Waller et al.,[8] with permission.)

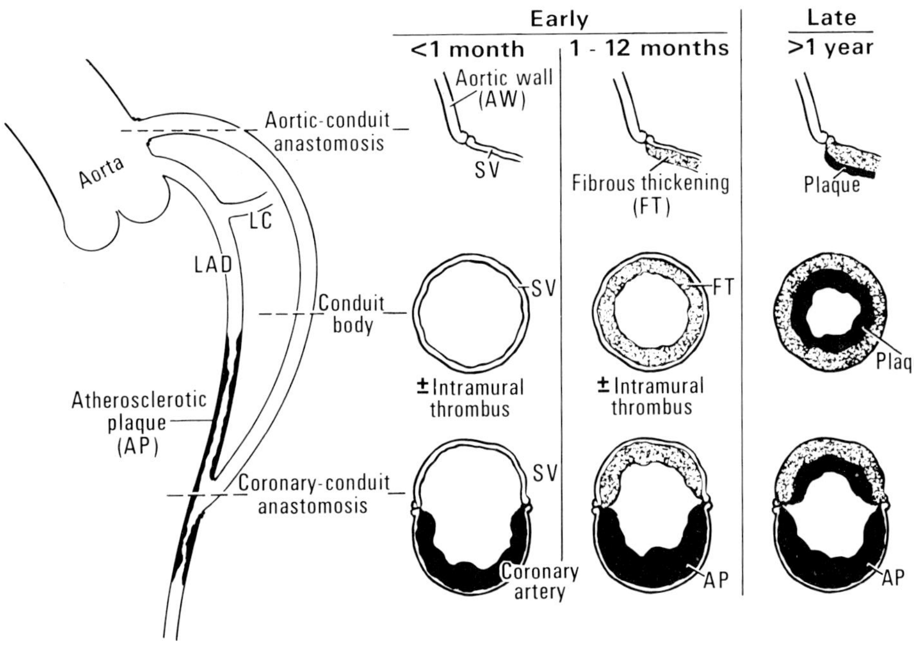

Figure 4–25. Diagram showing the anatomic features of the saphenous vein (SV) bypass graft–native coronary artery unit with luminal changes developing with increasing graft age. TBA would be most successful in areas containing some element of atherosclerotic plaque (that is, coronary-conduit anastomosis in the early and late grafts and the conduit body in the late grafts) and least successful in areas with primarily elastic tissue (that is, aortic anastomotic sites). LAD = left anterior descending coronary artery; LC = left circumflex coronary artery.

lesions in the graft body and at the aorta-graft anastomotic site, respectively (see Fig. 4–25). An anatomic factor supporting the relatively high success rate at dilating stenotic coronary-graft anastomotic sites is the presence of atherosclerotic plaque in the coronary portion of the anastomosis.[35] Stenoses in the graft body or aortic-anastomotic site are less likely to have the potential angioplasty advantage of associated atherosclerotic plaque unless the graft is more than 3 years old. An additional adverse factor for successful dilation at the aortic anastomotic site is the presence of aortic wall consisting of multiple layers of elastic fibers.

THROMBOLYSIS THERAPY FOR EVOLVING ACUTE MYOCARDIAL INFARCTION

Management of acute coronary thrombosis and evolving acute myocardial infarction (AMI) has included the use of *pharmacologic* (streptokinase, urokinase, tissue plasminogen activator), *mechanical* (balloon angioplasty, guidewire perforation), or *combined* therapies to reestablish coronary blood flow and limit infarct size. The use of intracoronary thrombolytic therapy to restore patency of occluded arteries in patients with AMI was first reported by Rentrop and colleagues[41] in 1979. The ability of this procedure to "lyse" the occluding thrombus during the early hours of myocardial infarction has been confirmed by numerous subsequent studies.[42–47] Streptokinase and urokinase were the first in a series of pharmacologic agents used for thrombolytic therapy. Intracoronary administration of streptokinase to patients with

AMI results in recanalization of 60 to 94 percent of occluded arteries,[48] but streptokinase is far from the perfect agent for the acute lysis of coronary thrombi. It is antigenic, it has a relatively long half-life, it has a low specificity for fibrin, and it induces a generalized lytic state.[49] Interest has focused on the development of new thrombolytic agents that would be more specific for fibrin clots and have less systemic bleeding complications. Tissue plasminogen activator (now available in recombinant form), urokinase-type plasminogen activator (pro-urokinase), and acylated streptokinase-plasmogen complex are being evaluated with a view toward achieving therapeutic coronary thrombolysis with increased safety. Hartzler and associates[50,51] using percutaneous TBA have taken a mechanical approach to acute coronary thrombolysis, avoiding the systemic lytic effects of currently available pharmacologic agents and treating the underlying severely stenosed coronary artery at the same procedure. Other strategies have combined both therapies using pharmacologic agents initially followed by TBA,[52–55] or TBA initially followed by smaller doses of streptokinase.[50,51]

Despite the widespread use of various forms of thrombolysis therapy, few necropsy observations regarding myocardium or coronary arteries have been reported in such patients.[4,3,48,54,56–66] With the exception of two patients,[43,54] all remaining observations thus far have been in patients receiving either streptokinase[56–63,65] or urokinase[64,66] thrombolysis therapy.

Personal Series

Clinical Observations. Between September 1982 and April 1986, I studied 16 patients at necropsy who had acute myocardial infarction and who underwent various forms of acute thrombolysis therapy shortly before death (Tables 4–1 through 4–3 and Figs. 4–26 through 4–42). The patients ranged in age from 44 to 66 years (average 52), and of the 16 patients, 14 (88 percent) were men. The location of the AMI was anterior (anteroseptal, anterior, anterolateral) in 13 patients (81 percent), and posterior ("inferior," posteroseptal, posterolateral) in the remaining three. The corresponding "infarct vessel" was the LAD in 12 patients, left main in one, and R in three. Five forms of thrombolytic therapy were employed: *streptokinase only* (seven patients) (see Figs. 4–26, 4–27), *percutaneous* (p) *TBA only* (four patients) (see Figs. 4–28, 4–29), *PTBA plus streptokinase* (three patients) (see Figs. 4–30 through 4–35), *streptokinase guidewire perforation* (one patient) (see Fig. 4–35), and *r-tissue plasminogen activator plus TBA* (one patient) (see Fig. 4–36 and Table 4–1). The interval from onset of symptoms of AMI to reperfusion ranged from 2.5 to 4.5 hours (average 3.8), with similar averages for each of the five subgroups. The thrombolysis therapy initially was angiographically successful in 12 patients but rethrombosis occurred in two patients. Of the 11 patients with streptokinase therapy, 10 received intracoronary administration of the drug, and one received it intravenously. The interval from reperfusion to death ranged from 1 to 96 hours (average 41 hours). Cause of death included progressive heart failure, systemic hypotension and shock (nine patients), sudden ventricular fibrillation (five patients), coronary artery rupture (one patient), and renal failure (noncardiac) (one patient).

Morphologic Observations

Myocardium. All 16 patients had *transmural* myocardial necrosis (see Table 4–2). Of the 11 patients with streptokinase thrombolysis therapy (alone or in combination with another mechanical form of thrombolysis therapy), 10 (91 percent) had *hemorrhagic myocardial infarcts* (Figs. 4–26, 4–27, 4–30 through 4–35). The single

Table 4–1. Certain Clinical Observations at Necropsy in 16 Patients with Acute Myocardial Infarction Undergoing Various Forms of Acute Thrombolysis Therapy

Observation	Streptokinase (S) Only (N = 7)	Percutaneous Transluminal Coronary Angioplasty (PTCA) (N = 4)	PTCA + S (N = 3)	S + Guidewire Perforation (N = 1)	r-Tissue-Plasminogen Activator + PTCA (N = 1)
1. Age (yr)	51–66(60)	52–63(57)	55–58(55)	44	45
2. Men:Women	7M:OW	4M:OW	3M:OW	W	W
3. Location AMI	5A, 2P	3A, 1P	3A	A	A
4. Infarct vessel	5LAD, 2R	3LAD, 1R	3LAD	LM	LAD
5. Form of thrombolysis therapy					
a. Mechanical	0	4	3	5W	1
b. Pharmacologic (dose) (units)	160,000–275,000 (215,000)(7 IC) (1.5 million)(1 IV)	0	50,000–80,000 (66,000) (3 IC)	80,000 IC	80 mg IC
6. Interval onset symptoms to reperfusion (hours)	2.5–4.5 (3.8)	3.5–4.5 (4.0)	3.5–4.5 (4.0)	3.5	3.5
7. Initial angiographically successful reperfusion	6[b]	4	2[a]	0	0
8. Interval reperfusion to death (hr)	16–96 (50)	1–260 (81)	16, 44.5 (2 pts)	—	12
9. Interval onset symptoms to death	20–99 (54)	5–264 (85)	20(31)-24da	24	16
10. Causes of death	6 PCHF 1 SVF	1 NC 3 VF	2 PCHF 1 VF	PCHF	CA Rupture

[a] Initially reperfused but then rethrombosis.
[b] Angiogram not performed in 1 patient with IV streptokinase but chest pain decreased and initially elevated ST segments decreased.
A = anterior, AMI = anterior myocardial infarction, CA = coronary artery, IC = intracoronary, IV = intravenous, LAD = left anterior descending, LM = left main, NC = noncardiac, PCHF = progressive congestive heart failure, SVF = sudden ventricular fibrillation, VF = ventricular fibrillation, W = guidewire.

patient with streptokinase infusion without hemorrhagic infarction did not have successful reperfusion, with total occlusion of the right coronary artery observed at necropsy (Fig. 4–37). Hemorrhagic infarction was defined as massive interstitial erythrocytic extravasation producing grossly visible hemorrhage (Figs. 4–27, 4–34). In contrast, focal areas of interstitial erythrocytes apparent only on microscopic examination did not produce grossly visible hemorrhage and was classified as "interstitial extravasated RBCs." Hemorrhagic infarction was also present in the single patient with r-tissue plasminogen activator thrombolysis (Fig. 4–36). Of the four patients with solely mechanical thrombolysis therapy with percutaneous TBA, *none had hemorrhagic infarction* (Fig. 4–28). The patients with streptokinase infusion (administered selectively or systemically) had variable total doses of streptokinase (50,000 to 1.5 million units) but had a similar average interval from onset of symptoms to clinical reperfusion compared with the patients with purely mechanical (PTBA) thrombolysis therapy (3.8 hours, 4.0 hours, respectively; see Table 4–2). The interval (hours) of clinical reperfusion to death also varied among the subgroups of patients with streptokinase infusion but was less than the subgroup with PTBA (31 hours, 81 hours, respectively). Each of the three patients with combined PTBA and streptokinase therapy had hemorrhagic infarction (see Figs. 4–30 through 4–35). *A common denominator for the patients with hemorrhagic infarction appears to be the lytic effects of pharmacologic reperfusion agents (streptokinase or tissue plasminogen activator) rather than reperfusion per se.*

Table 4–2. Left Ventricular Myocardial Observations at Necropsy in 16 Patients with Acute Myocardial Infarction Undergoing Various Forms of Acute Thrombolysis Therapy

Observation	Streptokinase (S) Only (N = 7)	Percutaneous Transluminal Coronary Angioplasty (PTCA) Only (N = 4)	S + PTCA (N = 3)	S + Guidewire (N = 1)	r-Tissue-Plasminogen Activator + PTCA (N = 1)
1. Type Transmural AMI					
a. Anemic	1*	4	0	0	0
b. Hemorrhagic	6	0	3	+	+
2. Histology of AMI					
a. Contraction band necrosis	6	4	3	+	+
b. Coagulation necrosis	7	3	3	+	+
c. Interstitial necrosis	6	3	3	+	+
d. Interstitial extravasated RBCs (0–4+)	4+ = 6 1+ = 1	1/2+ = 1 1+ = 1 0 = 2	4+ = 3	4+	4+
(1) Massive (grossly visible)	6	0	3	+	+
(2) Focal (microscopic only)	1	2	0	0	0
(3) Extravasated RBCs limited to necrotic zone	4/7	2/2	3/3	0	+

* Minute trace of hemorrhage present grossly.
AMI = acute myocardial infarction.

Table 4–3. Infarct Coronary Artery Observations in 16 Necropsy Patients with Acute Myocardial Infarction Undergoing Various Forms of Acute Thrombolysis Therapy

Observation	Streptokinase (S) Only (N = 7)	Percutaneous Transluminal Coronary Angioplasty (PTCA) Only (N = 4)	PTCA + S (N = 3)	S + Guidewire (N = 1)	r-Tissue-Plasminogen Activator + PTCA (N = 1)
1. Histology of infarct coronary artery					
a. Artery involved	5 LAD, 2R	3 LAD, 1R	3 LAD	LM	LAD
b. Residual thrombus	7	3	3	+	0
(1) Occlusive	4	2	1	0	0
c. Degree of underlying atherosclerotic plaque (% XSA)	5 > 75% 2 = 51–75%	1 > 75% 3 = 51–75%	2 > 75% 1 = 51–75%	>75%	51–75
d. Intraplaque hemorrhage	0	0	3	0	+
e. Intimal-medial "crack"	0	4	3	0	+*

* Coronary artery rupture with extension of medial "crack" to adventitia. LAD = left anterior descending, LM = left main, R = right, XSA = cross-sectional area.

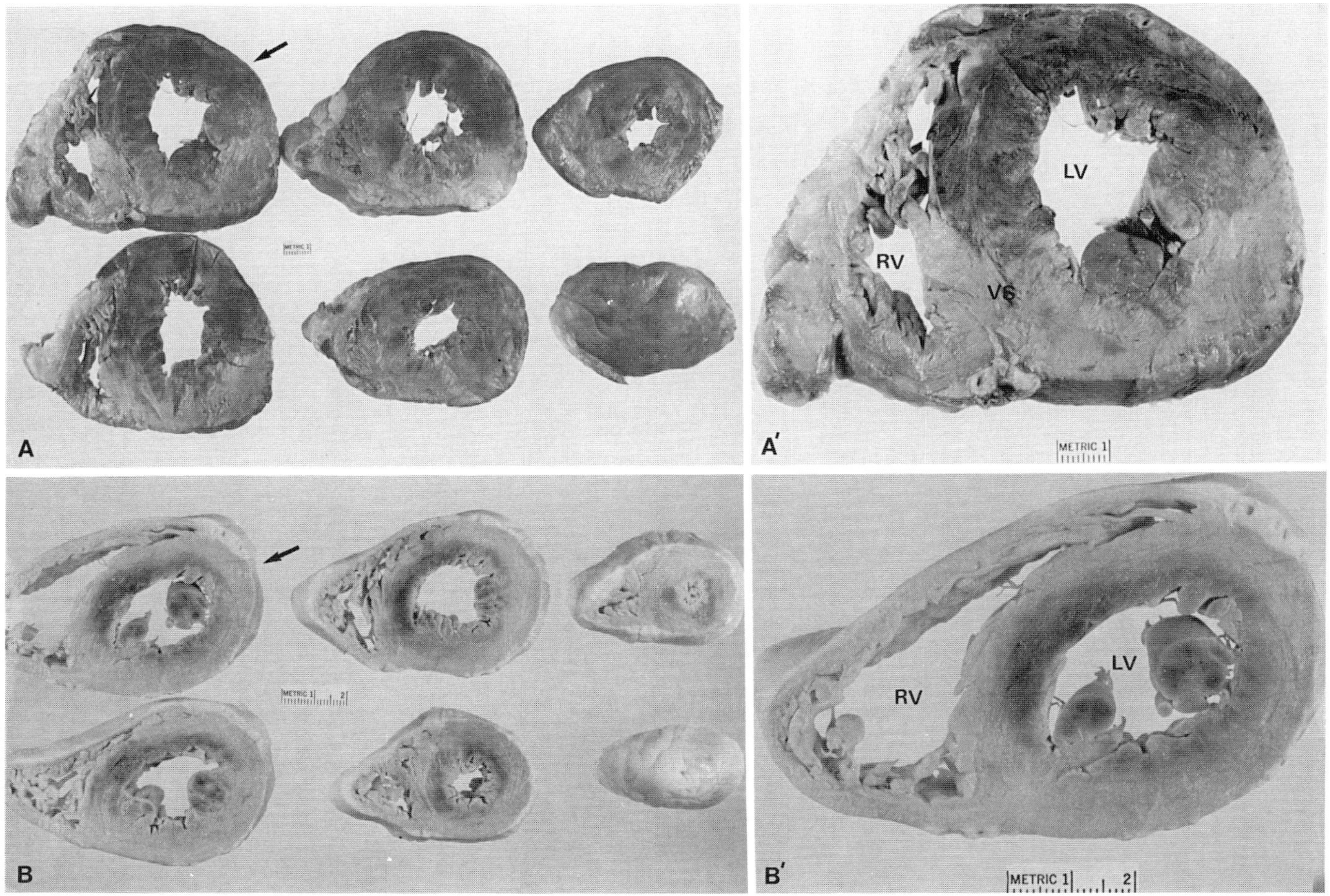

Figure 4 – 26. Thrombolysis therapy with streptokinase alone. *A, B,* Ventricular slices from hearts of two patients undergoing thrombolysis therapy with streptokinase infusion, showing extensive hemorrhagic infarction. *Arrows* indicate ventricular slice shown in *A′* and *B′*. LV = left ventricle, RV = right ventricle, VS = ventricular septum.

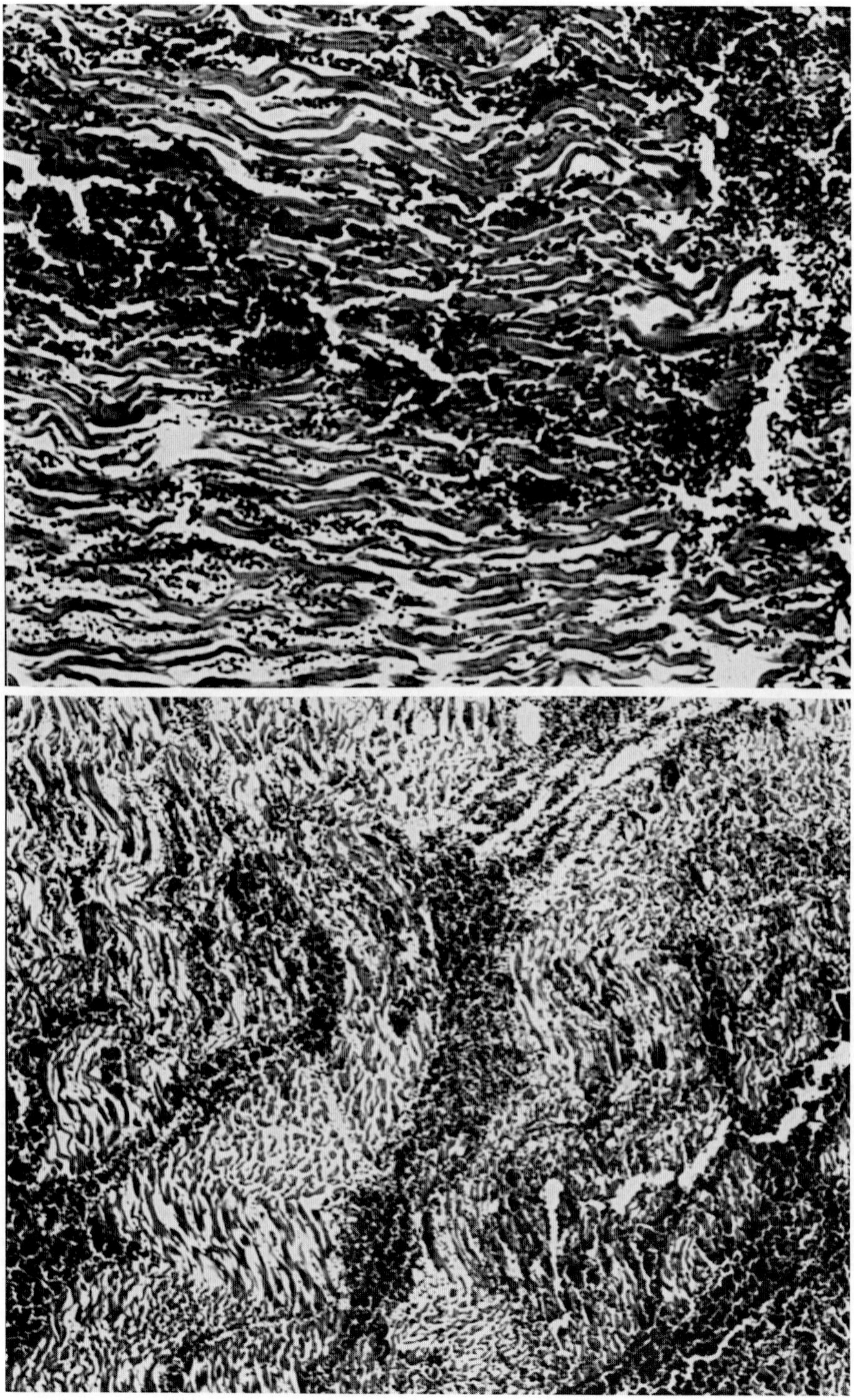

Figure 4–27. Histology sections from patients with streptokinase reperfusion showing extensive sheets of interstitial erythrocytes among necrotic myocardial fibers.

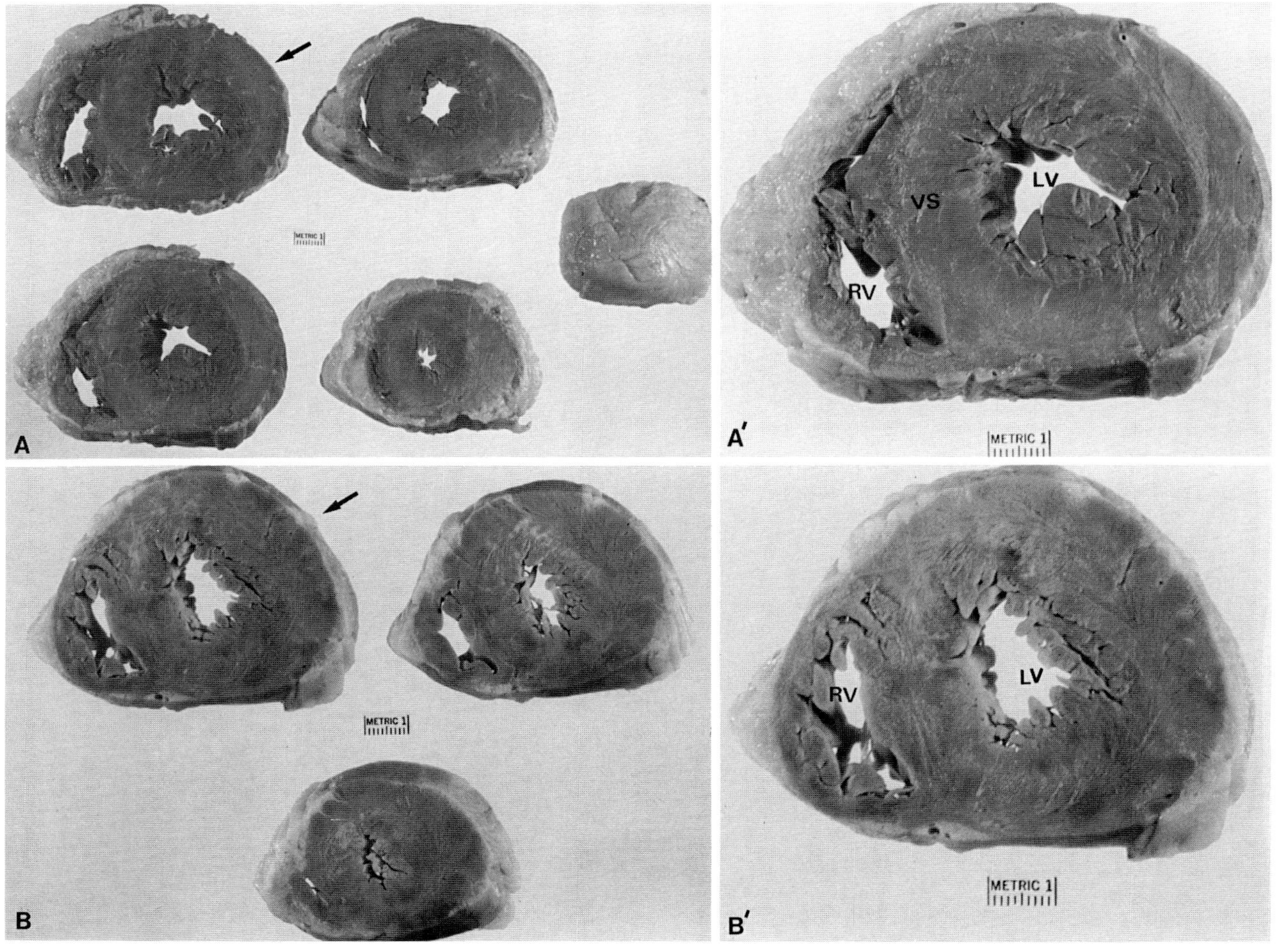

Figure 4–28. Thrombolysis therapy with percutaneous transluminal balloon angioplasty alone. *A, B,* Ventricular slices from hearts of two patients receiving thrombolysis therapy with balloon angioplasty showing no hemorrhagic infarction. *Arrows* indicate ventricular slice shown in *A′* and *B′*. (Abbreviations as in Fig. 4–26.)

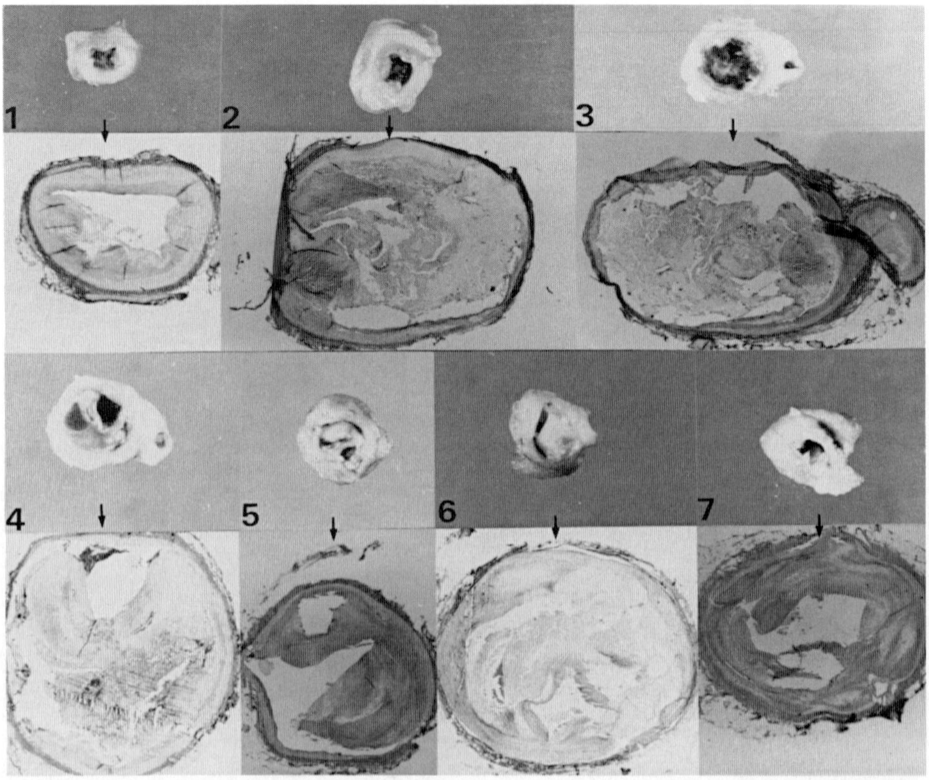

Figure 4–29. Composite of cross sections of left anterior descending coronary artery from patient A in Figure 4–28 showing atherosclerotic plaque "cracks" and localized medial dissection (segment 5) from balloon angioplasty. Segment 3 shows residual proximal thrombus. Histology sections correspond to macroscopic pictures.

Each of the four patients with purely mechanical thrombolysis therapy had angiographically successful reperfusion, and two of the four had mild and focal areas (1/2 to 1+/4+) of microscopic extravasated erythrocytes (see Table 4–2 and Fig. 4–29). These observations are in contrast to several experimental[63–73] and clinical reports[59,64,66] suggesting that the hemorrhagic infarction per se results purely from perfusion injury. Fujiwara and colleagues[66] commented that hemorrhagic infarction is probably due to the combined effects of reperfusion and large doses of thrombolytic agent (urokinase).

All 16 patients had coagulation and contraction band necrosis and interstitial necrosis in the central necrotic zone. Four patients (three streptokinase only, one streptokinase plus guidewire perforation; see Table 4–2) had *interstitial extravasated erythrocytes outside the infarction zone* (Fig. 4–40).

Infarct Coronary Artery. In 16 necropsy patients, the LAD was the "infarct artery" in 12 (75 percent), R in three (19 percent), and the left main in one (6 percent) (see Table 4–3); and 15 had residual thrombus at the site of previous occlusion (see Figs. 4–29 through 4–32, 4–42). Of the 15 arteries with residual thrombus, it was occlusive in seven (47 percent) (see Fig. 4–32). The degree of underlying atherosclerotic plaque present after thrombolysis therapy depended slightly on the form of therapy. All reperfusion arteries had greater than 50 percent cross-sectional area narrowing at the site of previous occlusion, and nine had 76 to

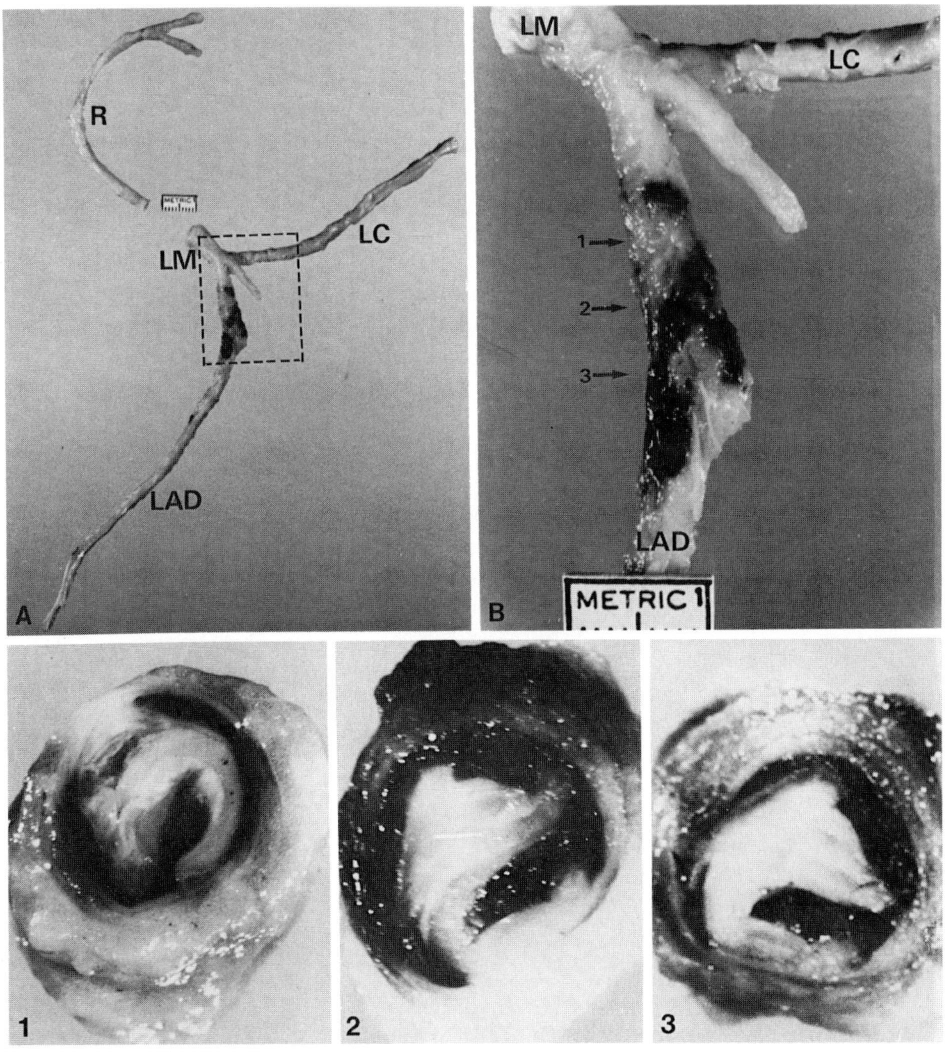

Figure 4-30. Thrombolysis therapy with combined balloon angioplasty plus streptokinase. *A, B,* Coronary arterial site of balloon angioplasty showing marked adventitial hemorrhage. Numbers in *B* correspond to sites of cross sections (*1-3*) along bottom of figure. *1,* Prominent atherosclerotic plaque "crack" with surrounding hemorrhage. *2, 3,* Marked bleeding into area of angioplasty severely narrows the coronary lumen. LAD = left anterior descending, LC = left circumflex, LM = left main, R = right.

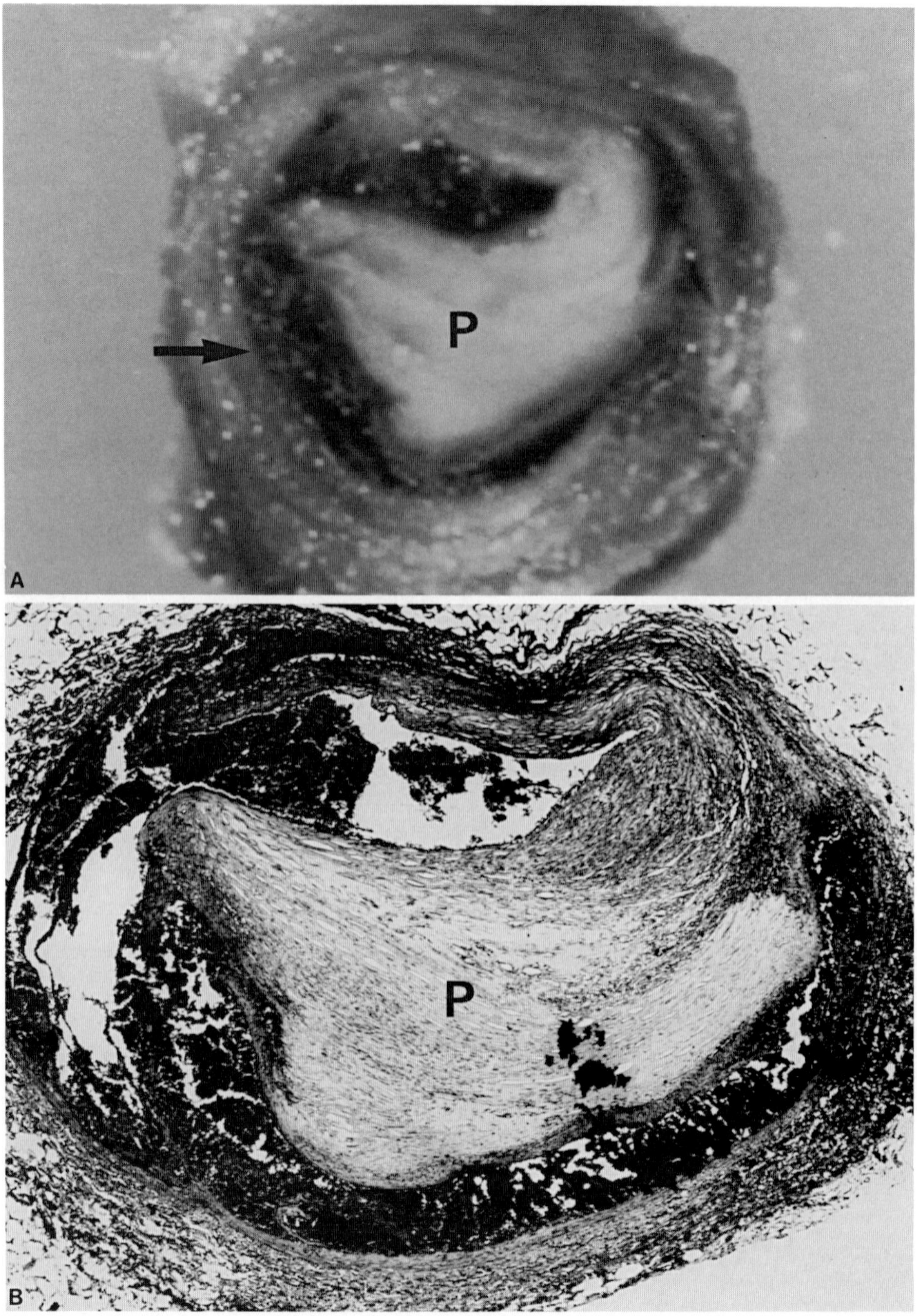

Figure 4–31. Close-up of angioplasty site shown in Figure 4–30. *A,* Prominent plaque (P) "crack" with surrounding hemorrhage *(arrow). B,* Histologic section of segment shows medial dissection and extensive adventitial blood.

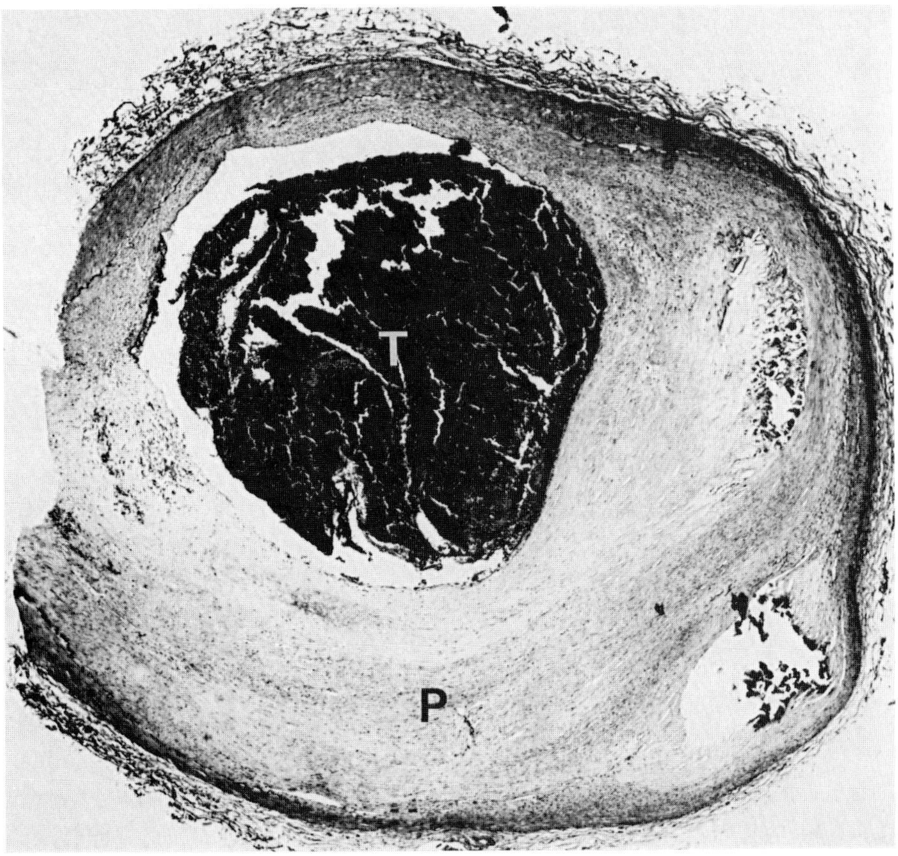

Figure 4–32. Residual occluding thrombus in patient illustrated in Figures 4–30 and 4–31. The artery is severely narrowed by atherosclerotic plaque (P) and thrombus (T).

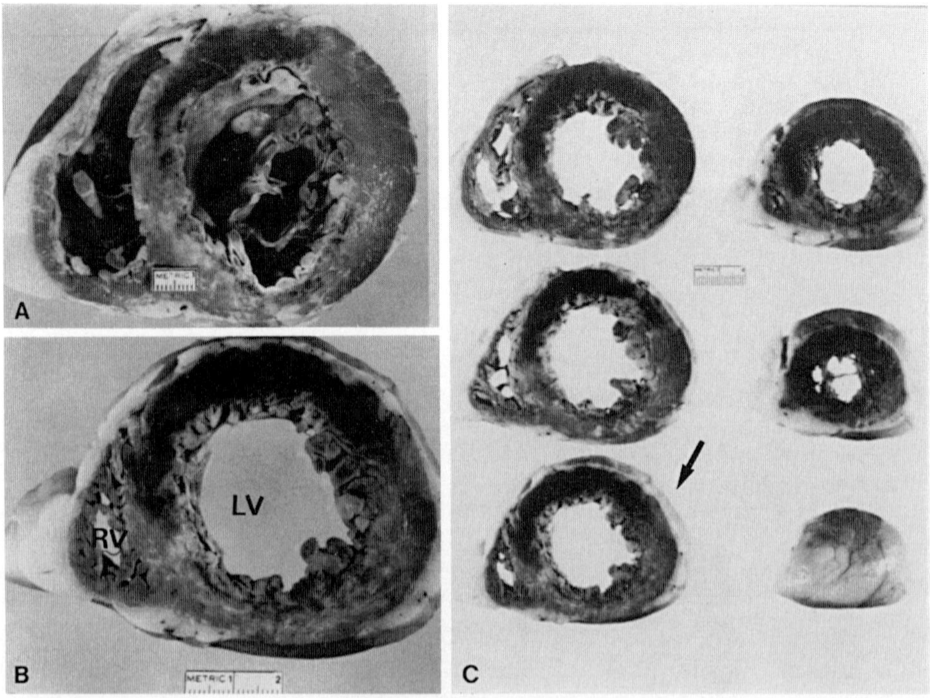

Figure 4–33. Ventricular myocardial slices from patient illustrated in Figures 4–30 through 4–32. Marked hemorrhagic infarction is present from base to apex. *Arrow* in *C* indicates close-up slice illustrated in *B*. LV = left ventricle, RV = right ventricle.

100 percent cross-sectional area narrowing (see Table 4–3). Of the eight patients with PTBA with or without lytic agents, five had narrowing 51 to 75 percent in cross-sectional area by plaque and three had greater than 75 percent narrowing. In contrast, of the eight patients with streptokinase infusion without PTBA, six had arteries greater than 75 percent narrowed in cross-sectional area by atherosclerotic plaque and two were narrowed 51 to 75 percent. Differences in the presence of intraplaque hemorrhage and plaque fracture were also dependent on the use of TBA with or without lytic agents (see Table 4–3) (see Figs. 4–29 through 4–31). Each of the eight patients with PTBA procedures had histologic evidence of intimal-medial plaque "fractures," "tears," or "cracks" (Figs. 4–29 through 4–31). In one patient, the fracture extended into the adventitia and caused coronary artery rupture. Of the eight arteries with evidence of TBA procedures, four had intraplaque hemorrhage in the area of TBA, and each of these patients had the additional use of a lytic agent (streptokinase in three, tissue plasminogen activator in one) (Figs. 4–30, 4–31). Intraplaque hemorrhage was absent in patients with streptokinase infusion alone. These observations suggest that the use of combined angioplasty and a lytic agent may produce localized bleeding at the site of TBA injury, which may produce additional coronary luminal narrowing.

Other Investigators

Despite the widespread use of various forms of acute thrombolysis therapy during evolving AMI, few reports describe necropsy findings in humans[43,54,56–66] (Fig. 4–43). Several reports describe causes of death but do not provide necropsy data.[48,50,85–96] Of 13 reports with necropsy data, 99 patients have been described who have received acute thrombolysis therapy (Table 4–4). Of these 99 patients, 66 (68 percent) received *streptokinase alone,* 31 (31 percent) *urokinase alone,* and two (2 percent) received *streptokinase plus PTBA.*[43,54] Detailed information on the two patients with combined pharmacologic and mechanical therapy was not provided. No reports to date have described necropsy findings in patients with pure mechanical thrombolysis therapy, tissue-plasminogen activator thrombolysis therapy alone or combined with PTBA.

Of the 99 previously reported patients at necropsy, clinical and morphologic information is incomplete (Table 4–4). In nine studies,[43,56–58,61,63–66] information was provided on the status of the myocardium. Of 93 patients, 43 (46 percent) had hemorrhagic infarction. Explanations for the lack of hemorrhage in the remaining hearts were not provided. Eleven reports[43,56–66] had some information on the status of the infarct artery: 28 had residual thrombus and 46 had underlying atherosclerotic plaque of varying amounts.

Fujiwara and colleagues[66] recently reported on the necropsy findings of 30 patients who had had selective intracoronary thrombolysis with urokinase. Three stages of infarcts were subgrouped based on number of hours after thrombolysis therapy. Hearts of patients in stage 2 (9 hours to 11 days after thrombolysis therapy) had hemorrhagic infarction (15 of 18 hearts). These authors concluded that myocardial hemorrhage increases gradually after thrombolysis, becoming moderately or markedly diffuse after 4 hours, and apparently is replaced by fibrous tissue after 3 to 4 weeks. The hemorrhagic infarction is due to the combined effects of reperfusion and large doses of urokinase.

Mathey and associates[59] described transmural, hemorrhagic myocardial infarction after intracoronary streptokinase in six patients dying 1 to 18 days after thrombolysis therapy. One patient had both anemic and hemorrhagic types of infarction — a large hemorrhagic infarct in the area of the recanalized LC coronary artery and an anemic infarct in the area supplied by the severely stenosed, nonreperfused LAD artery. In this patient, the speed of infarct healing was much delayed in the hemorrhagic compared with the anemic infarcted area.

Hemorrhagic Myocardial Infarction

Hemorrhagic myocardial infarction may be defined as grossly visible blood within myocardium, which histologically consists of massive sheets or pools of interstitial erythrocytes (see Figs. 4–26, 4–27, 4–33 through 4–36, 4–38, 4–39). Focal areas of scattered interstitial erythrocytes with an area of myocardial necrosis present histologically only do not produce the grossly visible hemorrhagic infarct. Hemorrhagic infarctions frequently coincide with reperfusion efforts (thrombolysis therapy,[43,48,54,56–66] aortocoronary bypass grafting[67,84]) during an evolving AMI. The degree of myocardial hemorrhage in revascularization operations is usually less than in the thrombolysis patients. In addition, the distribution of the hemorrhage in the revascularization cases is uneven because of the "non-reflow" phenomenon.[65,72] Clinical hemorrhagic myocardial infarction in AMI without intervening thrombolysis or revascularization therapy is distinctly unusual. At necropsy, of 119 personally examined necropsy patients with acute myocardial infarction without the aforementioned interventions, three (2 percent) had hemorrhagic infarctions. In one of these three patients, overwhelming sepsis with disseminated intravascular coagulation (DIC) developed surrounding the AMI during repair of an abdominal aortic aneu-

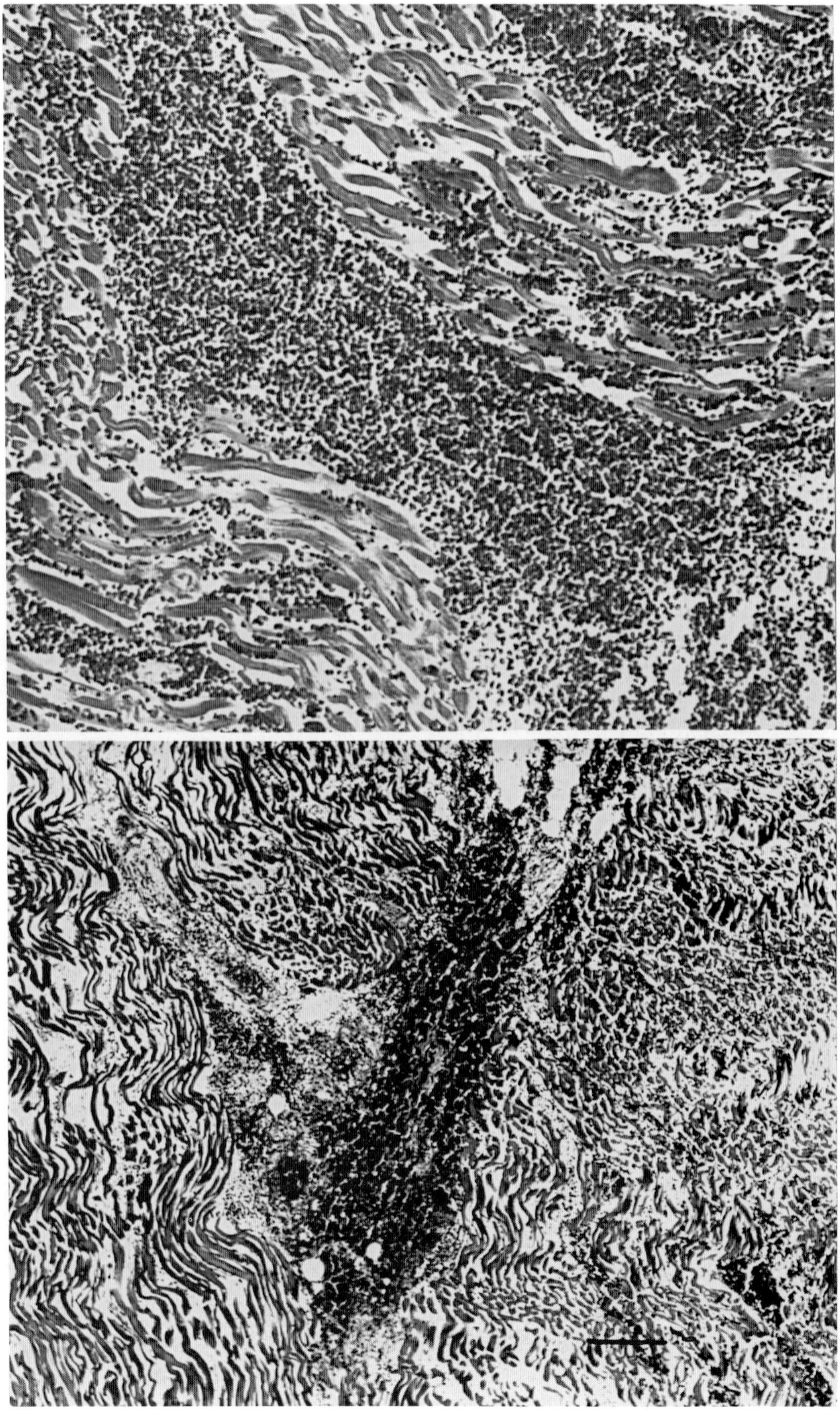

Figure 4 – 34. Histologic sections of ventricular myocardium from patient illustrated in Figure 4 – 33 show severe interstitial hemorrhage with marked myocardial necrosis.

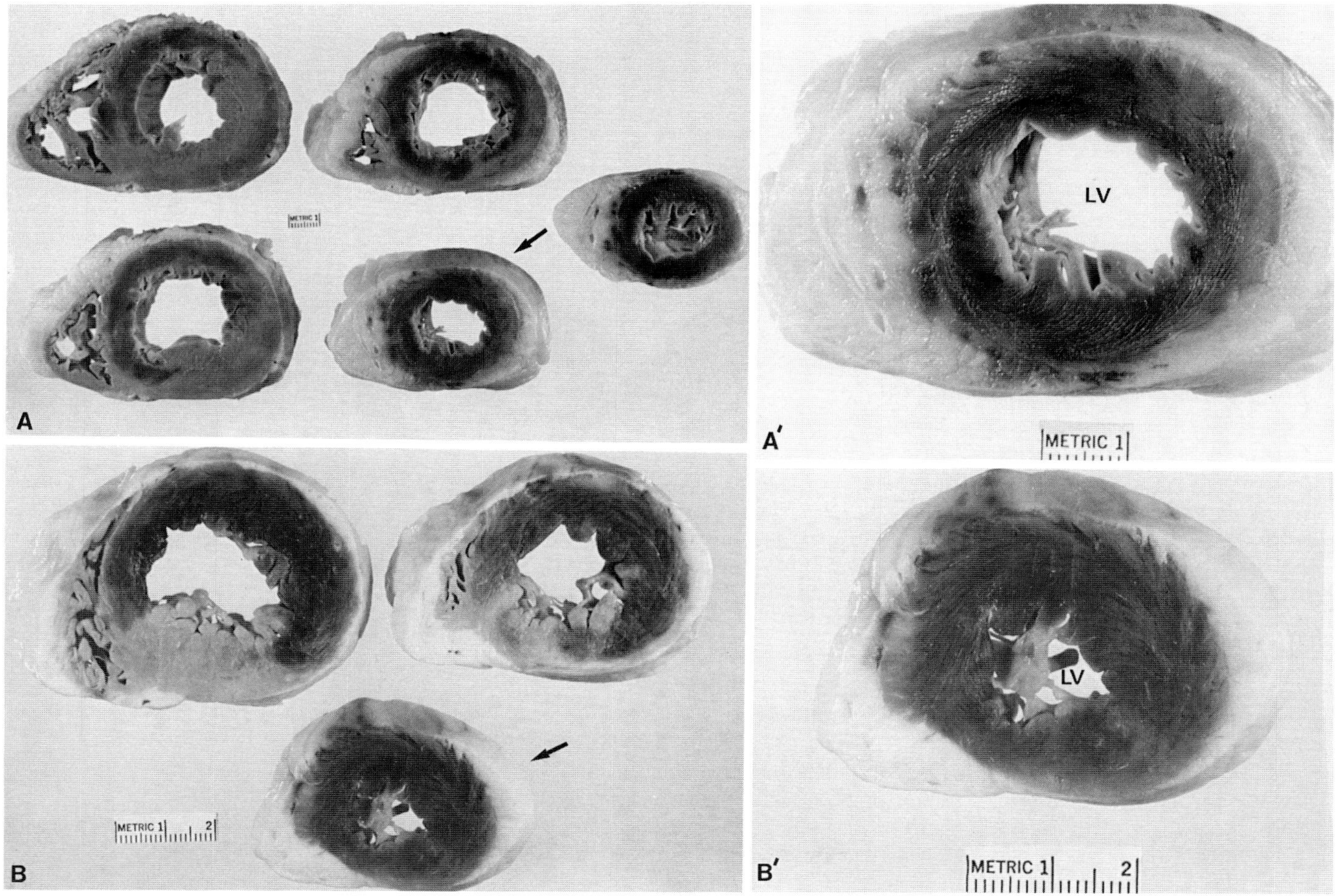

Figure 4–35. Thrombolysis therapy with combined balloon angioplasty and streptokinase. *A, B,* Two patients with combined therapy demonstrate severe hemorrhagic infarction. Compare these findings with those in Figure 4–26 (streptokinase alone) and Figure 4–28 (balloon angioplasty alone). *Arrows* indicate close-up slice in *A′, B′*. LV = left ventricle.

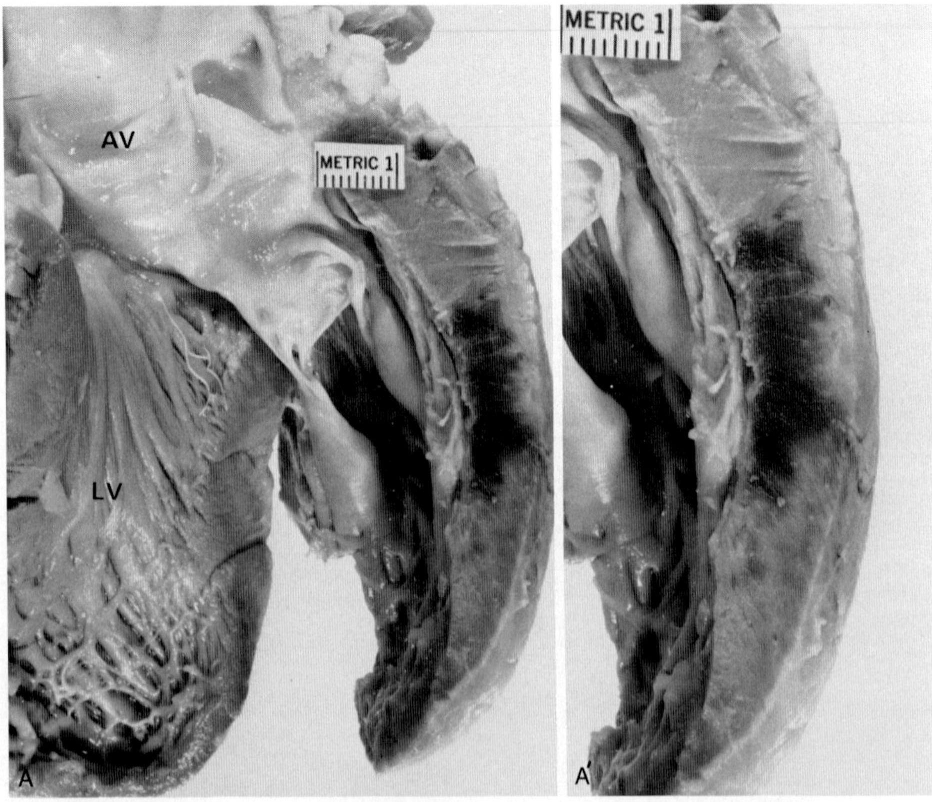

Figure 4–36. Thrombolysis therapy with r-tissue plasminogen activator and balloon angioplasty. *A, A′*. Hemorrhagic infarction present in anterior left ventricular (LV) free wall. The patient died with artery rupture. AV = aortic valve.

rysm (Fig. 4–38). The DIC process may have provided a "natural" reperfusion situation similar to the pharmacologically induced thrombolytic state during reperfusion therapy. Reasons for the remaining two hemorrhagic infarcts are unknown. Similarly, Mathey and colleagues[59] found hemorrhagic infarction in none of 200 patients at necropsy with fatal acute myocardial infarction without interventional therapy. Of 60 necropsy patients with AMI without thrombolysis therapy studied by Fujiwara and colleagues,[66] two (3 percent) had "moderate diffuse hemorrhage" (hemorrhagic infarction). Several other hearts (25 [42 percent]) had focal areas of interstitial hemorrhage observed histologically.[66] Occasionally, "anemic" AMI is observed at necropsy in patients with thrombolysis procedures. In the patients studied by Mathey and colleagues[59] and in one patient in the present series undergoing streptokinase therapy, hemorrhagic infarction was absent at necropsy (Fig. 4–37). In each of these patients, the "infarct vessel" was not reopened. In the patient in the present series, total occlusion of the right coronary artery by thrombus and plaque was found at necropsy.

Experimental. Experimental studies on various animals (rats, dogs, pigs) have been performed to define potential benefits and hazards of reperfusion. Results of these studies have been divergent in areas of hemorrhagic infarction, infarct size reduction or expansion, wall motion changes, and survival. The application of exper-

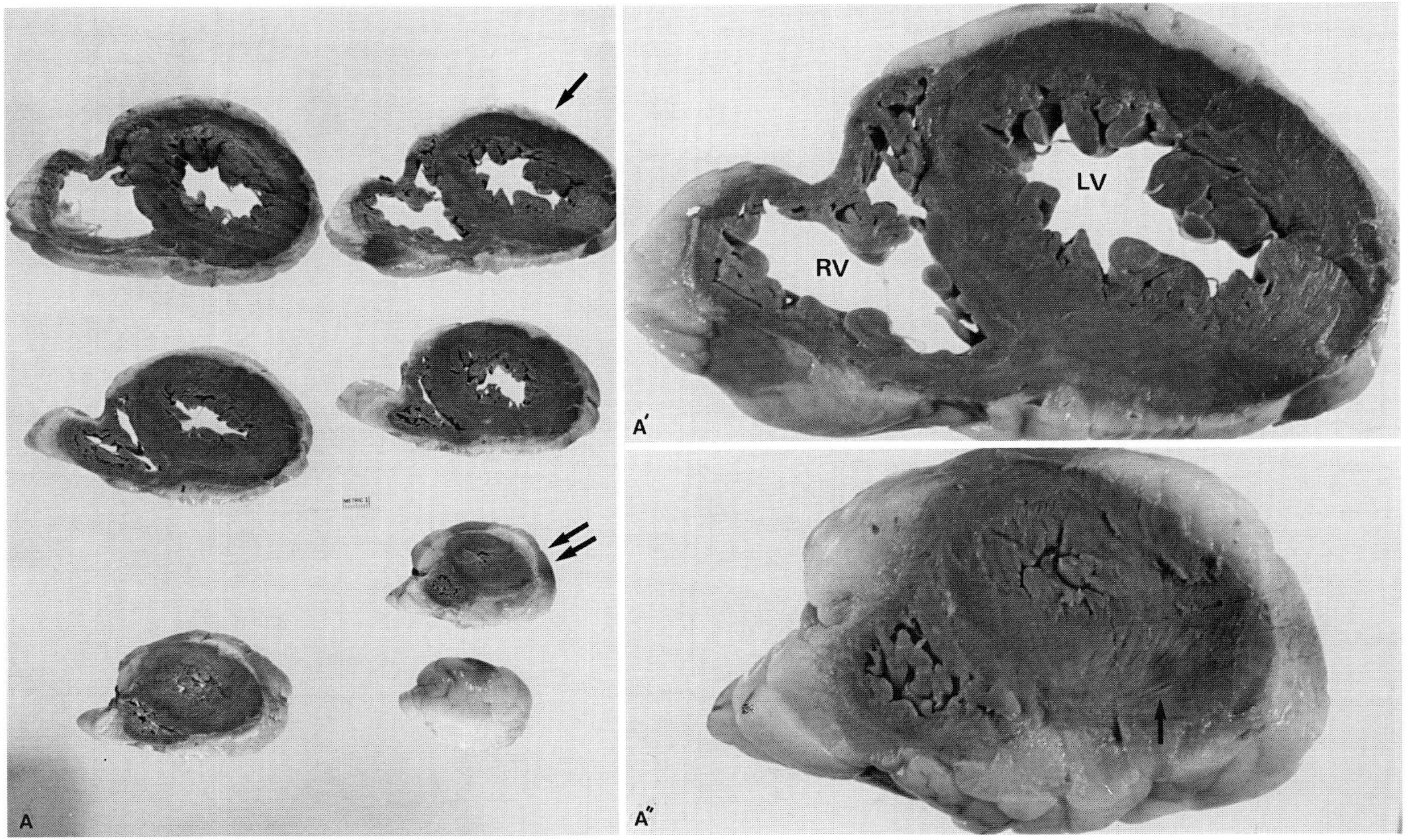

Figure 4–37. Thrombolysis therapy with systemic streptokinase. In contrast to Figures 4–26 and 4–35, which show hemorrhagic infarction with streptokinase therapy (solely or combined), the ventricular myocardium has only a hint of hemorrhage *(double arrow)* near the apex. Cross sections of the right coronary artery show total occlusion by atherosclerotic plaque and thrombus. The explanation for absent hemorrhagic infarction with the use of streptokinase is unsuccessful reperfusion. Slice with *single arrow* in *A* illustrated in *A′*, and slice with *double arrow* in *A* illustrated in *A″*. LV = left ventricle, RV = right ventricle.

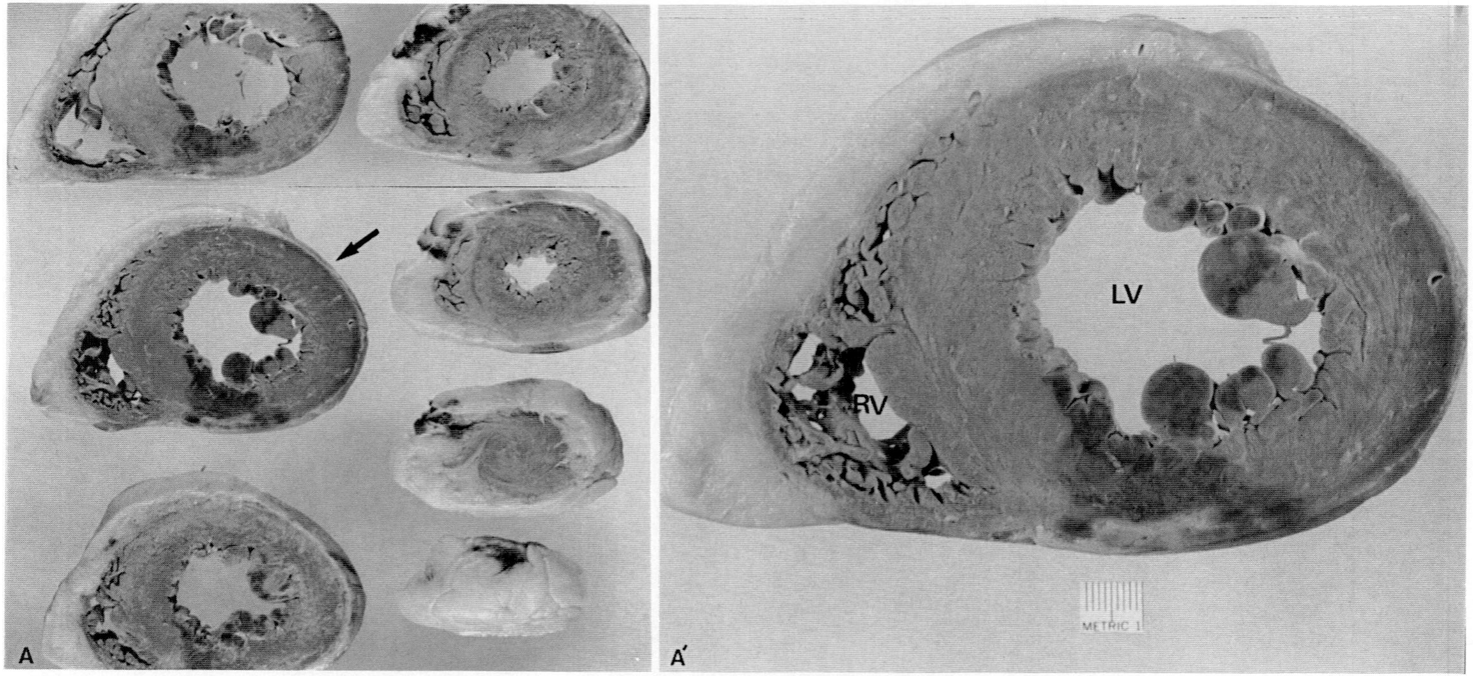

Figure 4–38. Hemorrhagic myocardial infarction in a patient *without* thrombolysis therapy who developed disseminated intravascular coagulation (DIC) from sepsis. The patient "reperfused" with the altered coagulation in the DIC process. *A′* represents close-up of slice indicated by *arrow* in *A*. LV = left ventricle, RV = right ventricle.

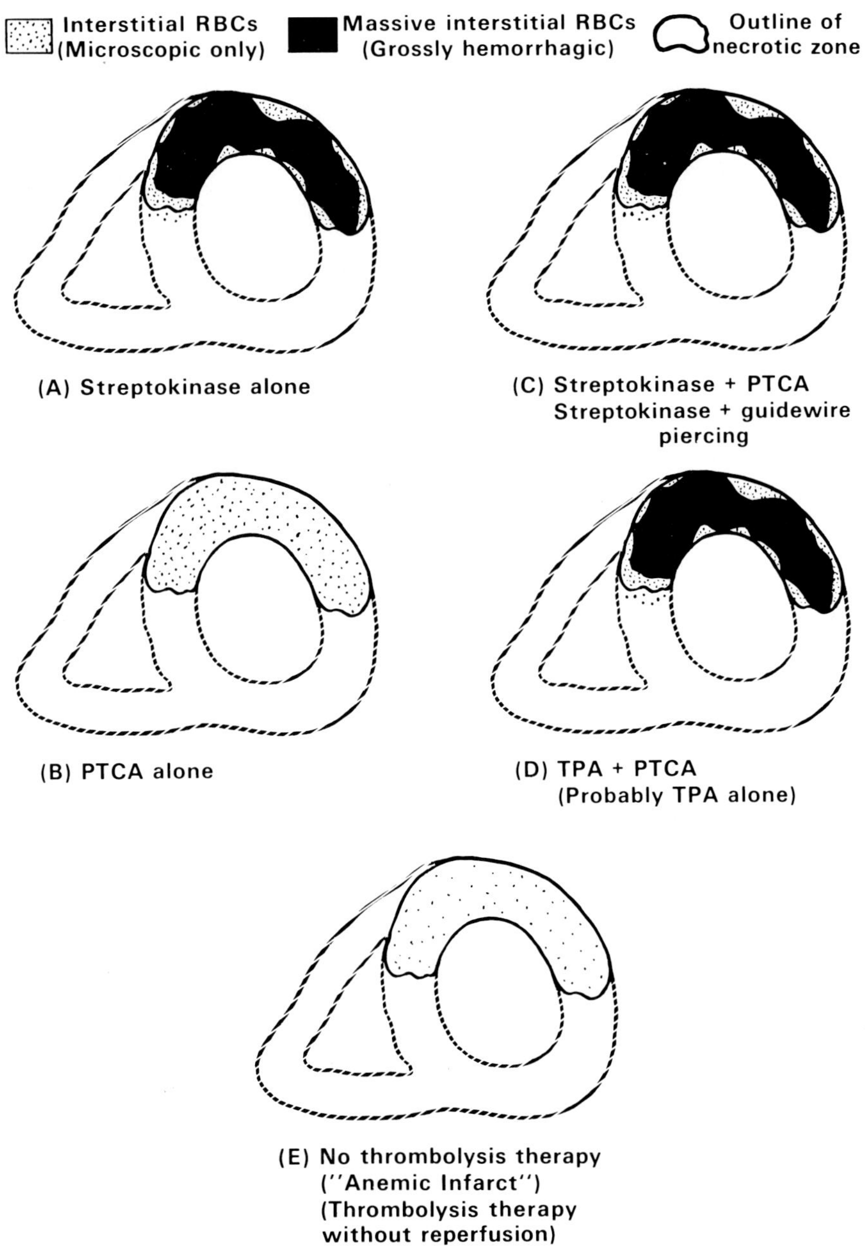

Figure 4-39. Diagram comparing the myocardial responses to various forms of thrombolysis therapy. Much of the hemorrhage is confined to the necrotic zone, but interstitial hemorrhage may be present in border zones, potentially compromising interstitial vascular channels. PTCA = percutaneous transluminal coronary angioplasty, TPA = tissue plasminogen activator.

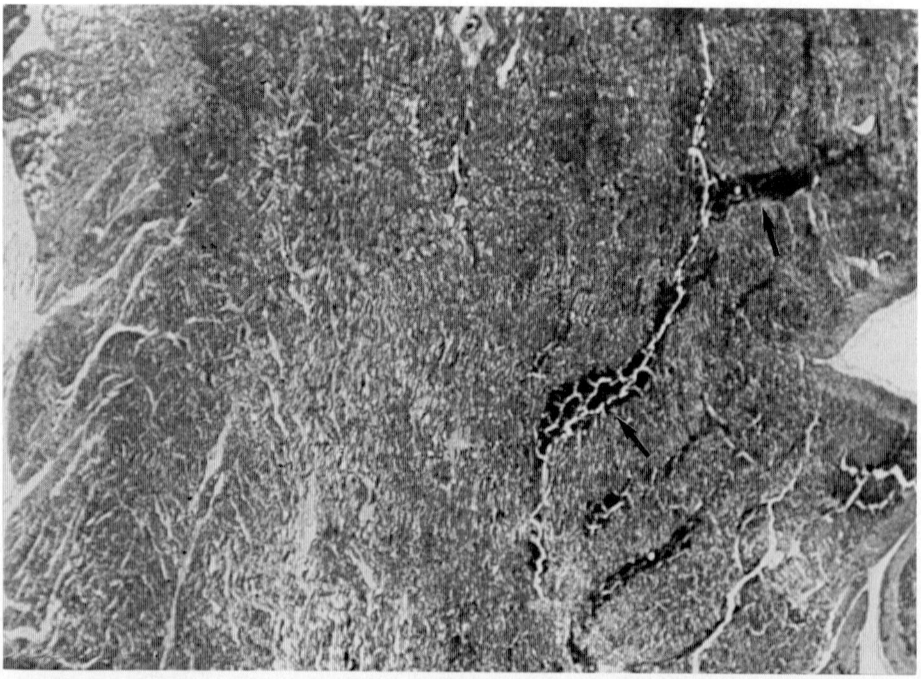

Figure 4–40. Histologic section near border zone of infarct, showing interstitial hemorrhage *(arrows)* and contraction bands.

imental studies to humans has its limitations with regard to animal model used, techniques (coronary ligation versus occlusion by atherosclerotic plaque and thrombus), collateral circulation, and nature of occlusion process (slow versus fast). Generally, hemorrhagic infarction in experimental animals has been confined to the area of necrosis, sparing the subepicardial zone (that is, "subendocardial infarction") and does not expand the infarct area.[70–71,76–83] Other investigators[68,69,74–75] have suggested that the hemorrhage is not strictly confined to the necrotic zone and that infarct expansion may occur with interstitial hemorrhage.

Experimental and Clinical Differences. At least two major differences exist between hemorrhagic infarcts observed in patients at necropsy and experimental animals undergoing reperfusion procedures. In human patients, the hemorrhagic

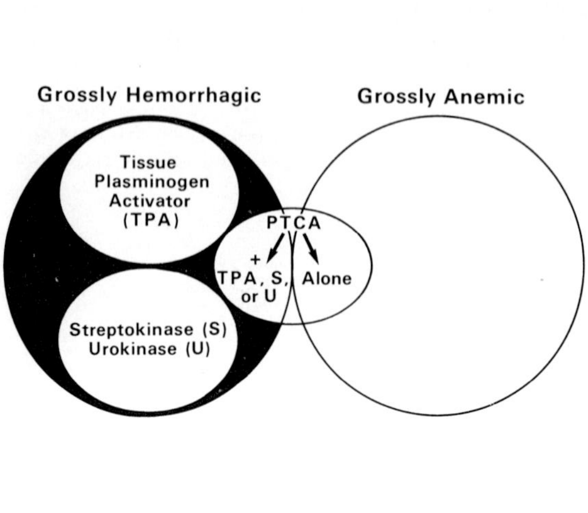

Figure 4–41. Myocardial response in acute myocardial infarction (AMI) with various forms of acute thrombolysis therapy. The *dark circle* represents hemorrhagic infarcts and the *white circle* indicates anemic infarcts. PTCA = percutaneous transluminal coronary angioplasty.

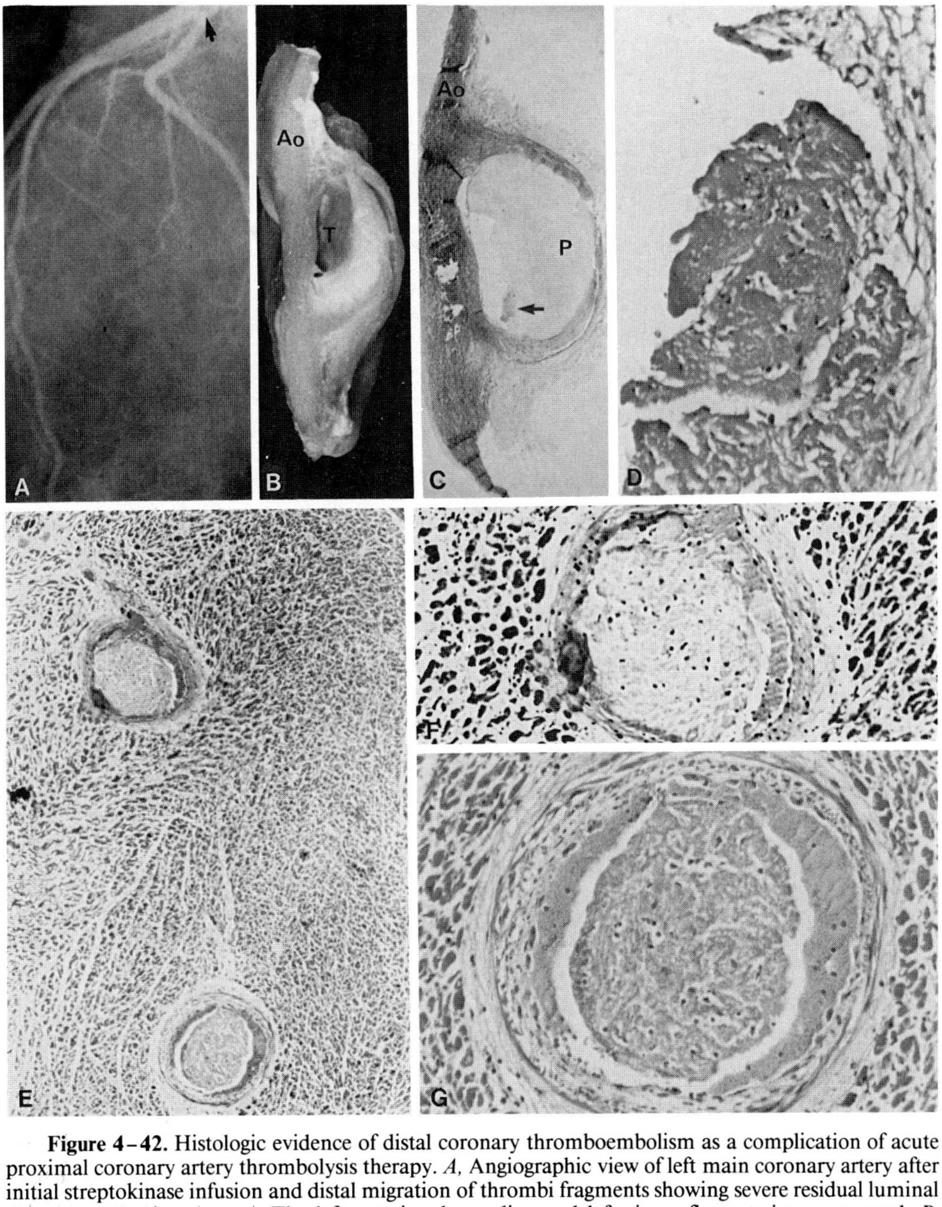

Figure 4-42. Histologic evidence of distal coronary thromboembolism as a complication of acute proximal coronary artery thrombolysis therapy. *A,* Angiographic view of left main coronary artery after initial streptokinase infusion and distal migration of thrombi fragments showing severe residual luminal diameter reduction *(arrow).* The left anterior descending and left circumflex arteries are normal. *B,* Microscopic view of cross-sectional view of the severely narrowed left main artery. The lumen is narrowed by atherosclerotic plaque and residual thrombus (T). Ao = aorta. *C,* Histologic cross section of segment shown in *B,* confirming the presence of underlying atherosclerotic plaque (P) and showing a residual amount of thrombus *(arrow). D,* High-powered view of thrombus shown in *C. E–G,* Photomicrographs of the anterolateral papillary muscle. *E,* Low magnification (×40, reduced 38 percent) showing two severely narrowed intramural coronary arteries. *F, G,* Higher magnification (×400, reduced 38 percent) of intramural coronary arteries shows the luminal narrowing is the result of thromboemboli. The occluding thrombus is similar in composition to that remaining in the left main coronary artery *(D).* (From Menke et al.,[90] with permission.)

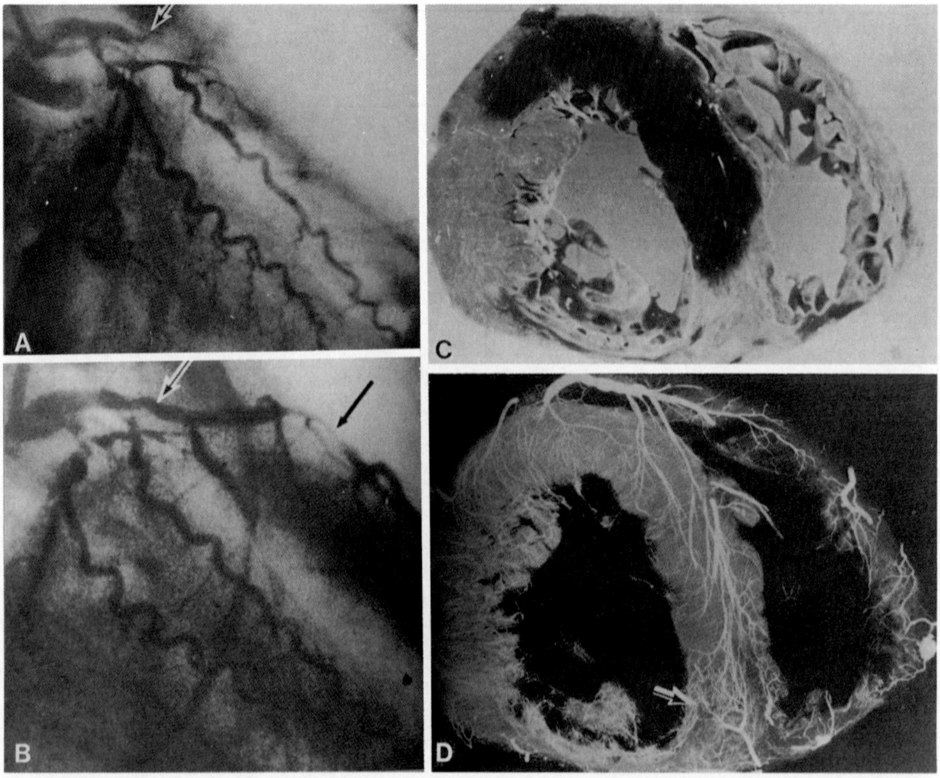

Figure 4–43. *A,* Coronary arteriogram showing complete occlusion *(arrow)* of left anterior descending artery prior to treatment with streptokinase. *B,* Coronary arteriogram taken after streptokinase administration showing reopening of lumen of left anterior descending artery at site of previous closure *(black and white arrow).* Note point of marked distal narrowing *(black arrow). C,* Upper surface of basal slice of ventricles showing severe hemorrhage (back) in anterior and septal regions of left ventricle. *D,* Roentgenogram of slice in *C,* illustrating left anterior descending artery (LAD) *(bottom)* and bed supplied by this vessel. Note correspondence to hemorrhagic region in *C. Arrows* indicate margins of bed of LAD. (From Kao et al.,[65] with permission.)

infarction is *transmural*[59] (transmural defined as damage greater than the inner one half of the free wall) and not subendocardial as has been described in experimental models.[73] In some patients, *extension of the hemorrhage into areas of noninfarcted tissue* has been reported[66] and was observed in four of our 16 patients at necropsy (Fig. 4–40). In contrast, most experimental models have found myocardial hemorrhage confined to the central necrotic zone, leaving a rim of nonhemorrhagic infarcted tissue.[71,73,79,81]

Clinical Evidence of Hemorrhagic Myocardial Infarction. To my knowledge, only two patients have been reported in whom the clinical diagnosis of hemorrhagic infarction was made following acute thrombolysis therapy.[64,93] Little and Rogers[93] reported angiographic evidence of intramyocardial contrast pooling (representing interstitial extravasation of erythrocytes) following successful streptokinase thrombolysis therapy. This patient subsequently deteriorated with infarction extension. No morphologic documentation of hemorrhagic infarction was provided. Yasuno and colleagues[64] reported an 83-year-old man with extravasated intramyocardial hemorrhage following urokinase thrombolysis treatment (Fig. 4–44). At necropsy, marked transmural hemorrhagic necrosis was observed in the area recognized clinically (Fig. 4–45). These patients suggest that variable degrees of myocardial hemorrhage probably occur in most patients undergoing reperfusion therapy but are not clinically appreciated. Interstitial extravasated erythrocytes may represent the morphologic-histologic equivalent of reperfusion ventricular arrhythmias. Yasuno and associates[64] suggested stopping thrombolytic agent administration if angiographic evidence of hemorrhagic infarction is observed.

Complications of Thrombolysis Therapy

Complications of pharmacologic, mechanical, or combined thrombolysis therapies include failure of clot lysis, systemic and localized bleeding (including hemorrhagic myocardial infarction), coronary artery dissection, delayed healing, and coronary embolism.[85–87] Failure of clot lysis, clot embolization, and delayed infarct healing will be discussed briefly.

FAILURE OF CLOT LYSIS. Limited angiographic observations and even fewer necropsy data are available in patients with "streptokinase-resistant" intracoronary thrombus. In 6 to 23 percent of patients with AMI undergoing thrombolysis therapy, totally occlusive intracoronary thrombus has been reported to persist despite the administration of streptokinase.[42,43,46,88] Necropsy studies of patients with totally occlusive thrombus resistant to streptokinase have been limited to two patients.[48,60] Mathey and associates[48] described a 71-year-old patient in whom 2 hours of intracoronary streptokinase infusion failed to reopen a totally occluded R coronary artery. At necropsy the artery had persistent occlusion due to thrombus superimposed on severe atherosclerotic plaque. Isner and colleagues[60] studied a 66-year-old woman with persistently occluded LAD despite 380,000 units of intravenous streptokinase. At necropsy, postmortem angiography showed a patent LAD but severe narrowing by atherosclerotic plaque. These authors interpreted this finding as evidence of "delayed" thrombolysis.

DISTAL EMBOLIZATION OF PROXIMAL CORONARY THROMBUS. Although angiographic evidence of distal coronary thromboembolism has been alluded to[51] or specifically excluded[89] during acute thrombolysis therapy, no previous report has documented at necropsy the final location or endpoint of fragments of thrombus angiographically observed to stream distally. We recently studied a 44-year-old patient at necropsy who had histologic evidence of distal embolization following proximal LM thrombolysis therapy.[90] Histologic sections of the anterolateral papillary muscle disclosed several intramyocardial coronary arteries occluded by thrombotic material identical in composition to that remaining in the left main artery (see Fig. 4–42). Two angiographic reports of thrombolysis therapy during acute myocardial infarction specifically mention distal coronary embolization.[51,89] In a study of 78 patients with acute myocardial infarction undergoing coronary angioplasty (with and without previous streptokinase infusion), Hartzler and colleagues[51] rarely observed distal coronary embolization, and when observed, it was without apparent clinical consequence. Gold and associates[89] performed coronary angioplasty in 28 patients with acute myocardial infarction immediately after intracoronary streptokinase infusion and reported no angiographic evidence of distal embolization of clot. Our patient had angiographic evidence of distal coronary embolism during streptokinase thrombolysis therapy, and at necropsy had multiple intramural vessels of the anterolateral papillary muscle occluded by thrombi.[90] Consequences of distal migration of

Table 4–4. Clinical and Morphologic Findings at Necropsy in 99 Patients from 13 Previous Reports With Acute Myocardial Infarction Undergoing Acute Thrombolysis Therapy (64 Streptokinase, 31 Urokinase, 2 Streptokinase + Percutaneous Transluminal Angioplasty (PTCA)

Observation	Schachenmayr, 1972[56] (N = 6)	Berry, 1975[57] (N = 27)	Verstraete, 1981[58] (N = 14)	Mathey, 1981[59] (N = 3)	Meyer, 1982[54] (N = 1)	Mathey, 1982[43] (N = 6)
1. Age (years)	43–67(59)	—	—	71,—	67	44–77(67)
2. Sex (Male/M):(Female/F)	5M:1F	—	—	—	M	4M:2F
3. Location AMI	—	—	8A,2P,3C,1UK	2A,1P	—	3P,3A[a]
4. Infarct vessel	1R,1LC,3LAD	—	—	2LAD,R	LAD	2R,1LC,3LAD
5. Int onset symptoms to reperfusion (hr)	—	—	—	—	—	1.7–3.5(2.9)
6. Angiographically successful thrombolysis	—	—	—	0	+	6
7. Int onset symptoms to death (days)	0.08–5(1.4)	—	—	2,—	2	1–9(6)
8. Thrombolysis method(s) (dose)	S(IV)	S(IV)	S(IV)	S	S	5S
a. Streptokinase (S) Urokinase (U)	1–5 mil	2.5 mil	1.45 mil	+	160,000	175,000–250,000
b. S + PTCA	0	0	0	0	+	1
9. Type acute myocardial infarct (AMI)						
a. Hemorrhagic	3	3(11%)[d]	3[n]	—	—	4
b. Anemic	2[i]	24(89%)	11	—	—	2
10. Histology of Infarct Coronary Artery						
a. Residual thrombus	4	11	9	1	—[f]	0(5)
(1) Occlusive				1	—	+(1)
b. Underlying atherosclerotic plaque	5	25	4	2	—	—

A = anterior, C = combination, Int = interval, IV = intravenous, LC = left circumflex, LAD = left anterior descending, mil = million, mo = months, P = posterior, R = right, UK = unknown.

[a] One patient had anterior and posterior infarcts of similar age, one with and one without reperfusion.
[b] Delayed thrombolysis—detected on postmortem coronary angiogram.
[c] 1.5 million units IV immediately followed by selective intracoronary infusion 2–4000 U/min.
[d] Reperfusion in only 3 of 7 patients including 1 of 2 with hemorrhage infarction.
[e] Intraplaque hemorrhage in 3, coronary artery dissection in 1.
[f] Simply described as "patient."
[g] Cardiac rupture.

occluding coronary thrombus fragmented during pharmacologic or mechanical thrombolysis therapy for evolving myocardial infarction remain unclear. Observing multiple occluded intramyocardial vessels in out patient suggests that the consequences of distal embolization may be similar to that of primary coronary embolism.[91,92] In primary coronary embolism, the *smaller* the embolus, the greater the chance the embolus will travel distally and lodge in a small coronary artery; conversely, the *larger* the embolus, the greater the likelihood it will travel proximally and lodge in a large coronary artery. An embolus so small that it lodges in a *single* intramural coronary artery and is only observed at necropsy by histologic examination is probably of little clinical or morphologic significance, whereas a larger embolus may occlude *multiple* intramural vessels and produce new or added clinical myocardial dysfunction. In the setting of an evolving myocardial infarction, migra-

Table 4–4. Clinical and Morphologic Findings at Necropsy in 99 Patients from 13 Previous Reports With Acute Myocardial Infarction Undergoing Acute Thrombolysis Therapy (64 Streptokinase, 31 Urokinase, 2 Streptokinase + Percutaneous Transluminal Angioplasty (PTCA) *(continued)*

Isner, 1983[60] (N = 1)	**Mattfeldt, 1984[61] (N = 7)**	**Harrison, 1984[62] (N = 1)**	**Hollander, 1984[63] (N = 1)**	**Yasuno, 1984[64] (N = 1)**	**Kao, 1984[65] (N = 1)**	**Fujiwara, 1986[66] (N = 30)**
66	32–70(56)	—	61	83	37	45–83(68)
F	5M:2F	—	M	M	M	17M:13M
A	—	—	A	P	A	21A,7P,2L
LAD	3LAD,3R,1LC	—	LAD	R	LAD	
	3.5–5.5(4.5)	—	1	2.5	5	2–9(4)
0[b]	3/7	—	+	+	+	
0.35	0.25–21(4.5)	—	0.54	0.62	1.2	4 hr–12 mo
	S	S	S	U	S	U
S						
380,000	7[c]	—	100,000	240,000	380,000	240,000–1.2 mil
0	0	—	0	0	0	0
—	2[d]	—	+[g]	+[h]	+	25(83%)[k]
—	5	—	0	0	0	5(17%)[l]
+	1	+	0	—	0	—[m]
0	1	+		—		
+	6/6[e]	—	+	+	+	—

[h] Angiographically recognized.
[i] Both died during administration of S with less than 1.3 million unions infused. One patient with hemorrhagic infarction had cardiac rupture.
[j] Of 27 hearts, 4 had cardiac rupture.
[k] Includes patients with slight, moderate, or marked bleeding (moderate or marked called hemorrhagic infarction).
[l] Three of 5 patients died within 3 hours of S, 2 patients died 12 and 24 mo after S therapy.
[m] Uncertain if post S findings represent angiographic or autopsy findings.
[n] Of 14 patients, 7 had myocardial rupture.

tion of a single small fragment of occluding thrombus into the distal portion of the "infarct artery" is likely to be clinically "silent" or clinically inseparable from the ongoing infarction and produce little additional myocardial damage. Migration of a single larger fragment of thrombus may lodge more proximally in the "infarct artery" and result in continuation of myocardial necrosis already in progress. Alternatively, larger thrombi may fragment and occlude multiple intramyocardial arteries producing secondary thrombus of the epicardial coronary vessel feeding the obstructed arterioles, or compromise collateral flow from other major coronary arteries, or both. In either situation, extension of myocardial necrosis may occur.

Delayed Infarct Healing. Discussion continues as to whether the presence of hemorrhage within zones of necrosis delays[59] or accelerates[76] healing of infarcted tissue or whether its presence expands or accelerates myocardial necrosis.[69] Mathey

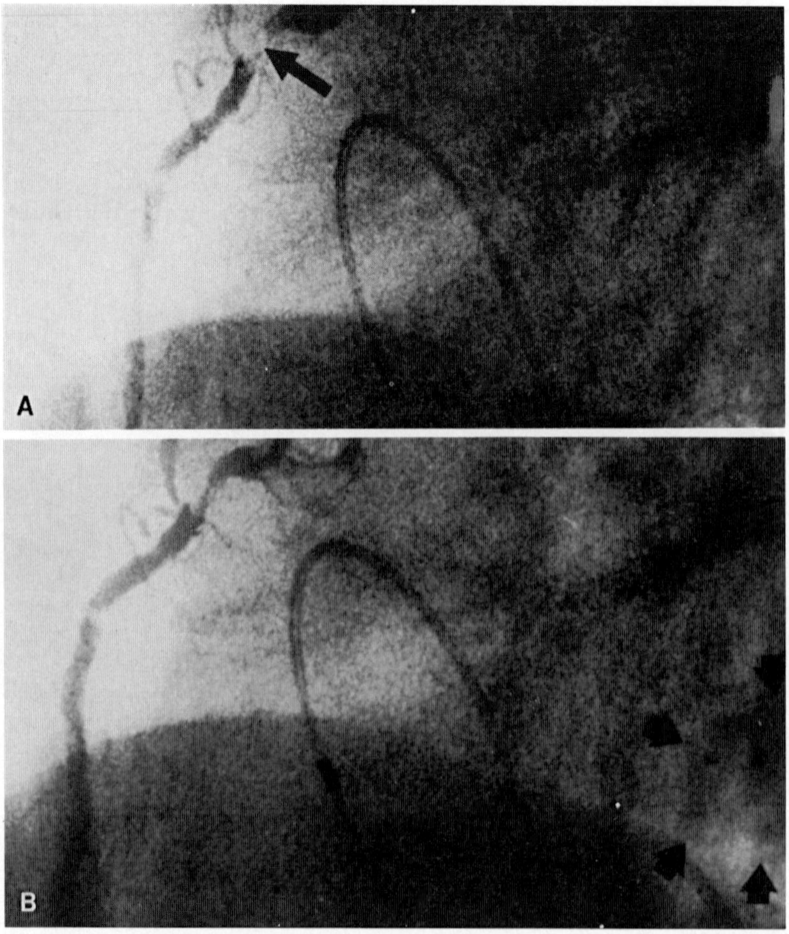

Figure 4–44. Angiographic recognition of myocardial hemorrhage. *A,* The initial right coronary arteriogram in the left anterior oblique projection showing subtotal occlusion at the proximal portion *(arrow)* and delayed distal flow. *B,* The arteriogram after nitroglycerin infusion showing extravasation of the contrast medium at the inferoposterior wall of the left ventricle *(arrows).* (See Fig. 4–45.) (From Yasuno et al.,[64] with permission.)

and colleagues[59] described a patient with two infarcts of equal age in whom one infarct artery was reperfused and the other was not. At necropsy, both hemorrhagic and anemic infarcts, respectively, were present, and there were histologically clear-cut differences in the removal of necrotic tissue and replacement by connective tissue between the hemorrhagic and anemic infarcts. In the hemorrhagic infarct, repair processes were completely lacking after 18 days, whereas the anemic infarct showed typical resorption and repair by granulation tissue. This difference indicated marked delay in the usual infarct healing process. In addition, comparison of infarct size (area) indicated the anemic infarct was much smaller than the reperfused hemorrhagic infarct (4 cm^2 versus 30 cm^2, respectively).[59]

LASER IRRADIATION

Rapid advances are being achieved in the use of lasers (*l*ight *a*mplification by *s*timulated *e*mission of *r*adiation) in the therapy of coronary and peripheral atherosclerosis.[94,95] Many types of lasers are being investigated, including neodymium-doped-yttrium aluminum garnet (Nd-YAG), argon, CO_2, and "excimer." Variation in biologic tissue response appears dependent on a number of factors, including physical characteristics of both the laser energy source and the target lesion. As pointed out by Isner and Clarke,[95] laser irradiation appears to be a logical extension of therapies developed for treatment of coronary atherosclerosis: bypass grafting *"bypasses"* the obstruction, balloon angioplasty *"remodels"* the plaque obstruction, and lasers *"eliminate"* atherosclerotic plaque by converting plaque from a solid-phase matter to a water (or blood) - soluble gas. "Laser offers the promise of a percutaneous, definitive therapy for atherosclerosis."[95] Perforation of the coronary artery wall represents the current principal factor in limiting routine clinical use of lasers in humans. Morphologic consequences of laser radiation of coronary atherosclerotic plaque consists of a charred crater lining and underlying photocoagulated tissue. In addition, full-thickness laser injury may alter the adventitia or cause artery rupture or both.[94] Laser recanalization of atherosclerotic plaque results in removal of plaque by directed energy that is absorbed and converted into heat in the target tissue. The irradiated tissue evaporates, becomes carbonized (charred) or desiccated, or becomes thermally injured sufficiently to cause necrosis.[94] The net result is vessel luminal

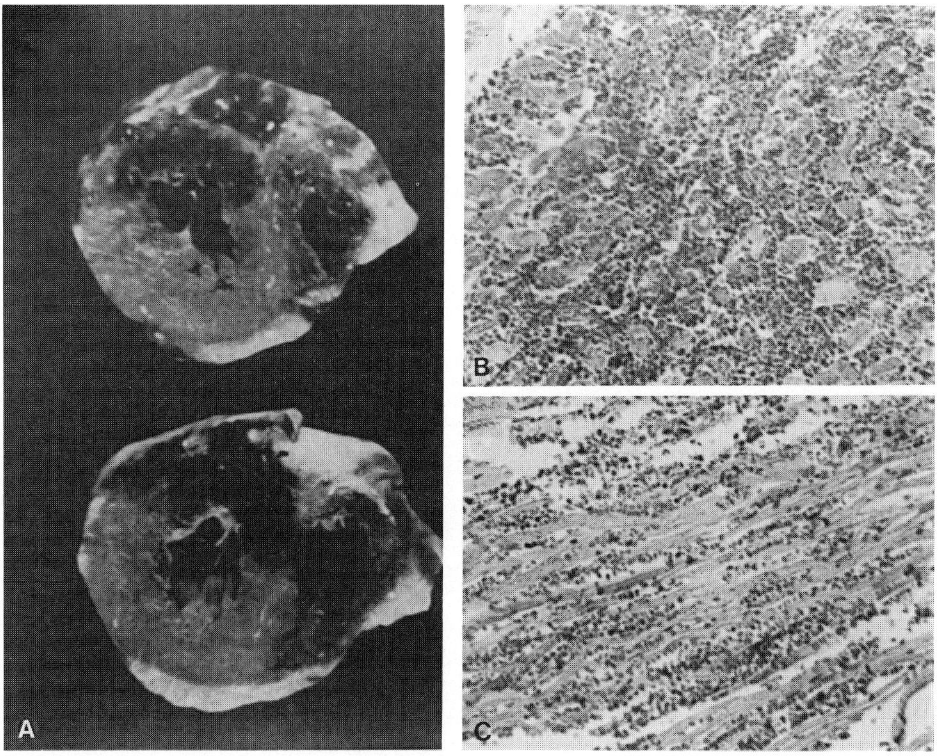

Figure 4–45. Necropsy documentation of angiographically recognized hemorrhagic infarction during streptokinase thrombolysis therapy. *A,* Transverse slices of the heart from the patient. Severe hemorrhagic transmural infarction is seen in the inferoposterior wall of the left ventricle. *B, C,* Microscopic findings in the hemorrhagic infarction. Note coagulation necrosis of the myocytes and marked bleeding. (Hematoxylin-eosin stain; magnification ×200, reduced 12 percent.) (See Fig. 4–44.) (From Yasuno et al.,[64] with permission.)

expansion. The tissue that first absorbs the incident laser beam is explosively evaporated, resulting in a plaque crater.[94] Most early laser reaction probably represents thermal degradation rather than molecular photo dissociation, inasmuch as the gaseous byproducts of laser-irradiated plaque have been identified as hydrocarbon fragments.[94] Tissue not evaporated may persist as charred material. Hyalinized, fibrotic, and calcified plaque result in greater debris compared with more lipid-laden ("fatty") plaques.[94] Chronic changes of postirradiated lesions show endothelialization in the evaluated area and focal aneurysmal dilation of the sites where medial injury has occurred.[94] In experimental models, the laser-induced crater is still evident several weeks later.

Most recent attempts at eliminating vessel wall perforation have involved the use of laser sources capable of vaporizing the plaque without causing thermal injury to surrounding tissues. Many of the lasers employed thus far have been "continuous wave lasers"[95] that result in lesions with gross charring at the edges of the laser crater with polymorphous lacunae. Isner and colleagues[95,96] have reported the absence of these undesirable changes in tissues irradiated with "pulsed" ultraviolet light from an excimer laser. Gross and light microscopic signs of thermal injury can be eliminated by pulsed energy delivery of any wavelength, given high peak power density and low repetition rate.[95,96] In 30 atherosclerotic coronary segments irradiated by Isner and colleagues,[15] none showed gross, light microscopic, or ultrastructural evidence of pathologic injury seen with continuous wave irradiation (Fig. 4–46). Similar results were achieved after excimer laser irradiation of 30 samples of myocardium and calcified aortic valve tissue. These exciting observations have major potential clinical benefits, but further technical advances are needed before laser recanalization becomes clinically applicable.

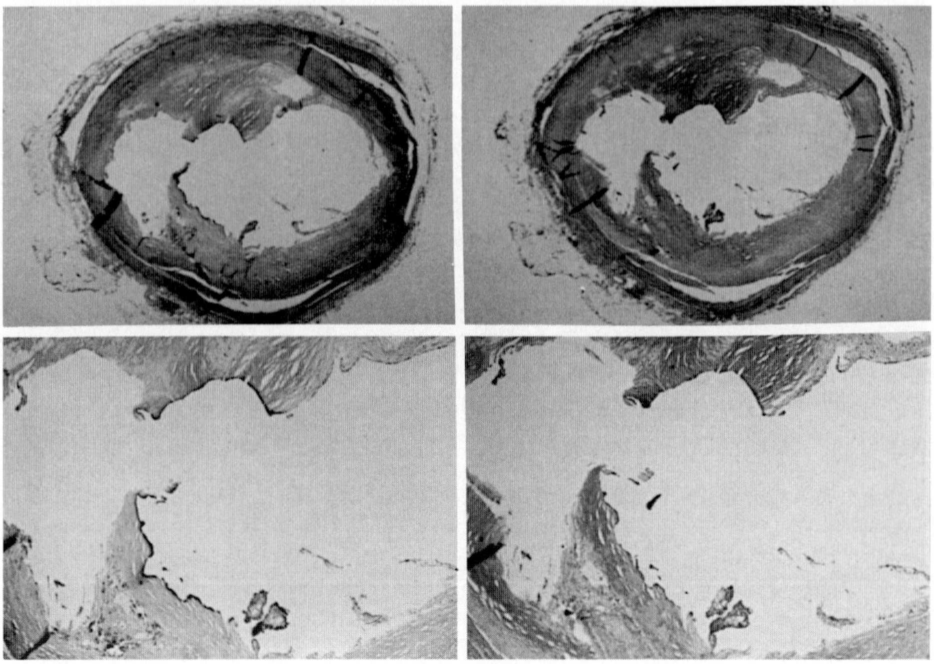

Figure 4–46. Light microscopic findings after excimer laser irradiation of atherosclerotic coronary artery plaque. There is a superficial zone of linear discoloration at the perimeter of the neolumen; otherwise, no remarkable alterations are observed. *Top,* Verhoeff's elastic tissue stain *(left)* and Richardson's stain *(right),* original magnification ×10; (reduced 20 percent). (From Isner et al.,[96] with permission.)

VENTRICULAR ENDOCARDIAL RESECTION AND CATHETER ABLATION FOR CHRONIC VENTRICULAR ARRHYTHMIAS

Even with the vast array of pharmacologic agents available for treatment of recurrent ventricular arrhythmias, the clinical results have been disappointing.[76] Surgical treatment with direct excision or ablation of a focus of ventricular tachycardia has emerged as an alternative to pharmacologic therapy.[97–103] As a result, surgical pathologists are now receiving resected endocardial tissue for histologic evaluation (Fig. 4–47). Endocardial resection procedure (ERP), described by Josephson and colleagues,[99] is at present the most commonly used technique. However, *endocardial* resection may fail to eliminate the arrhythmia because ventricular arrhythmias arise from *myocardial* or *subepicardial* layers of the ventricular wall.[103] For this reason, endocardial shocks delivered through transvenous catheters have been used to improve results.[102–104]

Endocardial Resection

Operative excision of portions of ventricular endocardium and underlying myocardium in patients with chronic, recurrent sustained ventricular tachycardia often eliminates the ventricular tachycardia (Fig. 4–47). Morphologic-histologic features of operatively excised left ventricular subendocardial regions have been described by Fenoglio and colleagues.[105] Bundles of apparently viable myocardial fibers embedded in dense fibrous tissue were identified throughout the endocardial resections from each of 23 patients.[105] The cell bundles were separated from one another by fibrous tissue but extended uninterrupted to the margins of the surgical resection. In 14 patients, Purkinje fibers were identified beneath the thickened endocardium, whereas the remaining bundles were composed of ventricular muscle. The Purkinje fibers appeared to have normal ultrastructure, and ventricular cells had both normal and abnormal ultrastructural changes. The abnormal muscle cells were characterized by loss of contractile elements, aggregates of dilated sarcoplasmic reticulum, and osmiophilic dense bodies. Fenoglio and associates[105] suggested the abnormal structure and arrangement of the surviving cardiac fibers in resected endocardium may be responsible for the abnormal electrophysiologic function that results in ventricular tachycardia.

Silver and colleagues[106] recently reported late necropsy findings in a 51-year-old man receiving endomyocardial resection for recurrent ventricular tachycardia 19 months earlier. Ventricular tachycardia was successfully ablated, but the patient died from postoperative wound infection. At necropsy, the ventricular resection site was covered with snowy-white thickened endocardium, which consisted of collagen fibers and elastic fibers similar to the acquired form of endocardial fibroelastosis.

Catheter Ablation

Catheter ablation of ventricular arrhythmias resistant to medical therapy appears to be a promising technique. High-energy catheter-delivered discharges are used to damage the previously mapped ventricular focus. Endocardial shocks produce local myocardial necrosis, the extent of which depends on the dose of energy delivered. Experimental models[106] have noted discrete transmural wedge-shaped zones of necrosis without perforation at necropsy. To date, five patients have had catheter ablation of ventricular tachycardia by endocardial shocks.[102,104,108] All of the patients had episodic, drug-resistant ventricular tachycardia, and in all, endocardial shocks prevented recurrence of clinical ventricular tachycardia. We recently exam-

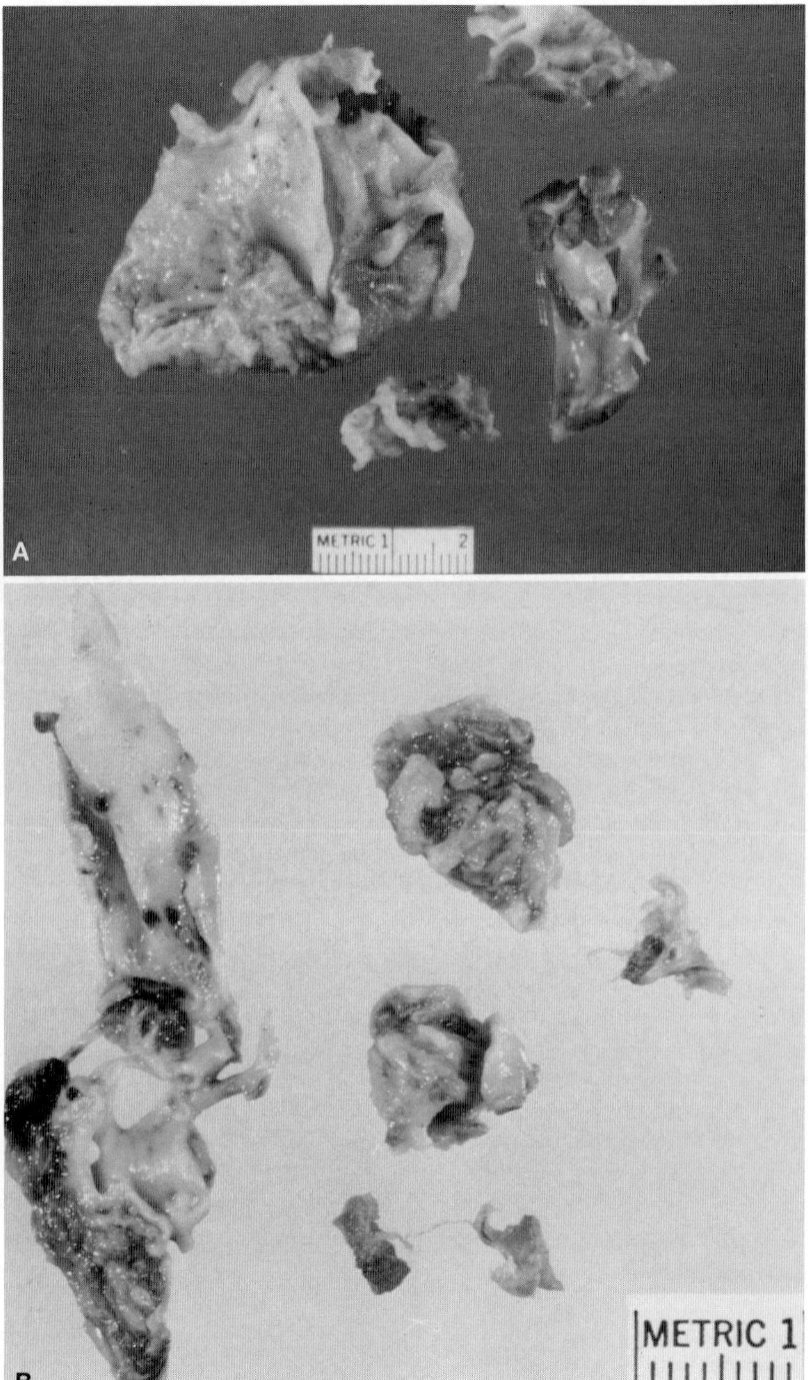

Figure 4–47. Operatively excised ventricular endocardium from two patients *(A, B)* with chronic ventricular arrhythmia following myocardial infarction. The site of tachycardia was mapped at surgery before endocardial resection.

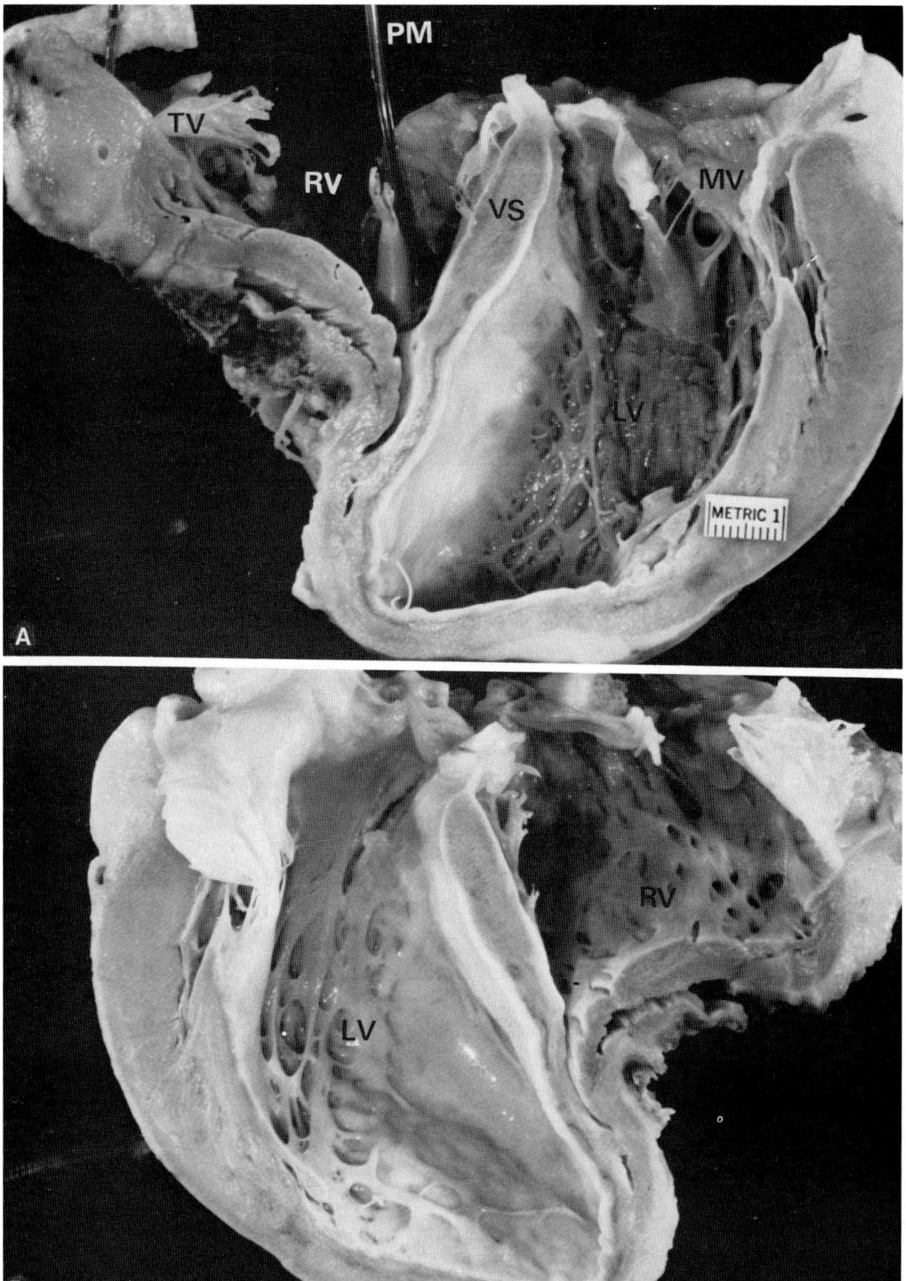

Figure 4–48. Explanted heart (transplant patient) from a patient undergoing catheter ablation therapy from recurrent ventricular tachycardia. The catheter shocks were delivered along the right (RV) and left (LV) ventricular surfaces of the ventricular septum (VS). There is marked endocardial fibrosis *(whitish area). A, B,* Tomographic views of right (RV) and left (LV) ventricle. Note the healed myocardial infarction involving the ventricular septum with marked endocardial thickening (pearly white LV lining). MV = mitral valve, PM = pacemaker catheter, TV = tricuspid valve.

ined the explanted heart of a patient receiving catheter ablation prior to cardiac transplantation (Fig. 4–48). Despite several catheter shocks, the arrhythmia frequency was reduced but not eliminated. Catheter ablation appears to eliminate the irritable focus by creating a localized ventricular myocardial infarct. The extent of myocardial necrosis resulting from multiple endocardial shocks may contribute to the development of congestive heart failure.

TEMPORARY VENTRICULAR ASSIST DEVICES

Temporary left and right ventricular assist devices are currently being used in patients unable to be separated from cardiopulmonary bypass or those with severe myocardial dysfunction. Relatively little morphologic information is available from these patients. Schoen and colleagues[109] initially reported pathologic findings in 21 patients receiving temporary left ventricular assist pump support (Model X pump in 20 patients, Model XI in one patient). Patients received the device following isolated valve replacement, coronary artery bypass grafting, or combined procedures. The duration of left ventricular support was 1 to 190 hours (average 61). Myocardial biopsies were obtained at the time of ventricular assist device implantation. Correlation of myocardial biopsies taken at pump implantation in 15 patients and necropsy findings in nonsurvivors suggested that myocardial dysfunction has a reversible component that appears related to diminished compliance (probably edema), severe but reversible ischemic myocardial injury, or both.[109] None of the patients studied had evidence of thromboemboli, biomaterials-emboli, or other pump-related complications. Schoen and associates[110] recently updated their findings in evaluation of 41 patients, distributed among four centers who had left (33 patients), right (five), or bilateral (three) temporary ventricular assist devices. Cardiac failure had occurred in 39 postoperative patients (following aortocoronary bypass [23], valve replacement [four], both [nine], or other [three]). Death of 35 nonsurvivors was due to myocardial necrosis (14), hemorrhage (nine), cerebrovascular accidents (three), infection (three), and other (six). Mean duration of support in all patients was 62 hours. In 16 patients (40 percent) who improved, cardiac assist duration was mean 127 hours (range 44 to 264), compared with mean 19 hours (range 1 to 120) in 25 who did not. Of 17 patients in whom duration of support exceeded 72 hours, 15 (88 percent) improved, 11 were weaned, and six survived long-term. Tissue examination (in 33 patients) by biopsy at pump implantation or autopsy revealed coagulation or contraction band myocyte necrosis, with or without hemorrhage, in 26 patients; of these, 10 improved and six were long-term survivors. Pump-related complications (two) included one patient each with pulmonary embolism, most likely related to a cannulation site thrombus, and an aortic cannulation site infection. This study suggests that mechanical cardiac assist (1) may be accomplished with low complication rate; (2) should not necessarily be denied to patients with existing necrosis, because myocardial necrosis does not preclude improvement or survival; and (3) frequently leads to functional myocardial recovery if patients survive early noncardiac complications, often due to long duration of cardiopulmonary bypass.[110]

We recently examined the heart at necropsy from three patients receiving left (two) or right (one) ventricular assist devices for severe ventricular dysfunction following coronary artery bypass grafting or valve replacement (Fig. 4–49). In two of the three patients, the atrial cannula had thrombus in its tip. In addition, all three patients had variable degrees of atrial wall hemorrhage at sites of atrial collapse surrounding the cannulae (Fig. 4–49). In one patient, the hemorrhage appeared to encroach the

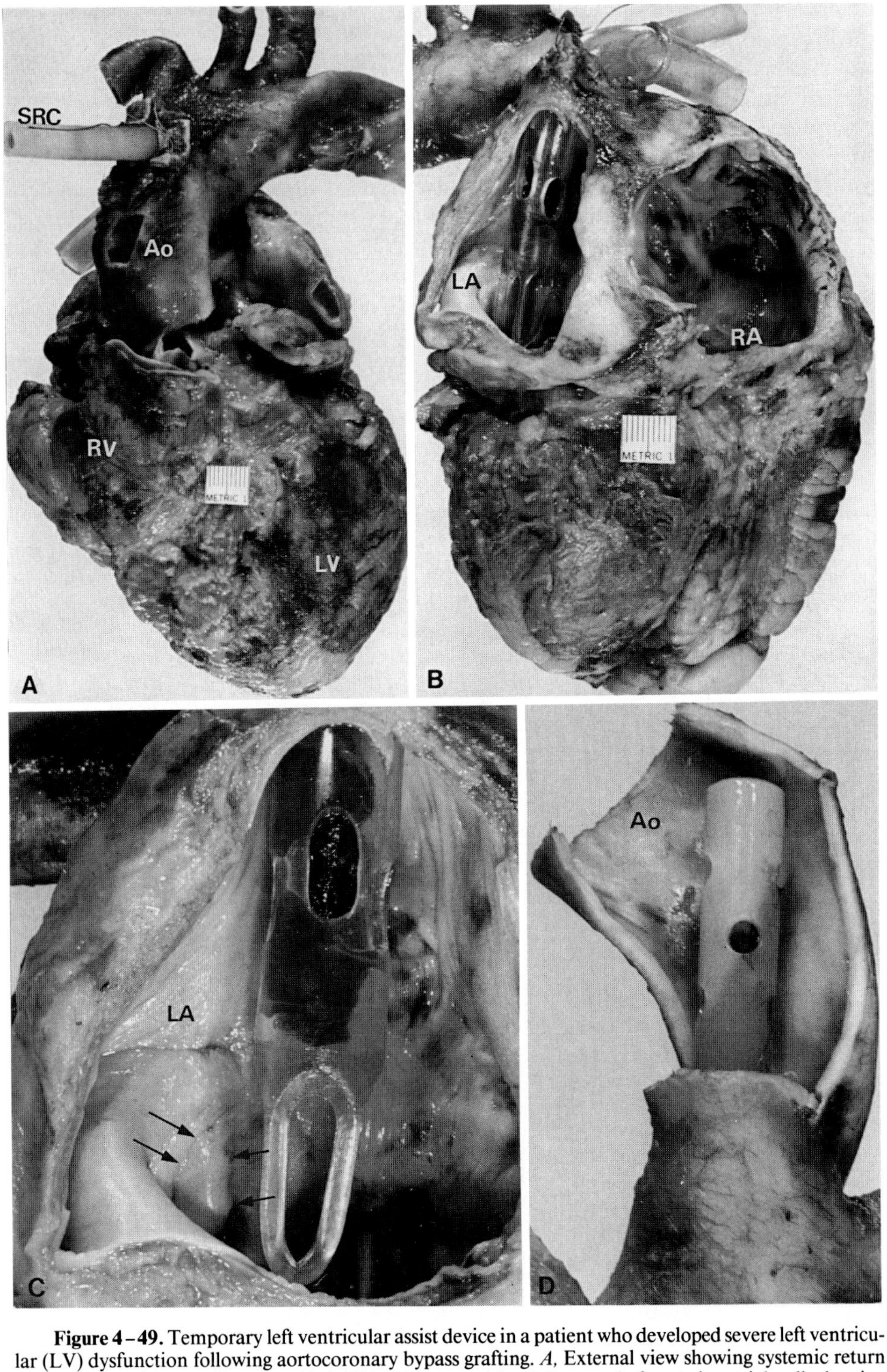

Figure 4-49. Temporary left ventricular assist device in a patient who developed severe left ventricular (LV) dysfunction following aortocoronary bypass grafting. *A,* External view showing systemic return cannula (SRC) in ascending aorta (Ao). RV = right ventricle. *B,* Removal of posterior atrial walls showing left atrial exit cannula in left atrium (LA). Note hemorrhage in atrial septum as viewed from right atrium (RA). *C,* Close-up of left atrial cannula showing tip thrombus and dimple of left atrial appendage, which has been sucked into cannula *(arrows)*. *D,* Close-up of systemic return cannula showing no thrombus or arterial wall damage.

AV node. Cannulae in the aorta or pulmonary trunk were free of thrombus, and the adjacent arterial walls were free of hemorrhage.

The pathogenesis of the specific myocardial abnormality accounting for ventricular assist pump-induced reversibility of the early postoperative cardiac dysfunction remains unclear. Although the presence of myocardial necrosis itself does not appear to preclude a favorable hemodynamic response, the amount present on initial myocardial biopsies was associated with a poor prognosis.[109] Because repair of myocardial necrosis during left ventricular assist pump support is minimal, and because established areas of myocardial infarction are not affected by enhanced flows and pressures, the reversible functional abnormality must involve other factors (interstitial myocardial edema or hemorrhage) causing decreased compliance of otherwise viable myocardium.[109]

REFERENCES

1. Dotter, CT and Judkins, MP: Transluminal treatment of atherosclerotic obstruction: Description of new technic and a preliminary report of its application. Circulation 30:654, 1964.
2. Gruentzig, AR: Transluminal dilatation of coronary artery stenosis (letter). Lancet 1:263, 1978.
3. Gruentzig, AR, Senning, A, and Siegenthaler, WE: Nonoperative dilation of coronary artery stenosis. N Engl J Med 301:61, 1979.
4. Kent, KM, Bentivoglio, LG, Block, PC, et al: Percutaneous transluminal coronary angioplasty: Report from the Registry of the National Heart, Lung and Blood Institute. Am J Cardiol 49:2011, 1981.
5. Proceedings of the National Heart Lung and Blood Institute Workshop on the Outcome of Percutaneous Transluminal Coronary Angioplasty. Am J Cardiol 53:1C, 1984.
6. Anderson, HV, Roubin, GS, Leimgruber, PP, et al: Primary angiographic success rates of percutaneous transluminal coronary angioplasty. Am J Cardiol 56:712, 1985.
7. Ford, WB, Sholey, MH, Zikria, EA, et al: Percutaneous transluminal dilation of aortocoronary saphenous vein bypass grafts. Chest 79:529, 1981.
8. Waller, BF, Rothbaum, DA, Gorfinkel, HJ, et al: Morphologic observations following percutaneous transluminal balloon angioplasty of early and late aortocoronary saphenous vein bypass grafts. J Am Coll Cardiol 4:784, 1984.
9. Douglas, JS, Gruentzig, AR, King, SB, III, et al: Percutaneous transluminal coronary angioplasty in patients with prior coronary surgery. J Am Coll Cardiol 2:745, 1983.
10. Reeder, GS, Bresnahan, JF, Holmes, DR, et al: Angioplasty for aortocoronary bypass graft stenosis. Mayo Clin Proc 61:14, 1986.
11. Corbelli, J, Franco, I, Hollman, J, et al: Percutaneous transluminal coronary angioplasty in previous coronary artery bypass surgery. Am J Cardiol 56:398, 1985.
12. Block, PC, Myler, RK, Stertzer, S, et al: Morphology after transluminal angioplasty in human beings. N Engl J Med 305:382, 1981.
13. Waller, BF: Early and late morphologic changes in human coronary arteries after percutaneous transluminal coronary angioplasty. Clin Cardiol 6:363, 1983.
14. Waller, BF, Gorfinkel, HJ, Rogers, FJ, et al: Early and late morphologic changes in major epicardial coronary arteries after percutaneous transluminal coronary angioplasty. Am J Cardiol 53:42C, 1984.
15. Waller, BF, Dillon, JC, and Cowley, MH: Plaque hematoma and coronary dissection with percutaneous transluminal angioplasty (PTCA) of severely stenotic lesions. Morphologic coronary observations in 5 men within 30 days of PTCA. Circulation 68 (Suppl III):III-144, 1983.
16. Waller, BF, McManus, BM, Kishel, JC, et al: Status of the major coronary arteries 80 to 150 days after percutaneous transluminal coronary angioplasty. Analysis of 3 necropsy patients. Am J Cardiol 51:81, 1983.
17. Saffitz, JE, Rose, TE, Oaks, JB, et al: Coronary arterial rupture during coronary angioplasty. Am J Cardiol 51:902, 1983.
18. Essed, CD, Brand, MVD, and Becker, AE: Transluminal coronary angioplasty and early restenosis. Br Heart J 49:393, 1983.
19. Mizuno, K, Kurita, A, and Imazeki, N: Pathologic findings after percutaneous transluminal coronary angioplasty. Br Heart J 52:588, 1984.

20. Soward, AL, Essed, CE, and Serruys, PW: Coronary arterial findings after accidental death immediately after successful percutaneous transluminal coronary angioplasty. Am J Cardiol 56:794, 1985.
21. Baughman, KL, Pasternak, RC, Fallon, JT, et al: Transluminal coronary angioplasty of postmortem human hearts. Am J Cardiol 48:1044, 1981.
22. Block, PC: Histological and ultrastructural studies in animals. In Proceedings of the Workshop on Percutaneous Transluminal Coronary Angioplasty. DHEW Pub No (NIH) 80-2030, 1980, p 155.
23. Block, PC, Baughman, KL, Pasternack, RC, et al: Transluminal angioplasty: Correlation of morphologic and angiographic findings in an experimental model. Circulation 61:778, 1980.
24. Block, PC, Fallon, JT, and Elmer, D: Experimental angioplasty: Lessons from the laboratory. Am J Radiol 135:907, 1980.
25. Faxon, DP, Weber, VJ, Haudenschild, C, et al: Acute effects of transluminal angioplasty in three experimental models of atherosclerosis. Arteriosclerosis 2:125, 1982.
26. Castaneda-Zuniga, WR, Formarek, A, Todavarthy, M, et al: The mechanism of balloon angioplasty. Radiology 135:565, 1980.
27. Levine, S, Ewels, CJ, Rosing, DR, et al: Coronary angioplasty: Clinical and angiographic followup. Am J Cardiol 55:673, 1985.
28. Waller, BF: Coronary luminal shape and the arc of disease-free wall: Morphologic observations and clinical relevance. J Am Coll Cardiol 6:1100, 1985.
29. Saner, HE, Gobel, FL, Salomonowitz, E, et al: The disease-free wall in coronary atherosclerosis: Its relation to degree of obstruction. J Am Coll Cardiol 6:1096, 1985.
30. Vlodaver, Z and Edwards, JE: Pathology of coronary atherosclerosis. Prog Cardiovasc Dis 14:256, 1971.
31. Baroldi, G: Diseases of the coronary arteries. In Silver, MD (ed): Cardiovascular Pathology. Churchill Livingstone, New York, 1983, p 341.
32. Isner, JM and Fortin, RV: Frequency in nonangioplasty patients of morphologic findings reported in coronary arteries treated with transluminal angioplasty. Am J Cardiol 51:689, 1983.
33. Batayias, GE, Barboriak, JJ, Korns, ME, et al: The spectrum of pathologic changes in aortocoronary saphenous vein grafts. Circulation 56(Suppl II):II-18, 1977.
34. Bulkley, BH and Hutchins, G: Accelerated "atherosclerosis." A morphologic study of 97 saphenous vein coronary artery bypass grafts. Circulation 55:163, 1977.
35. Waller, BF and Roberts, WC: Amount of luminal narrowing in bypassed and nonbypassed native coronary arteries in necropsy patients dying early and late after aorto-coronary bypass operations. In Mason, DT and Collins, JT, Jr (eds): Myocardial Revascularization. Medical and Surgical Advances in Coronary Disease. York Medical Books, New York, 1981, p 503.
36. Ford, WB, Wholey, MH, Zikria, EA, et al: Percutaneous transluminal angioplasty in the management of occlusive disease involving the coronary arteries and saphenous vein bypass grafts. J Thorac Cardiovasc Surg 79:1, 1980.
37. Campeau, L, Lesperance, J, Corbara, F, et al: Aortocoronary saphenous vein bypass graft changes 5 to 7 years after surgery. Circulation 58 (Suppl I):I-170, 1978.
38. Lie, JT, Lawrie, GM, and Morris, GC, Jr: Aortocoronary bypass saphenous vein graft atherosclerosis. Anatomic study of 99 vein grafts from normal and hyperlipoproteinemic patients up to 75 months postoperatively. Am J Cardiol 40:906, 1977.
39. Smith, SH and Greer, JC: Morphology of saphenous vein-coronary artery bypass grafts. Seven to 116 months after surgery. Arch Pathol Lab Med 107:13, 1983.
40. Block, PC, Cowley, MJ, Kaltenback, M, et al: Percutaneous angioplasty of stenoses of bypass grafts or of bypass graft anastomotic sites. Am J Cardiol 53:666, 1984.
41. Rentrop, P, De Vivie, ER, Karsch, KR, et al: Acute myocardial infarction: Intracoronary application of nitroglycerin and streptokinase in combination with transluminal recanalization. Clin Cardiol 5:354, 1979.
42. Ganz, W, Buchbinder, N, Marcus, H, et al: Intracoronary thrombolysis in evolving myocardial infarction. Am Heart J 101:4, 1981.
43. Mathey, DG, Kuch, KH, Tilsner, V, et al: Nonsurgical coronary artery recanalization in acute transmural myocardial infarction. Circulation 63:489, 1981.
44. Reduto, LA, Smalling, RW, Freund, GC, et al: Intracoronary infusion of streptokinase in patients with acute myocardial infarction: Effects of reperfusion on left ventricular performance. Am J Cardiol 48:403, 1981.
45. Markis, JE, Malagould, M, Parker, A, et al: Myocardial salvage after intracoronary thrombolysis with streptokinase in acute myocardial infarction. N Engl J Med 305:777, 1981.

46. Rentrop, P, Blanke, H, Karsch, KR, et al: Selective intracoronary thrombolysis in acute myocardial infarction and unstable angina pectoris. Circulation 63:307, 1981.
47. Sobel, BE and Bergmann, SR: Coronary thrombolysis: Some unresolved issues. Am J Med 72:1, 1982.
48. The TIMI Study Group: The thrombolysis in myocardial infarction (TIMI) Trial: Phase I Findings. N Engl J Med 312:932, 1985.
49. Relman, AS: Intravenous thrombolysis in acute myocardial infarction. A Progress Report. N Engl J Med 312:915, 1985.
50. Hartzler, GO, Rutherford, BD, McConahay, DR, et al: Percutaneous transluminal coronary angioplasty with and without thrombolytic therapy for treatment of acute myocardial infarction. Am Heart J 106:965, 1983.
51. Hartzler, GO, Rutherford, BD, and McConahay, DR: Percutaneous transluminal coronary angioplasty: Application for acute myocardial infarction. Am J Cardiol 53:117C, 1984.
52. Serruys, PW, Wijns, W, Van den Brand, M, et al: Is transluminal coronary angioplasty mandatory after successful thrombolysis? Quantitative coronary angiographic study. Br Heart J 50:257, 1983.
53. Gold, HK, Cowley, MJ, Palacios, IF, et al: Combined intracoronary streptokinase infusion and coronary angioplasty during acute myocardial infarction. Am J Cardiol 53:122C, 1984.
54. Meyer, J, Marks, W, and Effert, S: Percutaneous transluminal coronary angioplasty immediately after intracoronary streptolysis of transluminal myocardial infarction. Circulation 66:905, 1982.
55. Papapiotro, SE, Machean, WAH, Stanley, AWH, Jr, et al: Percutaneous transluminal coronary angioplasty in acute myocardial infarction. Am J Cardiol 55:48, 1985.
56. Schachenmayr, W and Haferkamp, O: Der hamorrhagische Herzinfarkt. Dtsch Med Wschr 97:1172, 1972.
57. Berry, CL: Thrombolytic therapy and myocardial infarction. J Clin Pathol 28:352, 1975.
58. Verstraete, M, van de Loo, J, and Jesdinsky, HJ: Streptokinase in acute myocardial infarction. Acta Med Scand (Suppl) 648:7, 1981.
59. Mathey, DG, Schofer, J, Kuck, K-H, et al: Transmural, hemorrhagic myocardial infarction after intracoronary streptokinase. Clinical, angiographic and necropsy findings. Br Heart J 48:546, 1982.
60. Isner, JM, Konstam, MA, Fortin, RV, et al: Delayed thrombolysis of streptokinase-resistant occlusive thrombus: Documentation by pre and postmortem coronary angiography. Am J Cardiol 52:210, 1983.
61. Mattfeldt, T, Schwarz, F, Schuler, G, et al: Necropsy evaluation in seven patients with evolving acute myocardial infarction treated with thrombolytic therapy. Am J Cardiol 54:530, 1984.
62. Harrison, DG, Ferguson, DW, Collins, SM, et al: Rethrombosis after reperfusion with streptokinase: Importance of geometry of residual lesions. Circulation 69:991, 1984.
63. Hollander, G, Ozick, H, Anselmo, M, et al: Myocardial rupture following intracoronary thrombolysis therapy. NY State J Med 84:129, 1984.
64. Yasuno, M, Endo, S, Takakashi, M, et al: Angiographic and pathologic evidence of hemorrhage into the myocardium after coronary reperfusion. Angiology 35:797, 1984.
65. Kao, K-J, Hackel, DB, and Kong, Y: Hemorrhagic myocardial infarction after streptokinase treatment for acute coronary thrombosis. Arch Pathol Lab Med 108:121, 1984.
66. Fujiwara, H, Onodera, T, Tanaka, M, et al: A clinicopathologic study of patients with hemorrhagic myocardial infarction treated with selective coronary thrombolysis with urokinase. Circulation 73:749, 1986.
67. Lie, JT, Lawrie, GM, Morris, GC, Jr, et al: Hemorrhagic myocardial infarction associated with aortocoronary bypass revascularization. Am Heart J 96:295, 1978.
68. Bresnahan, GF, Roberts, R, Shell, WE, et al: Deleterious effects due to hemorrhage after myocardial reperfusion. Am J Cardiol 33:82, 1974.
69. Lang, T-W, Corday, E, Gold, H, et al: Consequences of reperfusion after coronary occlusion. Effects on hemodynamic and regional myocardial metabolic function. Am J Cardiol 33:69, 1974.
70. Cerra, FB, Lajos, TZ, Montes, M, et al: Hemorrhagic infarction: A reperfusion injury following prolonged myocardial ischemic anoxia. Surgery 78:1, 1975.
71. Jennings, RB and Reimer, KA: Factors involved in salvaging ischemic myocardium: Effect of reperfusion of arterial blood. Circulation 68 (Suppl I):I-25, 1983.
72. Reimer, KA and Jennings, RB: The wavefront phenomenon of myocardial ischemic death: Transmural progression of necrosis within the framework of ischemic bed size and collateral flow. Lab Invest 40:633, 1979.
73. Fishbein, MC, Y-Rit, J, Lando, U, et al: The relationship of vascular injury and myocardial hemorrhage to necrosis after reperfusion. Circulation 62:1274, 1980.

74. Banka, VS, Chadda, KD, and Helfant, RH: Limitations of myocardial revascularization in restoration of regional contraction abnormalities produced by coronary occlusion. Am J Cardiol 34:164, 1974.
75. Deloche, A, Fabiani, JN, Camilleri, JP, et al: The effect of coronary artery reperfusion in the extent of myocardial infarction. Am Heart J 93:358, 1977.
76. Althaus, U, Gwitner, HP, Bauer, H, et al: Consequences of myocardial reperfusion following temporary coronary occlusion in pigs: Effects on morphologic, biochemical and hemodynamic findings. Eur J Clin Invest 7:437, 1977.
77. Capone, RJ and Most, AS: Myocardial hemorrhage after coronary reperfusion on pigs. Am J Cardiol 41:259, 1978.
78. Kloner, RA, Rude, RE, Carlson, N, et al: Ultrastructural evidence of microvascular damage and myocardial cell injury after coronary artery occlusion: Which comes first? Circulation 62:945, 1980.
79. Fishbein, MC, Ganz, W, Y-Rit, J, et al: Relevance of hemorrhage after reperfusion in acute myocardial infarction. In Kaltenbach, M (ed): Transluminal Coronary Angioplasty and Intracoronary Thrombolysis. Springer-Verlag, Berlin, 1982, p 284.
80. Reimer, KA: Overview of potential mechanisms. In Wagner, GS (ed): Myocardial Infarction: Measurement and Intervention. Martinus Nijhoff Publishers, The Hague, Netherlands, 1982, p 387.
81. Kloner, RA, Ellis, SG, Lange, R, et al: Studies of experimental coronary artery reperfusion. Effects on infarct size, myocardial function, biochemistry, ultrastructure, microvascular damage. Circulation 68 (Suppl I):I-8, 1983.
82. Kloner, RA and Alker, KJ: The effect of streptokinase on intramyocardial hemorrhage, infarct size and the no-reflow phenomena during coronary reperfusion. Circulation 70:513, 1984.
83. Roberts, CS, Schoen, FJ, and Kloner, RA: Effect of coronary reperfusion on myocardial infarct healing and hemorrhage. Am J Cardiol 52:610, 1983.
84. Hutchans, GM and Bulkley, BH: Correlation of myocardial contraction band necrosis and vascular patency. Lab Invest 36:642, 1977.
85. Health and Public Policy Committee, American College of Physicians: Thrombolysis for evolving myocardial infarction. Ann Intern Med 103:463, 1985.
86. Lo, YSA: Intravenous versus intracoronary streptokinase in acute myocardial infarction. Clin Cardiol 8:609, 1985.
87. Little, WC: Thrombolytic therapy of acute myocardial infarction. Curr Prob Cardiol 8(9):7, 1983.
88. Schwarz, F, Schuler, G, Katus, H, et al: Intracoronary thrombolysis in acute myocardial infarction: Duration of ischemia is a major determinant of late results after recanalization. Am J Cardiol 50:933, 1982.
89. Gold, HK, Cowley, MJ, Palacios, IF, et al: Combined intracoronary streptokinase infusion and coronary angioplasty during acute myocardial infarction. Am J Cardiol 53:122C, 1984.
90. Menke, DM, Jordan, MD, Aust, CH, et al: Histologic evidence of distal coronary thromboembolism: A complication of acute proximal coronary artery thrombolysis therapy. Chest 90:614, 1986.
91. Roberts, WC: Coronary embolism: A review of causes, consequences and diagnostic considerations. Cardiovasc Med 3:699, 1978.
92. Waller, BF, Dixon, DS, Kim, RW, et al: Embolus to the left main coronary artery. Am J Cardiol 50:658, 1982.
93. Little, WC and Rogers, EW: Angiographic evidence of hemorrhagic myocardial infarction after intracoronary thrombolysis with streptokinase. Am J Cardiol 51:906, 1983.
94. Lee, G, Lee, MH, Ikeda, RM, et al: Effects of laser radiation on the morphology of human coronary atherosclerotic disease. In Waller, BF (ed): Cardiac Morphology. Vol 2, No. 4, WB Saunders, Philadelphia, 1984, p 621.
95. Isner, JM and Clarke, RH: Laser angioplasty: Unraveling the Gordian knot. J Am Coll Cardiol 7:705, 1986.
96. Isner, JM, Donaldson, RF, Deckelbaum, LI, et al: The excimer laser: Gross, light microscopic and ultrastructural analysis of potential advantages for use in laser therapy of cardiovascular disease. J Am Coll Cardiol 6:1102, 1985.
97. Morady, F, Scheinman, MM, Hess, DS, et al: Electrophysiologic testing in the management of survivors of out-of-hospital cardiac arrest. Am J Cardiol 51:85, 1983.
98. Guiraudon, GM, Fontaine, G, Frank, R, et al: Encircling endocardial ventriculotomy: A new surgical treatment for life-threatening ventricular tachycardias resistant to medical treatment following myocardial infarction. Ann Thorac Surg 26:438, 1978.
99. Josephson, ME, Horowitz, LN, and Harken, AH: Endocardial excision: A new surgical technique for the treatment of ventricular tachycardia. Circulation 60:1430, 1979.

100. Waldo, AL, Arciniegas, JG, and Klein, H: Surgical treatment of life-threatening ventricular arrhythmias: The role of intraoperative mapping and consideration of the presently available surgical techniques. Prog Cardiovasc Dis 23:247, 1981.
101. Horowitz, LN, Harken, AH, Kastor, JA, et al: Ventricular resection guided by epicardial mapping for treatment of recurrent ventricular tachycardia. N Engl J Med 302:489, 1980.
102. Harzler, GO: Electrode catheter ablation of refractory focal ventricular tachycardia. J Am Coll Cardiol 2:1107, 1983.
103. Cox, JL: The status of surgery for cardiac arrhythmias. Circulation 71:413, 1985.
104. Puech, P, Gallay, P, Grolleau, R, et al: Traitement par electrofulguration endocavitaire d'une tachycardie ventriculire par dysplasie ventriculaire droite. Arch Mal Coeur 77:826, 1984.
105. Fenoglio, JJ, Jr, Pham, TD, Harken, AH, et al: Recurrent sustained ventricular tachycardia: Structure and ultrastructure of subendocardial regions in which tachycardia originates. Circulation 68:518, 1983.
106. Silver, MA, Cohen, AI, Katz, NM, et al: Cardiac morphologic findings late after partial left ventricular endomyocardial resection for recurrent ventricular tachycardia. Am J Cardiol 54:233, 1984.
107. Chapman, PD, Klopfenstein, S, Troup, PJ, et al: Evaluation of a percutaneous catheter technique for ablation of ventricular tachycardia in a canine model. Am Heart J 110:1, 1985.
108. Belhassen, B, Miller, HI, and Landiado, S: Catheter ablation of incessant ventricular tachycardia refractory to external cardioversions. Am J Cardiol 55:1637, 1985.
109. Schoen, FJ, Bernhard, WF, Khuri, SF, et al: Pathologic findings in postcardiotomy patients managed with a temporary left ventricular assist pump. Am J Surg 143:508, 1982.
110. Schoen, FJ, Palmer, DC, Bernhard, WF, et al: Clinical temporary assist: Pathologic findings and their implications in a multi-institutional study of 41 patients. J Thorac Cardiovasc Surg (in press).

CHAPTER 5

Effects of Coronary Laser Radiation

Garrett Lee, M.D.
Ming C. Chan, M.D.
Jorge M. Garcia, M.D.
Augusto D. Pichard, M.D.
Paul J. Corso, M.D.
Hamner Hannah III, M.D.
Robert L. Reis, M.D.
Dean T. Mason, M.D.

The idea of using laser light to eliminate coronary atherosclerotic plaque has continued to interest and stimulate the scientific community, as judged by the ever-increasing number of ongoing investigations, scientific presentations, and articles published in the past few years. The development of very thin and flexible optical fibers to transmit the laser energies has made it possible to deliver the intense coherent light into the coronary and peripheral arteries, to rid them of diseased obstructions. This concept is appealing, because current therapeutic options such as the bypass procedure and transluminal coronary angioplasty do not accomplish the actual physical removal of the atherosclerotic plaque. The bypass operation also necessitates anesthetizing the patient, opening the chest cavity, and harvesting vein grafts from the legs. The purpose of this chapter is to review the progress of laser technology in the coronary and peripheral arteries in experimental studies and provide an update on laser recanalization in human trials.

EXISTING TECHNOLOGY

The existing technology for laser recanalization of atherosclerotic arteries is far from ideal. The basic system is comprised of a laser and a delivery catheter that encompasses an optical fiber that transmits the laser light.[1] Currently, four different lasers (Table 5–1) have been used and shown to be capable of vaporizing plaque: (1) the argon laser, which emits photons with wavelengths of 488 to 514 nm (blue-green portion of the electromagnetic spectrum); (2) the neodymium-doped-yttrium-alumi-

Table 5–1. Lasers Used in Recanalizing Obstructed Arteries

Type of Laser	Wavelengths (nm)	Power Output	Flexible Delivery System
Argon	488–514	1–20 W	Quartz fiber
Nd-YAG	1060	Up to 100 W	Quartz fiber
CO_2	10600	Up to 100 W	Not available (silver chloride fiber semi-flexible)
Excimer	193, 248, 308, 351	Up to 10^8 W pulsed mode	Not available (308, 351 nm can be transmitted through quartz fiber)

num-garnet (Nd-YAG) laser, which is a solid-state laser that emits photons with a wavelength of 1060 nm (in the near infrared part of the spectrum); (3) the carbon dioxide (CO_2) laser, which emits photons with wavelength of 10,600 nm (in the middle infrared portion of the spectrum); and (4) the excimer laser, which uses rare gas halide as its lasing medium and emits photons with wavelengths in the ultraviolet part of the spectrum, that is, argon fluoride (193 nm), krypton fluoride (248 nm), xenon chloride (308 nm), and xenon fluoride (351 nm). However, despite the variety of lasers, the ideal wavelength that is selectively absorbed by the plaque but not any other normal tissue has not yet been found.

Ideally, the laser energies are transmitted through a flexible, thin, nontoxic optical fiber confined to a small-diameter catheter, which is capable of entering the coronary artery to destroy plaque obstruction. Current commercially available fibers used to transmit laser energies are made of quartz silica. These fibers can transmit argon, Nd-YAG, and portions of the ultraviolet wavelength (that is, 351 nm). Delivery systems for carbon dioxide and other ultraviolet wavelengths are in various stages of development and are not readily available. Fibers made of thallium halides, which transmit the carbon dioxide laser beam, are quite brittle and toxic; however, fibers made of silver chloride appear to be flexible and nontoxic, but have a 30 percent loss over their 1 meter length.[2] Finally, there is also a fiberoptic delivery system that transmits laser energies to a metal cap attached to its distal end. When the laser is activated, the metallic tip can be heated to very high temperatures (greater than 200°C), which can effect vaporization by its mere contact with diseased plaque.[3]

LASER RADIATION: IN VITRO STUDIES

Effect on Human Cadaver Plaque

Initial studies have shown that argon, Nd-YAG, and carbon dioxide laser radiation can vaporize human cadaver coronary atherosclerotic plaque.[4–7] When the laser is directed upon an area of plaque, the plaque absorbs the light energy which is transformed to thermal energy, and the area of plaque becomes vaporized, producing charring around its vaporized surrounding (Fig. 5–1). The process of laser vaporization can generate gaseous products and minute particles that effluoresce from the focal point of the beam. Analysis of the gas products reveals water vapor, carbon dioxide, nitrogen, hydrogen, and light hydrocarbon fragments.[8,9]

The ability of a laser to penetrate plaque depends on the absorptive characteristics of certain materials within the plaque, which is comprised primarily of lipid, hyaline, and calcium, in order of their increasing densities. Rapid vaporization can be achieved with plaque containing material of lower densities such as lipid-laden deposits, whereas high-density deposits such as calcified plaque usually retard laser penetration. Moreover, a greater extent of charred remnants may be found in the vaporized channel of calcified plaque than in hyalinized plaque obstructions. In lipid-laden plaque-occluded coronary arteries, no charred debris is found in its laser-treated passageway.

When the laser beam is transmitted through an optical fiber, the energy intensity is greater, the closer the target plaque lesion is to the tip of the quartz fiber. When directed coaxially along the central axis of the vessel, the plaque can be dissolved adjacent to the stenotic lumen, and by this repeated lasing process, can widen the diameter of the stenotic channel. Additionally, in completely blocked vessels, the beam can be directed to clear a new passageway within the plaque obstruction.

In addition to the physical characteristics of plaque materials that affect laser absorption, the depth of penetration and area (or volume) of plaque vaporization depend on wavelength of the laser used, power intensity, duration of exposure, size of the beam, distance from fiber tip to target lesion, and the surrounding medium (blood, saline, or perfluorocarbon blood substitutes) of the plaque. In general, the higher the power intensity or the longer the exposure time, or the more focused the beam, the greater the plaque vaporization or depth of penetration.

As previously mentioned, argon, Nd-YAG, and carbon dioxide lasers can effect tissue or plaque vaporization, but each laser wavelength behaves differently in different surrounding media. Argon light is readily absorbed by blood owing to its hemoglobin pigment but is usually transmitted through clear aqueous tissue. The Nd-YAG laser transmits through water better than the carbon dioxide laser, but not as well as the argon laser. Carbon dioxide energies are easily absorbed by water in soft tissue and can remove soft superficial layers. Several studies have demonstrated that optical

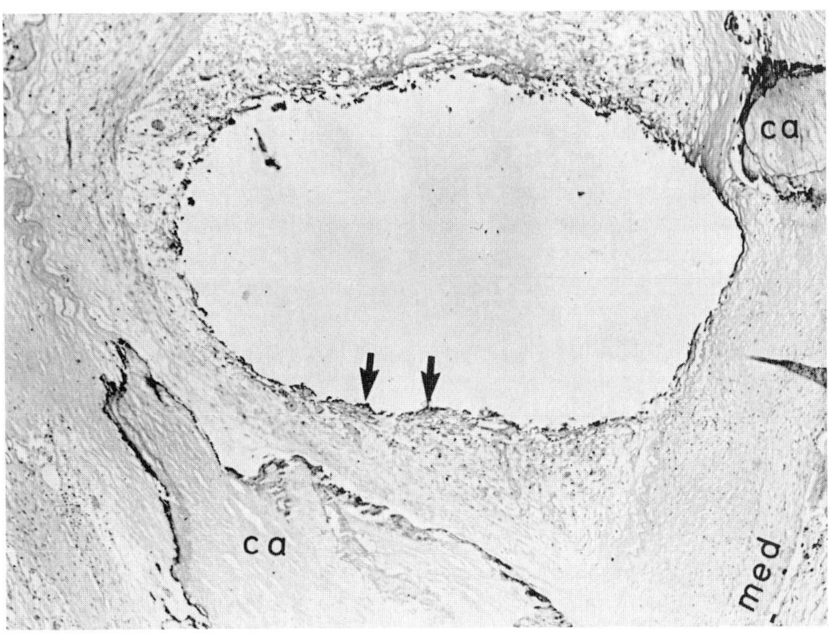

Figure 5–1. Cross-sectional view of argon laser-treated human epicardial coronary artery previously occluded by atherosclerotic plaque. Note vaporized area and carbonized rim *(arrows)* surrounding this area (med = medial wall, ca = calcified area of plaque).

fiber delivery of argon or Nd-YAG energies penetrated plaque better under dry conditions (air) than under wet ones (saline, blood, or perfluorocarbon blood substitutes).[5,10,11]

THERMAL VERSUS PHOTOCHEMICAL ABLATION

Argon, Nd-YAG, or carbon dioxide continuous-wave laser radiation vaporizes plaque by a thermal mechanism, creating a charred rim around the vaporized crater. It has not been definitively shown that such charring produces a greater likelihood of thromboembolic complications. The excimer laser, which emits ultra-violet light, may have the advantage of producing photochemical ablation of the atheroma with little or no thermal injury; the photon energy is converted to electrical excitation, which breaks long-chain polymer molecules into smaller volatile fragments. Thus, the depth of penetration varies with the cumulative number of ultraviolet pulses, while the diameter of the lased channel and its surroundings remain largely unchanged.[12,13] Recently it has been shown that other laser wavelengths can indeed ablate tissue without thermal injury by using high peak powers and low repetition rates.[14]

Laser-Assisted Balloon Angioplasty

Laser may have a complementary role with balloon angioplasty in revascularizing arteries with atherosclerotic disease.[15] In severely obstructed coronary arteries that do not permit the passage of the angioplasty catheter, laser energies directed onto the stenotic obstruction via a thin flexible quartz fiber were demonstrated to increase the vascular lumen by vaporizing atherosclerotic plaque. Even in totally obstructed arteries, the laser produced a newly vaporized channel large enough to accommodate the passage of an angioplasty catheter. The latter was used to dilate and expand the stenotic coronary lumen further by causing stretching and microscopic tears in the intimal, medial, and adventitial wall layers, splitting the plaque, and possibly compressing the atheromatous material.[16–18]

Since laser has been used successfully in vascular repair and anastomosis, this method may also have a place following plaque disruption by balloon angioplasty.[19] The laser-induced fusion of disrupted plaque and arterial wall layers was demonstrated by the Nd-YAG laser. Thus, the combined use of laser and balloon angioplasty may increase luminal size and improve luminal geometry, thereby reducing frequency of arterial restenosis or reclosure.

Dissolution of Plaque By Laser-Heated Metal Cap

The laser-heated metal cautery cap, developed by Xintec Corporation (Oakland, California), avoids the risk of a direct free laser beam inadvertently straying from the target area and causing vascular damage. Studies on atherosclerotic cadaver vessels show that the metal cautery cap can dissolve atherosclerotic lesions instantaneously upon physical contact.[3] The depth of penetration varies with the duration of contact and the physical characteristics of the obstructive material.

LASER RADIATION: IN VIVO STUDIES

Microscopic Examination

Laser exposure via flexible fiber upon atherosclerosis in animal models fed a hyperlipidemic diet demonstrates findings nearly identical to those seen in in vitro studies using diseased human cadaver arteries. In atherosclerotic rabbits, argon laser energies (3 to 6 joules) transmitted via quartz fiber into the diseased aorta induced a vaporized plaque area that was surrounded by a carbonized lining.[20] Subjacent to this lining was a zone of coagulation necrosis whereby lacunae (tiny gas pockets) may be seen. The tissue beyond the latter area was left intact and unaffected by the laser. Similarly, laser radiation of rabbit aortic atheromatous plaque was also achieved with the infrared optical fiber made of silver chloride capable of transmitting carbon dioxide laser energy (15 watts, 1 sec or less).[2] The 1-meter-long flexible fiber was inserted into the right iliac artery and passed to the diseased atheromatous aorta. Again, an area of thermal injury occurred on the surface of the plaque.

In atherosclerotic monkeys, the intravascular insertion of the laser-heated metal cautery cap in the aortic or iliac artery can produce an area of plaque ablation that, within 3 months, scarred and reendothelialized without thinning of the vessel wall.[21] The healing course after plaque vaporization was also carefully followed for up to 8 weeks in atherosclerotic aortas of swine fed a fatty diet.[22] Two days following treatment, platelet-fibrin thrombi covered the vaporized crater. By 2 weeks, the crater was still depressed, but the surface had rapidly endothelialized, with some fibrin and platelets remaining. By 8 weeks, the lased site was still visible as a reendothelialized crater. Importantly, thrombogenic complications did not occur in either the monkey or the swine experiments.

Hazards of Laser

Studies in arteries of animals also uncovered many hazards of laser such as perforations, aneurysms, debris, and thrombosis.[20,23] In experiments in which a flexible laser fiber was passed into the dog coronary artery, argon energies approximating those used to vaporize plaque resulted in coronary perforation.[24] The outcome is usually cardiac tamponade, causing hemodynamic and electrical instability. Histologic examinations usually show coronary perforation and vascular hemorrhages. When laser injury extended beyond the coronary artery into the cardiac muscle, myocardial necrosis and hemorrhage were also present.

Vascular wall aneurysms can be seen in some live rabbits previously fed an atherogenic diet, and some had extensive arterial medial wall injury due to laser treatment.[20] Occasionally, intravascular lasing may lead to thrombosis, possibly by exposing subintimal structure causing platelet aggregation and fibrin deposition.

Targeting Plaque for Laser Treatment

Inside the blood vessel, the precise placement of the laser fiber upon the atherosclerotic plaque is required in order to avoid vascular damage including perforation and aneurysm formation. One method is to visualize the plaque obstruction directly with an angioscope prior to activating the laser.[25,26] With a clear view of the target, the laser light can be directed for controlled thermal ablation. Furthermore, plaque and thrombus obstructions may be distinguished.[27] The latter distinction may be noteworthy, because different energy densities may be needed for laser penetration. Moreover, angioscopy provides a topographic view and cross-sectional picture of stenoses not observed by angiography. Visualization of the proximal segments of diseased coronary arteries has been successfully attempted during cardiac catherization.[28] In the operative setting, single-plane angioscopic cross-sectional stenotic lumens correlated well with calculated angiographic luminal narrowings.[29]

Early multichannel imaging devices have been tested with efficacy in peripheral arteries of live dogs.[30] The prototype used in clogged arteries implanted with human cadaver atherosclerotic segments consisted of a catheter with channels to (1) view the diseased obstruction, (2) house the quartz fiber, and (3) deliver flush solution (saline, perfluorocarbon blood substitutes, or contrast dye) or remove particulate debris, gas, or blood by suction. A balloon around the distal catheter tip can also be inflated to halt the flow of blood momentarily. Thus, this prototype device is a demonstration of the feasibility of simultaneous in vivo visualization and laser vaporization of atheromatous disease.

Other means of targeting plaque for laser therapy include the passage of laser quartz fiber under fluoroscopic[20] or ultrasonic[31] guidance. Moreover, the use of a steerable guidewire permits the coaxial passage of the laser delivery system onto the plaque within a convoluted artery.[32]

CLINICAL STUDIES (TABLE 5-2)

Peripheral Vascular Disease

In an early study using percutaneous transluminal laser angioplasty in the clinical setting, a 7 French balloon catheter was modified by inserting a 200 μ diameter core fiber mode made of silica down its main channel.[33] The balloon was used to position the fiber so that it would be coaxial to the vascular lumen. This modified catheter was inserted through an 8 French sheath placed percutaneously in the common femoral artery and passed downward under fluoroscopy at the 90 percent obstructed left profunda femoral artery of a 62-year-old man with claudication. With an argon laser coupled to the silica fiber, a power of 2 watts was applied to bore through the stenosis, and 7 watts were used during withdrawal of fiber to enlarge the stenotic lumen. The total duration was 26 seconds. The patient was symptomatically improved on followup after 6 months, and, although postoperative angiographic documentation was lacking, improvement of blood flow was detected using a Doppler flowmeter.

In a second study, another modified balloon catheter containing a 200 μ diameter quartz fiber was used to improve the stenotic or occluded peripheral artery channel of three patients (one popliteal and two femoral arteries).[34] The catheter system was cooled by using a diluted blood perfusate comprised of 3 g/100 ml/min hemoglobin and circulated at a rate of 20 ml/min at a temperature of 20°C. In these patients, a Nd-YAG laser was coupled to the fiber and a power of 12 watts was used (three firings of 30 to 50 seconds). Although no vascular perforations occurred in any of these cases, followup results and complications were not reported.

In a third trial, argon laser recanalization was performed in the diseased peripheral (iliac, femoral, and popliteal) arteries of 16 patients.[35] A guiding catheter was inserted percutaneously into the common femoral artery over a guidewire to the site of total occlusion or through the partial obstruction. At the proximal end of the

Table 5–2. Laser Recanalization in Humans

Reference Number	Laser Used	Delivery System	Energy Parameters	No. of Pts.	Diseased Artery(ies)	Comments
33	Argon	Catheter with quartz fiber	2–7 W 26 sec	1	Profunda femoral	Procedure completed without complication.
34	Nd-YAG	Catheter with quartz fiber	12 W 30–50 sec × 3	3	Femoral, popliteal	Three arteries had laser improved channel. No major complications reported.
35	Argon	Catheter with quartz fiber	24–2904 J	16	Iliac, femoral, popliteal	Eight of 16 artery segments had laser improved channels. Complications included perforation, dissection, pain, spasm, and thrombosis.
36	Argon	Angioscopic catheter with quartz fiber	1–5 W 9 sec	5	Superficial femoral	Laser improved channel from 0 to 0.5–3 mm; perforation occurred at 3 cm from entry site.
37	Argon	Quartz fiber with metal cap	6–8 W 2–5 sec pulses	5	Femoral, popliteal	Laser improved channel from 0.6 to 1.9 mm; balloon angioplasty followed laser treatment.
38	Argon	Catheter with quartz fiber	60–1231 J	5	Coronary	Four of 5 recanalized artery segments occluded at followup. One artery had perforation.
39	CO_2	Needle probe	Not reported	3	Coronary	Five of 6 arteries recanalized by laser and no residual stenosis among patent arteries.

guiding catheter was a Y connector that allowed the fiber to be inserted through one port and saline perfusate through the other. The delivery system was composed of a 400 μ silica fiber with metallic marker. In total occlusion, the delivery system was passed through the guiding catheter until the fiber tip extended 1 to 2 mm beyond the catheter and directly into the occlusion. Under direct fluoroscopic visualization using contrast dye injections, the catheter was advanced into the lesions. In partial obstructed vessels, the laser was activated as the fiber or catheter was withdrawn. Total energies used ranged from 24 to 2904 joules, depending on the lesion. The totally or partially obstructed lumen was improved in 8 of 16 patients treated with laser recanalization. In all but three patients, laser recanalization was followed by percutaneous balloon angioplasty to further enlarge the lumen. Complications included mechanical or laser perforation (three patients), dissection (two), pain during laser activation (7), spasm (four), and thrombosis (one). The latter three complications were believed to be related to the high total energies used, generating high temperatures at the lased site.

In an intraoperative study, an optical fiber probe (1 or 2 mm tip diameter) coupled to an argon laser was applied under angioscopic guidance to recanalize occluded superficial femoral artery in five patients just prior to bypass graft surgery.[36] Laser power output varied between 1 and 5 watts for an average duration of 9 seconds. After lasing, the treated arterial segment was excised for histologic studies. Of the five arteries treated by the laser probe, all had smooth recanalized channels with minimal charring between 0.5 and 3 mm in diameter. However, every artery demonstrated perforation at 3 cm from the entry site.

In still another investigation, a laser-heated metallic cap was passed percutaneously and applied in severely atherosclerotic peripheral arteries to create a small channel prior to the balloon angioplasty procedure.[37] Five diseased arteries were treated by an argon laser-heated metallic tip probe (6 to 8 watts, 2 to 5 sec pulses). The mean luminal diameter was reportedly increased from 0.6 to 1.9 mm following laser treatment and to 3.3 mm following balloon angioplasty. Vascular perforation by laser was not reported.

Coronary Artery Disease

In a preliminary study, argon laser energies were applied in native coronary stenotic arteries of five patients during open-chest saphenous vein bypass surgery. All patients had significant stenotic lesions (80 to 95 percent) in the left anterior descending (two patients) and right coronary arteries (three patients).[38] A catheter with an 85 μ quartz fiber delivered argon laser energies to the area of obstruction proximal to the bypass graft site. Total energies of 60 to 1231 joules were applied, and there was one mechanical or laser perforation. One patient had severe thermal damage (1231 joules) to the medial wall, and an excisional biopsy was carried out. At follow-up within 1 month, all but one of the lased native vessels were occluded.

In another report, laser endarterectomy was performed in six coronary arteries of three patients undergoing bypass surgery.[39] Atherosclerotic plaque was vaporized using a hand-held carbon dioxide laser. A laser probe needle, 3 inches long with an inner diameter of 0.9 mm, was inserted into the diseased coronary artery. At restudy 1 week later, five of six lased arteries were patent with little residual stenosis. All bypass grafts remained patent, and arterial perforation was not observed.

FUTURE TECHNOLOGY

Much of the technology of the future will be concentrated on improving the safety and efficacy of laser recanalization, specifically the fiberoptic delivery of laser energies onto the plaque obstruction without damaging the vascular wall. Multichannel fiberscopes to vaporize and lase the diseased lesion simultaneously need greater flexibility, ability to angulate, and be smaller in design so as to pass into the coronary arteries.

The application of specific agents and dyes to stain plaque so as to enhance laser absorption by the plaque will also need exploration.[5,40] Application of fluorescein and Sudan black dyes onto the obstruction permits greater thermal injury to the plaque than either saline or blood. Furthermore, hematoporphyrin derivative (HpD), an agent used in the photoradiation therapy of cancer, can be selectively taken up by atherosclerotic plaque.[41,42] In animals with atherosclerosis treated with intravenous HpD, a fiberoptic catheter delivering a low-power beam from a tunable dye laser driven by an argon laser destroyed the pathologic tissue by causing a photochemical reaction. However, further research is needed to determine whether HpD therapy can be applied in human atherosclerotic obstructions.

CONCLUSION

Inasmuch as there are approximately 4.5 million Americans with angina pectoris or history of myocardial infarction, or both, and the annual economic loss for Americans, as a result of disability, runs into multibillions of dollars, the quest continues for modes of treatment that are safe, effective, less invasive, and inexpensive. Laser recanalization fulfills many of these needs, and its potential is only beginning to be realized. Through a tiny flexible fiber, laser can be transmitted inside the artery to vaporize atherosclerotic plaque obstruction. The goal of advancing this technology is to replace the costly intraoperative bypass procedure and its inherent extended length of recovery. During the process of achieving this goal, it is hoped that it can be used in conjunction with open-chest surgery by laser recanalizing occluded bypass grafts or diseased native arteries, thereby eliminating the extraction of vein grafts from the extremities. Additionally, it may be applied to assist balloon angioplasty in producing a vaporized channel large enough to accommodate the passage of a balloon catheter, or be used to thermally fuse the disrupted plaque and tears within the arterial wall following balloon angioplasty. However, early in vitro and in vivo studies reveal the current limitations and potential risks of the technology and recent clinical trials reflect these concerns. Therefore, much more research and technical advances are needed before laser recanalization can become an accepted therapeutic modality for obstructive vascular disease.

ACKNOWLEDGMENTS

The authors thank Dr. Andrew Kung and John Rink for their advice, the St. Mary's Foundation for its support, and Ms. Leslie Silvernail for her editorial assistance.

REFERENCES

1. Lee, G, Ikeda, RM, Chan, MD, et al: Recanalization of coronary atherosclerotic obstruction by laser radiation. Eur Heart J 6:91, 1985.
2. Eldar, M, Battler, A, Neufeld, HN, et al: Transluminal carbon dioxide laser catheter angioplasty for dissolution of atherosclerotic plaques. J Am Coll Cardiol 3:135, 1984.
3. Lee, G, Ikeda, RM, Chan, MC, et al: Dissolution of human atherosclerotic disease by fiberoptic laser-heated metal cautery cap. Am Heart J 107:777, 1984.
4. Lee, G, Ikeda, RM, Kozina, J, et al: Laser dissolution of coronary atherosclerotic obstruction. Am Heart J 102:1074, 1981.
5. Abela, GS, Normann, S, Cohen, D, et al: Effects of carbon dioxide, Nd-YAG and argon laser radiation on coronary atheromatous plaques. Am J Cardiol 50:1199, 1982.
6. Choy, DSJ, Stertzer, S, Rotterdam, HZ, et al: Laser coronary angioplasty: Experience with 9 cadaver hearts. Am J Cardiol 50:1209, 1982.
7. Lee, G, Ikeda, R, Herman, I, et al: The qualitative effects of laser irradiation on human arteriosclerotic disease. Am Heart J 105:885, 1983.

8. Isner, JM, Clarke, RH, Donaldson, RF, et al: Identification of photoproducts liberated by in vitro laser irradiation of atherosclerotic plaque, calcified cardiac valves and myocardium. Am J Cardiol 55:1192, 1985.
9. Kaminow, IP, Wiesenfeld, JM, and Choy, DSJ: Argon laser disintegration of thrombus and atherosclerotic plaque. Applied Optics 23:1301, 1984.
10. Lee, G, Chan, MC, Ikeda, RM, et al: The status and future of laser angioplasty. Seminars in Interventional Radiology 3:11, 1986.
11. Shelton, ME, Hoxworth, B, Shelton, JA, et al: A new model to study quantitative effects of laser angioplasty on human atherosclerotic plaque. J Am Coll Cardiol 7:909, 1986.
12. Grundfest, W, Litvack, F, Forrester, J, et al: Pulsed ultraviolet lasers provide precise control of atheroma ablation. Circulation 70(Suppl II):35, 1984.
13. Isner, JM, Clarke, RH, Donaldson, RF, et al: The excimer laser: Gross, light microscopic, and ultrastructural analysis of potential advantages for use in laser therapy of cardiovascular disease. Circulation 70(Suppl II):35, 1984.
14. Deckelbaum, LI, Isner, JM, Donaldson, RF, et al: Use of pulsed energy delivery to minimize tissue injury resulting from carbon dioxide laser irradiation of cardiovascular tissues. J Am Coll Cardiol 7:898, 1986.
15. Lee, G, Chan, MD, Ikeda, RM, et al: Applicability of laser to assist coronary balloon angioplasty. Am Heart J 110:1233, 1985.
16. Lee, G, Ikeda, RM, Joye, JA, et al: Evaluation of transluminal angioplasty of chronic artery stenosis. Value and limitations assessed in fresh human cadaver hearts. Circulation 61:77, 1980.
17. Block, PC, Baughman, KL, Pasternak, RC, et al: Transluminal angioplasty: Correlation of morphologic and angiographic findings in an experimental model. Circulation 61:778, 1980.
18. Lee, G, Ikeda, R, Joye, JA, et al: Pathoanatomic changes achieved by transluminal coronary angioplasty. In Mason, DT and Collins, JJ, Jr (eds): Myocardial Revascularization. Medical and Surgical Advances in Coronary Disease. Yorke Medical Books, New York, 1981.
19. Hiehle, JF, Bourgelais, DBC, Shapshay, S, et al: Nd:YAG laser fusion of human atheromatous plaque-arterial wall separations in vitro. Am J Cardiol 56:953, 1985.
20. Lee, G, Ikeda, RM, Theis, JH, et al: Acute and chronic complications of laser angioplasty. Vascular wall damage and formation of aneurysms in the atherosclerotic rabbit. Am J Cardiol 53:290, 1984.
21. Theis, JH, Lee, G, Chan, MC, et al: Laser treatment of atherosclerosis in the monkey: Reendothelialization without thrombosis effected by fiberoptic metal cap. J Am Coll Cardiol 7:212A, 1986.
22. Gerrity, RG, Loop, FD, Golding, LAR, et al: Arterial response to laser operation for removal of atherosclerotic plaques. J Thorac Cardiovasc Surg 85:409, 1983.
23. Lee, G, Ikeda, RM, Chan, MC, et al: Limitations, risks and complications of laser recanalization: A cautious approach warranted. Am J Cardiol 56:181, 1985.
24. Lee, G, Seckinger, D, Chan, MC, et al: Potential complications of coronary laser angioplasty. Am Heart J 106:1577, 1984.
25. Lee, G, Ikeda, RM, Dwyer, RM, et al: Feasibility of intravascular laser irradiation for in vivo visualization and therapy of cardiocirculatory diseases. Am Heart J 103:1076, 1982.
26. Lee, G, Ikeda, RM, Stobbe, D, et al: Laser irradiation of human atherosclerotic obstructive disease: Simultaneous visualization and vaporization achieved by a dual fiberoptic catheter. Am Heart J 105:163, 1983.
27. Shure, D, Gregoratos, G, and Moser, KM: Fiberoptic angioscopy: Role in the diagnosis of chronic pulmonary arterial obstruction. Ann Intern Med 103:844, 1985.
28. Spears, JR, Spokojny, AM, and Marais, J: Coronary angioscopy during cardiac catheterization. J Am Coll Cardiol 6:93, 1985.
29. Lee, G, Garcia, JM, Corso, PJ, et al: Correlation of coronary angioscopy to angiographic findings in patients with coronary artery disease. Am J Cardiol 58:238, 1986.
30. Lee, G, Ikeda, RM, Stobbe, D, et al: Intraoperative use of dual fiberoptic catheter for simultaneous in vivo visualization and laser vaporization of peripheral atherosclerotic obstructive disease. Cathet Cardiovasc Diagn 10:11, 1984.
31. Bommer, WJ, Lee, G, Rebeck, K, et al: Two-dimensional echocardiography of argon-laser vapor trails: Monitoring of catheter position and prevention of potential complications. Circulation 68:259, 1983.
32. Lee, G, Chan, MC, Ikeda, RM, et al: Intravascular steerable guidewire for fiberoptic laser-heated metal cautery cap in dissolution of human atherosclerotic coronary disease. Am Heart J 110:1304, 1985.

33. Ginsburg, R, Kim, DS, Guthaner, D, et al: Salvage of an ischemic limb by laser angioplasty: Description of a new technique. Clin Cardiol 7:54, 1984.
34. Geschwind, H, Boussignac, G, Teisseire, B, et al: Percutaneous transluminal laser angioplasty in man. (Letters to the Editor.) Lancet 1:844, 1984.
35. Ginsburg, R, Wexler, L, Mitchell, RS, et al: Percutaneous transluminal laser angioplasty for treatment of peripheral vascular disease. Clinical experience with 16 patients. Radiology 156:619, 1985.
36. Abela, GS, Seeger, JM, Fenech, A, et al: Laser recanalization of peripheral arteries in man: A preliminary report. Circulation 72(Suppl III):303, 1985.
37. Sanborn, TA, Cumberland, DC, Tayler, DI, et al: Human percutaneous laser thermal angioplasty. Circulation 72(Suppl III):303, 1985.
38. Choy, DSJ, Stertzer, SH, Myler, RK, et al: Human coronary laser recanalization. Clin Cardiol 7:377, 1984.
39. Livesay, JJ, Leachman, DR, Hogan, PJ, et al: Preliminary report on laser coronary endarterectomy in patients. Circulation 72(Suppl III):302, 1985.
40. Chan, MC, Lee, G, Seckinger, DL, et al: Pretreatment with vital dyes to enhance or attenuate argon laser energy absorption in blood vessels. Circulation 70(Suppl II):298, 1984.
41. Spears, JR, Serur, J, Shropshire, D, et al: Fluorescence of experimental atheromatous plaques with hematoporphyrin derivative. J Clin Invest 71:395, 1983.
42. Hundley, RF, Spears, JR, and Weinstein, R: Photodynamic cytolysis of arterial smooth muscle cells in vitro: Implications for laser angioplasty. J Am Coll Cardiol 5:408, 1985.

PART 2

Pathology of Myocarditis and Cardiomyopathy

CHAPTER 6

Biopsy Diagnosis of Myocarditis*

Charles C. Marboe, M.D.
John J. Fenoglio, Jr., M.D.

The term "myocarditis" as a descriptive phrase has a clear meaning: inflammation in the myocardium. It is the clinical correlation and meaning for this histologic observation that has a varied and confusing history. The term was introduced by Sobernheim[1,2] in 1837 and after Virchow's publication of *Cellular Pathologie* in 1858 enjoyed wide application, becoming synonymous with all "nonvalvular heart disease." The association with certain infectious diseases (scarlet fever and typhus) was recognized by Romberg in 1891, and the entity of isolated idiopathic interstitial myocarditis was described by Fiedler[3] in 1899. However, many detailed accounts of "myocarditis" are, in retrospect, recognized to be descriptions of acute myocardial infarcts, and early descriptions of "chronic myocarditis" also include the effects and results of vascular disease in the heart. Indeed, the risk factors for "myocarditis" included those we now recognize for atherosclerosis. Failure to differentiate the effects of ischemia from infectious or idiopathic events stemmed from an inability to recognize the pathology of ischemic necrosis in the myocardium. Relief from this ever-increasing application of "myocarditis" came with the keen insight of Herrick,[4] who recognized and, in 1912, wrote about the clinical effects of acute coronary thrombosis and the associated acute infarct of the myocardium. With this discovery seemingly explaining inflammation in the myocardium, the term "myocarditis" fell into disrepute and became a nonentity, with rare exceptions in rheumatic fever and diphtheria. This change allowed accurate and specific diagnosis of ischemic heart disease and redirected clinical interest to its study, which to this day has flourished in clinical-pathologic correlations. With the better definition of infarct pathology and its clinical correlates, however, in 1941 Saphir[5] was able to define histologically cases that had no clinical correlate typical of ischemic disease. He could then study the clinical aspects of this group and finally attempt a classification of myocarditis based on etiology. Saphir, however, also realized that there was a "gap between the abundance of anatomic changes in the myocardium and their apparent clinical insignificance," and conversely that "there is sometimes definite clinical evidence of myocar-

*Supported in part by grant HL 26588 from the National Heart, Lung, and Blood Institute.

ditis. . . . Ironically enough, such a diagnosis is rarely, if ever, confirmed by a pathologist." The correlation of anatomic evidence with clinical evidence in myocarditis has long been a problem. Burch and Ray[6] in 1948 outlined the clinical manifestations of myocarditis and, although concentrating on acute disease, recognized acute and chronic types of inflammation having different clinical courses. In 1931 Boikan[7] described a "myocarditis perniciosa" with a course of greater than 4 months' duration, and in 1960 Kline and Saphir[8] detailed the anatomic and clinical aspects of what they titled "chronic pernicious myocarditis." Once ischemic causes for myocardial inflammation were separated from myocarditis, researchers saw the remaining cases as heterogeneous and have been drawn to subclassify these cases, in the hopes of both gaining understanding and providing useful information to aid in the care of patients with "myocarditis."

DIAGNOSTIC CRITERIA FOR ENDOMYOCARDIAL BIOPSY

The study of human myocarditis accelerated following the introduction of the endomyocardial bioptome in 1962.[9] Anatomic confirmation of clinically suspected myocarditis was suddenly possible prior to postmortem examination. Studies of the natural history of histologically confirmed myocarditis began, and the contribution of clinically unsuspected myocarditis to entities such as dilated cardiomyopathy was assessed. While these studies have flourished, the problem of the imperfect correspondence of clinical and pathologic diagnosis has persisted.

The sudden onset of congestive heart failure in previously asymptomatic persons having no evidence of valvular or coronary heart disease may be due to myocarditis; endomyocardial biopsy is frequently performed to confirm this diagnosis. Histologically defined myocarditis has been diagnosed in 17 to 30 percent[10–12] of patients with clinically suspected myocarditis and in 41 percent of patients with acute (duration less than 6 months) dilated cardiomyopathies.[13] In one study[14] of idiopathic dilated cardiomyopathy, the incidence of inflammatory cell infiltrates in the myocardium was even higher—63 percent—with half the patients having congestive heart failure of more than 6 months' duration and half with symptoms for 1 week to 4 months; in another study,[10] only 12 percent of patients with dilated cardiomyopathy were diagnosed on biopsy as having myocarditis. In unselected series of endomyocardial biopsies, myocarditis is present in 6 to 43 percent of patients.[15–19]

There are many possible causes of this wide variation in reported rates of myocarditis and the disparity between clinical and pathologic diagnosis of myocarditis. The lack of specific symptoms and noninvasive tests may lead to the clinical overdiagnosis of the disease. Limitations in the biopsy technique, including the focal nature of the disease, the limited size of the biopsy tissue, the number of pieces taken, and the timing of the biopsy in relation to maximal myocardial inflammation may contribute to failure of the biopsy to confirm the presence of myocarditis. Finally, the criteria for the morphologic diagnosis of myocarditis may be too imprecise to yield clinically useful information.

Technical Considerations

Myocarditis may be a focal disease, and efforts must be made to minimize the likelihood of a falsely negative biopsy. Sample size is one consideration; the modified Caves-Schultz-Stanford bioptome avulses a relatively large piece of endomyocardium, whereas other devices, such as the disposable Cordis or pediatric Olympus or Machida or the King's or left ventricular bioptomes retrieve smaller fragments. The most important factor in sampling is the number of pieces taken at the time of biopsy. We now recommend, whenever myocarditis is strongly suspected, that six individual pieces of tissue be examined. This may not always be possible for clinical or technical reasons, but we agree with the recommendation[20] that three is the minimum number of pieces that should be obtained. Special studies, to be described subsequently, are encouraged for teaching or research purposes, but optional for diagnosis; it is important, however, that sections from those pieces be examined by light microscopy or that additional pieces be taken to meet the minimum number of pieces reviewed under the microscope. We study ribbons of tissue from three different levels in the paraffin block of tissue. A good connective tissue stain such as Masson's trichrome is essential for assessment of the amount and distribution of interstitial tissue and aids in identification of damaged or degenerating myocytes. The elastic van Gieson stain of Miller[21] has been advocated[22] as a more appropriate stain for the specific demonstration of collagen. Blanks for special stains are cut from the block at the time the routine sections are cut, avoiding loss of tissue in trimming for recuts.

The amount of clinical information known by the pathologist when first examining the slides is a matter of personal preference. However, no diagnosis should be rendered, and none should be expected by a cardiologist, unless certain basic clinical details have been reviewed. These details are pertinent in ruling out other processes that histologically mimic myocarditis. The information must include age, sex, duration of symptoms, ejection fraction (preferably not by echocardiogram), arrhythmias, echocardiographic or catheterization data on ventricular size and function, status of coronary arteries (by angiogram) and presence of risk factors for atherosclerosis, history of myocardial infarct, recent viral illness, recent pregnancy, drug history (including alcohol consumption, pressor administration, hypersensitivity-reaction-associated drugs, controlled substances, immunosuppressives and chemotherapeutic agents), and other systemic illnesses (particularly infectious or autoimmune).

Definition

Myocarditis is characterized by an inflammatory infiltrate that is directly associated with myocyte damage; this characteristic occurs in the absence of changes typical of ischemic damage associated with vascular disease. This definition, including special studies, and the effect of the factors that may produce false-negative or false-positive results, will be discussed hereafter.

The Inflammatory Infiltrate

The extent and composition of the inflammatory infiltrate should be described. The distribution and intensity of the infiltrate is best judged at low-power examination and may be classified as diffuse or focal (patchy) and semiquantitatively as mild, moderate, or severe. The cellular components of the infiltrate should be characterized.

In some instances of acute myocarditis, polymorphonuclear leukocytes are present, but lymphocytes and macrophages usually predominate. Eosinophils are rarely seen, and their presence should stimulate thorough searches of the biopsy for parasites and of the medical record for possible drug-associated hypersensitivity. Myocardial damage associated with hypereosinophilic states should be ruled out.

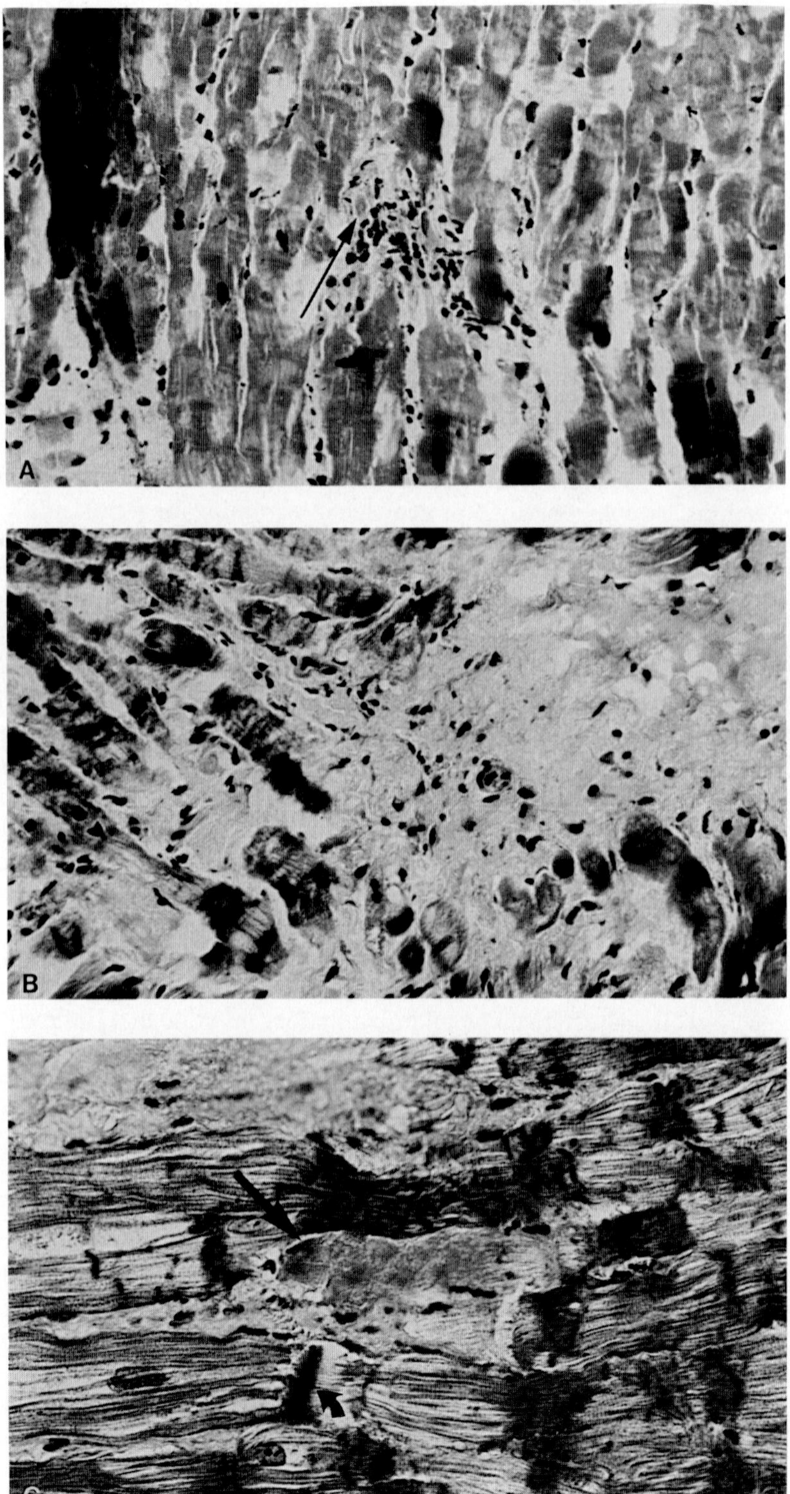

Figure 6–1. See legend on facing page.

Giant cells may be present in some florid cases of idiopathic myocarditis and may be present in sarcoidosis and hypersensitivity, rheumatic and rheumatoid myocarditis, as well as in myocardial infection by tuberculosis or fungi. Granulomas may be present in these latter entities as well as in visceral larva migrans, Trichinella spiralis, and rarely in Schistosoma mansoni infection,[23] Chagas' disease, and foreign body reaction around echinococcal cysts.

Myocyte Damage

Myocyte damage is integral to the diagnosis of myocarditis and helps differentiate it from other cardiac infiltrates such as those associated with lymphoma or infectious mononucleosis. The damage may consist of necrosis with myocyte debris, degeneration with altered staining characteristics (often better seen as a blue-grey appearance on Masson's trichrome) or vacuolization, a ragged frayed appearance of the margins of the myocyte,[24] or disruption of the cell with infiltration of lymphocytes (Fig. 6–1). If the degeneration has the appearance of coagulative necrosis and there are polymorphonuclear leukocytes in the accompanying infiltrate, ischemic damage or pressor effect or even seeding of the myocardium by septic emboli must be considered. The staining irregularities and apparent disruption of myocytes by contraction-band artifact should not be mistaken for myocyte degeneration. Contraction bands are virtually ubiquitous in endomyocardial biopsies.

The histologic appearance of the myocardium adjacent to damaged myocytes in myocarditis is a topic of some debate. The "Dallas criteria"[20] (described in detail later) suggest that myocarditis be superimposed on a background of normal myocardium. This finding is used to avoid confusion with focal infiltrates and myocyte damage in cardiomyopathies, in which there is interstitial fibrosis and myocyte hypertrophy. In our experience, however, patients who initially have clear-cut "active myocarditis with fibrosis" on a background of otherwise-normal myocardium may have subsequent biopsies that show marked hypertrophy of myocytes and interstitial fibrosis. The presence of hypertrophy may simply reflect the timing of the biopsy in the course of myocarditis.

CLASSIFICATION

Using the aforementioned diagnostic criteria, "myocarditis" is a pathologic term that can be both specific and generic. It *specifically* refers to inflammation and myocyte damage, of the nonischemic type, in the myocardium. It is *general* to the extent that many factors may cause this histologic reaction. The classification of myocarditis has generally been based on either of two approaches: chronology or etiology. The chronologic classification schemes[6,7,16,25] rely on histologic distinctions, and they correlate clinical course with pathologic features. The goal is to make the

---

Figure 6–1. *A,* In active myocarditis, inflammatory infiltrates are associated with myocyte damage. Here, portions of myocardial fibers have been reduced to debris *(arrow).* (Hematoxylin-phloxine-saffron [HPS] stain; magnification ×250, reduced 10 percent.) *B,* In another area of the same biopsy there is healing with fibrosis and persistence of some inflammatory cells, which appear to be engulfing myocyte debris. (HPS stain; magnification ×250, reduced 10 percent.) *C,* Myocyte damage may take different forms. In an additional focus in the same biopsy, this degenerating myocyte, with altered staining characteristics, was present *(long arrow).* The contraction band artifact so commonly seen in endomyocardial biopsies is prominent here *(short arrow).* (Masson trichrome stain; magnification ×400, reduced 10 percent.)

biopsy useful in determining an individual patient's prognosis. With this approach,[16] we identified three clinicopathologic groups of patients with biopsy-proven myocarditis and labeled them "acute," "rapidly progressive," and "chronic," without reference to etiology or pathogenesis. It is very difficult to know the complete natural history of the disease, for the appearance of symptoms may be insidious, developing only at variable periods after the true onset of the disease. The advantage of this chronologic form of classification is its ability to offer suggestions to the cardiologist and patient about the probable course of the disease and the likelihood of response to immunosuppressive therapy. The limitation of the scheme is its reliance on relatively subtle distinctions in histology to differentiate the "rapidly progressive" from the "chronic" myocarditis groups. With the Dallas classification,[20] both groups are subsumed under "active myocarditis with fibrosis." The histologic distinction between the groups lies in the greater extent of damage and the numerous patches of fibrosis, consisting of a central fibrous scar surrounded by looser connective tissue (granulation tissue) with fibroblasts, capillaries, and mononuclear inflammatory cells, seen in the cases that subsequently follow a "rapidly progressive" course to death, usually in 2 years. This aggravated form of myocarditis has been previously recognized; Boikan[7] and Kline and Saphir[8] described an identical pathologic and clinical form of myocarditis, which they classified as "chronic pernicious myocarditis."

Burch and Ray[6] also preferred the clinical utility of the simple division of myocarditis into "acute" and "chronic" clinicopathologic forms, which "differ essentially in degree and/or severity of muscle destruction, rapidity of course, severity of clinical manifestations and gravity of prognosis." Similarly, Lustock and coworkers[25] classified myocarditis by clinical course into "acute," "recurrent," and "chronic" (persistent) types that had varied pathology. The subacute stage included lymphocytes, monocytes, and fibroblasts with edema and areas of early fibrosis. The Lustock group thought the Burch and Ray classification concentrated solely on the clinical severity of the initial illness and neglected the features of recurrence and chronicity often present in myocarditis. To most authors choosing a chronologic or pathologic classification, the schemes based on etiologic considerations prove "unwieldy because of the multiplicity and complexity of underlying causes."[25]

One example of an etiologic classification was proposed by Gore and Saphir[26] in 1947. They divided myocarditis by etiology into those following infectious diseases (with or without endocarditis); those associated with specific agents, chemical or hypersensitivity; and isolated (unassociated with any known illness). The grouping was not considered sharp and distinctive, nor was it complete; limitations of medical knowledge prevented cataloging of entities such as sarcoid heart disease and infectious mononucleosis. One strength of this etiologic classification is the recognition that many diseases may be complicated by myocarditis, and, to the extent that these diseases are treatable, some instances of myocarditis might be prevented. It should also be noted that the authors reported in an era when they thought it crucial to stress "the importance of overcoming the prevailing prejudice against the diagnosis of myocarditis. . . ."

The most recent classification scheme[20] was developed by a group of eight pathologists in 1984 in conjunction with the American College of Cardiology annual meeting in Dallas, Texas. This system relies on morphology alone and sets forth histopathologic criteria for the diagnosis of myocarditis but does not comment on natural history, etiology, or implications for therapy. Briefly outlined, the classification is as follows: Active myocarditis is defined as a "process characterized by an inflammatory infiltrate of the myocardium with necrosis and/or degeneration of adjacent myocytes not typical of the ischemic damage associated with coronary artery disease." As the system has no inherent suppositions about the time course of myocarditis, separate terminologies were proposed for the initial and all subsequent biopsies. On initial endomyocardial biopsy, the possible diagnoses are (1) active myocarditis with or without fibrosis; (2) borderline myocarditis, in which an inflammatory infiltrate but no myocyte necrosis is present (this is a controversial group and rebiopsy may be indicated); and (3) no myocarditis. All subsequent biopsies are classified as ongoing (persistent) myocarditis with or without fibrosis, resolving (healing) myocarditis with or without fibrosis, or resolved (healed) myocarditis with or without fibrosis. The microscopic description should include (1) a subclassification of the inflammatory infiltrate by cell type (lymphocytic, neutrophilic, eosinophilic, and so on); (2) the amount and distribution of the infiltrate (mild, moderate, or severe and focal, confluent, or diffuse, respectively, as outlined previously);[27] and (3) the amount and distribution of fibrosis, if present, including its type as endocardial, replacement, or interstitial.

The denotation "borderline myocarditis" has the greatest potential for confusion. As mentioned earlier, it includes biopsies in which there is a scant, interstitial mononuclear cell infiltrate, but no myocyte necrosis. The paraffin blocks from these cases should be recut at multiple deeper levels, with the hope of demonstrating definite "active myocarditis" adjacent to the infiltrates. If no myocyte damage can be found and there is a strong clinical suspicion of myocarditis, repeat biopsy is recommended to attempt to overcome what may be sampling error. Preliminary experience suggests that in this situation, rebiopsy will document active myocarditis in the majority of persons with borderline myocarditis on initial biopsy. Special studies, such as immunohistochemical staining of lymphocytes in the biopsy, do not appear to be as helpful as rebiopsy in these cases.

It is recommended by the Dallas group that biopsy reports be phrased in this histologic terminology, after careful consideration to exclude lesions that may mimic myocarditis. This will provide uniform diagnostic criteria reflecting the morphology of the disease as seen on biopsy. The clinical correlations and prognostic implications of these histologic findings are yet to be determined; but with this standard terminology, valid comparison of different medical centers' experience should be possible.

Most cases of myocarditis in humans are presumed to be viral in etiology and autoimmune in pathogenesis. As noted subsequently in the section on special studies, techniques in molecular biology may enhance the identification of associated viruses such as coxsackievirus B. Excellent studies in animal models[28–31] are the basis for the presumed autoimmune mechanism of myocardial damage, and we anticipate that in the next decade the application of the tools of molecular biology and immunology will facilitate studies in humans to test the applicability of the models. In the absence of proven etiology, the descriptive diagnoses of the Dallas histopathologic scheme are strongly recommended and encouraged. Uniform diagnostic criteria will facilitate comparison of material from different centers and encourage multicenter studies, which will be crucial in testing the efficacy of present and new forms of therapy. The clinical utility and correlations of the histopathologic groups defined by the Dallas criteria are not yet determined. For example, we have identified three clinical subgroups within the group of "active myocarditis with fibrosis": one group experiencing "spontaneous" improvement with standard medical therapy (digitalis, diuretics, peripheral vasodilator therapy),[32] and the two groups previously designated[16] as "rapidly progressive" and "chronic" myocarditis. Special studies and further subclassification by routine light microscopy should be continued in the attempt to separate groups by prognosis and response to treatment.

DIFFERENTIAL DIAGNOSIS

In some instances there are histologic features in the endomyocardial biopsy that will suggest an etiology for myocarditis. There may also be features that can help identify lesions that mimic myocarditis. When a specific type of myocarditis is identified or an etiology for myocarditis is determined, the diagnosis may be phrased in a manner analogous to the specific heart muscle diseases, such as "Toxoplasma heart disease," or as a combination of Dallas' histologic terminology with the etiology, such as "active myocarditis with fibrosis, secondary to Toxoplasma gondii."

Ischemic Damage and Pressor Effects

These two forms of myocardial damage must be distinguished from myocarditis. The histology of ischemic damage is well known now in postmortem specimens, and the key features must be recognized in biopsy specimens. In the acute phase, coagulation necrosis of myocytes is accompanied by an infiltrate of polymorphonuclear leukocytes at the periphery of the lesion. The distribution of the lesions may be helpful in diagnosis; acute ischemic necrosis may be subendocardial in distribution, but infarcts with necrosis and reactive inflammation seldom involve the endocardium and subendocardium other than in association with overlying mural thrombus.

Organizing lesions contain histiocytes, hemosiderin, and granulation tissue, and increasing amounts of fibrous tissue as healing occurs. A biopsy from the edge of the lesion may resemble myocarditis. This is one reason a patient's risk factors for atherosclerosis and the status of extramural coronary arteries should be known prior to a final diagnosis. We survey the biopsy for evidence of small (intramyocardial) vessel disease and the distribution of fibrous tissue, which may, if it is perivascular, interfascicular, and subendocardial, suggest ischemic damage. In the setting of a history of myocardial infarct, of demonstrated coronary artery disease or evidence of ischemic damage in the biopsy, we are very reluctant to make a diagnosis of myocarditis. Biopsies with infiltrates and myocyte necrosis from patients in this clinical setting are often diagnostic dilemmas.

The inflammation and myofibrillar degeneration associated with catecholamine toxicity has been well described.[33,34] Briefly, contraction bands are prominent in the early phase, and myocardial cell nuclei become pyknotic and disappear. A basophilic, granular material may be present within cells and presumably is mitochondrial calcification. Interstitial cells are prominent, with a predominance of fibroblasts and histiocytes, but only occasional polymorphonuclear leukocytes. The lesions are sometimes in the immediate subendocardial zone. If patients with congestive heart failure have been treated aggressively with catecholamines prior to the biopsy, this toxicity must not be mistaken for myocarditis. The contribution of this form of damage due to endogenous catecholamine release to the pathogenesis of "idiopathic" cardiomyopathy has not been determined.

Hypersensitivity

Hypersensitivity myocarditis is characterized by a patchy interstitial inflammatory infiltrate with prominent eosinophils and only focal myocytolysis (Fig. 6–2).

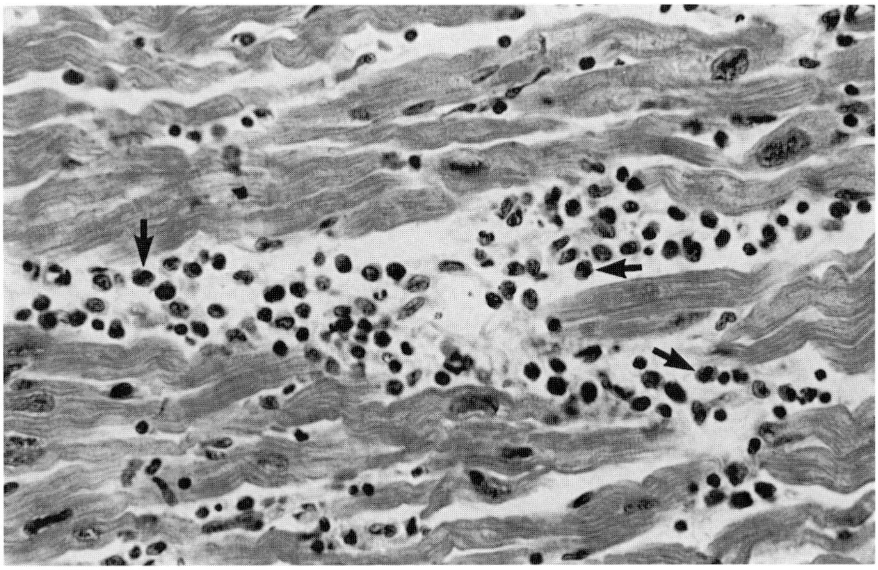

Figure 6-2. The inflammatory infiltrate in hypersensitivity myocarditis includes lymphocytes, plasma cells, monocytes, and eosinophils *(arrows)*. The infiltrate is predominantly interstitial and may also be perivascular. Focal myocytolysis is usually present; but disrupted, necrotic myocardial cells with smudging of cytoplasm and loss of nuclei are extremely uncommon. The myocarditis in this illustrated case was apparently associated with metolazone, a diuretic that is also a sulfonamide derivative. (HPS, magnification ×250.)

The infiltrate often has a perivascular distribution; vasculitis of the hypersensitivity type associated with drug therapy is seen in some patients, but necrotizing vessel lesions are not a feature of the disease.[35] There may be atypical lymphocytes in the infiltrate. Many drugs can be associated with hypersensitivity myocarditis. The presence of eosinophils in a biopsy should stimulate a thorough review of the patient's drug history, with particular attention to newer agents that may be chemically related to compounds known to be associated with hypersensitivity reactions, such as sulfonamides or methyldopa.

Giant Cell Myocarditis

This fulminant form of myocarditis is typically a fatal disease in young to middle-aged adults and has a distinctive histology. Multinucleated giant cells are present, particularly at the margin of zones of myocardial necrosis (Fig. 6-3). Recent studies with immunohistochemical techniques have shown the giant cells to contain intracellular enzymes[36] and bear surface antigens[37] consistent with macrophage rather than muscle cell lineage. The inflammatory infiltrate is rich in histiocytes and eosinophils, with lymphocytes also present; fibrosis is not present in acute disease but may appear in patients who survive. If significant endocardial fibrosis develops in subsequent biopsies, a form of endomyocardial fibrosis should be considered.

Toxic Myocarditis

In toxic myocarditis there is extensive myocyte necrosis, the infiltrate is predominantly neutrophilic, and lesions are at different stages of development in the biopsy. There may also be a necrotizing vasculitis in addition to the perivascular infiltrate.

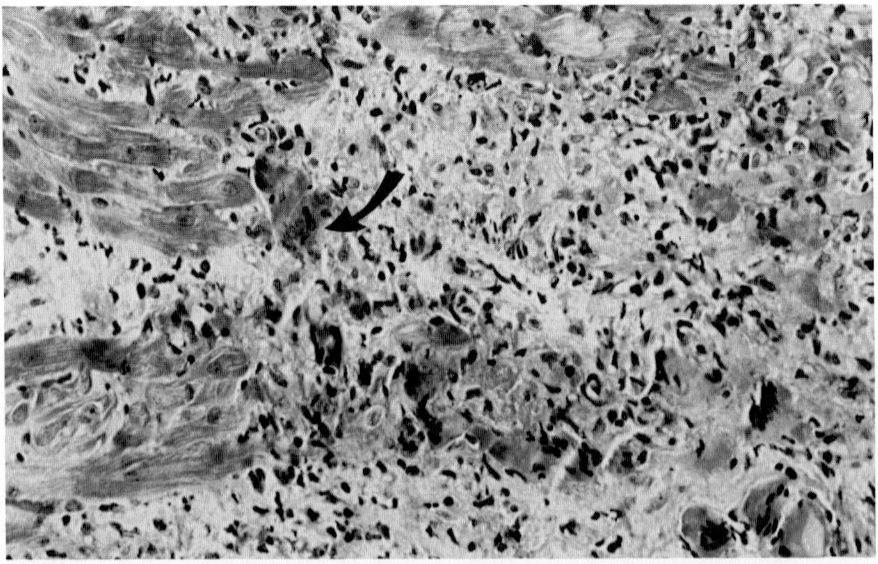

Figure 6–3. In this fulminant myocarditis, a giant cell *(arrow)* is present at the margin of a large area of myocardial necrosis. Immunohistochemical studies suggest a macrophage, rather than muscle cell, origin for these multinucleate cells. (HPS, magnification ×250.)

These features help distinguish this cumulative, dose-related form of myocardial damage from the myocarditis of the hypersensitivity type. Compounds that have been associated with toxic myocarditis include anthracyclines, arsenicals, carbon monoxide, catecholamines (described earlier), chloroquine, cyclophosphamide, emetine, hydrocarbons, lithium carbonate, phenothiazines, scorpion-sting toxin, and thyroid hormone, among others.

Collagen-Vascular Disease

Myocarditis may complicate systemic lupus erythematosus, juvenile or adult Still's disease, polymyositis-dermatomyositis, rheumatoid arthritis, Kawasaki disease, or giant cell arteritis. Adventitial fibrosis and a non-necrotizing mononuclear cell vasculitis involving small arterioles or, occasionally, small veins may be present. These findings differ from the typical vascular lesions of scleroderma, which include medial hypertrophy and an adventitial fibrosis, most prominent around small arteries and arterioles, with an "onion skin" appearance. The vessel lesions of panarteritis nodosa and rheumatoid arthritis are present in medium and large arteries, which are not seen in endomyocardial biopsies.

Sarcoid Heart Disease

Cardiac involvement in sarcoidosis can be identified in 13 to 27 percent of autopsied cases. Endomyocardial biopsy diagnosis of cardiac involvement in a patient with known sarcoidosis requires a noncaseating granuloma and negative special stains for organisms. However, the presence of an infiltrate without acute myocyte damage, in a patient with known sarcoidosis, may be considered "consistent with" cardiac involvement. Owing to the critical role of the granuloma, we take extra effort to find them in clinically suspected cases, and we will cut 10 to 15 slides through the paraffin-embedded tissue.[38]

Atypical Lymphoid Infiltrates

The heart may be involved by leukemias, lymphomas, or the atypical lymphocytes of Epstein-Barr virus infection. In these instances, the interstitial infiltrates may be focal rather than diffuse and are usually not associated with the myocyte necrosis typical of myocarditis.

SPECIAL STUDIES

Various special studies have been performed in an attempt to increase the diagnostic accuracy of the biopsy or to study the pathophysiology of myocarditis. These studies have generally included quantitation of tissue components or immunologic studies. One study concentrating on the infiltrating cell population determined the mean "normal" number of myocardial lymphocytes to be less than 5.0 per (×400) field; counts higher than that average for 20 fields are considered to represent active myocarditis.[39] This finding is consistent with the view that occasional interstitial lymphocytes may be present in biopsies of idiopathic cardiomyopathies[22,40,41] or in other nonmyocarditic hearts. It is our opinion, however, that in some instances the infiltrate in myocarditis may be focal and intense and associated with myocyte damage, yet over 20 microscopic fields do not surpass the five lymphocytes per field average. Furthermore, quantitation of cells may help diagnose "borderline" myocarditis but neglects the myocyte damage necessary for the diagnosis of "active" myocarditis.[42,43] The quest for quantitation to make diagnosis more reliable and reproducible is an important one, and it helps focus attention on the crucial histologic problem of distinguishing infiltrating cells from cells normally resident in the cardiac interstitium.

Other studies have quantified muscular and interstitial tissues in the myocarditic heart. In one such study,[22] performed on small (Konno-Sakakibara or King's College Hospital bioptome) endomyocardial biopsies, tissue with the diagnosis of myocarditis (infiltrate and myocardial fiber degeneration or necrosis) had significant increase in muscle fiber diameter compared with normal hearts, as well as in volume fraction of collagen (determined with elastic van Gieson stain) compared with normal controls and with biopsies with hypertrophy or hypertrophic cardiomyopathy. The volume fraction of the entire interstitium was not significantly different. Although these differences existed in the comparison of groups of patients, the extensive overlap and variance of results prevent the diagnostic use of these criteria in an individual patient. Biochemical assessments of collagen content of endomyocardial biopsy tissue has also been performed. In patients with dilated cardiomyopathy (the proportion associated with myocarditis is unstated), an increase in collagen content is closely correlated with an increase in left ventricular end-diastolic pressure and a decrease in ejection fraction.[44] In another study,[45] patients with biopsy or clinical evidence of myocarditis were identified and followup biopsies without active inflammation studied quantitatively. These pieces of tissue contained increased interstitial tissue (assessed by Masson's trichrome) compared with controls (patients with tumor prior to chemotherapy). A degenerative change within myocytes, myofilament loss, has been semiquantitatively evaluated, and in myocarditis the severity of the myofilament loss may be related to prognosis.[46] Mortality at 18-month followup is predicted by the severity of the loss, independent of clinical class and left ventricular ejection fraction. Quantitative studies have also been applied in the study of Chagas' disease-related myocarditis.[47]

Immunologic studies have described components of humoral or cellular immunity in endomyocardial biopsy tissue or in peripheral blood. None of these tests has a proven diagnostic use, but they have aided the identification of infiltrating cells and do offer clues to the pathogenesis of myocarditis. Immunoglobulins are bound in endomyocardial biopsy tissue from patients with myocarditis; in cases of active myocarditis, there is C3 with or without IgG.[48,49] In followup biopsies, these direct immunofluorescent findings closely follow histologic findings; deposition of immune complexes recurred when myocarditis recurred.[50] One center also reports bound IgM and/or IgA and C3 complexes in left and right ventricular biopsies from patients with active myocarditis but not in control subjects without primary cardiac disease. Biopsies from patients with resolving perimyocarditis or pericardial effusion or dilated cardiomyopathy are less likely to contain bound complexes of immunoglobulin and complement[51] than are those from patients with active perimyocarditis. There is a close association between the presence of IgG and/or complement and the presence of more than five infiltrating cells (lymphocytes and macrophages) per high power field.[46] The presence of immunoglobulin deposition in active and inactive rheumatic carditis is well known.[52–54] The binding of immunoglobulin in the heart is not, however, limited to instances of myocarditis. Immunoglobulin and complement may be present in endomyocardial fibrosis,[55] various chronic myocardial diseases,[56] and idiopathic cardiomyopathy.[57]

The recent development of monoclonal antibodies against cell surface antigens on distinct populations of lymphocytes has allowed the phenotyping of the inflammatory infiltrate in myocarditis. We have demonstrated that in idiopathic, presumably viral, myocarditis the mononuclear cell infiltrate is composed of almost equal proportions of macrophages and lymphocytes.[58,59] The distribution of cell types has been confirmed at another center.[49] In the more rapidly progressive form of myocarditis[16] (one subset of patients with active myocarditis with fibrosis), the lymphocytes are almost equally divided between cytotoxic/suppressor and helper phenotypes whereas in patients with a more chronic myocarditis, lymphocytes of the cytotoxic/suppressor phenotype predominate.[58,59] With double-staining immunofluorescence techniques, we have shown that many (14 to 100 percent) of these infiltrating lymphocytes are activated and bear surface Ia (HLA-DR) or Tac antigen and are not just resting peripheral blood T lymphocytes that happen to be passing through the myocardium. The differences in ratios of helper to cytotoxic/suppressor T lymphocytes in situ in the two clinical groups of patients with active myocarditis with fibrosis were not large enough to be useful diagnostically. In addition, these cell-phenotyping studies did not predict response to conventional or immunosuppressive therapy. We have also studied a patient with active rheumatic carditis and seen a predominance of T helper cells in situ, prior to steroid treatment.[54] The various ratios of infiltrating inflammatory cells in situ suggest that there may be varied pathophysiologic mechanisms in myocarditis. It is crucial to continue studies of the inflammatory infiltrate within the myocardium, as this population contains the immunologic effector cells in greatest concentration. There are many immunologically mediated diseases in which the peripheral blood does not reflect ratios of cell types present at the actual site of tissue damage.[60,61] It must also be noted that the cell surface phenotype of lymphocytes does not necessarily correlate with cell function.[62] Routine use of immunohistochemical techniques to aid in the identification and counting of infiltrating lymphocytes is not necessary, although it may help identify some patients with cases of "borderline" myocarditis. Careful review of well-prepared specimens is adequate to identify myocarditis by the Dallas criteria. The most useful information will be gained only with studies of the functional properties of cells from within the myocardium. In this regard, the ability to grow and clone lymphocytes from endomyocardial biopsies from patients with myocarditis offers a new avenue for research.[63,64] The functional ability of these cells to kill appropriate targets or to regulate other cells' activities may be studied. In addition, preliminary studies[63] demonstrating gene rearrangements have suggested clonal expansion of lymphocytes, raising the possibility of identifying the antigen(s) that these cells recognize.

The potential disparity between peripheral blood and events in the myocardium must be considered in the interpretation of studies of peripheral blood lymphocytes or circulating antibodies in myocarditis. Circulating lymphocytes have been studied by flow cytometry in idiopathic dilated cardiomyopathy and myocarditis. Although there appears to be no alteration from normal ratios in cardiomyopathy,[65,66] one preliminary report[66] observed a selective decrease in cytotoxic/suppressor phenotype cells in active myocarditis, with normalization of ratios after (? immunosuppressive) treatment.

There have been many excellent studies of circulating antibodies directed against various components of the myocardium, such as the sarcolemma, myolemma, actin, myosin, interfibrillary substance, collagen, endothelium, and mitochondria. The antimyolemmal antiobodies present in acute myocarditis associated with coxsackievirus B, influenza, and mumps are generally not present in cytomegalovirus myocarditis. These antibodies have cytolytic activity when mixed with complement in a vital adult rat cardiocyte assay.[67] This finding has suggested a diagnostic utility for these studies in known cases of myocarditis; but it will be difficult to prove a pathogenic role for the antibodies. In addition, the presence of any or all of these antibodies is not specific for active myocarditis; persons with resolving and resolved perimyocarditis, systemic lupus erythematosus, pericardial effusion, idiopathic dilated cardiomyopathy, sarcoidosis, coronary artery disease, endocarditis, and post-cardiac injury syndrome may have the same circulating antibodies.[68]

One special technique that holds great promise for the study of myocarditis is the application of methods from molecular biology to the study of endomyocardial biopsy tissue. Using coxsackievirus B cDNA hybridization probes, two groups have demonstrated coxsackievirus B2 and B3 genomic RNA in 8 of 16 and 2 of 13 biopsies with active or healed myocarditis and dilated cardiomyopathy, respectively.[69,70] This method has extraordinary sensitivity to define virus genome in single cells; copies of genome are present in both myocardial cells and interstitial cells. One advantage of the technique is its ability to detect a virus RNA sequence that is highly conserved in all six coxsackievirus B serotypes, making the probe group-specific. These methods will allow the study of possible etiologic associations, in contrast to previous unsuccessful attempts to isolate infectious virus from, or demonstrate viral antigens in, biopsy tissue.

NATURAL HISTORY AND RESPONSE TO THERAPY

Natural History

Endomyocardial biopsy has provided histologic confirmation of myocarditis prior to death and has facilitated studies of the natural history of the disease. The "incubation" period from viral infection to development of symptoms remains largely undefined in humans, but the subsequent course of disease is being studied in both acute and chronic forms. The findings from these studies have important implications for prognosis and therapy.

Acute idiopathic myocarditis generally resolves spontaneously or proves lethal. Whether the improvement noted a few months after the initial, severe disease is permanent is not yet clear and requires careful followup studies with reproducible, objective assessments of ventricular function. A recent study[71] of the short-term history of 15 patients with biopsy-proven myocarditis followed for 9 to 54 weeks (mean of 16 weeks) found that three had spontaneous clearing of the infiltrate and a normal left ventricular ejection fraction (LVEF) at followup. Of the 12 patients with persistent histologic myocarditis, one improved and 11 had a diminution or no change in ejection fraction.

Our studies of long-term followup in patients with a chronic form of "active myocarditis with fibrosis" have identified an even larger proportion of patients who improve on standard medical therapy.[32] Seven of 13 patients with biopsy-confirmed myocarditis, followed for 9 to 81 months (average of 34 months), improved their ejection fraction by more than 5 percent. However, two of these seven subsequently demonstrated an unexplained deterioration of function; one underwent transplantation and the other died. In those patients who increased their ejection fractions, the improvement was usually present within 3 months of biopsy diagnosis and often after 1 month of conventional supportive therapy. With this information, we have decided to treat patients with myocarditis supportively for at least 3 months before considering immunosuppressive therapy. The timing of immunosuppressive therapy is an additional variable: should treatment be started immediately after diagnosis or only after supportive therapy has failed? Unfortunately, we cannot predict on the basis of histologic criteria which patients will respond to immunotherapy. This form of long-term followup study must be completed for other histologic forms of myocarditis. The studies outlined previously are for patients with the chronic form of active myocarditis with fibrosis; our studies have also indicated a group of patients who do not appear to respond to immunosuppression. This group has a more rapidly progressive disease[16] of shorter duration (average 23 months from onset of symptoms to transplant or death) that is almost always lethal and is not affected by immunosuppressive therapy. It should be noted that the histology for this latter group is also included under "active myocarditis with fibrosis" by the Dallas classification.

Therapy and Correlation of Structure with Function

With the recognition that myocarditis is an immunologically mediated disease, there was a rationale for immunosuppressive therapy in addition to standard, supportive measures. The endomyocardial biopsy was suggested as an objective means of assessing the effects of such therapy.[11] If the biopsy is to be an accurate tool for this assessment, it must be sensitive and specific, and there should be good correlation of structure (judged by histology) with function (as measured clinically). The limitations of the sensitivity and specificity of the biopsy have been discussed earlier. At least two groups have looked at the correlation of structure (classifying myocarditis by the Dallas criteria into active, resolving, or resolved) with function (LVEF); in neither of the studies was there a good association of "appropriate" histology with change in ejection fraction. The group at the Massachusetts General Hospital[72] studied 17 patients with acute onset of heart failure, with a diagnostic biopsy, and repeat biopsy after 6 to 12 weeks of treatment that included immunosuppression in

15 patients and conventional therapy for heart failure in all patients. We[73] studied 29 patients with the chronic form of active myocarditis with fibrosis, with an average followup of 29 months from initial, diagnostic biopsy. A total of 66 followup biopsy results were examined; all patients were treated supportively, and 16 also received prednisone alone or with azathioprine. The histology of the followup biopsy did not predict clinical response, with or without immunosuppressive therapy: of 21 instances when the biopsy showed ongoing disease, the ejection fraction was actually improved in six; in 45 instances when the biopsy showed resolving or resolved disease, the LVEF was unimproved in 28. Clinical improvement or deterioration may occur without the "appropriate" change in biopsy histology: of the 23 biopsies taken when the LVEF was improved (increase of more than 5 percent over previous determination), six showed ongoing disease; of 43 biopsies taken when there was no improvement in LVEF, 28 showed resolved or resolving disease.

In some instances, a repeat biopsy can help resolve this dilemma, but we now suspect that changes in therapy may be better determined by objective clinical factors, such as LVEF by MUGA, than by biopsy histology. One possible conclusion to be drawn from these observations is that the mechanism of cardiac dysfunction in myocarditis may be independent of light-microscopic evidence of active inflammation or myocyte necrosis. Routine histology of the biopsy by light microscopy may not be the standard for assessing the presence or activity of myocarditis. Other special studies, such as those mentioned earlier, or other physiologic or biochemical techniques may better predict clinical course and response to therapy in myocarditis.

The information previously presented on the incidence of "spontaneous" improvement in some patients with myocarditis has obvious implications for trials of therapy in this disease. Any such trial will require enough patients to allow for this high rate of spontaneous improvement. Most reports on therapy in myocarditis indicate improvement in some patients with immunosuppressive therapy but no clear difference from conventional therapy. A large multicenter trial is necessary to answer the question: Is there a significant difference between conventional supportive therapy and the same therapy with the addition of conventional immunosuppression (prednisone, azathioprine, and perhaps cyclosporin)? This question should be answered quickly, and if the answer is no, then research on other forms of treatment and immunotherapy should be started.

SUMMARY

In closing, we can only note that none of the classification schemes for myocarditis has been perfect for clinicians, pathologists, and researchers alike. The definition and classification protocol offered by the "Dallas" group is based solely on histology, but we urge its use by physicians and other researchers as a means of imposing some standardization on the study of myocarditis. The question of optimum treatment, particularly immunosuppressive therapy, has never been definitively answered, but it is now clear that a large, multicenter randomized trial is the only proper method to search for such an answer. Standard nomenclature is a prerequisite for this study. In the meantime, the clinical correlates and prognostic utility of these histologic categories may be defined; these morphologic groupings will probably be shown to be clinically heterogeneous. In the end, we hope a hybrid clinical-pathologic scheme for the diagnosis and classification of myocarditis will be forged. Such a protocol, ideally, will allow the correlation of structure with function and also realiably predict clinical behavior and response to treatment so that someday we may be able to both counsel and cure persons with myocarditis.

ACKNOWLEDGMENT

We deeply appreciate the expert secretarial assistance of Karen Brower and the photographic expertise of Alfred T. Lamme, F.B.P.A.

REFERENCES

1. Sobernheim, JF: Praktische Diagnostik der inneren Krankheiten mit vorzuegleicher Ruecksicht auf pathologische Anatomie. Hirschwald, Berlin, 1837.
2. Mattingly, TW: Changing concepts of myocardial disease. JAMA 191:33, 1965.
3. Fiedler, A: Ueber akute interstitielle Myokarditis, In Festschinft des Stadtkrankenhauses. Dresden-Friedrichstadt, 1899.
4. Herrick, JB: Clinical features of sudden obstruction of the coronary arteries. JAMA 59:2015, 1912.
5. Saphir, O: Myocarditis, a general review with an analysis of 240 cases. Arch Pathol 32:1000, 1941; 33:88, 1942.
6. Burch, GE and Ray, CT: Myocarditis and myocardial degeneration. Bull Tulane Medical Faculty 8:1, 1948.
7. Boikan, WJ: Myocarditis perniciosa. Virchow Arch 282:46, 1931.
8. Kline, IK and Saphir, O: Chronic pernicious myocarditis. Am Heart J 59:681, 1960.
9. Sakakibara, S and Konno, S: Endomyocardial biopsy. Jpn Heart J 3:537, 1962.
10. Nippoldt, TB, Edwards, WD, Holmes, DR, Jr, et al: Right ventricular endomyocardial biopsy. Mayo Clin Proc 57:407, 1982.
11. Mason, JW, Billingham, ME, and Ricci, DR: Treatment of acute inflammatory myocarditis assisted by endomyocardial biopsy. Am J Cardiol 45:1037, 1980.
12. Aretz, HT, Chapman, C, and Fallon, JT: Morphologic and immunologic findings in patients with clinically suspected myocarditis. Circulation 68:III-27, 1983.
13. Dec, GW, Jr, Palacios, IF, Fallon, JT, et al: Active myocarditis in the spectrum of acute dilated cardiomyopathies. N Engl J Med 312:885, 1985.
14. Zee-Cheng, CS, Tsai, CC, Palmer, DC, et al: High incidence of myocarditis by endomyocardial biopsy in patients with idiopathic congestive cardiomyopathy. JACC 3:63, 1984.
15. Olsen, EGJ: Morphological evaluation (histologic, histochemical, and ultrastructural) of endomyocardial biopsies. In Bolte, H-D (ed): Myocardial Biopsy: Diagnostic Significance. Springer-Verlag, Berlin, 1980.
16. Fenoglio, JJ, Jr, Ursell, PC, Kellogg, CF, et al: Diagnosis and classification of myocarditis by endomyocardial biopsy. N Engl J Med 308:12, 1983.
17. Parrillo, JE, Aretz, HT, Palacios, IF, et al: The results of transvenous endomyocardial biopsy can frequently be used to diagnose myocardial diseases in patients with idiopathic heart failure. Circulation 69:93, 1984.
18. Billingham, ME and Mason, JW: Endomyocardial biopsy diagnosis of myocarditis and changes following immunosuppressive treatment. In Bolte, H-D (ed): Viral Heart Disease. Springer-Verlag, Berlin, 1984.
19. Ursell, PC, Chevinsky, A, Weiss, MB, et al: Endomyocardial biopsy experience in 150 patients. In Fenoglio, CM (ed): Progress in Surgical Pathology. Masson, NY, 1983.
20. Aretz, HT, Billingham, ME, Edwards, WD, et al: Myocarditis: A histopathologic definition and classification. Am J Cardiovasc Pathol 1:3, 1987.
21. Miller, PJ: An elastin stain. Med Lab Technol 28:148, 1971.
22. Baandrup, U and Olsen, EGJ: Critical analysis of endomyocardial biopsies from patients suspected of having cardiomyopathy. Br Heart J 45:475, 1981.
23. Gould, SE: Pathology of the Heart and Blood Vessels, ed 3. Charles C Thomas, Springfield, IL, 1968, p 825.
24. Olsen, EGJ: Histomorphological relations between myocarditis and dilated cardiomyopathy. In Bolte, H-D (ed): Viral Heart Disease, Springer-Verlag, Berlin, 1984, p 7.
25. Lustock, MJ, Chase, J, and Lubitz, JM: Myocarditis: A clinical and pathologic study of forty-five cases. Dis Chest 28:243, 1955.

26. Gore, I and Saphir, O: Myocarditis: A classification of 1402 cases. Am Heart J 34:827, 1947.
27. Edwards, WD: Myocarditis and endomyocardial biopsy. In Waller, BF (ed): Cardiology Clinics, Vol 2, No 4. WB Saunders, Philadelphia, 1984.
28. Woodruff, JF: Viral myocarditis: A review. Am J Pathol 101:425, 1980.
29. Huber, SA and Lodge, PA: Coxsackievirus B-3 myocarditis in Balb/c mice—Evidence for autoimmunity to myocyte antigens. Am J Pathol 116:21, 1984.
30. Paque, RE and Gauntt, CJ: Cellular and humoral responses in the induction and expression of viral-induced myocarditis. In Robinson, JA and O'Connell, J (eds): Myocarditis: Precursor of Cardiomyopathy. Collamore Press, DC Heath & Co, Lexington, MA, 1983.
31. Gauntt, CT, Arizpe, HM, Kung, JT, et al: Antimyocarditic activity of the guanine derivative BIOLF-70 in a Coxsackievirus B3-Murine model. Antimicrobial Agents and Chemotherapy, 1985.
32. Weiss, MB, Marboe, CC, Escala, E, et al: Natural history of untreated chronic myocarditis. Eur Heart J (in press).
33. Reichenbach, DD and Benditt, EP: Catecholamines and cardiomyopathy: The pathogenesis and potential importance of myofibrillar degeneration. Human Pathol 1:125, 1970.
34. McManus, BM, Fleury, TA, and Roberts, WC: Fatal catecholamine crisis in pheochromocytoma: Curable form of cardiac arrest. Am Heart J 102:930, 1981.
35. Fenoglio, JJ, Jr, McAllister, HA, Jr, and Mullick, FG: Drug related myocarditis. I. Hypersensibility myocarditis. Human Pathol 12:900, 1981.
36. Rabson, AB, Schoen, FJ, Warhol, MJ, et al: Giant cell myocarditis after mitral valve replacement: Case report and studies of the nature of giant cells. Human Pathol 15:585, 1984.
37. Theaker, JM, Gatter, KC, Heryet, A, et al: Giant cell myocarditis: Evidence for the macrophage origin of the giant cells. J Clin Pathol 38:160, 1985.
38. Ratner, SJ, Fenoglio, JJ, Jr, and Ursell, PC: Utility of endomyocardial biopsy in the diagnosis of cardiac sarcoidosis. Chest 90:528, 1986.
39. Edwards, WD, Holmes, DR, Jr, and Reeder, GS: Diagnosis of active lymphocytic myocarditis by endomyocardial biopsy: Quantitative criteria for light microscopy. Mayo Clin Proc 57:419, 1982.
40. Tazalaar, HD and Billingham, ME: Leukocytic infiltrates in idiopathic dilated cardiomyopathy: A source of confusion with active myocarditis. Lab Invest 52:67A, 1985.
41. Becker, AE: Cardiomyopathies. In Silver, MD (ed): Cardiovascular Pathology. Churchill Livingstone, New York, 1983, p 489.
42. Southern, JF, Gaynor, B, Howard, C, et al: Is immunoperoxidase staining of endomyocardial biopsies for interstitial inflammatory cells helpful in the diagnosis of myocarditis? Eur Heart J (in press).
43. Herskowitz, A, Beschorner, WE, Soule, LM, et al: The interpretation of the equivocal myocardial biopsy. Circulation 72:III-346, 1985.
44. Fischer, S and Bolte, H-D: Collagen content of myocardial biopsies related to cardiac function of patients with myocardial diseases. Circulation 66:II-117, 1982.
45. Unverferth, DV, Fetters, JK, Unverferth, BJ, et al: Human myocardial histologic characteristics in congestive heart failure. Circulation 68:1194, 1983.
46. Anderson, JL, Hammond, EH, Fowles, RE, et al: Predictive value of immunofluorescence and electron microscopic evaluation of endomyocardial biopsies in the diagnosis and prognosis of idiopathic heart muscle disease with or without inflammation. Eur Heart J (in press).
47. Oliveira, JSM: A natural human model of intrinsic heart nervous system denervation: Chagas' cardiopathy. Am Heart J 110:1092, 1985.
48. Aretz, HT, Chapman, C, and Fallon, JT: Morphologic and immunologic findings in patients with clinically suspected myocarditis. Circulation 68:III-27, 1983.
49. Hammond, EH and Anderson, JL: Cardiac immune complexes and mononuclear cell subsets in myocarditis: An endomyocardial biopsy study. Circulation 68:III-27, 1983.
50. Aretz, HT, Fallon, JT, Southern J, et al: Morphologic and immunologic findings in patients with clinically suspected and treated myocarditis—An endomyocardial biopsy study. Eur Heart J (in press).
51. Maisch, B, Buschel, G, Deeg, P, et al: Value of endomyocardial biopsy in inflammatory heart disease. Eur Heart J (in press).
52. Zabriskie, JB: Rheumatic fever: The interplay between host, genetics, and microbe. Circulation 71:1077, 1985.
53. Kaplan, MH, Bolande, R, Rakita, L, et al: Presence of immunoglobulins and complement in the myocardium in acute rheumatic fever. N Engl J Med 271:637, 1964.
54. Marboe, CC, Knowles, DM, II, Weiss, MB, et al: Monoclonal antibody identification of mononuclear

cells in endomyocardial biopsy specimens from a patient with rheumatic carditis. Human Pathol 16:332, 1985.
55. Van der Geld, H, Peetoom, F, Somers, K, et al: Immunohistological and serological studies in endomyocardial fibrosis. Lancet 2:1210, 1966.
56. Hatle, L and Melbye, OJ: Immunoglobulins and complement in chronic myocardial disease—A myocardial biopsy study. Acta Med Scand 200:385, 1976.
57. Das, SK, Callen, JP, Dodson, VN, et al: Immunoglobulin binding in cardiomyopathic hearts. Circulation 44:612, 1971.
58. Marboe, CC, Knowles, DM, II, Weiss, MB, et al: Characterization of the inflammatory infiltrate in human myocarditis—An endomyocardial biopsy study. In Bolte, H-D (ed): Viral Heart Disease. Springer-Verlag, Berlin, 1984.
59. Marboe, CC, Knowles, DM, II, and Fenoglio, JJ, Jr: Lymphocyte subsets in myocarditis: An endomyocardial biopsy study. Circulation 66:II-118, 1982.
60. Morris, PJ: Renal transplantation—1982, Transplant Proc 15:1022, 1983.
61. Ginns, LC, Goldenheim, PD, Burton, RC, et al: T-lymphocyte subsets in peripheral blood and lung lavage in idiopathic pulmonary fibrosis and sarcoidosis. Clin Immunol Immunopathol 25:11, 1982.
62. Thomas, Y, Rogozinski, L, Irigoyen, O, et al: Functional analysis of human T cell subsets defined by monoclonal antibodies. IV. Induction of suppressor cells within the OKT4 population. J Exp Med 154:459, 1981.
63. Kurnick, JT, Leary, C, Palacios, IF, et al: Characterization and culture of lymphocytic infiltrates from endomyocardial biopsies of patients with idiopathic myocarditis. Eur Heart J (in press).
64. Mayer, TG, Fuller, AA, Fuller, TC, et al: Propagation of specific T lymphocytes from human renal allograft biopsies. J Immunol 134:258, 1985.
65. Anderson, JL, Carlquist, JF, and Lutz, JR: HLA-A, B and DR typing in idiopathic dilated cardiomyopathy; a search for immune response factors. Am J Cardiol 53:1326, 1984.
66. Izumo, S, Abelmann, WA, and Morimoto, C: Peripheral T-cell subsets in patients with myocarditis and dilated cardiomyopathy. J Am Coll Cardiol 5:491, 1985.
67. Maisch, B, Trostel-Soeder, R, Stechemesser, E, et al: Diagnostic relevance of humoral and cell-mediated immune reactions in patients with acute viral myocarditis. Clin Exp Immunol 48:533, 1982.
68. DeScheerder, I, DeBuyzere, M, Algoed, L, et al: Characteristic anti-heart-antibody patterns in post-cardiac injury syndrome, endocarditis, and acute myocarditis. Eur Heart J (in press).
69. Archard, LC, Bowles, NE, Olsen, EGJ, et al: Detection of persistent Coxsackie B virus RNA in dilated cardiomyopathy and myocarditis. Eur Heart J (in press).
70. Kandolf, R, Arneis, D, Kirschner, P, et al: In situ detection of viral genomes in myocardial cells by nucleic acid hybridization: A novel approach to the diagnosis of viral heart disease. Eur Heart J (in press).
71. Strain, JE, Grose, RM, Cho, S, et al: Short-term natural history of untreated myocarditis. Circulation 72:III-110, 1985.
72. Dec, GW, Palacios, IF, and Falloon, JT: Does histology on repeat right ventricular biopsy predict improved ventricular function in patients treated for myocarditis? Circulation 72:III-109, 1985.
73. Marboe, CC, Schwartz, R, Adelson, D, et al: Active myocarditis with fibrosis: Poor correlation of ejection fraction with histology of follow-up biopsy. Eur Heart J (in press).

CHAPTER 7

Myocarditis and Dilated Cardiomyopathy: Different Stages of the Same Disease?

John T. Fallon, M.D., Ph.D.

A causal relationship between myocarditis and idiopathic dilated cardiomyopathy has long been suspected. However, until the application of endomyocardial biopsy, arguments for and against this relationship were based primarily on circumstantial evidence from clinical, serologic, epidemiologic, and morbid anatomic studies.[1-5] Recent studies using endomyocardial biopsy have demonstrated that myocarditis is associated with dilated cardiomyopathy, although not all patients having myocarditis present with or subsequently develop a dilated cardiomyopathy.[6-13] Endomyocardial biopsy provides not only a technique for the definitive diagnosis of myocarditis but also the opportunity to obtain insights into the etiology, pathogenesis, and natural history of myocarditis. In this chapter, the aim is to define and characterize dilated cardiomyopathy and myocarditis and to provide evidence from recent endomyocardial biopsy studies for their causal relationship, for the etiologic role of viruses, and for the participation of cellular immune mechanisms in the pathogenesis of these diseases.

DILATED CARDIOMYOPATHY—DEFINITION

Dilated, hypertrophic, and restrictive cardiomyopathies constitute the three major types of primary heart muscle disease.[2,14] Dilated cardiomyopathy is caused by loss of ventricular contractility and characterized by clinical signs and symptoms of ventricular failure, an enlarged heart, and a depressed ventricular ejection fraction (usually less than 40 percent). These clinical findings are present in a variety of cardiac diseases of known etiology, including ischemic heart disease, valvular disease, systemic diseases, toxic exposures, infections, nutritional deficiencies, and metabolic diseases. When no specific etiology is ascertained, the patient is classified as having "idiopathic" dilated cardiomyopathy. In several instances, associated clinical conditions are used to characterize the cardiomyopathy further—for example, familial, peripartum, and alcoholic cardiomyopathies—but these conditions are also idiopathic forms of dilated cardiomyopathy. Another possibly useful but arbitrary subdivision of idiopathic dilated cardiomyopathy is based on time, that is, acute (or recent) onset idiopathic dilated cardiomyopathy and chronic idiopathic dilated cardiomyopathy—with the division being at 6 months of symptoms. Thus, the terms "acute dilated cardiomyopathy" and "chronic dilated cardiomyopathy" are derived.[7]

Dilated cardiomyopathy is not a specific pathologic entity. The hearts of patients with clinical evidence of dilated cardiomyopathy are most often characterized by an increased organ weight with biventricular and biatrial dilation. The ventricular walls are of normal thickness or are thinned. The coronary arteries and the valves are not intrinsically diseased, but evidence of secondary mitral or tricuspid regurgitation, or both, may be present. Intracavitary mural thrombi and patch endocardial fibrosis are common. Microscopic examination of the ventricular myocardium often reveals nonspecific findings of myocyte hypertrophy and degeneration; varying degrees of interstitial, replacement, and/or perivascular fibrosis with or without chronic inflammation;[15] and subendocardial myofibrillar lysis. Dilated cardiomyopathies do not have specific diagnostic morphologic findings, even by electron microscopy or sophisticated morphometric analysis.[4,16–18] Some cases of dilated cardiomyopathy reveal few histologic changes except for myocyte hypertrophy.[4,19] It is not surprising, therefore, that the application of endomyocardial biopsy for the routine evaluation of patients with idiopathic dilated cardiomyopathy yields a low percentage of specific diagnostic findings.[20] This is especially true for the chronic idiopathic dilated cardiomyopathy in which myocardial degenerative changes or reparative processes, or both, may overshadow or mask etiologically specific morphologic changes. Therefore, the ability to examine myocardial tissue at an early stage of the clinical process (that is, at the stage of acute dilated cardiomyopathy) may help to provide clues to the etiology and pathogenesis of dilated cardiomyopathy.

MYOCARDITIS—DEFINITION

In contrast to dilated cardiomyopathy, myocarditis is not easily defined or characterized clinically (see Chapter 6). Patients having myocarditis may present with acute dilated cardiomyopathy, ventricular arrhythmias, acute myocardial infarction syndrome, or a restrictive cardiomyopathy. Furthermore, cardiogenic shock, sudden death, and/or chronic idiopathic dilated cardiomyopathy may occur during or following an episode of myocarditis.

Myocarditis is a pathologic term that, simply defined, means inflammation of the myocardium. However, this broad or generic definition has caused confusion. Thus, the Dallas criteria (developed by a group of eight pathologists in 1984) defines *idiopathic* myocarditis as a "process characterized by an inflammatory infiltrate of the myocardium with necrosis and/or degeneration of adjacent myocytes not typical of the ischemic damage associated with coronary artery disease."[21] In addition to excluding myocardial infarction, several other known causes of myocardial inflammation are excluded: hypersensitivity reactions, infections, toxic processes, vasculitides, and malignant infiltrates. However, the pathologist is still left with a morphologically diverse group of pathologies under the heading of "idiopathic myocarditis." The most common type is lymphocytic myocarditis, but some types are primarily eosinophilic, granulomatous, or mixed. Furthermore, the infiltrates may vary in intensity and may be focal, multifocal, or diffuse. Thus, like idiopathic dilated cardiomyopathy, idiopathic myocarditis is also a nonspecific pathologic entity.

VIRAL MYOCARDITIS

The association of myocarditis and dilated cardiomyopathy was initially supported by observations during epidemics of coxsackievirus B infection. During these epidemics, as many as 12 percent of infected patients manifested some clinical sign, symptom, or positive laboratory test of cardiac involvement.[1,2] The majority of such affected individuals remained asymptomatic and recovered uneventfully without evidence of subsequent myocardial dysfunction. However, a few of these patients subsequently developed a dilated cardiomyopathy. Similarly, serologic studies in patients with dilated cardiomyopathy have implicated virus in the etiology of dilated cardiomyopathy.[2,9,22] Do these patients really have "myocarditis"? Furthermore, even assuming such patients have myocarditis, what etiologic or pathogenetic role does the concomitant viral infection play?

Viral cultures of myocardial tissue obtained by endomyocardial biopsy from patients with biopsy-proven myocarditis or dilated cardiomyopathy are almost always negative, even when either the clinical history or serologic studies indicative of recent viral infection are present.[6,10] Furthermore, immunocytochemical studies of myocardial tissue have repeatedly failed to demonstrate the presence of viral antigens in patients with myocarditis and chronic dilated cardiomyopathy.[4] Therefore, human myocarditis appears to be rarely if ever due to replicating virus.

Recent cDNA hybridization studies using a quantitative slot blot technique have demonstrated the presence of coxsackievirus B viral RNA sequences in 14 of 27 endomyocardial biopsies from patients with myocarditis or dilated cardiomyopathy and the absence of such RNA sequences in 11 biopsies from patients with unrelated diseases.[23] These findings suggest the possibility that coxsackievirus B may persist in the myocardium of patients with myocarditis and may in some way be responsible for the subsequent development of dilated cardiomyopathy. If confirmed, this evidence for persistent coxsackievirus B infection will have major therapeutic implications.

EXPERIMENTAL MYOCARDITIS AND DILATED CARDIOMYOPATHY

Experimentally, myocarditis and dilated cardiomyopathy are established and well-characterized sequelae of viral infection.[24] Briefly, coxsackie/EMC infection in mice/hamsters results in a systemic viremia 24 and 72 hours postinoculation. Viral replication occurs in myocytes between 72 hours and 96 hours after infection. Mononuclear cells, predominantly macrophages, infiltrate the myocardium between 5 and 10 days postinoculation. Neutralizing antibody titers rise within 5 days; and by 14 days, virus or viral antigen, or both, can no longer be detected in the myocardium. During the initial infection, cytotoxic T lymphocytes are produced that are capable of lysing virus-infected myocytes. These T cells account for approximately 80 percent of the cells in the myocardium at 2 weeks postinoculation. Depending on age, sex, strain, size of inoculum, and other variables, a percentage of animals die during the acute phase of viral infection from overwhelming viremia, cardiogenic shock, and/or arrhythmias. Surviving animals may be unaffected; however, some of the survivors succumb to sudden death or develop a dilated cardiomyopathy and die with congestive heart failure and its complications weeks to months later.

In strains of animals that develop dilated cardiomyopathy following an acute viral myocarditis, the T lymphocytes appear to mediate continued myocyte necrosis in the apparent absence of virus. These cytotoxic T lymphocytes exhibit specificity for both virus-infection and H_2 antigens on the infected cell surface, although the myocytic antigen responsible for T-cell cytolysis is unknown.[25] EMC myocarditis in *nude* mice, which are athymic and lack mature T lymphocytes, causes less congestive heart failure than in either normal mice or lymphocyte-reconstituted nude mice.[26] In fact, cellular infiltration and myocardial necrosis are minimal on day 14 in the athymic mouse model and other models where mature T lymphocytes are depleted. Thus, T lymphocytes may be responsible for the subsequent development of dilated cardiomyopathy in these experimental models. It is uncertain, however, whether the direct cytotoxic effects of the T lymphocytes are responsible for the loss of myocardial function or whether secondary products (interleukins, interferon, or other mediators) are responsible for a "non-necrotic" loss of myocardial function. Humoral mechanisms have not been shown to be involved in this "delayed" reaction but are not yet fully examined.

ENDOMYOCARDIAL BIOPSY—CLINICOPATHOLOGIC STUDIES

Since the introduction of endomyocardial biopsy, it has been shown that the correlation between a clinical diagnosis of myocarditis and a pathologic diagnosis of myocarditis is poor. In patients with a presumptive clinical diagnosis of myocarditis who have a dilated cardiomyopathy, endomyocardial biopsy more often than not reveals normal myocardium or only nonspecific changes of myocyte hypertrophy and interstitial or replacement fibrosis. As pointed out in a previous chapter, a lymphocytic myocarditis is demonstrated in only about 20 percent of such patients but ranges in various published reports from 0 to 63 percent.[3] This disparity has led some investigators to discredit the endomyocardial biopsy as a worthwhile diagnostic technique.[27] Although most biopsies are negative for myocarditis, clearly one fifth are positive for the presence of inflammation and myocyte degeneration/necrosis. We should not despair regarding the relatively low percentage of biopsies with myocarditis in patients with dilated cardiomyopathy. Rather, we should be encouraged that an identifiable and potentially treatable disease is present in some of these patients.

It may be possible to increase the frequency of positive biopsies through a better understanding of the pathogenesis of myocarditis gained from long-term clinical and pathologic examination of select groups of patients. We have reported the clinical features and biopsy findings of 27 patients with acute-onset idiopathic dilated cardiomyopathy and a mean followup of 18 ± 4 months.[7] Eleven patients had unequivocal myocarditis on endomyocardial biopsy. Of these, two died, four improved, and five developed chronic dilated cardiomyopathy. The remaining 16 patients without biopsy confirmation of myocarditis had a similar course on followup: six died, six improved, and four developed chronic dilated cardiomyopathy. The rate of positive biopsies for myocarditis in these patients with acute dilated cardiomyopathy was significantly influenced by when the biopsy was performed with respect to the onset of symptoms: 89 percent for 0 to 4 weeks, 70 percent for 4 to 12 weeks, and 38 percent for 12 to 26 weeks after onset. Moreover, this study also demonstrated a lack of correlation between the classic clinical criteria for myocarditis and the likelihood of myocarditis on biopsy.

The empirical use of immunosuppressive agents to treat biopsy-proven myocarditis in patients with acute dilated cardiomyopathy was introduced only 6 years ago.[28] In 82 patients with biopsy-proven myocarditis, immunosuppression resulted in improvement in 60 percent.[3] Improvement often (although not always) is associated with resolution of the myocarditis on biopsy.[6,7] We have followed 21 patients with acute dilated cardiomyopathy who had initial biopsies positive for myocarditis and who were treated with immunosuppressive therapy. Followup clinical evaluation, endomyocardial biopsy, and left ventricular ejection fraction were obtained 81 ± 17 days after the initial biopsy. Overall, there was significant improvement in NYHA class from 3.7 to 2.0 ($p < 0.03$) and in ejection fraction from 0.22 ± 0.02 to 0.35 ± 0.03 ($p = 0.0005$). Eight followup biopsies revealed ongoing or healing myocarditis, whereas 13 revealed healed myocarditis. There was no significant difference in the improvement of either group. A few studies have also reported that patients who improve on immunosuppression may relapse when therapy is terminated but improve again with reinstitution of treatment.[6,7,28] This course suggests that an "autoimmune" process akin to cardiac transplant rejection is occurring in some patients.

At present, a definite diagnosis of myocarditis requires endomyocardial biopsy. Because the clinical diagnosis alone appears to be even more insensitive than endomyocardial biopsy, a means of screening patients with clinically suspected myocarditis prior to endomyocardial biopsy would be helpful. Gallium-67 scans were introduced as a method for noninvasively detecting an inflammatory infiltrate in the myocardium.[29] However, these scans do not appear to be sensitive enough to be of practical use as a screening tool. Because myocarditis also involves myocyte necrosis, we have used indium-111 labeled monoclonal antimyosin antibody gamma imaging to detect myocardial necrosis in patients referred for endomyocardial biopsy to rule out myocarditis.[30] Of 28 patients with clinically suspected myocarditis, nine had positive scans and positive biopsies, eight had positive scans and negative biopsies, and 11 had negative scans and negative biopsies. No patients had a negative scan with a positive biopsy. Thus, more than half the patients with a positive antimyosin scan had biopsy-proven myocarditis, whereas a negative scan was highly indicative of the absence of myocarditis on endomyocardial biopsy. The finding of eight patients with positive scans and negative biopsies again points out the possible insensitivity of endomyocardial biopsy but may also be due to the nonspecificity of this imaging technique for myocarditis per se.

ENDOMYOCARDIAL BIOPSY—IMMUNOLOGICAL STUDIES

Immunocytochemical studies have shown that many of the infiltrating cells in biopsies of patients with myocarditis are T lymphocytes.[31,32] These T lymphocytes are "activated," that is, they respond to interleukin-2 stimulation and can be cultured from the myocardium.[32] The T lymphocytes cultured from myocardial biopsies are composed of both T4 and T8 subsets, the ratio of one to another being patient dependent. These T lymphocytes produce lymphokines and are cytotoxic in lectin-mediated assays. Their cytotoxicity is HLA restricted just as the cytotoxic T lymphocytes in the mouse are H_2 restricted. Furthermore, the cultured T lymphocytes are often oligoclonal, as evidenced by restriction fragment length polymorphism analysis of the beta chain of the T-cell receptor gene, suggesting that these T cells are directed toward specific antigens.[33] Whether these are self-antigens or neo-antigens (for example, persistent coxsackievirus B) is unknown at this time.

The role of humoral immune reactions in the development of dilated cardiomyopathy is unresolved. Antimyocardial antibodies of various types are present in 10 to 30 percent of patients with dilated cardiomyopathy. However, antibody titers do not correlate well with disease activity or clinical course. This finding suggests a reactive rather than a pathogenic significance. Some studies[34] have shown that antimyolemmal antibodies in sera of patients with dilated cardiomyopathy can be absorbed and their cytolytic activity blocked by appropriate viral antigens. Others[35] have found an inverse correlation between the amount of immunoglobulin demonstrable in endomyocardial biopsies of dilated cardiomyopathy patients and the ejection fraction, but this finding has never been confirmed.

Circulating lymphocyte subsets have been quantitated in patients with myocarditis and dilated cardiomyopathy.[36,37] Decreased suppressor and natural killer cell activities have been found in some patients, but such studies have not been well controlled.[35]

CONCLUSIONS

Pathologically defined myocarditis and clinically observed dilated cardiomyopathy are stages of the same disease. The evidence that myocarditis precedes and/or accompanies acute dilated cardiomyopathy is irrefutable. Recent clinical endomyocardial biopsy studies reveal that although some patients with acute dilated cardiomyopathy recover spontaneously or with immunosuppressive therapy, many develop chronic dilated cardiomyopathy. However, myocarditis is unlikely to be the only cause of dilated cardiomyopathy.

Table 7-1 shows a framework of the hypothesized pathogenesis of dilated cardiomyopathy. The etiology of this sequence may be a viral infection involving the heart and resulting in a persistence of virus in myocytes. Genetically determined cellular immune reactions are evoked by the initial infection and are maintained because of an autoimmune process or the persistence of a viral neo-antigen. Cytotoxic T lymphocytes either directly or indirectly produce myocardial dysfunction, resulting in loss of myocardial contractility and ultimately the development of dilated cardiomyopathy.

Endomyocardial biopsy may be an imperfect test, but it has provided pathologic documentation of myocarditis and the tissue samples for the cDNA hybridization and T-lymphocyte studies that have important pathogenetic and therapeutic implications (Table 7-2). Realization of the deficiencies of endomyocardial biopsy in diagnosing myocarditis and dilated cardiomyopathy, the development of newer screening tests for myocarditis, and further molecular biologic and immunologic

Table 7-1. Pathogenesis of Chronic Dilated Cardiomyopathy via Myocarditis

VIRAL INFECTION
↓ Virus (dose and strain)
MYOCARDIUM (age, sex, physiologic state)
↓ Inflammatory and humoral response
(ACUTE) MYOCARDITIS
↓ Persistent T-lymphocyte activity (genetics)
LYMPHOCYTIC MYOCARDITIS
↓ Impairment of myocardial contractility
ACUTE DILATED CARDIOMYOPATHY
↓ Irreversible loss of myocytes and structural changes
CHRONIC DILATED CARDIOMYOPATHY

Table 7-2. Endomyocardial Biopsy Evidence for Myocarditis Causing Dilated Cardiomyopathy

1. Serial biopsy progression from myocarditis to dilated cardiomyopathy
2. Clinical and biopsy improvement with use of immunosuppressive therapy
3. Recovery of oligoclonal T lymphocytes from myocardium of patients with myocarditis and dilated cardiomyopathy
4. cDNA hybridization demonstration of coxsackievirus B within myocytes from patients with dilated cardiomyopathy and myocarditis

studies of the tissues provided by endomyocardial biopsy will undoubtedly provide us with even greater insight into this often-confusing disease process.

ACKNOWLEDGMENTS

I am grateful to all my collaborators at the Massachusetts General Hospital who have been involved in these studies, but especially to Drs. J. F. Southern, I. F. Palacios, J. T. Kurnick, and G. W. Dec. I also wish to thank Ms. Gail Arbuthnot for her patience and assistance with the preparation of this manuscript.

REFERENCES

1. Abelmann, WH: Myocarditis. N Engl J Med 275:832; 944, 1966.
2. Johnson, RA and Palacios, I: Dilated cardiomyopathies of the adult. N Engl J Med 307:1051; 1119, 1982.
3. Kereiakes, DJ and Parmley, WW: Myocarditis and cardiomyopathy. Am Heart J 108:1318, 1984.
4. Rose, AG and Beck, W: Dilated (congestive) cardiomyopathy: A syndrome of severe cardiac dysfunction with remarkably few morphological features of myocardial damage. Histopathology 9:367, 1985.
5. Unverferth, DV: Etiologic factors, pathogenesis, and prognosis of dilated cardiomyopathy. J Lab Clin Med 106:349, 1985.
6. Daly, K, Richardson, PJ, Olsen, EGJ, et al: Acute myocarditis—role of histological and virological examination in the diagnosis and assessment of immunosuppressive treatment. Br Heart J 51:30, 1984.
7. Dec, GW, Palacios, IF, Fallon, JT, et al: Active myocarditis in the spectrum of acute dilated cardiomyopathies—clinical features, histologic correlates, and clinical outcome. N Engl J Med 312:885, 1985.
8. Edwards, WD, Holmes, DR, and Reeder, GS: Diagnosis of active lymphocytic myocarditis by endomyocardial biopsy. Quantitative criteria for light microscopy. Mayo Clin Proc 57:419, 1982.
9. MacArthur, CGC, Tarin, D, Goodwin, JF, et al: The relationship of myocarditis to dilated cardiomyopathy. Eur Heart J 5:1023, 1984.
10. Parrillo, JE, Aretz, HT, Palacios, I, et al: The results of transvenous endomyocardial biopsy can frequently be used to diagnose myocardial diseases in patients with idiopathic heart failure—endomyocardial biopsies in 100 consecutive patients revealed a substantial incidence of myocarditis. Circulation 69:93, 1984.
11. Shanes, JG, Krone, RJ, Tsai, CC, et al: Mild myocardial inflammation presenting as congestive cardiomyopathy responsive to immunosuppression. Am Heart J 107:798, 1984.
12. Zee-Cheng, CS, Tsai, CC, Palmer, DC, et al: High incidence of myocarditis by endomyocardial biopsy in patients with idiopathic congestive cardiomyopathy. J Am Coll Cardiol 3:63, 1984.
13. Nippoldt, TB, Edwards, WD, Holmes, DR, et al: Right ventricular endomyocardial biopsy—clinicopathologic correlates in 100 consecutive patients. Mayo Clin Proc 57:407, 1982.
14. Abelmann, WH: Classification and natural history of primary myocardial disease. Prog Cardiovasc Dis 27:73, 1984.
15. Tazelaar, HD and Billingham, ME: Leukocytic infiltrates in idiopathic dilated cardiomyopathy. A source of confusion with active myocarditis. Am J Surg Pathol 10:405, 1986.

16. Anderson, KR, Sutton, MGS, and Lie, JT: Histopathological types of cardiac fibrosis in myocardial disease. J Pathol 128:79, 1979.
17. Baandrup, U and Olsen, EGJ: Critical analysis of endomyocardial biopsies from patients suspected of having cardiomyopathy I: Morphological and morphometric aspects. Br Heart J 45:475, 1981.
18. Dick, MR, Unverferth, DV, and Baba, N: The pattern of myocardial degeneration in nonischemic congestive cardiomyopathy. Human Pathol 13:740, 1982.
19. Keren, A, Billingham, ME, Weintraub, D, et al: Mildly dilated congestive cardiomyopathy. Circulation 72:302, 1985.
20. Mason, JW: Endomyocardial biopsy: The balance of success and failure. Circulation 71:185, 1985.
21. Aretz, HT, Billingham, ME, Edwards, WE, et al: Myocarditis, a histopathologic definition and classification. Am J Cardiovasc Pathol 1:3, 1987.
22. Cambridge, G, MacArthur, CGC, Waterson, AP, et al: Antibodies to Coxsackie B viruses in congestive cardiomyopathy. Br Heart J 41:692, 1979.
23. Archard, LC, Bowles, NE, Olsen, EGJ, et al: Detection of persistent Coxsackie B virus RNA in dilated cardiomyopathy and myocarditis. Eur Heart J 8, 1987.
24. Woodruff, JF: Viral myocarditis—a review. Am J Pathol 101:427, 1980.
25. Huber, SA, Job, LP, and Woodruff, JF: Lysis of infected myofibers by Coxsackievirus B-3 immune T lymphocytes. Am J Pathol 98:681, 1980.
26. Kishimoto, C, Kuribayashi, K, Masuda, T, et al: Immunologic behavior of lymphocytes in experimental viral myocarditis: Significance of T lymphocytes in the severity of myocarditis and silent myocarditis in BALB/c-nu/nu mice. Circulation 71:1247, 1985.
27. Ferrans, VJ and Roberts, WC: Myocardial biopsy: A useful diagnostic procedure or only a research tool? Am J Cardiol 41:965, 1978.
28. Mason, JW, Billingham, ME, and Ricci, DR: Treatment of acute inflammatory myocarditis assisted by endomyocardial biopsy. Am J Cardiol 45:1037, 1980.
29. Robinson, J, O'Connell, J, Henkin, RE, et al: Gallium-67 imaging in cardiomyopathy. Ann Intern Med 90:198, 1979.
30. Haber, E. Yasuda, T, Palacios, IF, et al: Antimyosin antibody imaging in the diagnosis of acute myocarditis. Eur Heart J 8, 1987.
31. Cassling, RS, Linder, J, Sears, TD, et al: Quantitative evaluation of inflammation in biopsy specimens from idiopathically failing or irritable hearts: Experience in 80 pediatric and adult patients. Am Heart J 110:713, 1985.
32. Kurnick, JT, Leary, C, Palacios,IF, et al: Culture and characterization of lymphocytic infiltrates from endomyocardial biopsies of patients with idiopathic myocarditis. Eur Heart J 8, 1987.
33. Stamenkovic, I, Kurnick, JT, Leary, C, et al: Clonality of T-lymphocytes cultured from endomyocardial biopsies of patients with myocarditis. Circulation 74:II-143, 1986.
34. Maisch, B: Surface antigens of adult heart cells and their use in diagnosis. Basic Res Cardiol 80 (Suppl 1):47, 1985.
35. Bolte, HD: Immunological defects—precursors of myocarditis and dilated cardiomyopathy? J Mol Cell Cardiol 17 (Suppl 2):69, 1985.
36. Fowles, RE, Bieber, CP, and Stinson, EB: Defective in vitro suppressor cell function in idiopathic congestive cardiomyopathy. Circulation 59:483, 1979.
37. Anderson, JL, Carlquist, JF, and Hammond, EH: Deficient natural killer cell activity in patients with idiopathic dilated cardiomyopathy. Lancet 2:1124, 1982.

CHAPTER 8

Immunopathologic Basis of Myocardial Injury

Bruce M. McManus, M.D., Ph.D.
Charles J. Gauntt, Ph.D.
Randal S. Cassling, M.D.

Immunologic mechanisms are presumed important in human lymphocytic myocarditis. However, much of what we know in this regard is circumstantial and only vaguely substantiated. Other human diseases, including trypanosomiasis, rheumatic heart disease, and hepatitis B, have been used to suggest and support the concept of microorganism-initiated, immunologically sustained, organ-selected inflammatory processes in humans. With all of the problems inherent in animal models, the murine coxsackievirus and encephalomyocarditis virus models have provided insights into the immunologic bases of disease and host and viral genetic heterogeneity in determination of host responses, tissue necrosis, inflammation, dysfunction, disability, and death. In this chapter, we will outline the evidence of an immunologic component in murine and human myocarditis and suggest directions to resolve the uncertainties about the *immunologic injury paradigm* in myocarditis.

Inflammatory cell infiltration and myocyte necrosis represent the end result of several forms of injury to the heart. This injury may be on the basis of ischemia, trauma, toxin exposure, infection, or connective tissue diseases. Beyond ischemic causes of myocardial injury, the next most prominent category of inflammatory processes involving the heart is that known or suspected to be due to infectious agents, mainly bacteria, fungi, and viruses. Currently, most clinical cases of myocarditis in free-living humans are suspected to be of viral etiology. Typically, the clinical diagnosis of myocarditis in humans is considered after a person presents with a recent "viral illness" and one or all of the clinical sequelae of "infection," inflammation, and necrosis—congestive heart failure, conduction system abnormalities, or arrhythmias. A specific infectious etiology is found infrequently, despite the enthusiasm for identifying such a possibility.

The discovery of the coxsackievirus group A and B families in the 1940s and later of their association with "myopericarditis" sparked renewed interest in myocarditis. The RNA genome-containing picornaviruses, especially the coxsackieviruses group

B (CVB), make up the most significant proportion of serologically positive human infections. Since the recognition that coxsackieviruses may infect the heart, many other viruses have been linked serologically to myocarditis in humans.[1]

ANIMAL MODELS

In light of the clinical relevance of coxsackievirus infections in people, and the similarity of histologic changes produced by coxsackieviruses in myocarditis in animal models and in humans, the majority of experimental myocarditis work has used CVB. Owing to the small number of human cases of community-acquired lymphocytic myocarditis with a strong infectious association and the typically late clinical presentation, the students of myocarditis have been obliged to use animal models. Many animal models have been used to study the mechanism of induction of CVB myocarditis, including the mouse [including the nude mouse[2]], hamster,[3] rat, cynomolgus monkey,[4] baboon,[5] and swine. Larger mammals have allowed easier evaluation of the hemodynamic, echocardiographic, and electrocardiographic consequences of virus-induced myocarditis. Also, they have provided a genetic background closer in proximity to humans.

Despite the favorable large-animal model characteristics, the majority of investigations have been performed using a murine model with different attributes. Although less phylogenetically related to humans, the genetic background of the mouse including H-2 and non-H-2 genes is well characterized. The virus-infected mouse has already provided much of our knowledge regarding general immunologic mechanisms, information that can be applied in efforts to understand human myocarditis. As alluded to earlier, the use of mice and hamsters evolved primarily because of the similarities in pathologic cardiac lesions in these animals and humans. The availability of large numbers of rodents for experiments and the reproducibility in the course of the disease has also contributed to their selection.

Basic studies with CVB-rodent models have sought to explain several elements of the disease that affect severity and probable outcome. A "classic" view evolved in the 1960s that cell necrosis was secondary to virus-induced cell lysis.[1] This paradigm has not been found entirely true, recognition of its inadequacies having depended on more sophisticated, recently developed experimental methods. Currently, investigative efforts are focused on the nature of the immunologic parameters that are believed to play a major role in myocardial lesion formation—infective, injurious, and immunologic properties of the viruses, and host genetic, age, stress, and gender-related susceptibilities. Despite our incomplete understanding of immunologic reactivities of the host against CVB, and CVB interactions with host cells, clinical trials of immunotherapeutic agents in mice and humans have been undertaken. We will briefly review the data obtained with animal models of CVB-induced myocarditis in an attempt to explain the variable success of immune-intervention therapy. For earlier reviews of studies on basic mechanisms of viral myocarditis, the reader has several excellent choices.[1,6–10]

Host Immunologic Responses in Murine Myocarditis

Pioneering studies on the mechanisms of CVB-induced murine myocarditis have shown that the *severity* of virus-induced myocarditis depends on *age* of the animal at inoculation, *strain* of mouse used, *gender* of mouse, and *virus variant*.[1,6–10]

These studies showed that after oral or intraperitoneal induction of a CVB myocarditis, virus and destructive lesions are detected not only in heart tissue but also in the liver, spleen, and pancreas. Virus titers are maximal around days 3 to 5 postinoculation (p.i.) in pancreas and heart tissues, prior to appearance of myocarditic lesions on days 5 to 6 p.i. Virus titers decline from day 5 p.i. onward, and in most murine models virus becomes undetectable by day 14 p.i. The central question—whether primary viral myocytolysis or secondary immune reactivities cause the majority of pathologic lesions in acute myocarditis in an adolescent mouse model—was answered in a series of classic experiments by Woodruff and Woodruff.[11] Mice depleted of T lymphocytes by thymectomy, immunodepletion, or lethal irradiation and then challenged with CVB3 harbored virus in heart tissues but had little or no inflammatory cell infiltrate and little subsequent scar tissue formation. Very few necrotic myofibers could be detected in vivo in T-cell-depleted mice, suggesting that most myocardial damage was secondary to cellular immune processes.

What cell population(s) in fetal, neonatal, and adolescent heart tissues become(s) infected? An examination of heart sections from CVB3-inoculated adolescent mice prior to mononuclear cell infiltration reveals the presence of myocytes undergoing necrosis, a finding suggestive of direct myocyte infection by virus and concomitant myocytolysis.[1] However, only fibroblasts cultured from adolescent tissues have been shown to replicate CVB3, and replication occurs in the absence of cytopathologic changes.[12] Fetal or neonatal murine myofibers,[13,14] neonatal cardiac endothelial cells,[15] and neonatal skin fibroblasts[12,16] can replicate CVB3. Skin and cardiac fibroblast cultures may contain virus for up to 12 days p.i. in adolescent tissues. The significance of the latter is uncertain; however, infection may elicit a greater subsequent immunologic response owing to sustained replication of CVB3 in cardiac fibroblasts or may allow for a source of virus for sustained direct viral injury.

More recent work on the immunopathologic basis of acute CVB3-induced myocarditis has established several facts. Heart tissues from myocarditic mice inoculated with a myocarditic CVB3 strain contain salt-extractable antigen(s) that immunospecifically reacts with peritoneal leukocytes from virus-inoculated myocarditic mice in vitro.[17] This antigen(s) preparation (? viral-altered tissue antigen, ? tissue neo-antigen, ? cross-reactive antigen, ? anti-idiotypic antibody) does not contain detectable CVB3 viral antigens,[17] nor does it induce neutralizing antibody to CVB3.[18] Similar immunoreactive antigen(s) cannot be detected in normal heart tissues or in spleen or liver tissues from mice with CVB3-induced myocarditis.[17] As already implied, this neo-antigen(s) has not been identified but may be a virus-induced cell antigen(s). One nonmyocarditic CVB3 variant ($CVB3_o$) does not induce the immunoreactive heart tissue antigen(s), even though the virus replicates in heart tissues.[19] However, additional studies with another amyocarditic CVB3 variant (ts5R) have found that ts5R induces immunoreactive heart tissue antigen(s) in vivo. Thus, additional host factors may be involved in the complex process leading to myocarditis.[20]

One such probable host factor is subsets of functional T lymphocytes. Indirect evidence, obtained in experiments that used low-dose cyclophosphamide to reduce preferentially *suppressor* T lymphocytes in vivo, suggests that induction of T suppressor cells during CVB3 infection may ameliorate the disease.[20,21] Transfer of the presumed T suppressor cells (lyt 2+) from mice inoculated with the amyocarditic $CVB3_o$ variant into mice challenged with a myocarditic CVB3 variant provides some protection against myocarditis.[21]

Several kinds of experiments have demonstrated that CVB3-induced acute myocarditis is a result of reactions of cytotoxic T lymphocytes (CTLs) with antigens in heart tissue of myocarditic mice. At issue is the nature of the antigens being recognized by the CTLs. Apparently, one kind of antigen(s) is virus-induced, as CTLs from CVB3-induced myocarditic mice can recognize and preferentially lyse CVB3-infected neonatal myofibers,[13,14,22] endothelial cells,[15] or skin fibroblasts[16,20,23,24] in vitro.

Adoptively transferred CTLs obtained from CVB3-inoculated mice and selectively adsorbed to virus-infected cells in vitro[15,16,25,26] or to anti–Thy 1– or anti–lyt 2+–coated dishes[26] can induce myocarditis in thymectomized T–lymphocyte–deficient CVB3-inoculated mice. However, adoptive transfer of spleen cells from mice inoculated with the amyocarditic $CVB3_0$ variant into mice inoculated with the myocarditic CVB3 virus resulted in an inhibition of myocarditis.[27] Thus, induction of a CTL population by the amyocarditic viruses $CVB3_0$[27] or ts5R[20] (in absence of myocarditis) requires an additional factor to eventuate in myocarditis. CVB3 infection may involve viral-induction of a population of "autoreactive" CTLs that recognize antigen(s) on uninfected neonatal myofibers.[25] Transfer of this latter population of "autoreactive" CTLs, enriched by adsorption to uninfected myofibers, into thymectomized mice induces more severe myocarditis than transfer of CTLs that recognize antigen(s) on virus-infected myofibers.[25]

Activated natural killer (NK) cells of the host may ameliorate CVB3-induced myocarditis. Infection of mice with CVB3 induces maximal activation of NK cells between 2 and 4 days p.i. with virus.[28] Immunodepletion of mice of NK cells prior to CVB3 inoculation results in increased virus titers in heart tissues and more severe myocarditis.[28] Thus, the proposed role for NK cells in murine myocarditis is lysis of virus-infected cells to effect a reduction in tissue virus titers. Earlier work[1] has suggested that macrophages and virus-specific neutralizing antibody eliminate virus; these factors likely contribute, along with NK cells, to early immunologic processing of virus by an infected murine host. Additionally, CVB3 infections induce moderate titers (approximately 1280 units/ml) of interferon with similar kinetics as NK cell activation; the heat lability (56°C 30 min) and lack of neutralization by antiserum directed against interferon beta suggest this interferon is the gamma species.[155]

Yet another mechanism has been proposed to account for the acute myocarditis induced by CVB3 in DBA/2 mice.[29] A comparative study of immune responses in DBA/2 and Balb/c species of mice during acute myocarditis has shown that virus titers in heart tissues are equivalent, and CTLs that recognize both uninfected and virus infected myofibers are generated. Antithymocyte or anti-Ia antibodies will prevent CVB3-induced myocarditis in both murine strains. Both virus-inoculated murine strains produce autoantibodies that react with normal heart tissue; however, complement depletion of the two strains with cobra venom prevents myocarditis in DBA/2 but not Balb/c mice. The latter result suggests that a portion of the myocardial damage in DBA/2 mice is mediated more directly by humoral immune mechanisms.

Female mice develop less severe myocarditis than male mice in response to CVB3 inoculation.[13,22] Female mice appear to activate NK cells more efficiently and maintain these activated cells longer than male mice.[14]

Although less studied, the encephalomyocarditis-murine model of myocarditis is in general agreement with the CVB-murine models of myocarditis on the central role of T lymphocytes in mediating disease.[30,31]

Recent studies on the antigen(s) recognized by virus-induced CTL used dual fluorescence to show that only CVB3-infected fibroblasts in a culture display a surface change that is detectable by the binding of the lectin *ulex europaeus* agglutinin I (UEAI) and soybean agglutinin and the internal presence of viral capsid antigens. Only 12 to 25 percent of cells in either murine neonatal skin or adolescent heart fibroblasts are simultaneously positive for UEAI binding and capsid antigens. Infected skin fibroblasts bind a maximum amount of UEAI at 72 hours postinfection, a time when these infected cultures best serve as targets for virus-induced sensitized CTL.[156] The amount of UEAI bound to interferon beta–treated infected cells that have reduced virus yields is diminished. Fibroblasts infected with the amyocarditic ts5R virus show reduced UEAI binding, suggesting one possible explanation for the amyocarditic nature of the virus. In vitro data on CVB3-infected fibroblasts show that they do not undergo any cytopathologic change and can exhibit the UEAI-binding change for days. Because the nonenveloped CVB3 is not known to induce any glycoproteins, the UEAI-binding antigen(s) is proposed to be of cellular origin.

The Viruses

The body's defenses against viremia and virus multiplication during the initial state of viral infection include macrophages, NK cells, and gamma interferon.[32] In the murine model of viral-induced myocarditis, the viremia is present for approximately 3 days, whereas the peak myocardial titers of virus are present between 3 and 5 days. Usually, virus cannot be detected in the myocardium after 10 to 14 days, but on rare occasions it may be present for several weeks after exposure.[2]

Virus receptors on host plasma membranes are major determinants of virus infectivity. These receptors are organ- and host species–specific, as well as virus subgroup–specific.[33] This multilevel specificity partially explains the selective tissue "tropism" displayed by each virus. Thus, tropism is largely genetically determined.

Among the more than 18 common viruses that can cause or are linked to human or animal myocarditis, considerable evidence has accumulated to implicate coxsackieviruses B1–B5 in serious inflammatory cardiac disease in children and adults.[1,8,10] The CVBs are classified within the picornavirus family along with the polioviruses, coxsackieviruses group A, echoviruses, and rhinoviruses. They are small (29 to 33 nm), nonenveloped, icosahedral particles containing RNA genomes. Laboratory strains[19,34–39] and clinical isolates[40–43] of CVB consist of heterogeneous populations relative to biologic and antigenic surface properties. Although minor biologic markers for myocarditic[40,42] and cardiotropic[41] properties of coxsackievirus B4 (CVB4) in murine models have been reported, a major biologic marker covariant with myocarditis-inducing capability has not been found to explain the immune picture of myocarditis. In an attempt to study virus variants derived from a mutant myocarditic coxsackievirus B3 (CVB3) parent virus, revertants of temperature-sensitive mutants were obtained.[20,44,45] Major biologic marker differences were not detected between amyocarditic and myocarditic variants in mouse models, although differences in nucleic acid sequences were suggested by oligonucleotide fingerprint mapping.[45] Because of high mutation rates (10^{-4} per incorporated nucleotide) among these viruses,[40,46] it may not be possible to identify definitively a nucleotide sequence(s) associated with myocarditis capabilities in mice until viral, double-stranded cDNA sequences that are stable (to mutation), complementary, and molecularly cloned can be examined. The latter possibility is at hand, as CVB3 has been molecularly cloned.[47,48] In summary, variants of CVB4 and CVB3 have been unsuccessfully examined for major biologic markers descriptive of myocarditis or amyocarditic capabilities. A careful study of the nucleotide sequence(s) of the RNA genomes and the secondary and tertiary structure of the genomes will define these descriptors of virulence.

Working Paradigm—Immune Mechanisms in the Mouse

Composite data (Fig. 8–1) obtained with CVB3 adolescent murine models of acute myocarditis suggest the following scenario: Virus replicates in several organs during the initial 3 to 4 days p.i. and then persists in the heart and pancreas for an additional 10 days. During the initial period, gamma-interferon is induced and NK cells are activated. NK cells provide some protection by reducing virus titers in heart tissues. Viral infection of cells in heart tissues, perhaps myocytes and likely fibroblasts, results in the appearance of new antigens. At this point it is not known whether the immunoreactive antigen(s) that is salt-extracted from infected mouse heart tissues is related to the virus-induced change(s) detectable by UEAI binding on the surface of infected fibroblasts. Two kinds of CTL responses are evoked by virus infection of heart tissue cells. One type of CTL recognizes an as yet uncharacterized virus-induced antigen(s), while a second type of CTL recognizes an antigen(s) on the surface of uninfected neonatal cardiac myofibers. These two CTL populations presumably exert lytic activity against infected, and perhaps uninfected, cells. The targeting of infected and uninfected cells is not well understood; however, the end result is lysis of myocytes and subsequent formation of scar tissue.

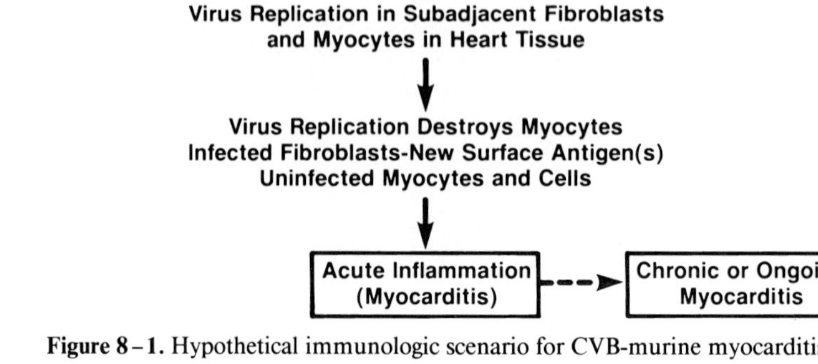

Figure 8–1. Hypothetical immunologic scenario for CVB-murine myocarditis.

Other Considerations in the Mouse

The Thymus

Although the thymic T lymphocyte has been demonstrated to have a role in murine-CVB3 myocarditis, other studies with athymic mice have shown that a CVB3-induced inflammatory response can occur in the absence of T lymphocytes. Athymic or nude mice lack mature thymocytes and should thus serve as models of CVB3-induced myocarditis in T lymphocyte–depleted mice. Comparative studies of athymic mice and their hairy euthymic counterparts have not resulted in a consensus of opinion. No difference in CVB3 titers in heart tissues, extent of myocytolysis, or extent of mononuclear cell inflammation[49] has been observed in two studies;[49,50] however, CVB3 titers in heart tissue were similar,[50] or persist in heart tissues of the nude mice for up to 28 days compared with 7 days for euthymic mice.[50] A third study, previously mentioned,[2] showed that virus persisted for up to 94 days in nude mice but for only 14 days in euthymic mice. Myocarditis was detected in both groups each time the tissue was examined; however, it was not found in nude mice until 14 days p.i. In yet other reports,[51,52] the hearts of CVB3-inoculated nude mice showed myocardial inflammation that was less intense than that of hearts of euthymic mice. The differing results reported in these studies may be due to genotypic differences in virus strains or in mice. Nevertheless, the data as a whole suggest that monocyte-macrophage cells are sufficient, in the absence of mature T lymphocytes, to produce an inflammatory response.

Age

Age of the mouse at the time of infection is a known determinant of the severity of myocarditis or the outcome of infection.[1] Infant mice often die following CVB inoculation, including after inoculation with temperature-sensitive mutants of CVB3.[49] Adult mice generally exhibit less severe myocarditis than adolescent mice.[1] A recent study[53] with a CVB4-murine infant heart disease model illustrates the role of the thymic T cells in neonatal myocarditis. Infant mice surviving a CVB4 challenge (21 percent) developed transmural ventricular necrosis, fibrosis, and ventricular aneurysm. Administration of antithymocyte serum before infection delayed virus elimination, increased mortality, and increased pathologic lesions—that is, the lesions included more extensive myofiber necrosis and mineralization, even though leukocyte infiltration was decreased.[53] Thus, in the CVB4 infant murine model, T-cell function(s) is apparently needed for elimination of virus; when elimination is impaired, myocardial injury is more severe.

Physical Stress

Stress is a factor known to exacerbate many viral infections. A clever early study[54] on the effects of exercise (swimming) on CVB3-induced cardiomyopathy showed that when 3-week-old CVB3-infected mice were forced to swim for 30 minutes twice a day for up to 3 weeks, mortality increased significantly. Half of these deaths were due to congestive heart failure, most occurring while swimming. Hearts were dilated, hypertrophied, inflamed, necrotic, and calcified. Virus titers in heart tissues were increased over 500-fold in mice forced to swim. Mice inoculated with CVB3 at 2 weeks of age were forced to swim for 9 days as already described and then were followed for 15 months.[55] This short exercise period during infection significantly increased mortality, and only the forced swimmers (compared with infected nonswimming mice) had atrial enlargement with mural thrombi, myocardial fiber disintegration, and heavy calcium deposits in the myocardium with ultimate replacement of myocardium by fibrous scar. It is of interest that exercise alone may enhance release of T lymphocytes from the thymus.[56] A more recent study by Lerner and colleagues[57] used ^{51}Cr-labeled lymphocytes and xeroradiography to assess the effect of forced swimming on CVB3-induced acute dilated cardiomyopathy. Three-week-old mice, infected with CVB3 and forced to swim, had a fourfold greater number of T lymphocytes of blood origin directed to the heart when compared with CVB3-infected mice not forced to swim. These studies suggest that exercise in CVB3-infected juvenile mice in some manner enhances movement of T lymphocytes from the blood to a heart that is replicating virus in significantly higher titers.

Gender

Gender of the CVB-inoculated mouse also affects the severity of myocarditis induced, with male mice generally exhibiting more severe myocarditis than female mice.[1] A few strains of mice have been found in which the female mice are more sensitive to CVB3-induction of myocarditis than are the males.[45] Of course, investigators have asked why there is a gender difference. Several studies indicate that females do not produce cytotoxic T lymphocytes specific for virus-infected targets during infection but rather continue to produce cells with characteristics of NK cells.[13,22,58] By contrast, females in the first and last thirds of pregnancy develop more severe myocarditis than their nonpregnant counterparts in response to CVB3 infections.[59] The enhanced myocarditis is accompanied by increased virus titers in the heart and increased cytotoxic T-lymphocyte reactivities against both infected and uninfected myofibers. Pregnant females depleted of T lymphocytes do not develop significant myocarditis. Because progesterone was increased during the last third of the pregnancy, progesterone was administered to castrated males and castrated females. This maneuver increased virus titers in the heart, increased cytotoxic T-lymphocyte reactivities to virus-infected myofibers, and increased myocarditis. The mechanism of action of progesterone in this model is not known; however, immune responses in a number of strains of male mice with a high sensitivity to androgens were depressed.[60]

Drugs

Studies of therapy in acute murine viral myocarditis have in part confirmed the complex interplay of immunologic reactions that contribute to the disease. Early work[1,61] showed that administration of corticosteroids during the acute phase of murine viral myocarditis significantly exacerbated the disease. The nonsteroidal anti-inflammatory drug ibuprofen significantly exacerbated CVB3-induced myocarditis, that is, both myocyte necrosis and inflammation were worse.[62] Cyclosporine, a widely used immunosuppressive agent in allotransplantation, caused a significant increase in myocardial necrosis, mortality, and enhanced virus persistence in heart tissues if given early during acute CVB3-induced myocarditis.[63] On the other hand, levamisole, a drug that restores cell-mediated immune responses in an immunodepressed or immune-deficient host, exacerbated CVB3-induced murine myocarditis.[64] This drug appeared to increase blastogenic activity of T lymphocytes, altered T-lymphocyte distribution in the body, and increased T-lymphocyte reactivities. Studies with beta-interferon in the CVB3-murine model established that interferon was a beneficial line of defense against virus-induced disease if present within 24 hours of infection.[32] Paradoxically, the absence of interferon around 3 days after infection, as cleared by the administration of anti-beta-interferon antisera, resulted in a reduced number of myocardial lesions.[32]

B10LF-70, a substituted guanine derivative, reduced the number of CVB3-induced myocardial lesions if administered at the time of virus infection.[65] This drug had minimal antiviral activity in vivo but was likely to be effective as an immunomodulatory agent: NK cell activity was increased, and CTL reactivity against virus-infected target cells was reduced. In the encephalomyocarditis virus murine model of myocarditis, successful therapy with the antiviral drug, ribavirin, was achieved.[66] Treatment with this drug in the acute disease reduced cardiac tissue levels of virus, reduced inflammation and the number of gross myocardial lesions, and promoted survival. In contrast, the effect of prednisolone on encephalomyocarditis virus-induced myocarditis was similar to that of prednisone on CVB3-induced murine myocarditis, that is, it exacerbated the course of the acute disease.[67]

Chronic Models

Chronic animal studies of virus-induced myocarditis have been limited in the past; however, exciting models have been established recently.[68–70] Several parameters of infection and disease activity were measured in a survey of murine species to determine the influence of the major histocompatibility complex (MHC) on CVB3 induction of disease. The data suggested that production of disease was not under control of the major histocompatibility complex, a conclusion previously reached by Gauntt and colleagues.[45] Some strains had high mortality rates, others developed acute myocarditis, and yet others developed a continuing chronic myocardial disease.[68–70] Mice with chronic disease produced heart-specific myocardial autoantibodies and had mononuclear cells both within foci of repair after myocyte necrosis and in a distinctive, diffuse interstitial pattern. Whether the autoantibodies have an active role in the chronic disease process or whether they will be useful only as diagnostic indicators of disease is not clear.

An encephalomyocarditis virus model in DBA/2 mice was established to determine whether electrocardiographic abnormalities could be detected in mice with chronic myocarditis over a course lasting 220 days.[71] Atrial complexes, ventricular premature complexes, and complete atrioventricular block were detected in 13, 17, and 53 percent of mice with myocarditis, respectively. Arrhythmias were detected in the later stages of the study period. On the basis of their observations, the authors suggested that people with new arrhythmias and without other clinical manifestations may be manifesting signs of previous viral myocarditis.[71]

Hamsters are susceptible to coxsackievirus B3–induced myocarditis, although mortality is high.[1] More recent studies of animals surviving coxsackievirus B1 inoculation (28 percent) show that some hamsters develop ventricular premature complexes and ventricular aneurysms.[72] Left ventricular aneurysms as a complication of myocarditis have also been found in mice inoculated with coxsackievirus B1 or B4.[73] Hamsters inoculated with CVB3 develop acute myocarditis and may progress to death or recovery; if they recover, left ventricular function may return to near normal or may deteriorate with progression to congestive heart failure.[74] It is of interest that myocardial lesions in the CVB3-hamster model of myocarditis do not calcify[75] whereas those lesions in murine models of CVB myocarditis typically do.

Chimpanzees and cynomolgus monkeys can serve as animal models for induction of myocarditis by the CVB.[1] The baboon also develops myocarditis following inoculation with CVB3.[5] Although less well studied than the rodent models, these larger animals, along with swine, will provide opportunities to assess hemodynamic effects of myocarditis. Furthermore, the parallel experience of other investigators[76–78] in the use of rodents and monkeys to characterize myocarditis associated with Chagas' disease suggests that complementary chronic studies of CVB3-infected animals of different sizes and phylogenetic stock will be essential to our overall understanding.

Future Studies in Animal Models

Future studies in animal models should be directed toward identifying all cells participating in acute or chronic disease processes and their roles in the processes determined. We must extend earlier observations on lymphokines produced in response to viral antigens[17,18,44] and determine whether viral infection induces production of monokines and/or leukotrienes and whether these substances have a role in CVB3-induced myocarditis. Antigens on infected and uninfected heart tissue cells to which CTL responses are directed must be identified and characterized. Does the virus-induced antigen(s) represent an immunologic "stress" protein(s)? Persistence of virus or viral genome in heart tissue must be determined in order to understand chronic myocarditis.

As noted earlier, the genome of CVB3 has been cloned,[47,48] and early information on in situ hybridization and probes of mouse heart tissues with a viral (reovirus) probe has been published.[79] Thus, utility of molecular probes as diagnostic tools in CVB3 has been considered. Other immunologic methods of diagnosis, including assays for heart-specific enzymes or proteins and specific lymphocyte-response assays must be examined. Similarly, nuclear magnetic resonance imaging of normal versus myocarditic hearts, added to other studies of ventricular function, will enable characterization of the extent, distribution, and nature of lesional changes in acute and chronic myocarditis models. The animal models offer us possibilities for identifying and understanding the basic mechanisms operative in acute and chronic viral myocarditis, and we must take advantage of these opportunities. Furthermore, animal models must be used to assay potential therapies for myocarditis and dilated cardiomyopathy. Despite their limitations, couched mainly in their immunologic specificities, the various animals available can provide insight applicable to human myocarditis.

HUMAN DISEASE

The immunologic mechanisms of lymphocytic myocarditis in humans are far less clear than those in the mouse model. The leap of faith from the mouse, as the most studied model of coxsackievirus or encephalomyocarditis virus infection, to the human disease is troubled by several factors. The infrequency of primary lymphocytic myocarditis in general; the time point at which patients are seen *after* a "viral syndrome"; the uncommonness of documented, significant acute-to-convalescent rises in viral-specific antibodies; and the virtual failure to demonstrate virus by culture, fluorescence, or microscopy have made the tenability of community-acquired lymphocyte myocarditis as a predominantly viral or postviral disease less easy to accept. Furthermore, the generic definition of autoimmune disease as a problem of self-nonself immune tolerance has not yet been verified for human lymphocytic myocarditis. The following pieces of the puzzle stimulate more questions than they provide answers.

Human Studies

Models of Autoimmunity

As noted, the immunopathology of human myocarditis is just beginning to emerge. For clarity, but not without uncertainty, we define the suspected immunologic component of human myocarditis as that series of humoral and cellular events occurring after, but in continuity with, a known or likely viral trigger. An ever-broadening array of human autoimmune disorders is reflected in attacks on thyroid,[80] pancreas,[81-83] liver,[84] central and peripheral nervous systems,[85] joints and connective tissue,[86] bowel,[87] and blood elements,[88] and has bolstered the idea that at least some forms of myocarditis and cardiomyopathy may be attributable to humoral and/or cellular immune attack.

Perhaps the first suspicion that human myocardial injury could be immunologically mediated grew from the frequent observation of antiheart antibodies in human sera following rheumatic fever, postcardiotomy, and postmyocardial infarction syndromes; connective tissues diseases; idiopathic pericarditis; idiopathic dilated cardiomyopathy; and African endomyocardial fibrosis.[89]

The rheumatic fever model has been continuously studied.[89-92] A multitude of cardiocyte antigens[90,93,94] have been implicated as the antigenic determinant, cross-reactive with streptococcal antigens. Demonstration of in vitro cytotoxicity is yet lacking; however, such is the case for human infections with Trypanosoma cruzi as well.[95] In the latter infection, antilaminin antibodies have demonstrated cross-reactivity with trypomastigotes and amastigotes.[96] Other observations have suggested that an anti-ATPase antibody in myocarditis associated with Chagas' disease may modulate cardiocyte calcium fluxes and ventricular function.[97]

What is Human Myocarditis?

Studies of human lymphocytic myocarditis[98] have been hampered by the difficulty in defining the clinical syndrome of myocarditis and the histopathologic criteria for the diagnosis. As a result, numerous anecdotal studies have related immunologic data based on patients with idiopathic dilated cardiomyopathy, "healed" myocarditis, and active myocarditis, without clear distinction or relevant parallels among different patient subsets. Even more recent work[99] aimed at identifying viral genome in myocardium of failing hearts is fraught with the heterogeneity of patient material.

As noted, the marked variation in frequency of the diagnosis of myocarditis in humans illustrates the effect of the range of time from the onset of symptoms to diagnosis by morphologic methods, and the impact of variable patient presentations. In recent years, the majority of patients have undergone endomyocardial biopsy for elucidation of the cause of new onset of idiopathic congestive heart failure or left ventricular dysfunction, or idiopathic ventricular arrhythmias, or the presumptive diagnosis of myocarditis. Patients with idiopathic congestive failure account for the extremes of frequency of the histopathologic diagnosis of myocarditis (0 to 63 percent).[100-110] Those presenting with primary arrhythmias or syncope have similar but slightly narrower ranges of discrepancy (8.5 to 50 percent).[100,108,111,112] Previous investigators[100-104,112-114] have concluded that historic factors and viral culture add little to the histopathologic diagnosis. Furthermore, electron microscopy contributes less to the understanding of the inflammatory process than does light microscopy and provides information on a small tissue area at considerable expense in terms of time and money.[100] Evaluation of thick sections may be adjunctive in the identification of interstitial cells and fibrils, as well as in the assessment of myofibrillar loss and cytoplasmic vacuolization. Thus, light microscopy has been and remains the current standard for determination of the presence or absence of myocarditis and of the basis of the characteristic cellular infiltrate and the concomitant myocyte damage.

Quantitation of Inflammatory Cells in Myocardium

Beyond the recognition of the variety of infiltrating cells that might be present, investigators have successfully quantitated the infiltrate in myocarditis by a variety of light and immunohistochemical methods.[113,115-117] Edwards and colleagues[113] have suggested from their frequency distribution counts of lymphocytes in biopsy specimens from idiopathically failing or arrhythmic hearts that more than five lymphocytes per high-power field (×400) is indicative of myocarditis. Although immunofluorescent markers for different cell populations in the myocardium were used to characterize inflammatory infiltrates qualitatively,[118] the method, of course, is not quantitative. The method of immunocytochemical marking using avidin-biotin or other conjugates for the reaction of cell-surface antigens with specific antibodies has allowed for accurate quantitation of cellular infiltrates.[115-117] Also, the methodology allows for the phenotypic identification of cell subsets comprising various infiltrates.

Initial application of the immunocytochemical quantitation to myocardial lymphocytes in humans addressed the question as to how many and what kind of lymphocytes are present in uninflamed, nondilated hearts.[115] Fresh heart tissue from autopsies of male and female patients with a wide range of ages were sampled in the upper, mid, and lower right ventricular septal endomyocardium and the endomyocardium of the left ventricular free wall. The number of mononuclear cells reacting with monoclonal antibodies was similar in all sites sampled. This similarity included cells marking positively with OKT4, OKT8, and OKT11 (Ortho Diagnostics), as well as B1 (Coulter Immunology), HNK1 (Bectin-Dickinson, Inc.), and T200 (Hybritech). The majority of interstitial and mononuclear cells in all specimens expressed T cell markers, the phenotypic T helper cells (OKT4) being slightly more frequent than the T-suppressor/cytotoxic cells (OKT8). The ratio of the T helper to T suppressor/cytotoxic cells in the endomyocardium of hearts at autopsy was 1.44.

These and subsequent studies[116,117] on endomyocardial biopsy specimens from uninflamed and inflamed dilated hearts confirmed and extended the observation of Edwards and coworkers[113] regarding the normal number of cells in myocardium. The studies of Linder and colleagues[115] revealed an average of 8.9 T200 positive cells/mm^2 in noninflamed hearts obtained at autopsy and an average of 13.1 T200 positive cells/mm^2 in endomyocardial biopsy specimens from noninflamed, dilated hearts.[116] These numbers are consistently lower than the hematoxylin/eosin-stained cell counts in any given patient, with the intraobserver correlation between immunocytochemical and histologic mononuclear cell counts ranging from 0.90 to 0.99 in different material.[116,117] Thus, Linder and colleagues[115] estimated that the upper limit of normal for interstitial lymphoid and monocytic cells/mm^2, when the counts are made on hematoxylin/eosin-stained slides, may be 25 to 30 interstitial cells/mm^2. This number was *not offered as a criterion for diagnosis,* but rather as a guideline based on data that showed uninflamed autopsy hearts and endomyocardial biopsy specimens to have a mean and SEM of 17.5 ± 3.1 of positive cells in myocardium on hematoxylin/eosin-stained slides.

Immunoperoxidase-positive cells in the myocardium of 16 persons not believed to have myocarditis[116] were mainly T lymphocytes (OKT11) and monocytes/macrophages (MO2). The mean OKT4/OKT8 ratio of 1.0 in the biopsy specimens did not correlate with the ratio of peripheral blood markers of these same patients. However, the OKT4/OKT8 ratio in endomyocardial biopsy specimens of uninflamed hearts did correlate with that seen in myocardial sections taken at autopsy from people with no cardiac disease.

In contrast to those patients with uninflamed dilated hearts, one serially biopsied patient with active myocarditis had a markedly increased number of interstitial cells. The largest subset of cells was the suppressor/cytotoxic T cell population (OKT8), with a resultant OKT4/OKT8 ratio of 0.30 (1:3.8). At the same time, a marked absolute reduction in the macrophage/monocyte (MO2) series to only 0.1 cells/mm^2 was observed. As in uninflamed hearts, small populations of B cells and HNK cells were present. The patient's elevated tissue cell counts on hematoxylin/eosin-stained slides and by T200 immunocytochemistry far surpassed a cellular infiltration of 30 cells/mm^2 or 5 cells/HPF at magnification ×400. Serial biopsies with immunocytochemical quantitation revealed a marked diminution of lymphocytes with normalization of the helper/suppressor-cytotoxic ratios.[117] Of interest, the elevated number of OKT8 positive cells in inflamed myocardium in the experience of Cassling and colleagues[117] was consistent with earlier data of Zee-Cheng[101] and Hammond[118] and Marboe[119] and their colleagues.

Recently presented data from Southern and colleagues[120] extended the earlier observations on the immunohistochemical characterization of interstitial inflammatory infiltrates in failing hearts. In a single frozen fragment from 199 consecutive endomyocardial biopsy specimens from 160 patients, the authors reaffirmed that the histologic diagnosis of myocarditis was accompanied by a higher mean number of cells marking positive for leukocyte common antigen (DAKO) by the avidin-biotin immunoperoxidase technique. The increased number of positive cells in the patients with myocarditis corresponded quite well with previous work by Cassling and colleagues,[116,117] the mean number of cells by immunoperoxidase in the myocarditis being 30.2 and 50.9 cells/mm^2 when the myocarditis diagnosis was based on all biopsy material or solely on the frozen specimen, respectively. This mean number of cells far exceeds that seen in histopathologically normal biopsy material or material with apparently resolved myocarditis or nonspecific changes. All of the latter three categories had a mean number of cells/mm^2 of approximately 10, although some patients with normal or nonspecific histologic changes ranged up to the mean for inflamed hearts. Whereas the use of inflammatory cell counts as a sole indicator of myocarditis is not a reasonable approach, the apparent "false-negative" biopsy specimens on immunoperoxidase marking reported by Southern and colleagues[120] may indeed reflect the problem of overdiagnosis that is so common with simple histopathologic evaluation alone. Provided that one recognizes the need for a comprehensive evaluation of the tissue and realizes the pitfalls of diagnosis related to the multifocality of the inflammatory infiltrate[113,121-123] and the liability of "nondestructive" lymphocytic infiltrates in idiopathic dilated cardiomyopathy as a mimic of myocarditis,[124] the immunoperoxidase method, including a more specific battery of markers with minimum phenotypic crossover, is useful in the ongoing evaluation of inflammatory heart disease and its immunologic basis.

Tissue Culture of Human Myocardial Lymphocytes

Perhaps a more exciting and eventually more immunopathologically revealing approach has been recently applied to endomyocardial biopsy specimens by Kurnick and colleagues.[125] These investigators obtained infiltrating T lymphocyte populations from myocardium derived from 169 consecutive nontransplant endomyocardial biopsies from 135 patients. The cells were tissue cultured in the presence of human recombinant interleukin-2. Overall, 40 (24 percent) biopsy specimens from 33 patients gave rise to CD3+ cells. Phenotyping of 31 expanded cultures was performed by flow cytometry and revealed 19 CD4+ predominant cultures and 12 CD8+ predominant cultures. Sixteen of the expanded lymphocyte cultures were tested for lymphokine production, and all produced IL-2 and a macrophage stimulating factor (IL-0) in varying amounts. Each of the 14 cultures tested demonstrated variable degrees of cytotoxicity against NK target K562 cells and an NK-resistant tumor cell line. Of striking significance, yet to be confirmed and extended, neither the amount of lymphokine production nor the degree of cytotoxicity of the cultured lymphocyte populations correlated with the phenotypic predominance of the cultures. Further studies of activated T lymphocytes derived from human endocardial biopsy specimens will be necessary to clarify whether the specificity of the cell populations is intimately related to the pathogenesis of different forms of lymphocytic myocarditis. This investigative avenue deserves continued pursuit.

Peripheral Blood Lymphocytes

Studies of peripheral blood lymphocyte function in patients with myocarditis have been limited largely to T-suppressor cells.[126] A decrease in T suppressor cell activity has also been observed in idiopathic dilated cardiomyopathy,[126,127] in which others[128] found an increased T helper-to-suppressor ratio in peripheral blood. However, other investigators[129,130] have found no change in suppressor cell activity in association with idiopathic dilated cardiomyopathy. Studies by O'Connell and associates[131] are intriguing in that they relate alterations in peripheral blood suppressor cell function to patient genotype. They observed that myocarditis occurred in multiple family members of two families with idiopathic dilated cardiomyopathy, one of the families having members with diminished suppressor cell activity. Diminished NK cell function in peripheral blood has been observed in patients with idiopathic dilated cardiomyopathy,[132] and increased heterologous, myocyte-specific, lymphocyte-mediated cytotoxic activity has been reported in other patients with idiopathic dilated cardiomyopathy[133] and in primary myocarditis.[134] Recently, Franceschini and colleagues,[135] observed impaired blastogenic responses of peripheral lymphocytes of patients with idiopathic dilated cardiomyopathy to concanavalin A when compared with those of normal control subjects and of patients with coronary artery disease. Furthermore, the peripheral blood cytotoxic/suppressor lymphocytes were reduced in number in patients with dilated cardiomyopathy, and, correspondingly, the helper/suppressor cell ratio was significantly higher when compared with both control groups.

Autoantibodies and Immune Complexes

The issue of humoral autoimmunity as a mechanism of myocardial injury in myocarditis is unresolved. As noted earlier, several diseases, most prominently rheumatic fever, Chagasic myocardial disease, and postoperative and postpericardiotomy states are associated with myocardium-specific circulating autoantibodies. The generalizability of the autoantibody findings in rheumatic heart disease and in that induced by Trypanosoma cruzi, insofar as myocarditis is concerned, is unknown. Also, the specificity of the autoantibody findings has been obscured by the variable accuracy of the histopathologic diagnosis of myocarditis in patients with idiopathic heart failure. The strength of evidence that any of the antimyocyte antibodies, including those that react with sarcolemma or contractile proteins, can cause myocytolysis in vitro has been studied most intensively by Maisch and colleagues.[133,136,137] Recent work has raised the possibility that antibodies against intracellular mitochondrial antigens[138–142] play a role in the immunopathogenesis of dilated cardiomyopathy and virally induced heart disease. Thus far, studies of autoantibodies to membrane-related or intracellular antigens in the setting of idiopathic dilated cardiomyopathy or lymphocytic myocarditis support the view that most antibodies reflect the nonspecific process of myocardial injury rather than specifically altered myocardial antigens that can lead to the initiation or promotion of further myocardial injury. However, a subset of antibodies to components of myocytes, fibroblasts, or endothelium may yet prove to be immunopathogenic in humans.

Immunofluorescent studies[143,144] revealing variable amounts of immunoglobulins and complement in hearts biopsied for idiopathic failure have suggested a relationship with inflammatory disease activity. However, little attention has been given to immune complex subfractions and their possible relevance in primary or secondary aspects of myocardial injury in idiopathic dilated cardiomyopathy or myocarditis.[116,145] The activation of B cells as demonstrated in blastogenic studies[135] in patients with idiopathic dilated cardiomyopathy may be related to functional and quantitative defects of T cells, which are illustrated by reduced responses to concanavalin A.

Viral Genome in Human Hearts

The recent demonstration by Bowles and colleagues[99] that enterovirus-like nucleic acid sequences could be identified in 9 of 17 samples from patients with histologic evidence of active or healing myocarditis or dilated cardiomyopathy with inflammatory changes is a striking and, perhaps, somewhat surprising finding. The surprise relates to the fact that viral isolation from myocardium in otherwise serologically positive cases of coxsackievirus infection with accompanying myocarditis has not been successful. These authors used a large clone encompassing the viral RNA polymerase region of coxsackievirus B2 as a hybridization probe to test for the presence of viral nucleic acid sequence. This CVB sequence has been shown by others[146] to be useful as a relatively nonspecific hybridization probe to test for the detection of many enteroviral genomes other than the CVB. Similar approaches by Kandolf and colleagues[147] have been used to demonstrate enteroviral RNA sequences in infected cultured cells and in myocardial tissue sections of CVB3-infected mice using radiolabeled, cloned CVB3 cDNA as a diagnostic probe. They have also made preliminary application of this technique to human tissue. Tracy and colleagues[148] have presented preliminary evidence that suggests the human genome may harbor DNA copies of an enterovirus-like nucleotide sequence. They have demonstrated that nucleotide sequences in human DNA share enteroviral homology. The fascinating findings of Bowles and colleagues[99] and Kandolf and Hofschneider[157] demonstrating enterovirus RNA in cardiac tissue must be pursued to identify the origin of such RNA sequences and their coding capacity. These data may then finally implicate the long-term persistence of an enterovirus such as a CVB in myocardial disease. Such a process might implicate the viral gene copy in metabolic derangement as a mechanism for protracted heart failure in postmyocarditic patients. Much remains to be clarified, however.

Human Genetic Factors

Human genotype may influence the outcome of lymphocytic myocarditis through determinants of the major histocompatibility complex. This premise is not without precedent in numerous human diseases and certainly has been illustrated in the mouse.[124] In a recent study,[149] HLA DR4 and B27 antigens were more common in 37 patients with idiopathic cardiomyopathy than in controls, 54 versus 32 percent and 29 versus 3 percent, respectively.

Prospect

Despite widespread suspicion and human and animal evidence of immunologic alteration in association with tissue-proven primary (idiopathic) myocarditis, the respective roles of cellular and humoral immune dysfunction in the process of myocardial injury are still under active investigation. Several factors have prevented the clear establishment of the immune mechanisms in human myocarditis. The variability in the clinical and histopathologic diagnosis as well as the unlikelihood of investigating human myocarditis in its early course have left the early events enigmatic. The suggestive evidence that immunosuppressive therapy may ameliorate human myocarditis has come despite uncertainty about the precise mechanisms by which immunosuppressive therapy works in immune modulation. Much more work must be done in the application of immunologic, immunopathologic, and molecular biology techniques before the cellular, humoral, and genetic processes of the disease will be clear. Further understanding of the cell-surface receptors[150] on T lymphocytes will allow for eventual immune modulation, perhaps with a significant therapeutic impact on myocarditis. What effect the putative enterovirus-like sequences in human DNA might have on lymphocyte function is a pathway worth exploring. The manner in which immunologic processes interact with myocyte metabolism and myocyte function in the genesis of myocyte failure is also totally unknown. The use of various immunologic probes in studies of myocardial injury is just beginning.[151] The early events of tissue injury in idiopathic myocarditis may rely on yet-to-be clarified components of the acute inflammatory response including the humoral immune system and metabolites of the lipoxygenase pathway of arachidonic acid.[152,153] An upcoming multicenter trial of immunosuppressive therapy in biopsy-proven myocarditis in humans will concurrently address the clinical outcome[154] and the role of immunologic and genetic mechanisms in the myocarditic process, and will provide further opportunities for virologic and viral genomic studies of tissues from these patients.

ACKNOWLEDGMENT

The authors appreciate the review of this manuscript by Steven Tracy, Ph.D. They also wish to thank Janet Wilson and Lee Staples for preparation of the manuscript.

REFERENCES

1. Woodruff, JF: Viral myocarditis. A review. Am J Pathol 101:425, 1980.
2. Schnurr, DP, Cao, Y, and Schmidt, NJ: Coxsackievirus B3 persistence and myocarditis in N:NIH(S) II nu/nu and +/ nu mice. J Gen Virol 65:1197, 1984.
3. Morita, H, Kitaura, Y, Deguchi, H, et al: Experimental coxsackie B3 virus myocarditis in golden hamsters. II. Evaluation of left ventricular function in intact *in situ* heart 14 months after inoculation. Jpn Circ J 48:1097, 1984.
4. Hoshino, T, Kawai, C, and Tokuda, M: Experimental coxsackie B viral myocarditis in cynomolgus monkeys. Jpn Circ J 47:59, 1983.
5. Paque, RE, Gauntt, CJ, and Nealon, TJ: Assessment of cell-mediated immunity against coxsackievirus B3-induced myocarditis in a primate model *(Papio papio).* Infect Immunol 31:470, 1981.
6. Grist, NR and Bell, EJ: Coxsackie viruses and the heart. Am Heart J 77:295, 1969.
7. Burch, GE and Giles, TD: The role of viruses in the production of heart disease. Am J Cardiol 29:231, 1972.
8. Gear, JHS and Measroch, V: Coxsackievirus infections of the newborn. Prog Med Virol 15:42, 1973.
9. Lerner, AM and Wilson, FM: Virus myocardiopathy. Prog Med Virol 15:63, 1973.
10. Lansdown, ABG: Viral infections and diseases of the heart. Prog Med Virol 24:70, 1978.
11. Woodruff, JF and Woodruff, JJ: Involvement of T lymphocytes in the pathogenesis of coxsackievirus B3 heart disease. J Immunol 113:1726, 1974.
12. Lutton, CW and Gauntt, CJ: Coxsackievirus B3 infection alters plasma membrane of neonatal skin fibroblasts. J Virol 60:294, 1986.
13. Huber, SA, Job, LP, and Woodruff, JF: Sex-related differences in the pattern of coxsackievirus B3 induced immune spleen cell cytotoxicity against virus-infected myofibers. Infect Immunol 32:68, 1981.
14. Huber, SA, Job, LP, and Woodruff, JF: Lysis of infected myofibers by coxsackievirus B3-immune T lymphocytes. Am J Pathol 98:681, 1980.
15. Huber, SA, Job, LP, and Woodruff, JF: In vitro culture of coxsackievirus group B, type 3 immune spleen cells on infected endothelial cells and biological activity of the cultured cells in vivo. Infect Immunol 43:567, 1984.
16. Wong, CY, Woodruff, JJ, and Woodruff, JF: Generation of cytotoxic T lymphocytes during coxsackievirus B-3 infection. I. Model and viral specificity. J Immunol 118:1159, 1977.
17. Paque, RE, Gauntt, CJ, Nealon, TJ, et al: Assessment of cell-mediated hypersensitivity against coxsackievirus B3 viral-induced myocarditis utilizing hypertonic salt extract of cardiac tissue. J Immunol 120:1672, 1978.
18. Paque, RE, Straus, DC, Nealon, TJ, et al: Fractionation and immunologic assessment of KCL-extracted cardiac antigens in coxsackievirus B3 viral-induced myocarditis. J Immunol 123:358, 1979.
19. Gauntt, CJ, Trousdale, MD, LaBadie, DRL, et al: Properties of coxsackievirus B3 variants which are amyocarditic or myocarditic for mice. J Med Virol 3:207, 1979.
20. Lutton, CW, Gudvangen, RJ, Nealon, TJ, et al: Cellular immune responses in mice challenged with an amyocarditic variant of coxsackievirus B3. J Med Virol 17:345, 1985.
21. Estrin, M, Smith, C, and Huber, S: Antigen specific suppressor T cells prevent cardiac injury in Balb/c mice infected with a nonmyocarditic variant of coxsackievirus group B, type 3. Eur Heart J 7(Suppl E), 1987.
22. Huber, SA, Job, LP, Auld, KR, et al: Sex-related differences in the rapid production of cytotoxic spleen cells active against uninfected myofibers during coxsackievirus B-3 infection. J Immunol 126:1336, 1982.
23. Gauntt, CJ, Paque, RE, Trousdale, MD, et al: Temperature-sensitive mutant of coxsackievirus B3 (CVB3) establishes resistance in neonatal mice which protects them during adolescence against CVB3-induced myocarditis. Infect Immunol 39:851, 1983.
24. Kaplan, AS and Melnick, JL: Oral administration of coxsackie viruses to newborn and adult mice. Proc Soc Exp Biol Med 76:312, 1951.
25. Huber, SA and Lodge, PA: Coxsackievirus B-3 myocarditis in Balb/c mice. Evidence for autoimmunity to myocyte antigens. Am J Pathol 116:21, 1984.
26. Guthrie, M, Lodge, PA, and Huber, SA: Cardiac injury in myocarditis induced by coxsackievirus group B, type 3 in Balb/c mice is mediated by Lyt2+ cytolytic lymphocytes. Cell Immunol 88:558, 1984.
27. Huber, SA and Job, LP: Differences in cytolytic T cell response of Balb/c mice infected with myocarditic and nonmyocarditic strains of coxsackievirus group B, type 3. Infect Immunol 39:1419, 1983.

28. Godeny, EK and Gauntt, CJ: Involvement of natural killer cells in coxsackievirus B3-induced murine myocarditis. J Immunol 137:1695, 1986.
29. Huber, SA and Lodge, PA: Coxsackievirus B-3 myocarditis. Identification of different pathogenic mechanisms in DBA/2 and Balb/c mice. Am J Pathol 122:284, 1986.
30. Matsumori, A and Kawai, C: An experimental model for congestive heart failure following encephalomyocarditis virus myocarditis in mice. Circulation 65:1230, 1982.
31. Kishimoto, C, Kuribayashi, K, Masuda, T, et al: Immunological behavior of lymphocytes in experimental viral myocarditis: Significance of T lymphocytes in the severity of myocarditis and silent myocarditis in Balb/c-nu/nu mice. Circulation 71:1247, 1985.
32. Lutton, CW and Gauntt, CJ: Ameliorating effect of IFN-B and anti-IFN-B on coxsackievirus B3-induced myocarditis in mice. J Interferon Res 5:137, 1985.
33. Lonberg-Holm, K, Crowell, RL, and Philipson, L: Related animal viruses share receptors. Nature 259:679, 1976.
34. Richter, FA, MacPherson, LW, Campbell, JB, et al: Studies on intratypic variants of coxsackie B1 virus. Arch Gesamte Virusforsch 38:77, 1972.
35. Brown, F and Wild, F: Variation in the coxsackievirus type B5 and its possible role in the etiology of swine vesicular disease. Intervirology 3:125, 1974.
36. Jimes, S and Jamison, RM: Coxsackievirus B4: In vitro genetic markers and virulence. Arch Virol 77:1, 1983.
37. Hartig, PC, Madge, GE, and Webb, SR: Diversity within a human isolate of coxsackie B4: Relationship to viral-induced diabetes. J Med Virol 11:23, 1983.
38. Reagan, KJ, Goldberg, B, and Crowell, RL: Altered receptor specificity of coxsackievirus B3 after growth in rhabdomyosarcoma cells. J Virol 49:630, 1984.
39. Jimes, S, Jamison, RM, and Grafton, WD: Coxsackievirus B4: In vitro genetic markers and cardiovirulence. Arch Virol 81:345, 1984.
40. Prabhakar, BS, Haspel, MV, McClintock, PR, et al: High frequency of antigenic variants among naturally occurring human coxsackie B4 virus isolates identified by monoclonal antibodies. Nature 300:374, 1982.
41. Cao, Y, Schnurr, DP, and Schmidt, NJ: Differing cardiotropic and myocarditic properties of group B type 4 coxsackievirus strains. Arch Virol 80:119, 1984.
42. Cao, Y, Schnurr, DP, and Schmidt, NJ: Monoclonal antibodies for study of antigenic variation in coxsackievirus type B4: Association of antigenic determinants with myocarditic properties of the virus. J Gen Virol 65:925, 1984.
43. Jordan, GW, Bolton, V, and Schmidt, NJ: Diabetogenic potential of coxsackie B viruses in nature. Arch Virol 86:213, 1985.
44. Trousdale, MD, Paque, RE, Nealon, T, et al: Assessment of coxsackievirus in B3 *ts* mutants for induction of myocarditis in a murine model. Infect Immunol 23:486, 1979.
45. Gauntt, CJ, Gomez, PT, Duffey, PS, et al: Characterization and myocarditic capabilities of coxsackievirus B3 variants in selected murine strains. J Virol 52:598, 1984.
46. Holland, J, Spindler, K, Horodyski, F, et al: Rapid evolution of RNA genomes. Science 215:1577, 1982.
47. Tracy, S, Chapman, N, and Liu, H: Molecular cloning and partial characterization of the coxsackievirus B3 genome. Arch Virol 85:157, 1985.
48. Kandolf, R and Hofschneider, PH: Molecular cloning of the genome of a cardiotropic coxsackie B3 virus: Full-length reverse-transcribed recombinant cDNA generates infectious virus in mammalian cells. Proc Natl Acad Sci USA 82:4818, 1985.
49. Robinson, JA, O'Connell, JB, Roeges, LM, et al: Coxsackie B3 myocarditis in athymic mice. Proc Soc Exp Biol Med 166:80, 1981.
50. Schnurr, DP and Schmidt, NJ: Coxsackievirus B3 persistence and myocarditis in NFR nu/nu and +/nu mice. Med Microbiol Immunol 173:1, 1984.
51. Hashimoto, I and Komatsu, T: Myocardial changes after infection with coxsackie virus B3 in nude mice. Br J Exp Pathol 59:13, 1978.
52. Roesing, TG, Landau, BJ, and Crowell, RL: Limited persistence of viral antigen in coxsackievirus B-3 induced heart disease in mice. Proc Soc Exp Biol Med 160:382, 1979.
53. Khatib, R, Khatib, G, Chason, JL, et al: Alterations in coxsackievirus B4 heart muscle disease in ICR swiss mice by antithymocyte serum. J Gen Virol 64:231, 1983.
54. Gatmaitan, BG, Chason, JL, and Lerner, AM: Augmentation of the virulence of murine coxsackievirus B3 myocardiopathy by exercise. J Exp Med 131:1121, 1970.
55. Reyes, MP, Ho, KL, Smith, F, et al: A mouse model of dilated-type cardiomyopathy due to coxsackievirus B3. J Infect Dis 144:232, 1918.

56. Reyes, MP, Lerner, AM, and Ho, KL: Diminution in the size of the thymus in mice during forced swimming. J Infect Dis 143:292, 1981.
57. Reyes, MP, Smith, FE, and Lerner, AM: An enterovirus-induced murine model of an acute dilated-type cardiomyopathy. Intervirology 22:146, 1984.
58. Wong, CY, Woodruff, JJ, and Woodruff, JF: Generation of cytotoxic T lymphocytes during coxsackievirus B-3 infection. III. Role of sex. J Immunol 119:591, 1977.
59. Lyden, DC and Huber, SA: Aggravation of coxsackievirus, group B, type 3-induced myocarditis and increase in cellular immunity to myocarditis and increase in cellular immunity to myocyte antigens in pregnant Balb/c mice and animals treated with progesterone. Cell Immunol 87:462, 1984.
60. Cohn, DA: High sensitivity to androgen as a contributing factor in sex differences in the immune response. Arthrit Rheum 22:1218, 1979.
61. Lerner, AM: Coxsackie virus myocardiomyopathy. J Infect Dis 120:496, 1969.
62. Costanzo-Nordin, MR, Reap, EA, O'Connell, JB, et al: A nonsteroidal anti-inflammatory drug exacerbates coxsackievirus B3 murine myocarditis. J Am Coll Cardiol 6:1078, 1985.
63. O'Connell, JB, Reap, EA, and Robinson, JA: The effects of cyclosporine on acute murine coxsackie B3 myocarditis. Circulation 73:353, 1986.
64. Gudvangen, RJ, Duffey, PS, Paque, RE, et al: Levamisole exacerbates coxsackievirus B3-induced murine myocarditis. Infect Immunol 41:1157, 1983.
65. Gauntt, CJ, Arizpe, HM, Kung, JT, et al; Antimyocarditic activity of the guanine derivative BIOLF-70 in a coxsackievirus B3 murine model. Antimicrob Agents Chemother 27:184, 1985.
66. Matsumori, A, Wang, H, Abelmann, WH, et al: Treatment of viral myocarditis with ribavirin in an animal preparation. Circulation 71:834, 1985.
67. Tomioka, N, Kishimoto, C, Matsumori, A, et al: Effects of prednisolone on acute viral myocarditis in mice. J Am Coll Cardiol 7:868, 1986.
68. Wolfgram, LJ, Beisel, KW, Herskowitz, A, et al: Variations in the susceptibility to coxsackievirus B3-induced myocarditis among different strains of mice. J Immunol 136:1846, 1986.
69. Herskowitz, A, Beisel, KW, Wolfgram, LJ, et al: Coxsackievirus B3 murine myocarditis: Wide pathologic spectrum in genetically defined inbred strains. Hum Pathol 16:671, 1985.
70. Beisel, KW, Wolfgram, LJ, Herskowitz, A, et al: Variation in the susceptibility of congenic inbred mice to coxsackievirus B3-induced myocarditis among different strains of mice. J Immunol 136:1846, 1987.
71. Kishimoto, C, Matsumori, A, Ohmae, M, et al: Electrocardiographic findings in experimental myocarditis in DBA/2 mice: Complete atrioventricular block in the acute stage, low voltage of the QRS complex in the subacute stage and arrhythmias in the chronic stage. J Am Coll Cardiol 3:1461, 1984.
72. Hoshino, T, Matsumori, A, Kawai, C, et al: Ventricular aneurysms and ventricular arrhythmias complicating coxsackie virus B1 myocarditis of Syrian golden hamsters. Cardiovasc Res 18:24, 1984.
73. El-Khatib, MR, Chason, JL, and Lerner, AM: Ventricular aneurysms complicating coxsackie virus group B, types 1 and 4 murine myocarditis. Circulation 59:412, 1979.
74. Morita, H, Kitaura, Y, Deguchi, H, et al: Experimental coxsackie B3 virus myocarditis in golden hamsters. II. Evaluation of left ventricular function in intact in situ heart 14 months after inoculation. Jpn Circ J 48:1097, 1984.
75. Morita, H: Experimental coxsackie B3 virus myocarditis in golden hamsters. Light and electron microscopy findings in a long-term follow-up study. Jpn Circ J 45:713, 1981.
76. Frederici, EF, Abelmann, WH, and Neva, FA: Chronic and progressive myocarditis and myositis in C3H mice infected with Trypansoma cruzi. Am J Trop Med 13:272, 1964.
77. Kumar, R, Kline, IK, and Abelmann, WH: Immunosuppression in experimental acute and subacute myocarditis. Am J Trop Med 19:932, 1970.
78. Santos-Buch, CA: American trypanosomiasis: Chagas disease. Int Rev Exp Pathol 19:63, 1979.
79. Zahringer, J, Stangl, E, Aschauer, W, et al: Viral myocarditis: Molecular hybridization allows the detection of virus-RNA in heart muscle after virus infection. J Mol Cell Cardiol 17:83, 1985.
80. Burek, CL and Rose, NR: Cell-mediated immunity in autoimmune thyroid disease. Hum Pathol 17:246, 1986.
81. Yoon, JW: Viruses in pathogenesis of type I diabetes. Curr Probl Clin Biochem 12:11, 1983.
82. Brogren, CH, Baekkeskov, S, Dyrberg, T, et al: Role of islet cell antibodies in the pathogenesis of type I diabetes. Curr Probl Clin Biochem 12:65, 1983.
83. Gepts, W: Role of cellular immunity in the pathogenesis of type I diabetes. Curr Probl Clin Biochem 12:86, 1983.
84. Sherlock, S: Chronic hepatitis and cirrhosis. Hepatology 4:25s, 1984.

85. Zweiman, B and Lisak, RP: Cell-mediated immunity in neurologic disease. Hum Pathol 17:234, 1986.
86. Padula, SJ, Clark, RB, and Korn, JH: Cell-mediated immunity in rheumatic disease. Hum Pathol 17:254, 1986.
87. MacDermott, RP: Cell-mediated immunity in gastrointestinal disease. Hum Pathol 17:219, 1986.
88. Pini, M, Potli, R, and Dettor, AG: Porpora trombotica trombocitopenica. Descrizione di du casi e revisione della litteratura. Rec Prog Med 73:429, 1982.
89. Kaplan, MH and Frengley, JD: Autoimmunity to the heart in cardiac disease. Am J Cardiol 24:259, 1969.
90. Kaplan, MH, Meyeserian, M, and Kushner, I: Immunologic studies of heart tissue. IV. Serologic reactions with human heart tissue as revealed by immunofluorescent methods: Isoimmune, Wasserman, and autoimmune reactions. J Exp Med 113:17, 1961.
91. Zabriskie, JB: Mimetic relationships between group A streptococci and mammalian tissues. Adv Immunol 7:147, 1967.
92. Zabriskie, JB and Friedman, JE: The role of heart binding antibodies in rheumatic fever. Adv Exp Med Biol 161:457, 1983.
93. Kaplan, MH: Myosin: A link between streptococci and heart. J Immunol 80:268, 1958.
94. Krisher, K and Cunningham, MW: Differentiation of a myocardial sarcoplasmic antigen and cardiolifin. Science 227:413, 1985.
95. Santos-Buch, CA and Acosta, AM: Immunology of chagasic heart disease. In Zabriskie, JB, Engle, MA, and Villareal, H, Jr (eds): Clinical Immunology of the Heart. John Wiley & Sons, New York, 1981, pp 143–190.
96. Szarfman, A, Terranova, VP, Rennard, SI, et al: Antibodies to laminin in Chagas disease. J Exp Med 155:1161, 1982.
97. Acosta, AM, Sadigursky, M, and Santos-Buch, CA: Anti-striated muscle antibody activity produced by Trypanosoma cruzi. Proc Soc Exp Biol Med 172:364, 1983.
98. Aretz, HT, Billingham, ME, Fallon, JT, et al: Myocarditis—A histologic definition and working classification. Am J Cardiovasc Pathol 1:3, 1987.
99. Bowles, NE, Olsen, EGJ, Richardson, PJ, et al: Detection of coxsackie-B-virus-specific RNA sequences in myocardial biopsy samples from patients with myocarditis and dilated cardiomyopathy. Lancet 1:1120, 1986.
100. Nippoldt, TB, Edwards, WD, Holmes, DR, Jr, et al: Right ventricular endomyocardial biopsy. Clinicopathologic correlation in 100 consecutive patients. Mayo Clin Proc 57:407, 1982.
101. Zee-Cheng, CS, Tsai, CC, Palmer, DC, et al: High incidence of myocarditis by endomyocardial biopsy in patients with idiopathic congestive cardiomyopathy. J Am Coll Cardiol 3:63, 1984.
102. Baandrup, O and Olsen, EGJ: Critical analysis of endomyocardial biopsies from patients suspected of having cardiomyopathy. Part I: Morphological and morphometric aspects. Br Heart J 45:475, 1981.
103. Baandrup, O, Florio, RA, Rehahn, M, et al: Critical analysis of endomyocardial biopsies from patients suspected of having cardiomyopathy. Part II: Comparison of histology and clinical/haemodynamic formation. Br Heart J 45:486, 1981.
104. Parrillo, JE, Aretz, HT, Palacios, I, et al: The results of transvenous endomyocardial biopsy can frequently be used to diagnose myocardial disease in patients with idiopathic heart failure. Circulation 69:93, 1984.
105. Lewis, AB, Neustein, HB, Takahashi, M, et al: Findings on endomyocardial biopsy in infants and children with dilated cardiomyopathy. Am J Cardiol 55:143, 1985.
106. Daly, K, Richardson, PJ, Olsen, EGJ, et al: Acute myocarditis: Role of histological and virological examination in the diagnosis and assessment of immunosuppressive treatment. Br Heart J 51:30, 1984.
107. Fenoglio, JJ, Jr, Ursell, PC, Kellogg, CF, et al: Diagnosis and classification of myocarditis by endomyocardial biopsy. N Engl J Med 301:12, 1983.
108. Sugrue, DD, Holmes, DR, Jr, Gersh, BJ, et al: Cardiac histologic findings in patients with life-threatening ventricular arrhythmias of unknown origin. J Am Cell Cardiol 5:952, 1984.
109. O'Connell, JB, Henkin, RE, Robinson, JA, et al: Gallium-67 imaging in patients with dilated cardiomyopathy and biopsy-proven myocarditis. Circulation 70:58, 1984.
110. O'Connell, JB, Robinson, JA, Henkin, RE, et al: Immunosuppressive therapy in patients with congestive cardiomyopathy and myocardial uptake of Gallium-67. Circulation 64:780, 1981.
111. Strain, JE, Grose, RM, Factor, SM, et al: Results of endomyocardial biopsy in patients with sponta-

neous ventricular tachycardia but without apparent structural heart disease. Circulation 68:1171, 1983.
112. Vignola, PA, Kazutaka, A, Swaye, PS, et al: Lymphocytic myocarditis presenting as unexplained ventricular arrhythmias: Diagnosis with endomyocardial biopsy and response to immunosuppression. J Am Coll Cardiol 4:812, 1984.
113. Edwards, WD, Holmes, DR, Jr, and Reeder, GS: Diagnosis of active lymphocytic myocarditis by endomyocardial biopsy: Quantitative criteria for light microscopy. Mayo Clin Proc 57:419, 1982.
114. Aretz, HT, Chapman, C, and Fallon, JT: Morphologic and immunologic findings in patients with clinically suspected myocarditis. Circulation 68(Suppl III):27, 1983.
115. Linder, J, Markin, RS, Rogler, WC, et al: Immunohistochemical characterization of lymphocytes in ventricular myocardium. Arch Pathol 109:917, 1985.
116. Cassling, RS, Linder, J, Sears, TD, et al: Quantitative evaluation of inflammation in biopsy specimens from idiopathically failing or irritable hearts: Experience in 80 pediatric and adult patients. Am Heart J 110:713, 1985.
117. Cassling, RS, Linder, J, Rogler, WC, et al: Quantitative evaluation of lymphocyte subsets in failing and irritable hearts. Lab Invest 54:10A, 1986.
118. Hammond, EH and Anderson, JL: Cardiac immune complexes and mononuclear cell subsets in myocarditis: An endomyocardial biopsy study. Circulation 68:3, 1983.
119. Marboe, CC, Knowles, DML, Weiss, MB, et al: Characterization of the inflammatory infiltrate in human myocarditis—An endomyocardial biopsy study. In Bolte, HD (ed): Viral Heart Disease. Springer-Verlag, 1984, p 74.
120. Southern, JF, Kaynor, B, Howard, C, et al: Is immunoperoxidase staining of endomyocardial biopsies for interstitial inflammatory cells helpful in the diagnosis of myocarditis? Eur Heart J 7[Suppl E), 1987.
121. Dec, W, Palacios, I, Lee, DCS, et al: Dilated cardiomyopathy: Clinical features versus right ventricular biopsy in diagnosing acute myocarditis. Circulation 68 (Suppl III):28, 1983.
122. Mills, AS, Hastillo, A, and Hess, ML: Lymphocytic infiltration of the myocardium in idiopathic dilated cardiomyopathy: Underestimation of myocarditis with endomyocardial biopsy. Circulation 70 (Suppl II):401, 1984.
123. Unverferth, DV, Fetters, JK, Uretsky, B, et al: Right versus left heart biopsies—Different information. Circulation 70 (Suppl II):402, 1984.
124. Tazelaar, HD and Billingham, ME: Leukocytic infiltrates in idiopathic dilated cardiomyopathy: A source of confusion with active myocarditis. J Am Coll Cardiol 5:490, 1985.
125. Kurnick, JT, Leary, C, Palacios, IF, et al: Culture and characterization of lymphocytic infiltrates from endomyocardial biopsies of patients with idiopathic myocarditis. Eur Heart J 7(Suppl E), 1987.
126. Eckstein, R, Mempel, W, and Bolte, HD: Reduced suppressor cell activity in congestive cardiomyopathy and in myocarditis. Circulation 65:1224, 1982.
127. Fowles, RE, Bieber, CP, and Stinson, EB; Defective in vitro suppressor cell function in idiopathic congestive cardiomyopathy. Circulation 59:483, 1979.
128. Sanderson, JE, Koech, D, and Ojiambo, HP: T-lymphocyte subsets in idiopathic dilated cardiomyopathy. Am J Cardiol 55:755, 1985.
129. Gentle, T, Gammage, M, Lowry, PJ, et al: T-cell suppressor function in idiopathic congestive cardiomyopathy. Eur Heart J 7(Suppl E), 1987.
130. O'Connell, JB, Schervish, EW, Kowalczyk, D, et al: Suppressor cell function in idiopathic dilated cardiomyopathy. Eur Heart J 7(Suppl E), 1987.
131. O'Connell, JB, Fowles, RE, Robinson, JA, et al: Clinical and pathologic findings of myocarditis in two families with dilated cardiomyopathy. Am Heart J 107:127, 1983.
132. Anderson, JL, Carlquist, JF, and Hammond, EJ: Deficient natural killer cell activity in patients with idiopathic dilated cardiomyopathy. Lancet 2:1124, 1982.
133. Maisch, B, Deeg, P, Liebau, G, et al: Diagnostic relevance of humoral and cytotoxic immune reactions in primary and secondary dilated cardiomyopathy. Am J Cardiol 52:1072, 1983.
134. Maisch, B, Trostel-Soeder, R, Stechemesser, E, et al: Diagnostic relevance of humoral and cell-mediated immune reactions in patients with acute viral myocarditis. Clin Exp Immunol 48:533, 1982.
135. Franceschini, R, Messina, V, Petillo, A, et al: Humoral immunity and lymphocyte subpopulations in patients with dilated cardiomyopathy. Int J Cardiol 8:113, 1985.
136. Maisch, B: Cardiocytolysis by sera of patients suffering from acute perimyocarditis. In Bolte, HD (ed): Viral heart disease. Springer-Verlag, Basel, 1984, pp 121–130.
137. Maisch, B, Bauer, E, Cirsi, M, et al: Cytolytic cross-reactive antibodies directed against the cardiac

membrane of adult human myocytes in coxsackie B myocarditis—Analysis by western blot, immunofluorescence test and antibody mediated cytolysis of cardiocytes. Eur Heart J 7(Suppl E), 1987.
138. Schultheiss, HP, Kuhl, U, Ulrich, G, et al: The mitochondrion as antigen in inflammatory heart disease. Eur Heart J 7(Suppl E), 1987.
139. Klein, R, Seipel, L. Kleemann, U, et al: Relevance of antimitochondrial antibodies (anti-M7) in cardiac disease. Eur Heart J 7(Suppl E), 1987.
140. Reinauer, KM, Klein, R, Seipel, L, et al: Heartspecific antimitochondrial antibody (anti-M 7) in a patient with virus associated perimyocarditis. Eur Heart J 7(Suppl E), 1987.
141. Schulze, K, Becker, B, and Schultheiss, HP: Modulation of the energy metabolism of the myocardial cell by antibodies to the ADP/ATP carrier—Determination of the subcellular phosphorylation potentials of the ATP. Eur Heart J 7(Suppl E), 1987.
142. Ulrich, C, Kuhl, U, Janda, I, et al: Antibodies to the ADP/ATP-carrier of the inner mitochondrial membrane crossreact with cell surface antigens and induce a cytotoxic effect on isolated adult cardiac myocytes. Eur Heart J 7(Suppl E), 1987.
143. Anderson, JL, Hammond, EH, Fowles, RE, et al: Predictive value of immunofluorescence and electron microscopic evaluation of endomyocardial biopsies in the diagnosis and proposals of idiopathic heart muscle disease with or without inflammation. Eur Heart J 7(Suppl E), 1987.
144. Aretz, HT, Fallon, JT, Southern, J, et al: Morphologic and immunologic findings in patients with clinically suspected and treated myocarditis—An endomyocardial biopsy study. Eur Heart J 7(Suppl E), 1987.
145. Herzum, M, Maisch, B, and Kochiek, K: Circulating immune complexes in endocarditis and perimyocarditis. Eur Heart J 7(Suppl E), 1987.
146. Tracy, S: A comparison of homologies in the coxsackievirus B group: Use of fragments of the cloned coxsackievirus B3 genome as probes. J Gen Virol 65:2167, 1984.
147. Kandolf, R, Ameis, D, Kirschner, P, et al: In situ detection of viral genomes in myocardial cells by nucleic acid hybridization: A novel approach to the diagnosis of viral heart disease. Eur Heart J 7(Suppl E), 1987.
148. Tracy, S, Williams, L, and Chapman, NM: Discovery and characterization of enteroviral-like DNA sequences in human genomic DNA: Implications for viral persistence in chronic disease. Abstract, International Symposium on Inflammatory Heart Disease, Wurzburg, Germany, May, 1986.
149. Anderson, JL, Carlquist, JF, Lutz, JR, et al: HLA A, B and DR typing in idiopathic dilated cardiomyopathy; a search for immune response factors. Am J Cardiol 53:1326, 1984.
150. Desforges, JF: T-cell receptors. N Engl J Med 313:576, 1985.
151. Haber, E: Antibodies in cardiovascular diagnosis and therapy. Hosp Pract 15:147, 1986.
152. Emancipator, SN and Lamm, ME: Pathways of tissue injury initiated by humoral immune mechanisms. Lab Invest 54:475, 1986.
153. Maisch, B, Dienesch, C, and Wendl, I: Effect of leukotrienes on isolated vital cardiac cells—An in vitro model of cardiocytotoxic mediators in inflammation? Eur Heart J 7(Suppl E), 1987.
154. Mason, JW, Billingham, ME, and Ricci, DR: Treatment of acute inflammatory myocarditis assisted by endomyocardial biopsy. Am J Cardiol 45:1037, 1980.
155. Godeny, EK and Gauntt, CJ: Interferon and natural killer cell activity in coxsackievirus B3-induced murine myocarditis. Eur Heart J 7 (Suppl E), 1987.
156. Lutton, WC: Studies of pathogenic mechanisms of coxsackievirus B3 in a murine model of virus-induced myocarditis. Ph.D. Dissertation, May, 1986.
157. Kandolf, R and Hofschneider, PH: Molecular cloning of the genome of a cardiotropic Coxsackie B3 Virus: Full length reverse-transcriptase recombinant cDNA generates infectious virus in mammalian cells. Proc Natl Acad Sci USA 82:4818, 1985.

CHAPTER 9

Cardiac Transplantation

Margaret E. Billingham, M.D.

Cardiac transplantation can now be considered a therapeutic rather than an experimental procedure. In June 1986 the International Heart Transplantation Registry reported that there were 84 centers performing heart transplantation in the United States and more than 30 in other countries.[1] The actuarial survival rates after transplantation since the advent of cyclosporine is approximately 80 percent at 1-year. In the Stanford University Medical School experience with cyclosporine, of 213 1-year survivors, 87 percent were totally rehabilitated at 1 year; there was 65 percent survival at 5 years. The oldest living survivor at Stanford is 16 years post-transplantation, and the longest survivor is a Frenchman who is still living 18 years post-transplantation. Both patients receive regular conventional immunosuppressive treatment. These good results have now initiated a new era of cardiac transplantation in infants and young children. Those most likely to benefit from cardiac transplantation are young patients with end-stage heart disease (ejection fraction less than 20 percent, with progressive cardiac cachexia and declining functional ability) who have a very poor prognosis for survival (of less than 6 to 12 months) but who otherwise have reversible organ damage related to the heart disease.[2] Upper age limits for recipients of cardiac transplants range from 50 to 60 years, depending on the transplantation center.

This chapter will deal mainly with the pathology of the heart following cardiac transplantation and will touch only briefly on general pathology related to heart transplantation. It must be stated at the outset that the pathology of cardiac transplantation is influenced by the type of immunosuppressive regimen that is being used. Most centers are now using cyclosporine, usually in conjunction with azathioprine and prednisone. Because of the nephrotoxicity caused by cyclosporine, many centers are varying their immunosuppressive regimens to reduce the total amount of cyclosporine, by substituting azathioprine and prednisone. Cyclosporine is usually administered every 12 hours in doses calculated to produce trough serum levels (measured by radioimmunoassay) between 50 and 150 ng/ml.[2] Many of the histopathologic changes seen vary with the amount of cyclosporine given. There is also a cohort of patients who have survived from the precyclosporine era and who are being treated only with azathioprine and steroids, and for this reason the difference in the pathology of acute rejection between the two regimens will be outlined.

EARLY POST-CARDIAC TRANSPLANTATION PATHOLOGY

Cardiac pathology occurring in the early postoperative period (1 to 3 months post-transplant) can be considered under the headings of immediate failure of the heart, hyperacute rejection, reperfusion changes in the heart following transplantation, acute cardiac rejection, and infection.

Immediate Graft Failure

Very rarely, the donor heart will fail to function following cardiac transplantation before the patient has left the operating table. This can be caused by a number of surgical problems as well as by damage to the donor heart, either by the initial donor accident or by ischemic time if the heart has been obtained from a distant location and transported in the nonperfused state. Sometimes the right ventricle dilates, turns blue, and fails to contract adequately on the operating table. This failure may be due to increased pulmonary hypertension from the recipient's previous cardiac or pulmonary disease, or both, in which a nonhypertrophied normal right ventricle cannot overcome the pulmonary pressure. For this reason, recipients who have a pulmonary vascular wedge pressure of over 10 Wood units are not usually accepted. If the patient does not survive at this stage, the pathology of the right ventricle shows only interstitial edema and hemorrhage. The myocardium may show early ischemic damage, but the morphologic changes usually have not had time to develop. The heart should be inspected carefully for fibrin thrombi in the arterioles and small vessels.

Hyperacute Rejection

In over 400 cardiac transplants at Stanford, we have never seen a case of hyperacute rejection. This entity usually is a result of inaccurate cross-matching of the blood and of major histocompatibility differences of the donor and the recipient. The patient may survive a few hours following transplantation. The pathologic changes consist of marked interstitial hemorrhage, often with many neutrophils, depending on the length of survival. These changes are similar to those seen in animal models in which a histocompatibility mismatch between the donor and recipient is used deliberately. Once again, the small vessels contain fibrin thrombi and sludging of red cells blocking the capillaries. The changes are similar to a very acute myocardial infarct in which the changes are global rather than focal.

Reperfusion Injury

Reperfusion injury is encountered in all cardiac recipient hearts during the first week following cardiac transplantation. The changes are worse in those patients who have had prolonged ischemic time owing to distant procurement of the donor heart. The importance of these ischemic changes is due to the fact that they can be confused with acute rejection in the first or second cardiac biopsies following transplantation, unless the pathologist is aware of them. Because of the inevitable ischemic period of the donor heart, distantly procured or not, definite microscopic myocardial and vascular injury occurs following reperfusion of the heart at transplantation. The endothelial cells and small capillaries are damaged, as described in the classic experiments by Jennings and Wartman.[3] The first biopsy following cardiac transplantation, usually taken one week postoperatively, may show patchy ischemia and early focal damage of the myocardium, as shown in Figure 9–1. At 1 week there may be histiocytes around the edge of the damage, and neutrophils also may be seen. These changes are unlike the perimyocytic mononuclear infiltrate that occurs in acute rejection. The use of Masson's trichrome will highlight areas of damage of the myocardium due to reperfusion injury that have not yet developed an inflammatory infiltrate and that could be overlooked without the special stain (see Fig. 9–2).

In addition to reperfusion injury, changes in the myocardium can occur due to focal damage from catecholamine effect caused by pressor agents in the early postoperative period. In this case the predominantly focal damage is very characteristic and should not be confused with the more diffuse damage of acute rejection. It should also be noted that immediately following cadiac transplantation, small microinfarcts may occur in the myocardium as a result of air bubbles within the coronary arteries that have not been totally excluded when reperfusion was commenced; these findings also should not be confused with acute rejection.

Acute Cardiac Rejection

The sequential changes of the myocardium during acute cardiac rejection modified by immunosuppressive treatment has been worked out and described as a result of sequential endomyocardial biopsies in cardiac recipients by means of serial endomyocardial biopsies. Endomyocardial biopsy provides a safe, reliable morphologic index of acute rejection and plays an important role in the management of cardiac recipients. The technique and method of endomyocardial biopsy have been well described in numerous previous publications.[4,5] In August 1972, the technique was introduced into the clinical heart transplant program at Stanford University School of Medicine to monitor acute rejection in all the cardiac allograft recipients.[6] Re-

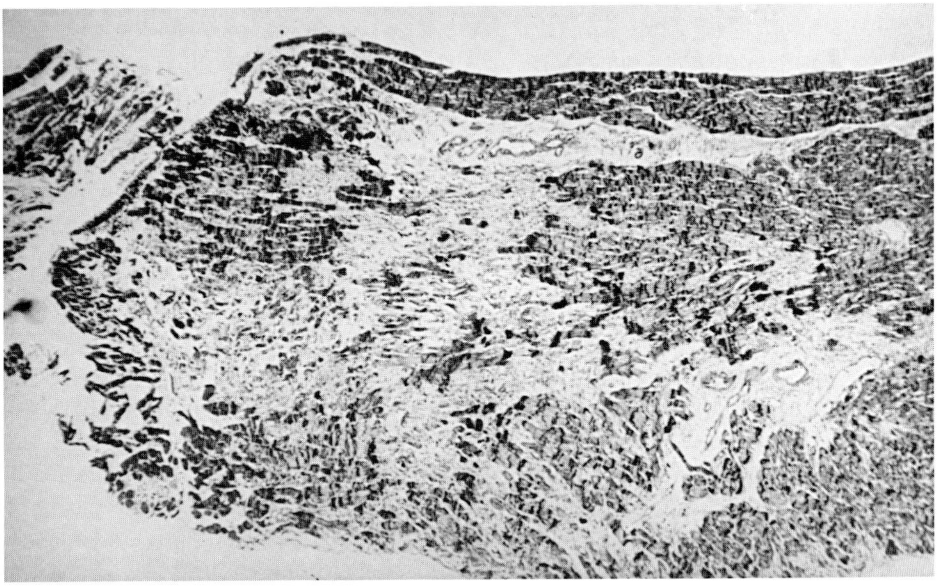

Figure 9–1. Endomyocardial biopsy 6 days after cardiac transplantation showing reperfusion injury. (Masson's trichrome stain; magnification ×40, reduced 23 percent.)

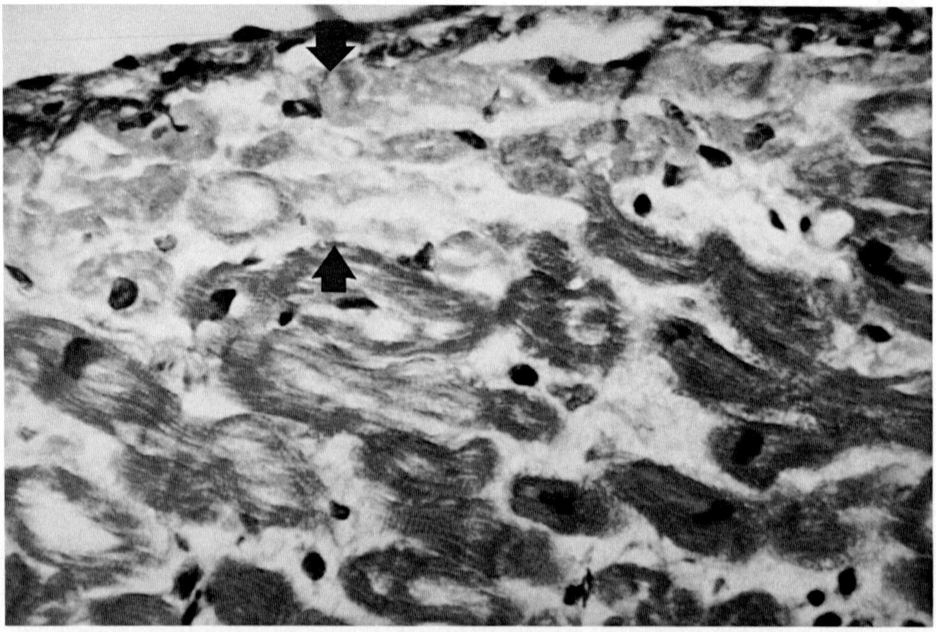

Figure 9–2. Portion of a cardiac biopsy showing early myocyte damage highlighted by Masson's trichrome stain *(between arrows)*. (Magnification ×200, reduced 23 percent.)

peated endomyocardial biopsies in any one patient are well tolerated, and many have undergone more than 20 serial biopsy procedures, with 38 being the maximum number of these procedures performed at Stanford. Although an invasive procedure, at Stanford it has caused no deaths and morbidity has been less than that for liver and renal transplants (0.3 percent).

Acute rejection cannot be ruled out without adequate sampling at each procedure. At Stanford, we require a minimum of three pieces for an adequate biopsy, but we usually obtain four to six pieces of myocardium to rule out acute rejection. We believe that adequate sampling with an adequately sized bioptome (9 French size of the catheter bioptome) is absolutely necessary to ensure good management of these patients. Some bioptomes such as the current disposable Cordis have only a 7 French catheter size and thus require six to eight pieces of tissue to be obtained for an adequate biopsy. Spiegelhalter and Stovin[7] have shown that using the larger bioptome there is still a 2 percent false-negative error for cardiac rejection with four pieces of tissue and a 5 percent false-negative error with three pieces. Hematoxylin and eosin stains are used to show up the mononuclear infiltrate. Masson's trichrome is used routinely to highlight early myocyte damage as well as fibrosis. Methyl-green pyronine stains may be useful in separating stimulated lymphoblasts in a new rejection episode from a resolving rejection following treatment when the mononuclear cells tend to be nonpyroninophilic. The pathologist should not confuse endothelial cells and fibroblasts, which are also pyroninophilic. Because the endomyocardial biopsies are usually no more than 3 mm in maximum dimension, at least three "step" levels of each specimen should be cut. The morphologic changes seen at different stages of acute rejection are shown in Table 9–1.

Table 9–1. Histopathologic Changes and Grading of Acute Cardiac Rejection

Hyperacute rejection	Global interstitial hemorrhage and neutrophils.
Mild acute rejection	Perivascular and/or endocardial and/or sparse interstitial infiltrate of pyroninophilic mononuclear cells. Myocyte necrosis is rare.
Moderate acute rejection	Increased perivascular and interstitial infiltrate of predominately mononuclear cells (eosinophils are seen with cyclosporine treatment). Perimyocytic infiltrates may cause focal myocyte necrosis.
Severe acute rejection	Interstitial hemorrhage with a mixed infiltrate of neutrophils and eosinophils. Vasculitis, edema, and myocyte necrosis are seen.
Resolving or resolved rejection	Decreased inflammatory infiltrate with fibroblasts and pigment-laden macrophages. Scars with trapped lymphocytes may be seen.

Mild Acute Rejection

Early or mild acute rejection is characterized by a sparse perivascular and/or endocardial infiltrate of large plump mononuclear cells with pyroninophilic cytoplasm. These cells may be sparsely distributed in the interstitium but are more commonly perivascular in location (Fig. 9–3). Myocyte necrosis is usually not obvious at this stage. The importance of making a diagnosis of a mild acute rejection lies in the fact that in our experience 50 percent of followup biopsies within 5 days will show a progression to moderate acute rejection in the cyclosporine-treated patients. In patients not treated with cyclosporine but with conventional therapy of azathioprine and steroids, it is important to treat mild acute rejection, because it can progress very rapidly, within 24 hours, to a life-threatening rejection. We therefore believe that

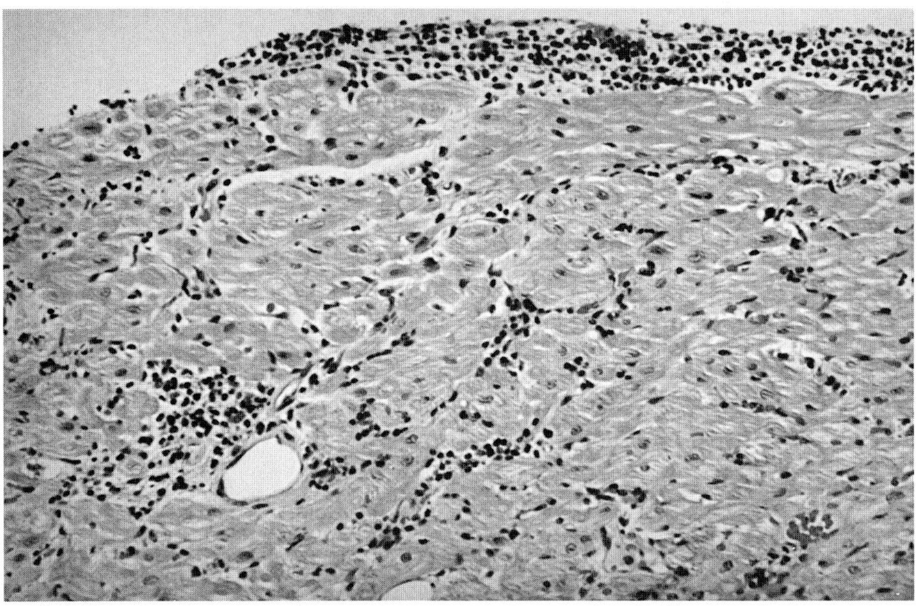

Figure 9–3. Endomyocardial biopsy showing mild acute rejection (perivascular and endocardial infiltrate. (Hematoxylin and eosin stain; magnification ×155, reduced 23 percent.)

this category of mild acute rejection is extremely important, regardless of the mode of treatment being used. At Stanford all mild acute rejection episodes are followed by a further biopsy within 5 days if the patient is receiving cyclosporine treatment.

Moderate Acute Rejection

At this stage, the mononuclear inflammatory infiltrate spreads into the interstitium and becomes perimyocytic. Where the infiltrate is most severe, there is usually adjacent myocyte damage, which may be focal or more extensive (Fig. 9–4). The infiltrate may still be perivascular and also endocardial in distribution. Although myocyte necrosis can usually be found at this stage, it is not necessary to have this finding to make a diagnosis of moderate acute rejection. The amount of infiltrate and the distribution of infiltrate is enough to make a diagnosis of moderate acute rejection. In the case of cyclosporine-treated patients, the interstitial infiltrate at this stage may also contain eosinophils. This eosinophilia appears to be related to the cyclosporine, inasmuch as it was not encountered in the precyclosporine era except when related to infections. Whenever eosinophils are seen, care should be taken to rule out an infectious agent evoking this response. The patient will usually reverse this moderate acute rejection readily, although it may take a week to 10 days in cyclosporine-treated patients. Conventionally treated patients normally reverse acute rejection within 36 to 48 hours following a steroid increase or antithymocyte globulin injection.

Severe Acute Rejection

Severe acute rejection is a relatively easy diagnosis for the pathologist to make on endomyocardial biopsy. There is a marked perivascular and interstitial inflammatory infiltrate with considerable myocyte necrosis. There is, in addition, marked interstitial hemorrhage, neutrophils, and sometimes eosinophils (Fig. 9–5). The

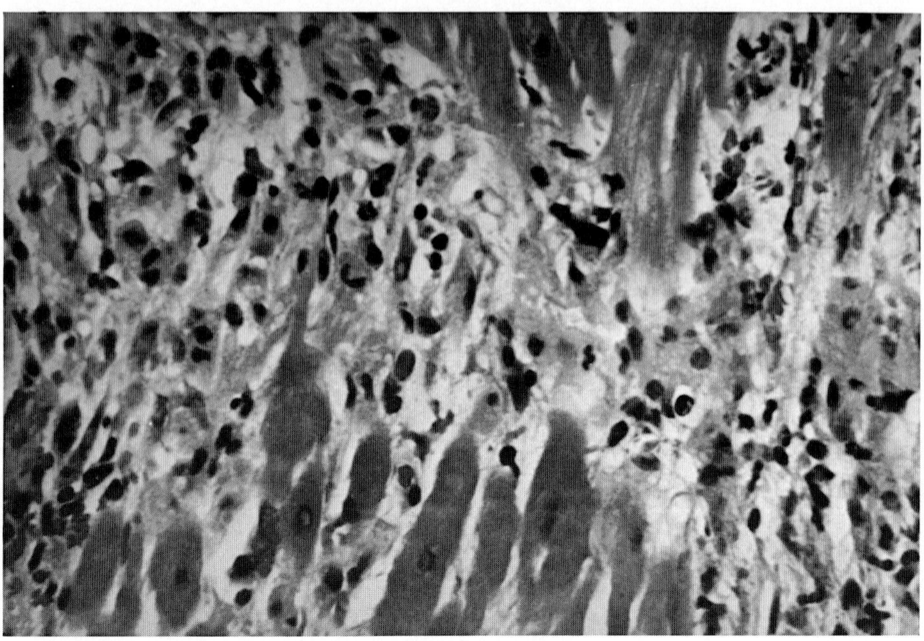

Figure 9–4. Endomyocardial biopsy showing moderate acute rejection with adjacent myocyte necrosis. (Hematoxylin and eosin stain; magnification ×300, reduced 23 percent.)

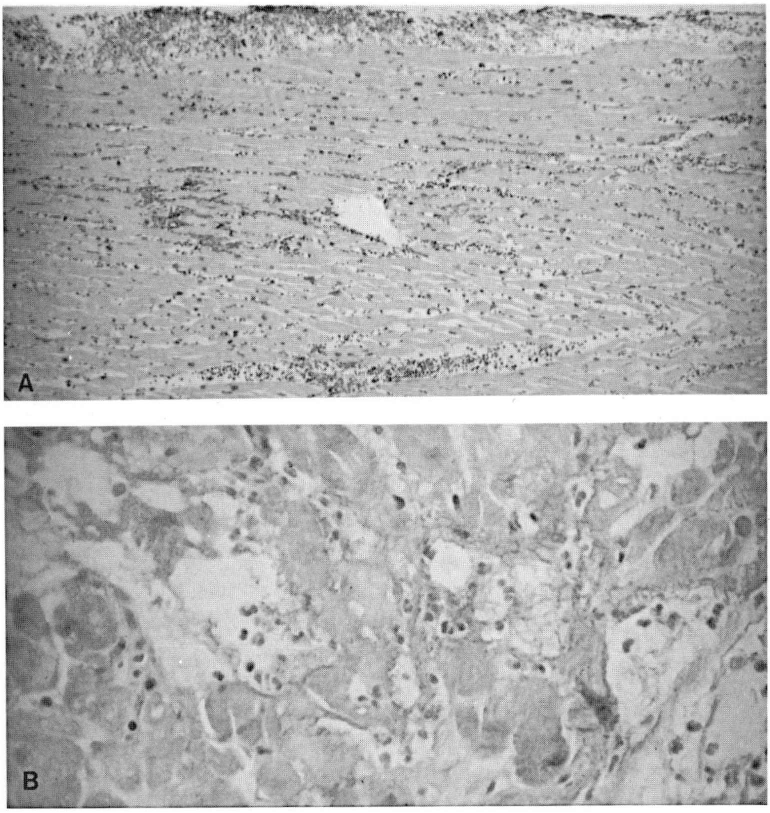

Figure 9–5. Endomyocardial biopsy showing severe acute rejection. *A*, subendocardial hemorrhage; *B*, neutrophilic infiltrate. (Hematoxylin and eosin stain; magnification ×155.)

hemorrhage results from the severe vasculitis that is usually present. Severe acute rejection is hard to reverse regardless of the immunosuppressive regimen but is more likely to be reversed successfully with cyclosporine. If the patient has been treated for a long time for ongoing acute rejection, sometimes severe acute rejection will result in more interstitial edema and hemorrhage than a lymphocytic infiltrate. This is encountered particularly in conventionally treated patients in whom there may be myelosuppression as well as lymphocytic suppression of the spleen and lymph nodes by the continuing high doses of steroids.

Resolving or Resolved Acute Rejection

This response occurs following successful treatment with conventional or cyclosporine drugs. The morphologic changes consist of a reduced interstitial infiltrate compared with the previous biopsy but, more importantly, there is early fibroblastic activity with young collagen formation and hemosiderin-laden macrophages. At this stage, therapy is usually tapered in whatever regimen the patient is following.

A resolved acute rejection will usually result in a small focal scar that may retain trapped lymphocytes within the fibrous tissue.

Pitfalls of Diagnosing Acute Rejection

In making the diagnosis of acute rejection by endomyocardial biopsy, the pathologist should be aware of several pitfalls. (1) The most common pitfall is that of previous biopsy sites. Although it might seem unlikely, anyone experienced with endomyocardial biopsies in cardiac recipients knows that many of the biopsies contain portions of previous biopsy sites. If the previous biopsy was recent, then the fibrin and granulation tissue present should alert the pathologist that this finding is not necrosis due to acute rejection. In a healing biopsy site, one of the most useful features is the myocyte disarray that is seen at the base of the biopsy site. (2) Of equal importance is the necessity of separating out an inflammatory infiltrate resembling acute rejection from that caused by infection causing a myocarditis. In this immunosuppressed cohort of patients, it is not uncommon to have an infection-induced myocarditis in the endomyocardial biopsies. In our experience we have detected cases of toxoplasmosis, cytomegalovirus (CMV), and even coccidioidomycosis on biopsies from cardiac transplants. One should be alerted to the infection by the presence of a mixed inflammatory infiltrate rather than the usual monotonous mononuclear infiltrate. If one cannot find an organism, it is wise to check the serum titers of the patient for toxoplasmosis and CMV as well as to consult with the clinicians managing the patient regarding the possibility of infection. It is one of the single most important dangers of reading the biopsies to confuse the diagnosis of acute rejection, which requires augmentation by immunosuppression, with that of an infection, in which case the added immunosuppression could have a fatal outcome. (3) Another pitfall is the "Quilty" effect. This term is used for the substantial focal endocardial infiltrates that may occur in cyclosporine-treated patients (Fig. 9–6). These infiltrates do not usually extend into the subendocardium. They consist of pyroninophilic T cells and are therefore likely to be due to the rejection phenomenon. However, this entity does not in itself cause any untoward reaction in the patient. At Stanford, we do not treat the "Quilty" effect with augmented immunosuppression, and usually it disappears spontaneously. If there is interstitial rejection

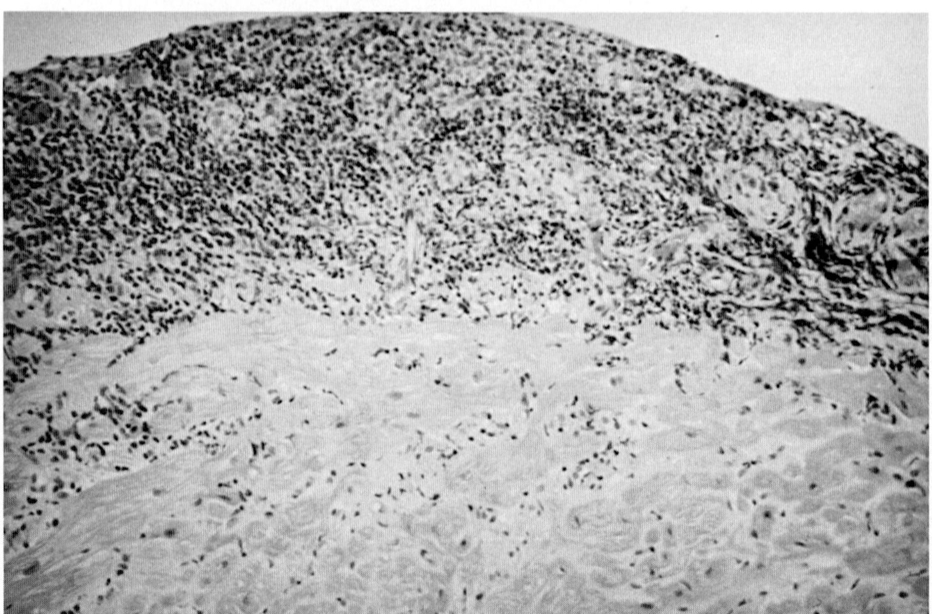

Figure 9–6. Subendocardial infiltrates ("Quilty" effect) seen in 10 percent of cardiac biopsies from cyclosporine-treated patients. (Hematoxylin and eosin stain; magnification ×155, reduced 23 percent.)

Table 9–2. Cyclosporine Immunosuppression Versus Azathioprine Immunosuppression

Cyclosporine	Azathioprine
Rejection develops slowly (4–5 days)	Rejection develops rapidly (24–36 hr)
Clinical signs often absent	Clinical signs (fever, gallop rhythm, ECG)
Slow reversal of rejection (2 wk)	Rapid reversal of rejection with therapy
Severe rejection often reversible	Severe rejection often not reversible
Eosinophils common in rejection	Eosinophils rare in rejection infiltrates
"Quilty" effect in 10% biopsies	Endocardial infiltrates ("Quilty" effect) very rare

as well as the "Quilty" effect, then the patient should be treated for the rejection, but the "Quilty" effect will not necessarily disappear. (4) The final pitfall is the fact that a biopsy to rule out acute rejection may include evidence of ischemia, in which neutrophils are usually prominent and the catecholamine effect already described usually occurs.

The Differences Between Conventional and Cyclosporine-Treated Acute Cardiac Rejection

These differences are outlined in Table 9–2. As can be seen, the major difference is that the usual clinical changes heralding a rejection process are not present in the cyclosporine-treated patients, except for a mild fever, which should always be investigated to rule out rejection as well as infection. It is for this reason that endomyocardial biopsies have to be repeated frequently in cyclosporine-treated patients, at least until such time as a reliable noninvasive procedure has been worked out. The biopsies are monitored concomitantly with cyclosporine levels in the serum. Should the serum levels fall below an optimal level, it is wise to do a biopsy to rule out acute rejection. Whenever there is a change in the amount of immunosuppression given or there is marked weight gain in the patient, which effectively reduces the serum level, then it is wise to perform an endomyocardial biopsy to rule out rejection. As shown in the table, reversal of acute rejection is rapid in patients receiving conventional therapy but may take 2 to 3 weeks with cyclosporine-treated patients. Severe rejection is sometimes reversible in cyclosporine-treated patients but is much more difficult to reverse in the conventionally treated patients. Eosinophils are found in the interstitial infiltrate at all stages of rejection in cyclosporine-treated patients, but they usually herald an infection involving the myocardium in conventionally treated patients. A fine perimyocytic fibrosis may be seen in cyclosporine-treated patients, but this finding is definitely dose-related and was much more common in the early days of cyclosporine treatment when the serum levels were much higher than they are today. Endocardial infiltrates or the "Quilty" effect is seen in approximately 10 percent of endomyocardial biopsies of patients treated with cyclosporine.[8] The etiology of the "Quilty" effect is not yet clear. It should be pointed out that nowadays there is a trend toward less cyclosporine and more azathioprine in many centers; therefore, the clear distinction between conventionally treated and cyclosporine-treated patients is becoming much more blurred, and the pathologist must be aware of the changes for both sets of treatment.

Immunoperoxidase Markers in Acute Rejection

In an attempt to characterize the phenotype of T lymphocytes for target-selective immunosuppression in acute rejection, many centers are now quantitating T cell subsets in serial biopsies. In our own experience at Stanford, we found that T cell subset demonstration was not useful in the management or prediction of acute rejection.[9] In brief, in our study we found that T4 and T8 lymphocytes were equally represented during acute rejection in cyclosporine-treated patients, which was in contrast to previous reports that in conventionally treated patients T8 lymphocytes were clearly predominant during rejection. The markers are useful for treatment with OKT3 antibodies but at present it is thought that this method can only be used once or twice in the same patient. In short, we have not found the immunoperoxidase markers useful in managing acute rejection. However, work is ongoing, particularly in other centers, and one should keep an open mind on this subject until more experience is obtained.

Other Methods of Identifying Acute Rejection

In cardiac allograft recipients, many methods are being studied at this time in order to try to find a reliable noninvasive method for monitoring acute rejection. Studies have been described that include the measurement of the isovolumic relaxation (IVR) calculated from an M-mode echophonocardiogram[10] showing that a 10 percent reduction in IVR was a criterion for moderate acute rejection: the correlation with the endomyocardial biopsy was fairly high for this method. Other studies that are being used to monitor acute rejection at some centers[11] include nuclear magnetic resonance (NMR), which may prove very valuable in this respect, different tissue signatures as obtained by echocardiogram, and also a method for monitoring the peripheral blood lymphoblasts in the serum known as cytologic immunologic marking (CIM). Care should be taken in using the noninvasive studies, some of which require much practice and experience to differentiate changes due to infections from those due to rejection. All noninvasive studies to monitor rejection, although desirable, are less specific than the endomyocardial biopsy. At present, even when noninvasive parameters are being used to monitor rejection, a positive result should be confirmed by an endomyocardial biopsy. An exception to this rule is, of course, the neonatal cardiac recipient in whom endomyocardial biopsy is impractical. Bailey and his group[12] have outlined clearly the criteria for the diagnosis of acute cardiac rejection in infants precluding the endomyocardial biopsy. A new marker for myocyte necrosis using antibody-specific methods and scintigraphy to mark focal myocyte necrosis with sarcolemmal disruption is also now being used as a possible marker for acute rejection with myocyte damage.[13] These are all good methods, but they are nonspecific inasmuch as myocyte damage can be caused by ischemia, catecholamine effect, infection, or acute rejection.

INFECTION

Acute infection is the most important cause of death in the cardiac recipient.[14] This complication can occur either early or in long-term survivors and has caused the death of 102 cardiac transplant recipients out of a total of 366 in the Stanford University Hospital series. The overall number of infections occurring in these patients is approximately the same in those treated with cyclosporine and those treated with azathioprine. In a study comparing 166 cyclosporine-treated patients with 99 azathioprine-treated recipients at Stanford, it was shown that during the first postoperative year there was approximately 4 percent less viral infection in cyclosporine-treated patients; over the subsequent years, however, this gap increased so that there was 10 percent less viral infection in cyclosporine-treated patients between the postoperative years 1 and 5. There is approximately 20 percent less fungal infection in cyclosporine-treated patients than in azathioprine-treated patients over a 5-year period. The gap with bacterial infections is less between the two groups (approximately 5 percent less bacterial infections in the cyclosporine-treated group over 5 years). The most common acute infections during the early postoperative period is with CMV and Toxoplasma gondii. It has been shown that when a heart from a CMV sero-positive donor is placed in a sero-negative recipient, the chances of conversion and infection after immunosuppression are quite high, and clinicians and pathologists alike should be alerted to this fact.

PATHOLOGY OF LONG-TERM CARDIAC TRANSPLANTATION SURVIVORS

In the late postoperative period, a number of potential complications can limit long-term survival. Acute rejection, as has been described in the early postoperative period, can still occur in the late postoperative period. Although episodes of acute rejection tend to be less after the first three postoperative months, occasionally acute rejection episodes will occur. These episodes are usually due to a reduction of immunosuppression either by design (e.g., to combat osteoporosis or nephrotoxicity) or inadvertently to a marked increase in patient weight, which reduces the amount of effective immunosuppression. It has been noticed that acute rejection may occur following a CMV infection, and it should always be looked for in this setting. Acute rejection occurring in the late postoperative period should be treated in the same way as acute rejection in the early postoperative period and should be easily reversible. The development of opportunistic infections, particularly fungal, is an inherent problem in organ grafting with high doses of immunosuppression. The range of organisms responsible for infections in cardiac recipients is extensive and is listed in Table 9–3. Infections in this group of patients may be seen in other organs of the body, including the brain and skin,[14] and will not be detailed in this chapter.

CHRONIC REJECTION OF THE TRANSPLANTED HEART

As in the case of transplanted kidneys, the term "chronic rejection" refers to changes in the small vessels of the organ. The coronary circulation in the transplanted heart is subject to the development of a rapidly progressive form of coronary artery disease in the allograft. This development takes the form of a concentric intimal proliferation often extending along the whole length of the vessel. Interestingly, this intimal proliferation also extends into the small intramyocardial, penetrating branches of the epicardial coronaries. This is important inasmuch as the small vessels may be affected before the concentric intimal proliferation is obvious on surveillance coronary angiography. The pathology of this disease is interesting in that it is different from naturally acquired atherosclerosis, which is usually more focal and contains disruption of the internal elastic membrane, with lipid-filled macrophages, calcium, and hemorrhage within these plaques. Although conventional focal lesions, such as those just described, can be seen in long-term survivors of cardiac transplantation, the concentric intimal proliferation is the more usual pattern. Because it affects the entire vessel length, angioplasty is less likely to be successful and coronary artery bypass cannot be performed. The lesion of chronic rejection, as seen in Figure 9–7,

Table 9–3. Stanford Cardiac Transplantation Infecting Organisms (December 15, 1980–July 1, 1986)

Type of Infecting Organism	Number
Fungal	
Aspergillus	16
Candida	10
Cryptococcus	3
Mucor	1
Yeast, unidentified	1
Viral	
CMV	25
titer rise only	35
Herpes simplex	55
Herpes zoster	23
EB	1
Protozoan	
Pneumocystis	7
Toxoplasma	3
Trichomonas	1
Nocardia	4

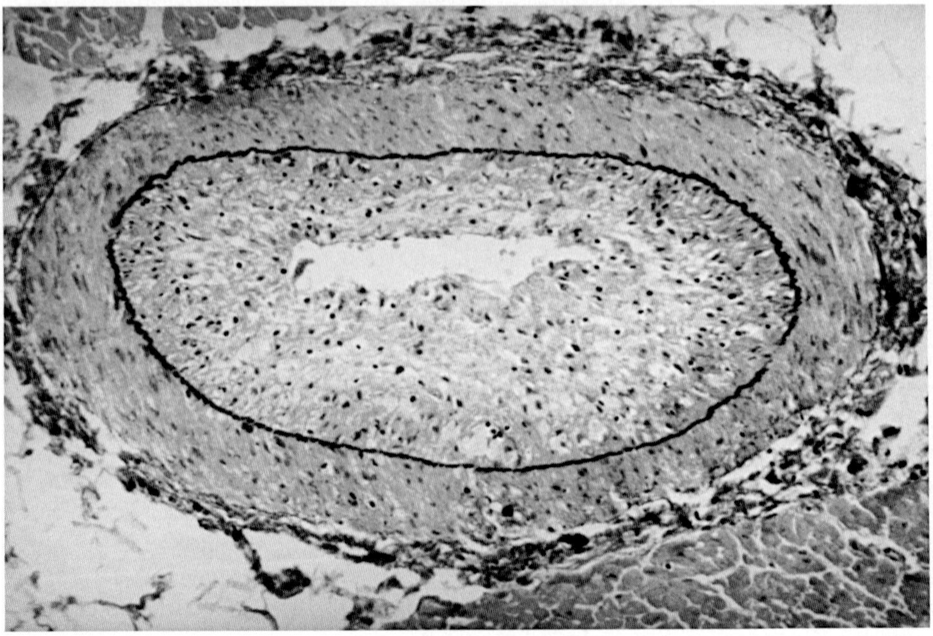

Figure 9–7. Chronic rejection: intimal proliferation in arteriole 1 year following cardiac transplantation. (Elastic van Giesen stain; magnification ×155, reduced 23 percent.)

shows almost intact internal elastic lamina and the marked intimal proliferation narrowing the lumen of the coronary artery. Chronic rejection is detectable to some extent by coronary arteriograms in 40 percent of transplant recipients by 2.5 years following cardiac transplantation.[2] This frequency does not appear to be different in cyclosporine-treated patients from that in the earlier azathioprine-treated group. Chronic coronary disease in recipient hearts leads to all the consequences of ordinary coronary artery disease, such as heart failure and sudden death. It is not usually associated with pain or angina pectoris, because of the lack of afferent reinnervation of the cardiac graft. An extensive autopsy study on 100 recipient hearts at Stanford[15] has shown that the underlying accelerated coronary artery disease does not seem to have any correlation with the number of acute rejection episodes suffered by the patient, with the age or sex of the donor heart, or with whether or not the cardiac recipient previously had coronary artery disease or cardiomyopathy with normal coronary arteries. Chronic rejection is one of the most discouraging aspects of cardiac transplantation at this time. Antiplatelet agents, diets, and other precautions have failed thus far to prevent this disease from occurring in some cardiac recipients, including the young patients.

Denervation of the Transplanted Heart

As far as we know, the transplanted heart remains denervated and is therefore not under the usual direct neural control of the autonomic nervous system. Serial cardiac biopsies studied by electron microscopy after transplantation show degeneration of the sympathetic and sensory nerves. The postganglionic parasympathetic nerves, however, remain intact indefinitely in the transplanted organ. At autopsy, sections through the atrioventricular groove will reveal many viable parasympathetic ganglion cells from which viable postganglionic fibers emanate. Cardiologic and physiologic studies have not indicated that reinnervation of the transplanted heart occurs.[16] Studies at Stanford have suggested that function of the transplanted heart at rest and during exercise depends on intrinsic cardiac mechanisms and on the response to circulating catecholamines released during activity.[17] It has also been shown that the resting heart rate of the denervated heart is 110 ± 10 beats per minute, and this high rate reflects the absence of normal vagal tone. The heart rate in response to dynamic exercise tends to be slower and tends not to achieve peak levels during maximum exercise compared with age-matched normal controls.[18,19]

Malignancies

It is well known that there is an increased risk of malignancies in recipients of organ transplants,[20] probably as a result of immunosuppression or chronic allo-antigen stimulation. The distribution of the tumors (hematologic, skin, and visceral) in the cardiac transplantation group of patients is similar to that in renal transplant patients. The lymphoproliferative malignancies have been of particular concern, inasmuch as there was an increased incidence of these diseases earlier in the program. Although occasional cases still occur, malignancies seem to be less of a problem now that lower doses of antithymocyte globulin and other immunosuppressives are being used. The etiology of these malignancies has raised considerable interest, and there are several good reports related to this subject.[21-23] The lymphoproliferative disorders tend to develop in younger patients given heart transplants for dilated cardiomyopathy. It has also been noticed that there is a predilection of these lymphoproliferative malignancies for the brain where they have responded to radiotherapy.[24] Tumors have been found extranodally in the gastrointestinal tract in cyclosporine-treated patients as well as at the site of injection of antithymocyte globulin in the thighs of cardiac recipients.

SUMMARY

Cardiac transplantation offers an excellent chance of long-term survival and functional rehabilitation for the carefully selected patient with end-stage heart disease. The part played by the pathologist in the care of these patients is crucial. It is vital to make the diagnosis of acute rejection before it becomes irreversible and also before it causes chronic damage to the coronary arteries. It is also vital that the pathologist does not either miss the diagnosis of an infectious myocarditis in the immunosuppressed patient or misdiagnose myocarditis as rejection, because the treatments for each one of these conditions are diametrically opposed. The role of the pathologist has become one of an important clinical colleague in the management and survival of patients with cardiac allografts.

REFERENCES

1. Solise, K and Kaye, MP: The registry of the international society of heart transplantation; 3rd official report—June 1986. J Heart Transplant 5:2, 1986.
2. Schroeder, JS and Hunt, SA: Cardiac transplantation: Where are we? N Engl J Med 315:961, 1986.
3. Jennings, RB and Wartman, WB: Reactions of the myocardium to obstruction of the coronary arteries. Med Clin North Am 46:3, 1962.
4. Caves, PK, Stinson, EB, Billingham, ME, et al: Diagnosis of human cardiac allograft rejection by serial biopsy. J Thorac Cardiovasc Surg 66:461, 1973.
5. Mason, JW: Techniques for right and left ventricular endomyocardial biopsy. Am J Cardiol 41:887, 1978.
6. Caves, PK, Stinson, EB, Billingham, ME, et al: Percutaneous transvenous endomyocardial biopsy in human heart recipients. Ann Thorac Surg 16:325, 1975.
7. Spiegelhalter, DJ and Stovin, PGI: An analysis of repeated biopsies following cardiac transplantation. Stat Med 2:33, 1983.
8. Billingham, ME: Endomyocardial biopsy detection of acute rejection in cardiac allograft recipients. Heart Vessels 1:86, 1985.
9. Weintraub, D, Masek, MA, and Billingham, ME: The lymphocytic subpopulations in cyclosporine-treated human heart rejection. Heart Transplant 4:213, 1985.
10. Dawkins, KD, Oldershaw, PJ, Billingham, ME, et al: Changes in diastolic function as a non-invasive marker of cardiac allograft rejection. Heart Transplant 3:286, 1984.
11. Ertel, W, Reichenspurner, H, Lersch, C, et al: Cytoimmunological monitoring in acute rejection and viral, bacterial or fungal infection following transplantation. Heart Transplant 4:390, 1985.
12. Bailey, LL, Nehlsen-Cannarella, SL, Doroshow, RW, et al: Cardiac allotransplantation in newborns as therapy for hypoplastic left heart syndrome. N Engl J Med 315:949, 1986.
13. Haber, E: Quantifying cell death in the myocardium: Myosin specific antibody in the evaluation of membrane defects. J Mol Cell Cardiol 17:53, 1985.
14. Mason, JW, Stinson, EB, Hunt, SA, et al: Infections after cardiac transplantation: Relation to rejection therapy. Ann Intern Med 85:69, 1976.
15. Billingham, ME, Masek, MA, Khanna, K, et al: Long-term cardiac allograft pathology in humans. Lab Invest 42:103, 1979.
16. Clark, DA, Schroeder, JS, Griepp, RB, et al: Cardiac transplantation in man: Review of first three years' experience. Am J Med 54:56, 1973.
17. Pope, SE, Stinson, EB, Daughters, GT, III, et al: Exercise response of the denervated heart in long-term cardiac transplant recipients. Am J Cardiol 46:213, 1980.

18. Stinson, EB, Griepp, RB, Schroeder, JS, et al: Hemodynamic observations 1 and 2 years after cardiac transplantation in man. Circulation 45:1183, 1972.
19. Savin, WM, Haskel, WL, Schroeder, JS, et al: Cardiorespiratory responses of cardiac transplant patients to graded, symptom-limited exercise. Circulation 62:55, 1980.
20. Penn, I: Malignant lymphoma in organ transplantation recipients. Transplant Proc 13:736, 1981.
21. Weintraub, J and Warnke, R: Lymphoma in cardiac allograft recipients: Clinical and histologic features and immunologic phenotypes. Transplant 33:347, 1982.
22. Cleary, ML and Sklar, J: Lymphoproliferative disorders in cardiac transplant recipients are multiclonal lymphomas. Lancet 2:489, 1984.
23. Cleary, ML Warnke, R, and Sklar, J: Monoclonality of lymphoproliferative lesions in cardiac transplant recipients: Clonal analysis based on immunoglobin-gene rearrangements. N Engl J Med 30:477, 1984.
24. Starzl, TE, Porter, KA, Iwatsuki, S, et al: Reversibility of lymphomas and lymphoproliferative lesions developing under cyclosporine steroid therapy. Lancet 1:583, 1984.

PART 3

Pathology of Valvular Heart Disease

CHAPTER 10

Evaluation of Operatively Excised Cardiac Valves

Bruce F. Waller, M.D.

GENERAL ASPECTS

Valvular heart disease is a term used to describe cardiac dysfunction produced by structural and/or functional abnormalities of single or multiple cardiac valves. Until recent years, most patients in the Western world with valvular heart disease had valvular lesions believed to be rheumatic in origin. In the last 20 to 30 years, however, it has been appreciated that rheumatic disease is only one of several causes of valvular heart disease, and depending on which geographic location in the world, it may not be the most common etiology. The recognition of multiple nonrheumatic causes of valve dysfunction has come about by the continued presence of valvular heart disease despite a gradually decreasing frequency of acute rheumatic fever and its cardiac valvular sequelae.

In recent years in the United States, there has been a decreasing number of patients seen at necropsy in whom valvular heart disease has followed its natural course. This decrease is for the most part a consequence of increased surgical therapy (cardiac valve replacement or repair) and is correspondingly associated with a sharp increase in diseased native cardiac valves seen by surgical pathologists. Indeed, at medical centers where extensive cardiovascular surgery is performed, the study of valvular heart disease is better done in the surgical pathology gross room rather than in the autopsy suite.

Morphologic evaluation of operatively excised native cardiac valves can lead to an etiologic diagnosis in most instances using a few simple gross observations and measurements (Table 10–1). *Routine histologic sectioning of all cardiac valves will add little, if any, additional information beyond the morphologic evaluation pertinent to the etiology or to therapy,* except in two instances: infective endocarditis and metabolic or inborn errors of metabolism.

In patients with operatively excised valves with infective endocarditis, it is necessary to examine the valve tissue histologically to determine the presence or absence of organisms and inflammatory infiltrates. In patients with operatively excised valves who also have metabolic or enzymatic abnormalities (Fabry's disease, mucopolysac-

Table 10–1. Morphologic Determination of Stenotic and Purely Regurgitant Cardiac Valves

Stenotic (With or Without Regurgitation)	Observation	Purely Regurgitant (No Element of Stenosis)
Increased	1. Valve weight	Normal
Diffuse	2. Fibrous thickening	Diffuse or focal
Heavy	3. Calcific deposits	Minimal (if any)
	4. Valve tissue loss (perforation, indentation)	
	or	
0	valve tissue excess	+
+/0	5. Commissural fusion	0
Rarely	6. Tissue vegetations	+/0
	7. Chordae tendineae	
+	Fused	0
0	Elongated	+
+	Shortened	0/+
0	Ruptured	+/0
0	8. Abnormal papillary muscles	+
1, 2, or 3	9. Number of semilunar cusps	2 or 3
Normal	10. Valve "anular" circumference	Increased

* Increased in floppy valves
+ = present, 0 = absent

charidoses, Whipple's disease, carcinoid syndrome), histologic evaluation of valve tissue will provide diagnostic information in establishing the etiology of valvular heart disease. Gross evaluation of operatively excised cardiac valves is the method used by several cardiovascular pathology centers.[1-5]

EVALUATION OF OPERATIVELY EXCISED VALVES

Morphologic Observations

Each submitted operatively excised valve should have the following 10 morphologic observations made (Table 10–1): (1) valve weight; (2) degree (mild to severe) of fibrous thickening; (3) degree (mild to severe) and extent (focal or diffuse) of calcific deposits; (4) valve tissue deficiency (loss; perforation or indentation, or both) or excess; (5) presence or absence and degree (mild to severe) of commissural fusion; (6) vegetation(s); (7) status of the chordae tendineae (fused, elongated, shortened, ruptured); (8) status of attached portions of papillary muscles; (9) number of semilunar cusps; (10) measurement of "anular" circumference of semilunar valves. Morphologic classification of *stenotic* versus *purely regurgitant* functional status of the excised valve can usually be determined from assessment of these 10 morphologic factors (Table 10–1). Determination of the functional status (stenotic versus purely regurgitant) of the excised valve(s) will then lead to etiologic differential diagnoses and classification of valvular heart disease (Table 10–2). While it is recognized that pulmonic valves are rarely[1] observed as operatively excised specimens,[6,7] the etiology of stenotic and purely regurgitant lesions is included for comparison with the aortic, mitral, and tricuspid valves.

Stenosis Versus Pure Regurgitation

Roberts[8] has emphasized the usefulness of establishing the type of valve dysfunction as either *stenotic* or *purely regurgitant* in determining the etiology of the valve dysfunction. Most stenotic valves have clinical evidence of some element of regurgitation, but by definition purely regurgitant valves have no element of stenosis. Although clinically and therapeutically useful, knowledge of whether a valve is both stenotic and regurgitant, or which hemodynamic lesion is dominant is less useful from an etiologic standpoint. For stenotic valves, the etiology of the vast majority can be categorized as either rheumatic or congenital (Table 10–2). On the other hand, if the valve dysfunction is purely regurgitant (no element of stenosis), the etiologic possibilities are numerous (Table 10–2).

Table 10–2. Etiology of Stenotic and Purely Regurgitant Lesions of the 4 Cardiac Valves

Stenosis (With or Without Regurgitation)	Pure Regurgitation (No Element of Stenosis)
Mitral	
A. Rheumatic	A. Rheumatic
B. Nonrheumatic	B. Nonrheumatic
1. Congenital	1. Floppy
	2. Endocarditis
	3. Papillary muscle dysfunction
	4. Congenital
	5. Idiopathic chordal rupture
	6. Carcinoid
	7. Trauma
	8. Hypereosinophilic syndrome
Aortic	
A. Rheumatic	A. Rheumatic
B. Nonrheumatic	B. Nonrheumatic
1. Congenital	1. Endocarditis
2. Degenerative	2. Syphilis
	3. Congenital
	4. Ankylosing spondylitis
	5. Aortic dissection
	6. Marfan's syndrome
	7. Systemic lupus erythematosus
	8. Trauma
Tricuspid	
A. Rheumatic	A. Rheumatic
B. Nonrheumatic	B. Nonrheumatic
1. Congenital	1. "Functional" (right ventricular systolic hypertension)
2. Carcinoid	2. Endocarditis
3. Endocarditis	3. Carcinoid
	4. Floppy
	5. Papillary muscle dysfunction
	6. Trauma
	7. Ebstein's anomaly
	8. Hypereosinophilic syndrome
Pulmonic	
A. Rheumatic	A. Rheumatic
B. Nonrheumatic	B. Nonrheumatic
1. Carcinoid	1. "Functional" (pulmonary artery systolic hypertension)
2. Congenital	2. Endocarditis
	3. Congenital
	4. Trauma (balloon-tip catheter)
	5. Carcinoid

STRUCTURE-FUNCTION CORRELATIONS

The most common morphologic alteration of an abnormal cardiac valve, regardless of etiology, is fibrous thickening (see Table 10–1). The *degree* (mild to severe) and *extent* (focal or diffuse) of fibrous thickening differ with the functional lesion and etiology. Stenotic valves always have severe and diffuse fibrous thickening and usually moderate to heavy amounts of calcific deposits (Figs. 10–1 through 10–4). Purely regurgitant valves, however, have mild to moderate degrees of focal fibrous thickening (except for purely regurgitant mitral valves of rheumatic etiology, which have diffuse fibrous thickening of the margins of closure). Purely regurgitant valves also have absent or minimal calcific deposits (Figs. 10–1 through 10–4). Because of extensive fibrous thickening and calcific deposits, stenotic cardiac valves are heavier than corresponding purely regurgitant valves. Stenotic valves usually have fusion of valve commissures with fibrous tissue or calcific deposits, or both, whereas purely regurgitant valves have minimal and usually absent commissural fusion. Stenotic atrioventricular valves usually have chordae tendineae abnormalities (shortened and fused chordae, normal papillary muscles, and normal anular circumferences) (see Fig. 10–1). Purely regurgitant valves also have chordae tendineae abnormalities (elongated or ruptured or both), but also may have abnormal papillary muscles and dilated anular circumferences (see Table 10–1).

Minimal if any structural valvular alterations may occur in certain purely regurgitant operatively excised valves. In purely regurgitant aortic valve lesions resulting from diseases primarily affecting the ascending aorta (e.g., syphilis, Marfan's syndrome, systemic hypertension, aortic dissection), the operatively excised aortic valve is morphologically normal or has minimal structural changes. Purely regurgitant tricuspid valves excised from patients with pulmonary hypertension (e.g., secondary to severe mitral stenosis) also may be anatomically normal except for dilated anular circumferences.[9,10]

FREQUENCY OF VARIOUS FUNCTIONAL LESIONS

Classification of 1885 stenotic and purely regurgitant operatively excised cardiac valves from 1537 patients aged 15 to 71 years[11,12] (Table 10–3) disclosed that stenotic valve lesions (isolated or combined with other valves) were more frequent (84 percent) than purely regurgitant lesions (isolated or combined) (16 percent). Of the 1885 operatively excised valves, 1571 were stenotic and 314 (17 percent) were purely regurgitant. The most frequently excised stenotic valve was the aortic valve (808 [51 percent]), followed by the mitral valve (759 [48 percent]) and the tricuspid valve (4 [1 percent]). The most frequently excised purely regurgitant valve was the aortic (150 [48 percent]), followed by the mitral (143 [45 percent]) and tricuspid valves (21 [7 percent]) (Table 10–3). No stenotic or purely regurgitant pulmonic valve was excised in this age group. Although multiple valve replacements occurred in 22 percent (335 patients), univalvular replacement was three times more common (78 percent [1212 patients]). Of 335 patients with multivalve replacement, 287 patients (86 percent) had *concordant* multivalvular lesions (all stenotic or all purely regurgitant) and 48 patients (14 percent) had *discordant* lesions (mixed stenotic and purely regurgitant valves).

Occasionally, classification of operatively excised valves into stenotic versus purely regurgitant lesions may require additional information from catheterization

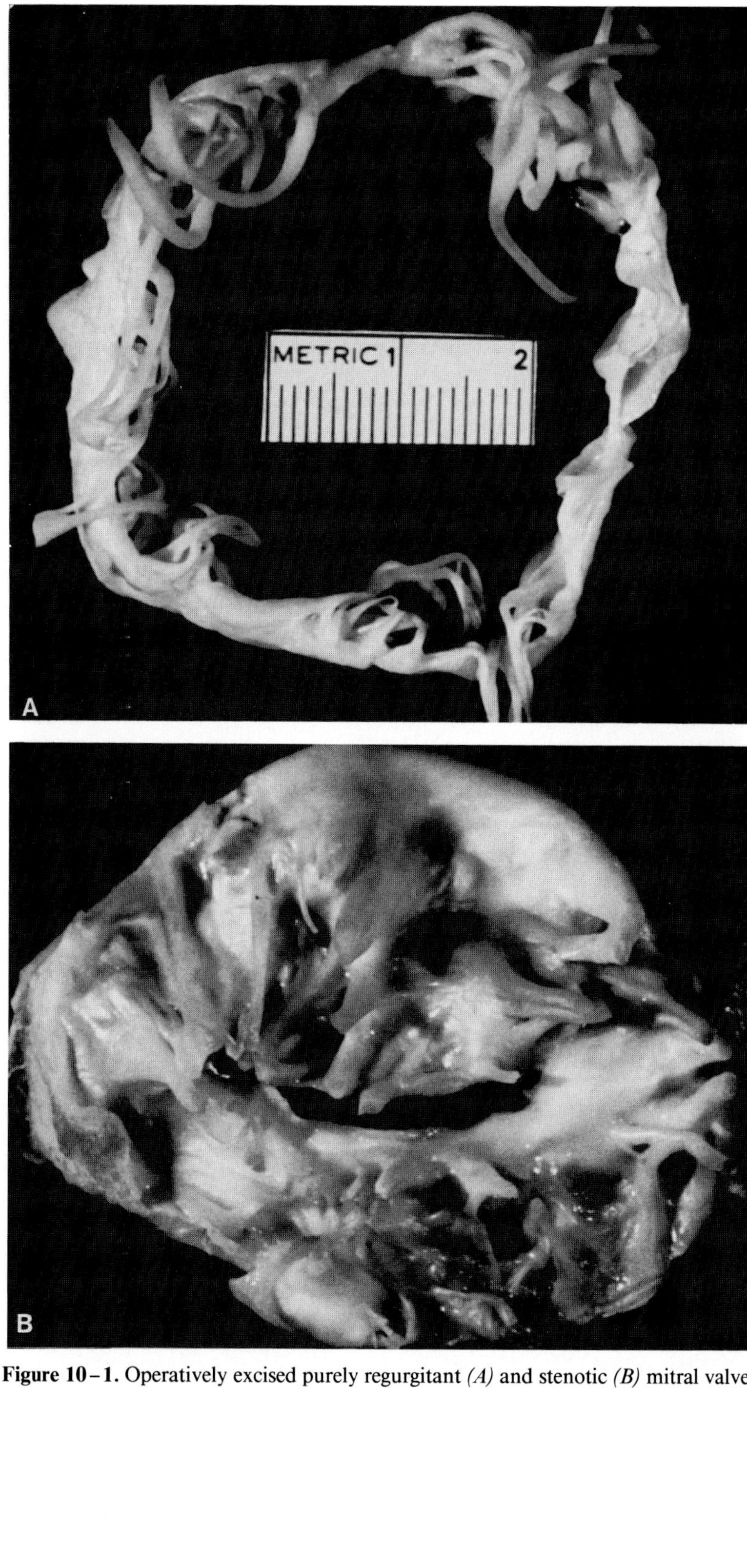

Figure 10–1. Operatively excised purely regurgitant *(A)* and stenotic *(B)* mitral valves.

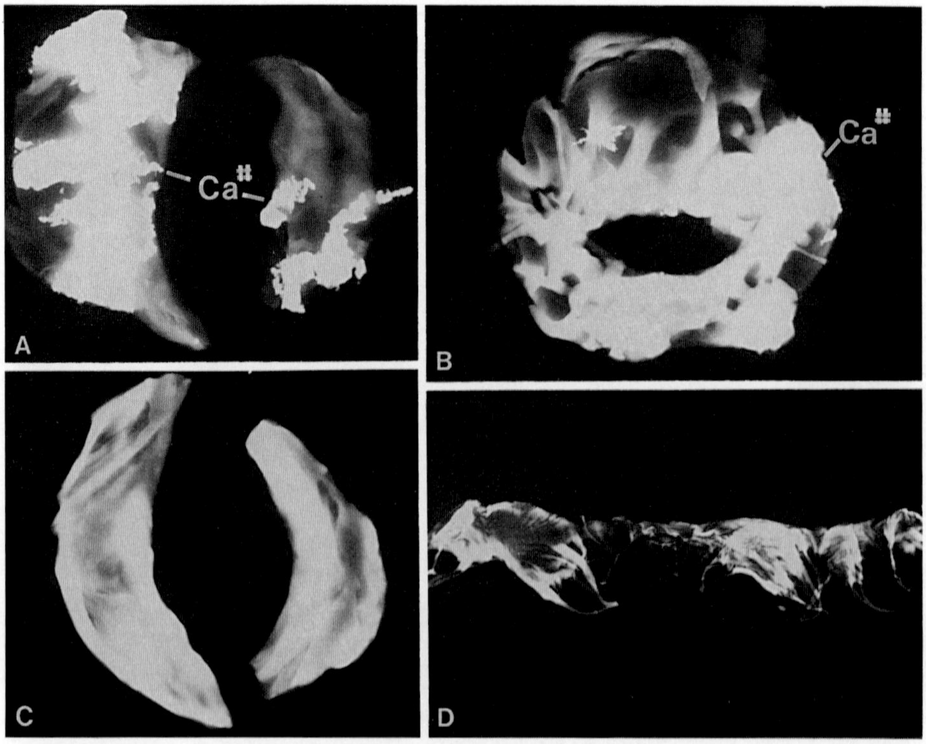

Figure 10–2. Amounts of calcific deposits (Ca#) in operatively excised stenotic aortic *(A)* and mitral *(B)* valves and purely regurgitant aortic *(C)* and mitral *(D)* valves. Stenotic valves have heavy Ca# deposits, as compared with those of purely regurgitant valves.

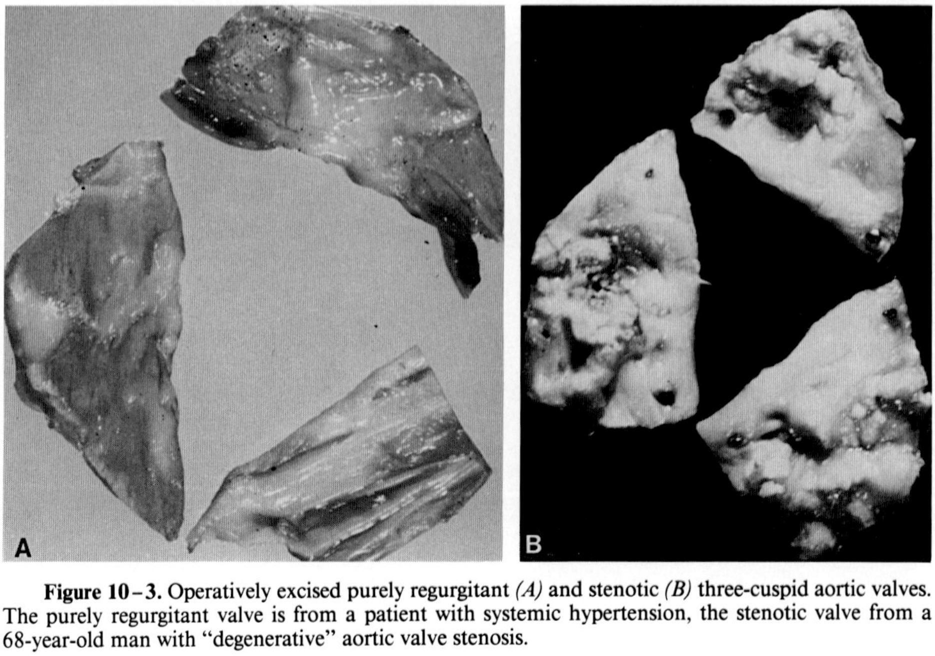

Figure 10–3. Operatively excised purely regurgitant *(A)* and stenotic *(B)* three-cuspid aortic valves. The purely regurgitant valve is from a patient with systemic hypertension, the stenotic valve from a 68-year-old man with "degenerative" aortic valve stenosis.

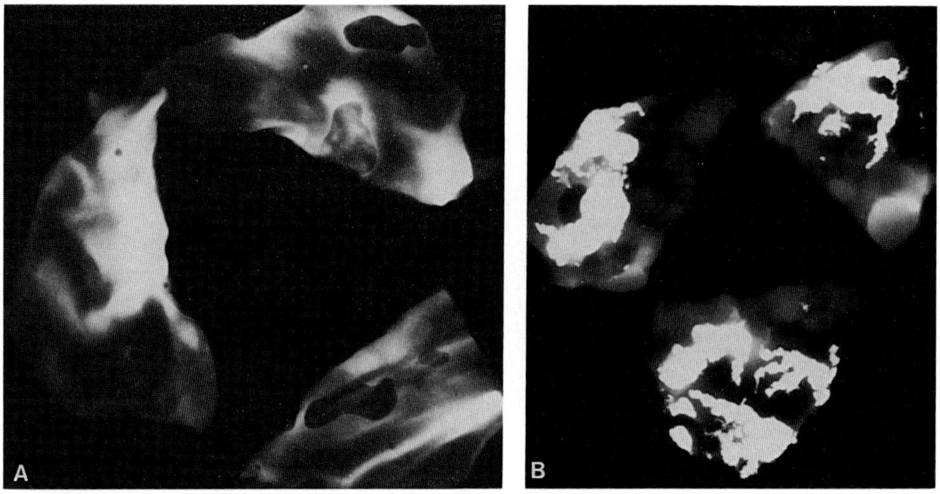

Figure 10–4. Radiographs of aortic valves in Figure 10–3. The purely regurgitant valve *(A)* has no calcific deposits, but the stenotic valve *(B)* has heavy calcific deposits.

data or information on the structural and functional status of a nonoperatively excised mitral valve. For both structural and functional classification, it is absolutely necessary to receive the entire excised valve specimen, so that proper morphologic assessment can be made.

Rose[13] recently examined 100 consecutive, surgically excised native cardiac valves and found that if the pathologist is given adequate information regarding the macroscopic appearance of the intact valve prior to excision, an etiologic diagnosis was possible in 81 percent of valves, compared with only 35 percent of valves without such information. Of interest was that for 62 percent of the patients, the surgeon gave

Table 10–3. Functional and Morphologic Classification of 1885 Operatively Excised Valves From 1547 Patients Aged ≥15 Yr, Between December 1962 and March 1986

Lesion	Number (%) Patients	Valves
1. Aortic stenosis (AS)	536 (35)	536 (29)
2. Mitral stenosis (MS)	438 (28)	(438) (23)
3. AS + MS	269 (17)	538 (28)
4. Mitral regurgitation (MR)	129 (8)	129 (7)
5. Aortic regurgitation (AR)	106 (7)	106 (6)
6. MS + AR	31 (2)	62 (3)
7. MS + tricuspid regurgitation (TR)	16 (1)	32 (2)
8. AR + MR	13 (1)	26 (1)
9. TR	3 (0.3)	3 (0.2)
10. MS + tricuspid stenosis (TS)	2 (0.2)	4 (0.2)
11. MS + AS + TS	2 (0.2)	6 (0.3)
12. MS + AS + TR	1 (0.1)	3 (0.2)
13. MR + TR	1 (0.1)	2 (0.1)
	1547 (100)	1885 (100)

no indication on the pathology request form as to the suspected etiology of the valve disease necessitating the operation. In only 15 percent of patients did the operation notes and the request form agree on the etiologic diagnosis. In 13 percent, however, the request form was more informative than the operation notes.[13]

ETIOLOGY OF VALVULAR HEART DISEASE BASED ON ASSESSMENT OF OPERATIVELY EXCISED CARDIAC VALVES

Stenotic Lesions

Aortic Valve

Stenotic aortic valves result from three major etiologies: *congenital, rheumatic,* and *degenerative* ("senile," "old age," "wear and tear") (Figs. 10–5 through 10–14). Congenital stenotic aortic valves may be *unicuspid* (Figs. 10–5, 10–6) or *bicuspid* (Figs. 10–5, 10–7 through 10–9). The unicuspid valve may have a dome-shaped orifice ("volcano-like," acommissural) or an eccentric-shaped orifice ("exclamation point," unicommissural) (Figs. 10–5, 10–6). Stenotic unicuspid aortic valves are most commonly excised from patients less than 30 years of age. Congenitally bicuspid aortic valves are probably the most frequently excised aortic valve between the ages of 25 and 50 years. Two types of bicuspid aortic valve occur in about equal frequency: anterior-posterior and right-left (Figs. 10–7 through 10–9). The anterior-posterior type has both coronary artery ostia arising from the anterior cusp, and the anterior cusps contains the raphe (false commissure) when a raphe is present. The right-left variety of bicuspid aortic valve has a coronary ostium arising from each of the sinuses and, when present, the raphe is always located in the right cusp.[11,12] Stenotic aortic valves of congenital origin usually contain heavy calcific deposits at an earlier age compared with stenotic three-cuspid aortic valves (Figs. 10–5, 10–8, 10–9).

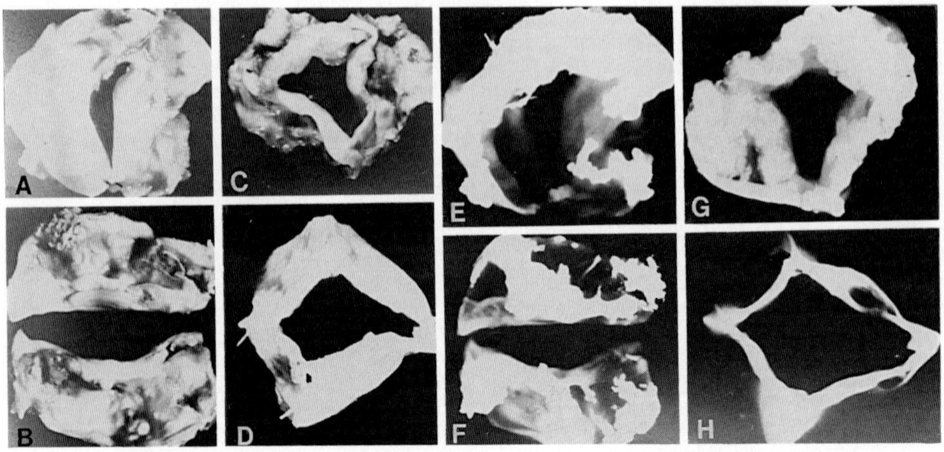

Figure 10–5. Four operatively excised aortic valves: *(A)* unicuspid (unicommissural), *(B)* bicuspid, *(C)* three-cuspid degenerative, *(D)* quadricuspid. Valves *A* through *C* are stenotic, and *D* is purely regurgitant. Corresponding radiographs of four aortic valves (*E* through *H*). The stenotic valves *E* through *G* have heavy calcific deposits, whereas the purely regurgitant valve *(H)* has no calcific deposits.

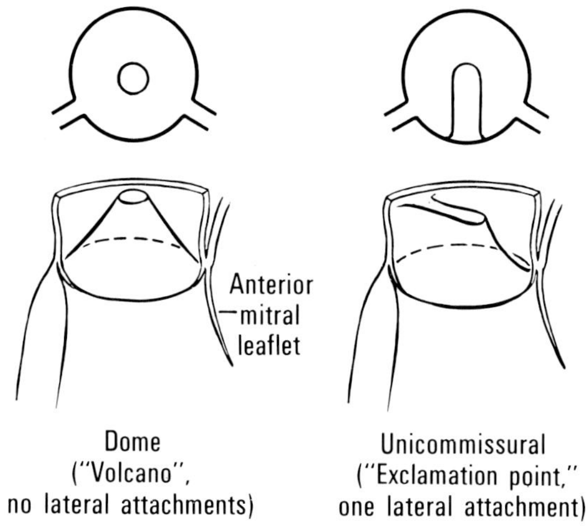

Figure 10–6. Types of congenital unicuspid aortic valves.

Congenital and *acquired* bicuspid aortic valves usually can be distinguished from simple cuspal measurements (Figs. 10–10 through 10–12). The circumferential distances between each commissure are about equal in normal three-cuspid aortic valves. In congenitally bicuspid aortic valves the distances between the two commissures are also about equal. Thus, in acquired bicuspid aortic valves, the cusp containing the fused commissure is at least twice as long as the remaining commissural length (Figs. 10–10 through 10–12). In severely calcified aortic valves, the distinction may not be possible.

Stenotic aortic valves of *rheumatic* origin are characterized by fusion of at least one and usually two or three commissures in the presence of an anatomically abnormal mitral valve (diffuse leaflet or margin of closure fibrous thickening). The classic stenotic aortic valve of rheumatic origin has extensive fusion of all three commissures producing a central triangular orifice (Figs. 10–10, 10–12).

The third etiology of aortic valve stenosis is *degenerative.* This valve is characterized by the following features: three-cuspid, absent commissural fusion, and nodular

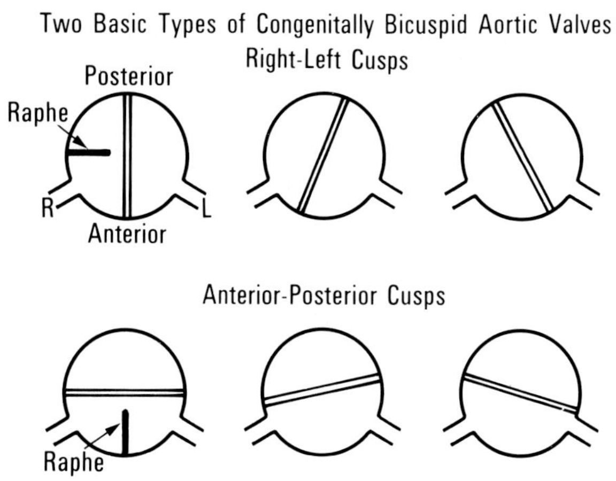

Figure 10–7. Types of congenitally bicuspid aortic valves.

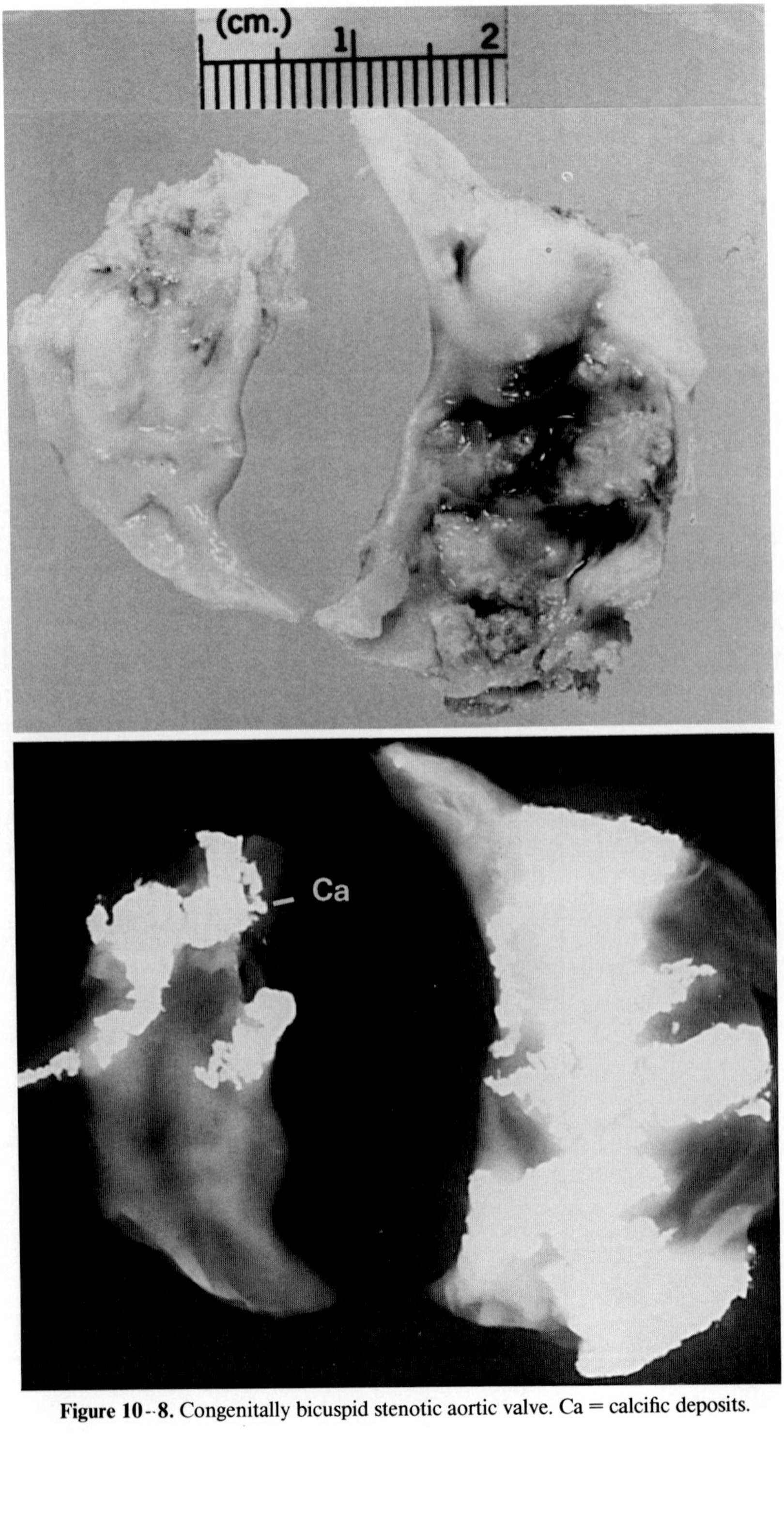

Figure 10-8. Congenitally bicuspid stenotic aortic valve. Ca = calcific deposits.

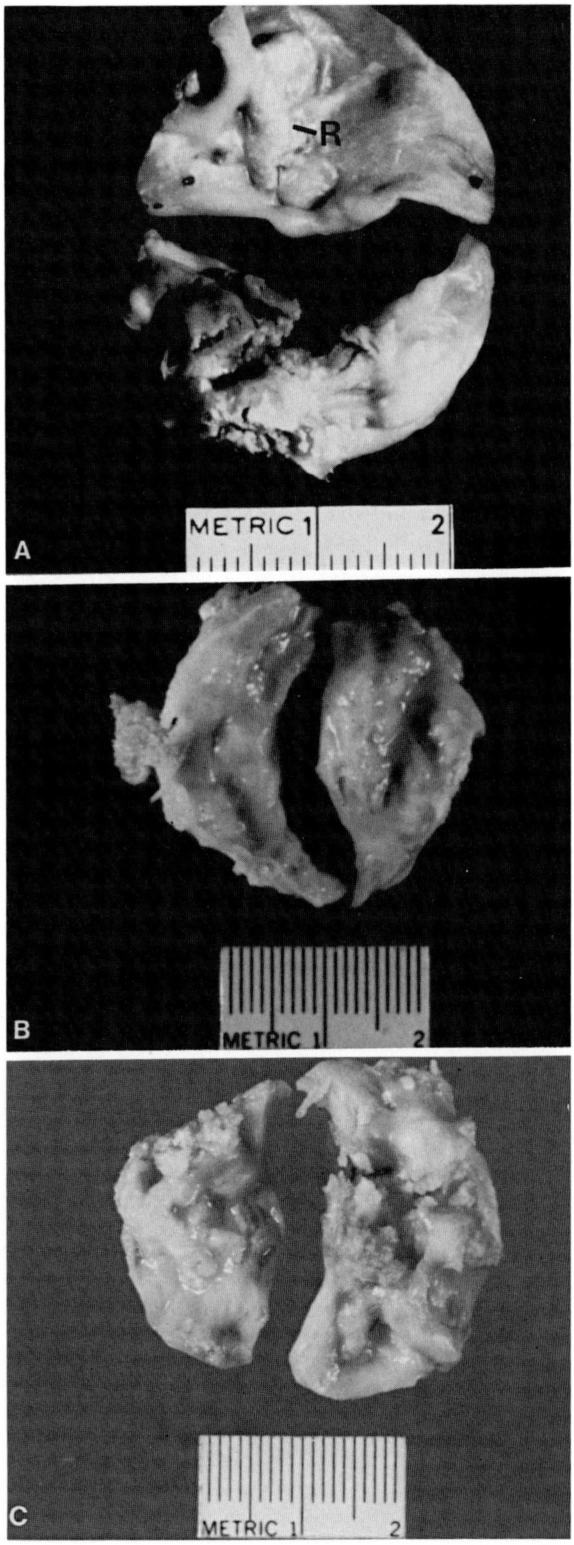

Figure 10-9. Three operatively excised stenotic congenitally bicuspid aortic valves. *A,* Anterior-posterior type. *B, C,* Right-left variety. All are heavily calcified. R = raphe (false commissure).

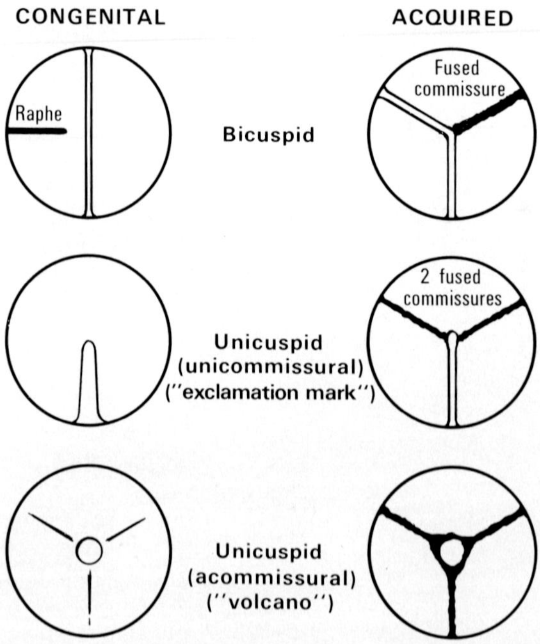

Figure 10–10. Comparison of congenital and acquired forms of bicuspid and unicuspid stenotic aortic valves. *Dark lines* = commissural fusion.

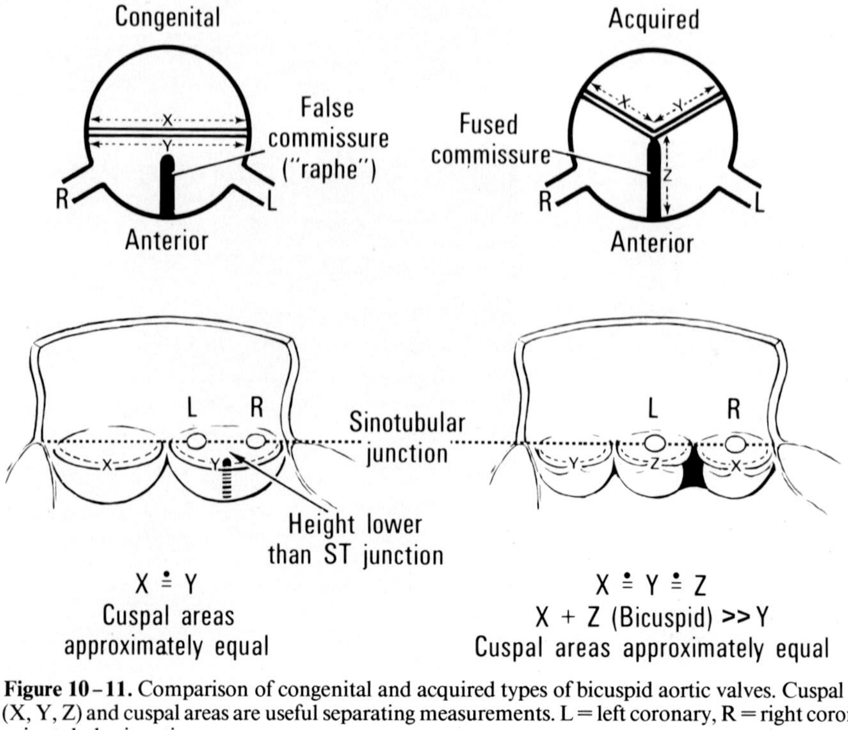

Figure 10–11. Comparison of congenital and acquired types of bicuspid aortic valves. Cuspal margins (X, Y, Z) and cuspal areas are useful separating measurements. L = left coronary, R = right coronary, ST = sinotubular junction.

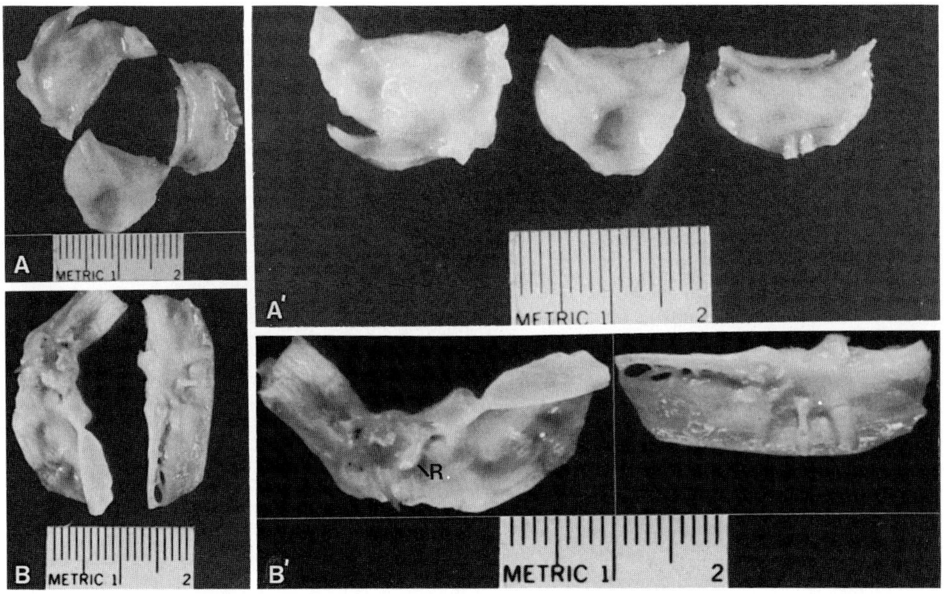

Figure 10–12. Cuspal measurements of normal three-cuspid aortic valve *(A,A′)* and congenitally bicuspid aortic valve *(B,B′)*. The cuspal margins of closure in each respective valve are nearly equal. Compare with Figure 10–11.

calcific deposits in two or three cusps. The vast majority of these valves come from patients aged 65 years and older (see Figs. 10–3 through 10–5).

Davies[2] reported the etiology of 187 operatively excised stenotic aortic valves (Fig. 10–13). In 113 patients (60 percent), the valve was congenital (specifically identified as bicuspid) in 104 of the 113 valves. An additional 31 (17 percent) valves were classified as rheumatic in origin, 22 (12 percent) degenerative, and 14 (7 percent) as "mixed" etiologies. Of the 187 valves, 7 (4 percent) were unclassifiable.

Subramanian and colleagues[3] recently reported the surgical pathology of pure aortic stenosis, analyzing 374 operatively excised valves during the years 1965, 1970, 1975, and 1980 (Figs. 10–13, 10–14). In this series, the aortic valves were classified as bicuspid, postinflammation (rheumatic for practical purposes), degenerative, or unicommissural. Of the 374 stenotic aortic valves, 171 (46 percent) were bicuspid, 130 (35 percent) postinflammatory (rheumatic), 38 (10 percent) degenerative, 21 (6 percent) unicommissural, and 14 (4 percent) indeterminate (Fig. 10–13). If one combines the bicuspid and unicuspid groups under the classification of "congenital," then the most common etiology for operatively excised stenotic aortic valves was congenital (52 percent) followed by postinflammatory (35 percent) and degenerative (10 percent). The authors also compared the various etiologies over a 4-year period (1965, 1970, 1975, and 1980). The frequency of postinflammatory etiology (rheumatic) remained about the same, whereas the frequency of congenital etiology decreased and degenerative etiology increased (Fig. 10–14).

Mitral Valve

The etiology of mitral stenosis is virtually limited to *rheumatic disease,* which accounts for over 98 percent of operatively excised mitral valves. Rarely, vegetation from active infective endocarditis may be large enough to obstruct the mitral valve

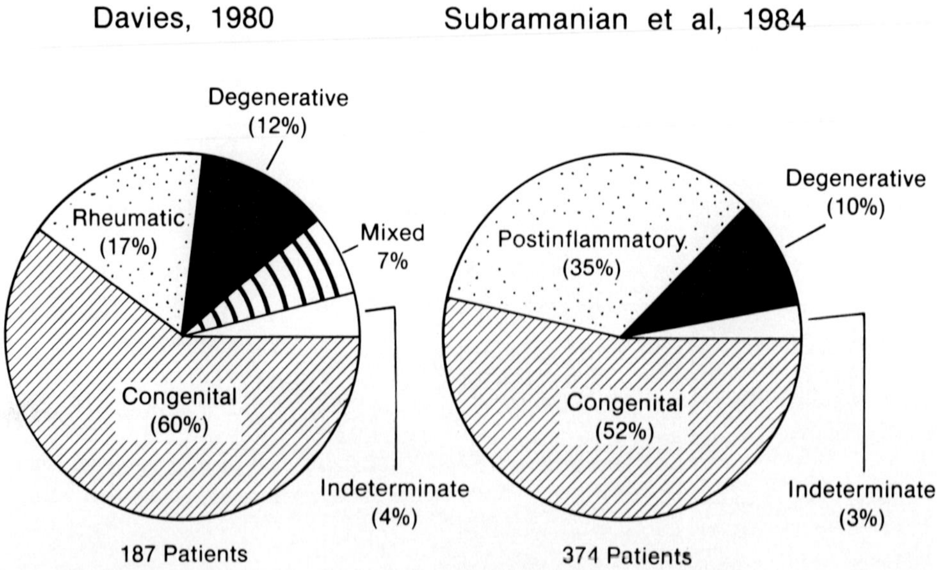

Figure 10–13. Etiology of operatively excised stenotic aortic valves. (Modified from Davies,[2] and Subramanian et al.[3])

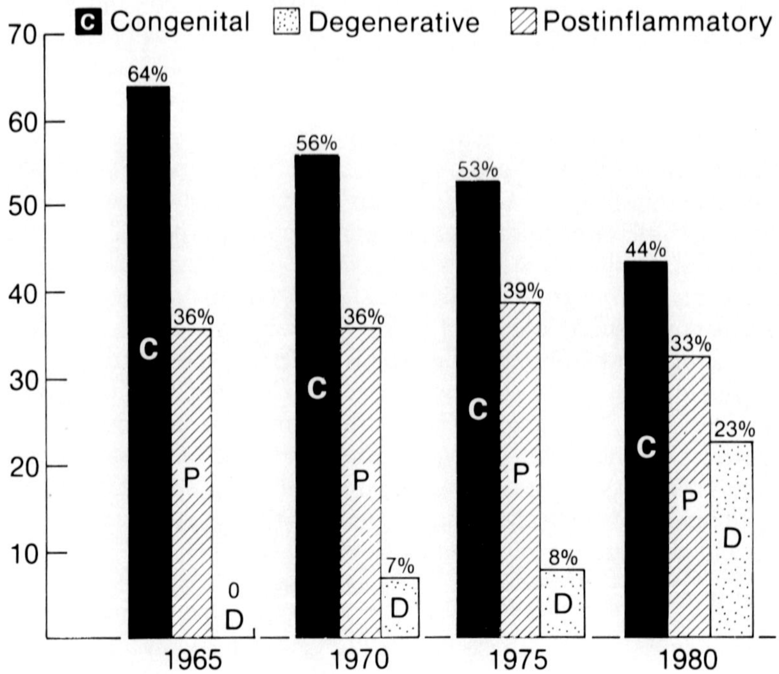

Figure 10–14. Comparison of etiology of operatively excised stenotic aortic valves and year of excision. (Modified from Subramanian et al.[3])

orifice. The rheumatic mitral stenotic valve is characterized by diffuse fibrous thickening of each leaflet, with calcific deposits of variable degree and fusion of both commissures (see Figs. 10–1, 10–2, 10–15). Commonly, the chordae tendineae are also thickened, shortened, and fused, further contributing to the stenotic orifice. Aschoff nodules may be encountered in operatively excised left atrial appendages (22 percent) or attached portions of papillary muscles (2 percent) in patients with stenotic mitral valves.[14] The presence and amount of calcific deposits in mitral valves have been directly correlated with the average end-diastolic pressure gradient across stenotic mitral valves measured at cardiac catheterization. Generally, as the amount of calcium increases, so does the pressure gradient increase.[15]

All of the 759 operative excised mitral valves from patients aged 15 years or older were rheumatic in etiology (Table 10–3). Recently, Olsen and colleagues[16] analyzed 452 cases of mitral stenosis at the Mayo Clinic. Of the 452 cases, 450 (99.5 percent) were classified as postinflammatory and 2 (0.5 percent) valves were congenital in etiology. Comparison of etiology over a 5-year period (1965, 1970, 1975, 1980, 1985) disclosed a decreasing frequency of postinflammatory operatively excised mitral valves: 25, 25, 25, 18, and 8 percent, respectively.

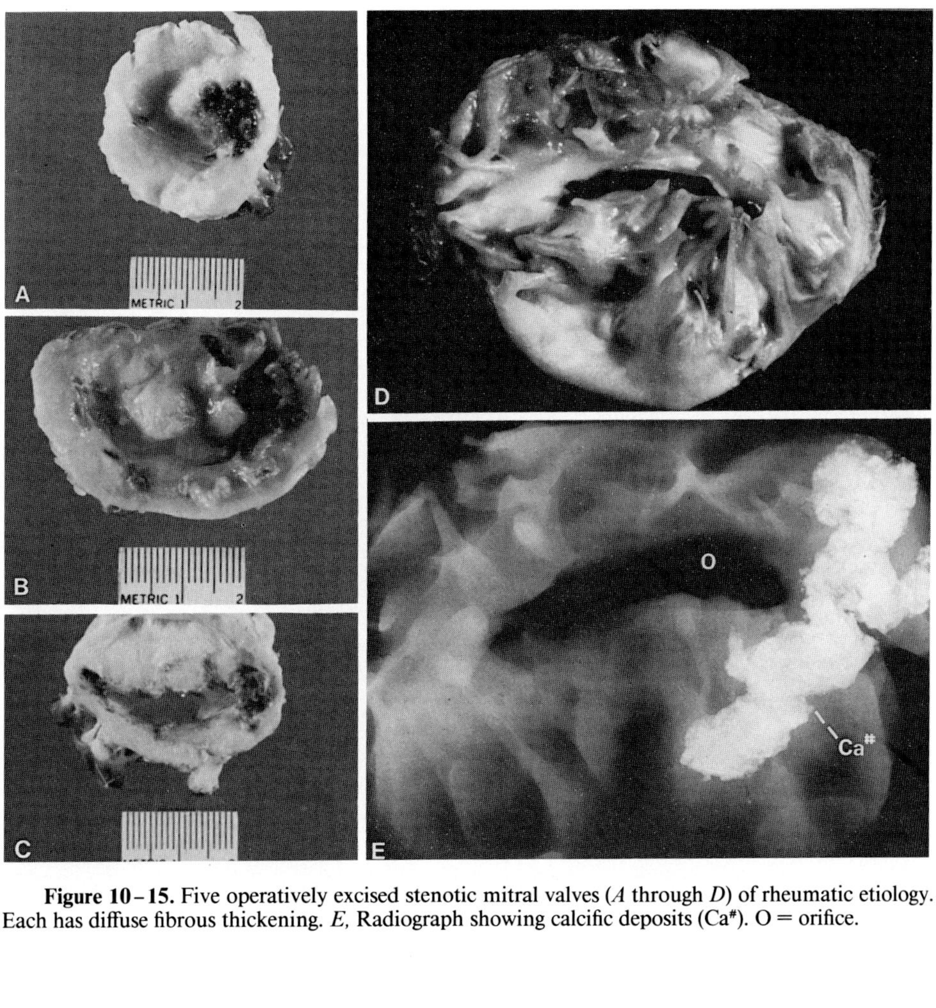

Figure 10–15. Five operatively excised stenotic mitral valves (*A* through *D*) of rheumatic etiology. Each has diffuse fibrous thickening. *E*, Radiograph showing calcific deposits (Ca#). O = orifice.

Tricuspid Valve

The etiology of stenotic tricuspid valves is limited to three abnormalities: *rheumatic* disease, *carcinoid* disease, and *congenital* malformations. Rheumatic tricuspid stenosis, in contrast to mitral stenosis, never occurs as an isolated lesion. All patients with rheumatic tricuspid stenosis have associated disease of the mitral valve and usually dysfunction of the aortic valve as well (Fig. 10–16). Rheumatic stenosis of the tricuspid valve is associated with diffuse fibrous thickening of the leaflets, with fusion of two and usually three commissures. The chordae tendineae may be thickened and shortened, but chordal changes are generally not as severe as in rheumatic mitral stenosis. Also, in contrast to many stenotic mitral valves, the leaflet thickening rarely is associated with calcific deposits. Carcinoid heart disease also may produce stenotic tricuspid valves requiring valve replacement.[17] The carcinoid plaque is a white, fibrous lesion that coats the valve without causing destruction of the underlying valve architecture. Characteristically, the coating occurs on the ventricular aspects of the tricuspid leaflets and may also cover the chordae tendineae. *Isolated* tricuspid stenosis is usually congenital in origin or may result from active infective endocarditis vegetations.

Between 1962 and 1986, of 1885 operatively excised valves only four (0.2 percent) were stenotic tricuspid valves and all four were rheumatic in etiology associated with stenotic mitral and aortic valves (Table 10–3).

Pulmonic Valve

Valvular pulmonic stenosis is caused by congenitally malformed valves, rheumatic disease, or carcinoid heart disease.[11,12] Only a few operatively excised pulmonic valves (isolated or combined with other valves) have been reported in patients aged 20 years and older.[6,7]

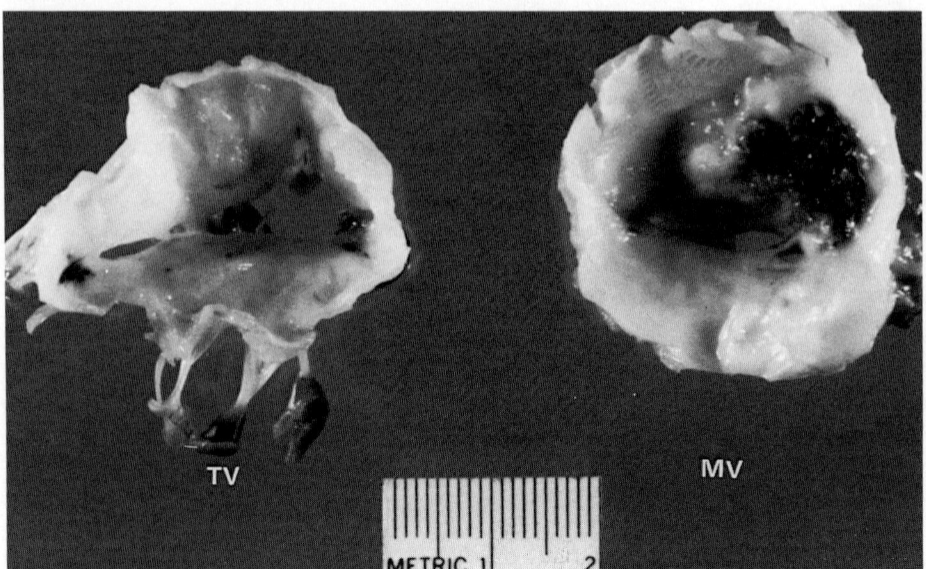

Figure 10–16. Operatively excised stenotic tricuspid *(left)* (TV) and mitral *(right)* (MV) valves from a patient with rheumatic heart disease.

Purely Regurgitant Lesions

In marked contrast to the relatively simple approach to etiology of stenotic valvular lesions, the etiology of purely regurgitant lesions are multiple (see Table 10–2, Figs. 10–17 through 10–56).

Aortic Valve

The various etiologies of *pure aortic regurgitation* can be subgrouped into those conditions primarily affecting the *aortic valve cusps,* primarily involving the *aorta,* and those conditions affecting *both* or *neither aorta and valve*[11,12] (Table 10–4, Figs. 10–17 through 10–25).

Diseases of the aortic valve account for over 75 percent of these conditions.[2,11,12,18] Conditions producing pure aortic regurgitation due to abnormalities of the aortic valve cusps include infective endocarditis on three-cuspid or congenitally bicuspid aortic valves, rheumatic, congenitally bicuspid aortic valves without superimposed infective endocarditis, trauma, and floppy aortic valves. The most frequent of these etiologies is rheumatic (Table 10–4, Figs. 10–17 through 10–22).

Aorta. Although the aortic valve is intrinsically normal, pure aortic regurgitation may result from various diseases affecting the ascending aorta (Table 10–4). Diseases of the ascending aorta account for the second most common cause of purely regurgitant aortic valves. Four major disease processes are found in this category: syphilis, Marfan's syndrome, aortitis, and laceration of aorta (dissection, trauma) (Figs. 10–23, 10–24). Occasionally, segments of operatively excised aorta accompanying the excised aortic valve permit histologic evaluation of the wall of aorta. In syphilis the aortic wall is thickened, whereas in Marfan's syndrome the aortic wall is characteristically thin with loss of medial elastic fibers and increased amounts of acid mucopolysaccharide material (Fig. 10–24).

Neither. Pure aortic regurgitation secondary to systemic hypertension is classified under the category of disease affecting *neither aorta nor valve* (Table 10–4, Figs. 10–24, 10–25).[19]

Both. Ankylosing spondylitis is the only disease process producing pure aortic regurgitation involving *both wall of aorta and aortic valve* (Table 10–4, Fig. 10–17).[20] The disease process in ankylosing spondylitis involves the wall of aorta behind the sinus of Valsalva (like Marfan's syndrome) and the proximal portion of the tubular segment of aorta (like syphilis), but also extends to involve the basal portion of the aortic valve cusp and onto the ventricular septum and anterior mitral valve leaflet. The aortic valve cusp becomes thickened and shortened.[20]

Of 106 patients with isolated, pure aortic regurgitation (Tables 10–3, 10–5), the etiology was *infective endocarditis* (50 [47 percent]), *congenitally bicuspid without superimposed infective endocarditis* (22 [21 percent]), *rheumatic* (with associated abnormal mitral valve) (15 [14 percent]), *aortic dissection* (12 [11 percent]), *prolapse* (2 [2 percent]), and one (1 percent) each *syphilis, radiation injury,* and *quadricuspid* (Figs. 10–18 through 10–22). Congenitally abnormal valves accounted for 44 (42 percent) of the specimens. These findings are in marked contrast to the series of 189 patients with isolated pure aortic regurgitation reported by Roberts and colleagues.[21] In this series, rheumatic etiology accounted for 94 (49 percent) of the aortic valves, and infective endocarditis was the second most frequent etiology (22 percent).

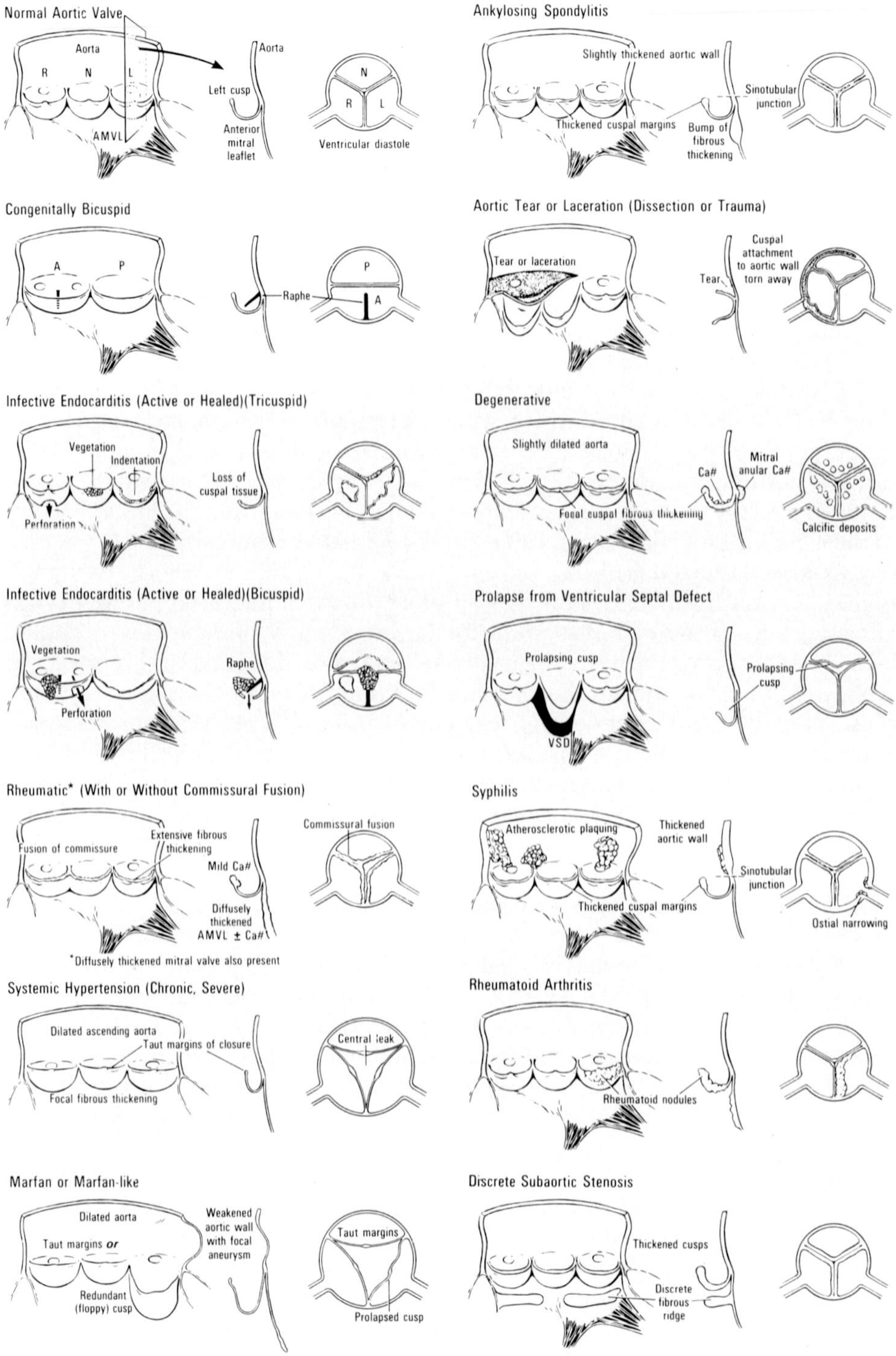

Figure 10–17. Various etiologies of pure aortic regurgitation.

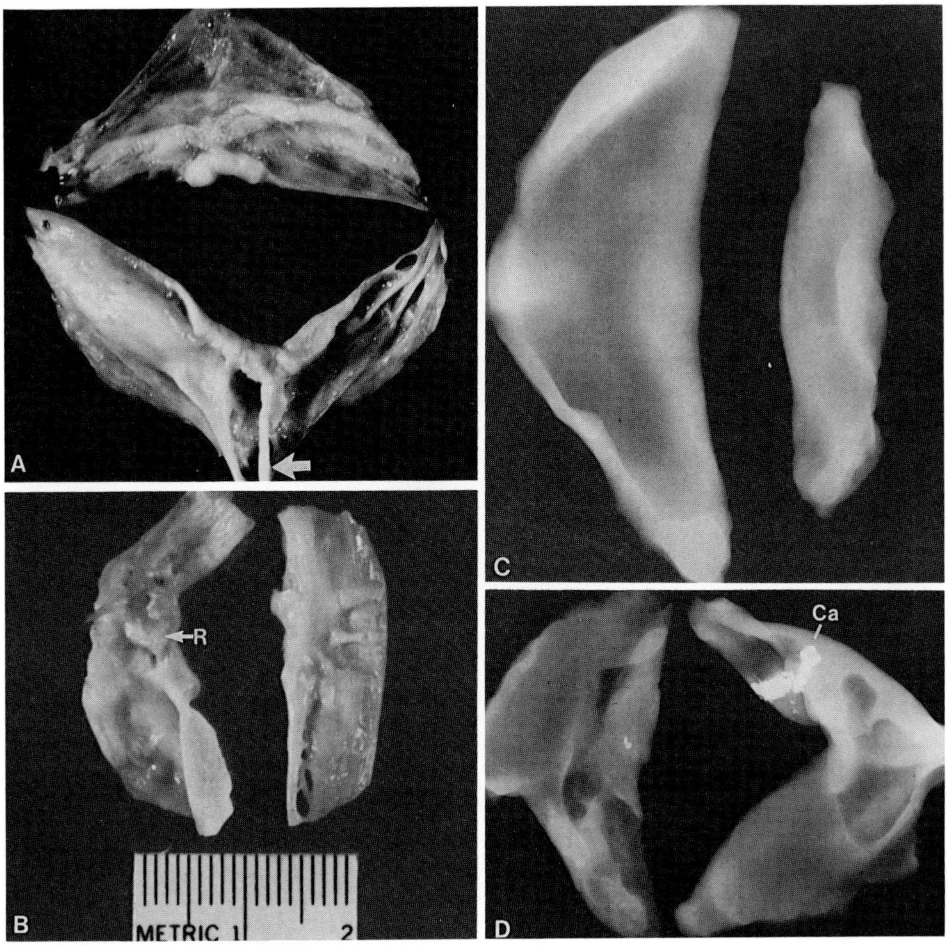

Figure 10–18. Operatively excised purely regurgitant congenitally bicuspid aortic valves from four patients (*A* through *C*). *A,* Raphe of bicuspid valve represented by thin strand to tissue *(arrow)* extending from the cusp to the aortic wall, which allowed the cusp to be held open during ventricular diastole. *B,* Raphe (R) in right cusp. *C, D,* Radiographs of two other purely regurgitant bicuspid valves showing no or minimal calcific deposits (Ca).

Mitral Valve

The etiology of *pure mitral regurgitation* may be classified into conditions altering certain components of the mitral valve apparatus: leaflets, chordae tendineae, anulus, papillary muscles, and commissures (Figs. 10–26 through 10–39). The structural alterations of purely regurgitant mitral valves of rheumatic etiology include diffuse fibrous thickening of at least the margins of closure, minimal if any calcific deposits, commissural fusion, and mild thickening of the chordae tendineae. *Nonrheumatic etiologies of pure mitral regurgitation account for the vast majority of operatively excised mitral valves in the United States.*[23]

Of 97 patients with operatively excised mitral valves for isolated, pure mitral regurgitation, nonrheumatic etiologies accounted for 97 percent: *floppy* (62 percent)

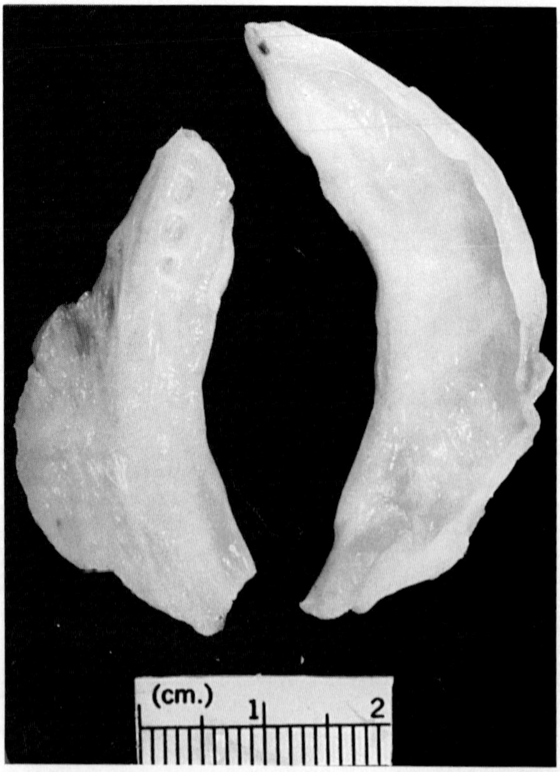

Figure 10–19. Operatively excised congenitally bicuspid aortic valve producing pure aortic regurgitation without superimposed infective endocarditis. The margins of closure are markedly unequal, allowing improper cuspal coaptation.

(Figs. 10–28, 10–29, 10–31 through 10–35), *papillary muscle dysfunction from atherosclerotic coronary disease* (30 percent) (Figs. 10–30, 10–31, 10–33 through 10–35), and *infective endocarditis* (Figs. 10–31, 10–37 through 10–39).[24] Morphologic distinction of floppy valves from other conditions of pure mitral regurgitation have included histologic and morphometric criteria. Although increased amounts of acid mucopolysaccharide material are present in many floppy valves, Waller and colleagues[23] found measurement of anular circumference (cm) and leaflet area (cm^2) a sensitive and highly specific method in detecting floppy from nonfloppy mitral valves (Figs. 10–32 through 10–35). Anular circumferences greater than 11 cm and leaflet areas greater than 11 cm^2 were always indicative of floppy mitral valves. Operatively excised floppy valves with associated ruptured chordae tendineae also had increased leaflet areas but had only a mild increase in anular circumference (greater than 10 cm but usually less than 11.5 cm). The increased leaflet area in floppy valves is the morphologic expression of leaflet "hooding," "redundancy," or "prolapse." Papillary muscle dysfunction from any conditions may produce severe acute or chronic mitral regurgitation requiring mitral valve replacement. One of the most common etiologies is atherosclerotic coronary disease with scarred papillary muscles.[23] The operatively excised mitral valve leaflets, anular circumference, commissures, and chordae tendineae are normal, but either or both of the attached portions of left ventricular papillary muscles are scarred and usually atrophied (Figs. 10–30, 10–33 through 10–36). Active or healed infective endocarditis causes pure mitral regurgitation by destroying leaflet tissue (perforation, indentation), by rupture of chordae tendineae, by producing vegetations that cause abnormal leaflet coaptation, or by various combinations (Figs. 10–37 through 10–39). Infection may occur on previously anatomically normal valves or may be superimposed on rheumatic or floppy mitral valves. Other rare causes of pure mitral regurgitation requiring mitral valve replacement include Libman-Sacks lesion of lupus erythematosus and hypereosinophilic syndrome. Olsen and associates,[16] in an analysis of 260 operatively excised purely regurgitant mitral valves, found floppy valves the most common etiology (38 percent) followed by *postinflammatory disease* (31 percent), *ischemia* (12 percent), *endocarditis* (6 percent), *idiopathic chordal rupture* (4 percent), *cardiomyopathy* (3 percent), *congenital anomaly* (3 percent), and *chronic aortic insufficiency* (1 percent). Of 16 patients with endocarditis, the underlying mitral valve was anatomically normal in 31 percent, postinflammatory in 31 percent, and floppy in 38 percent. During the 21 years spanned by the study, the frequency of postinflammatory mitral regurgitation progressively decreased from 45 percent in 1965 to 15

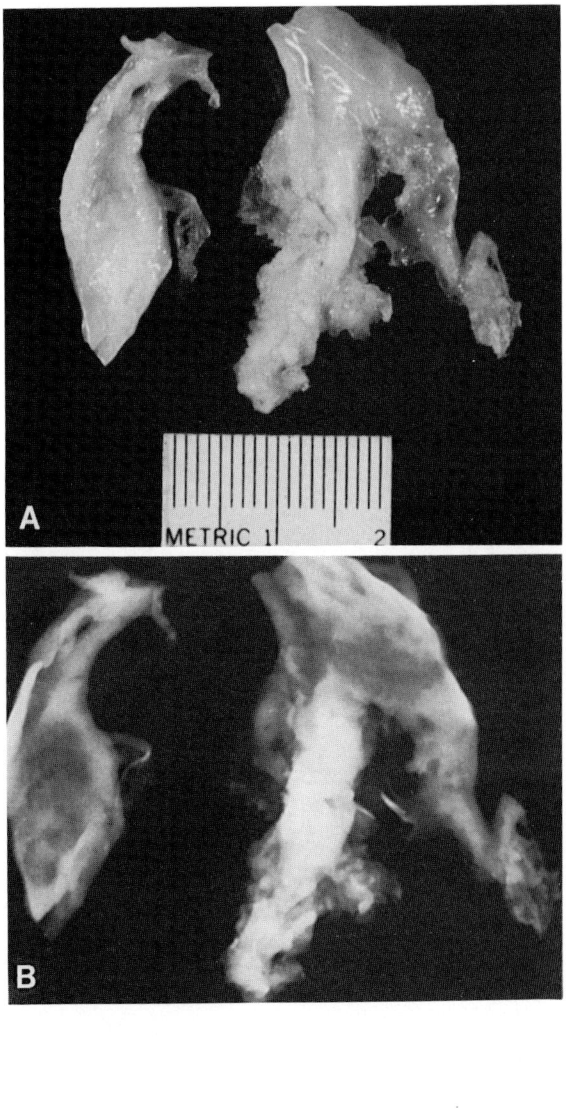

Figure 10–20. *A,* Operatively excised congenitally bicuspid aortic valve with superimposed active infective endocarditis producing pure aortic regurgitation. *B,* Radiograph discloses no calcific deposits.

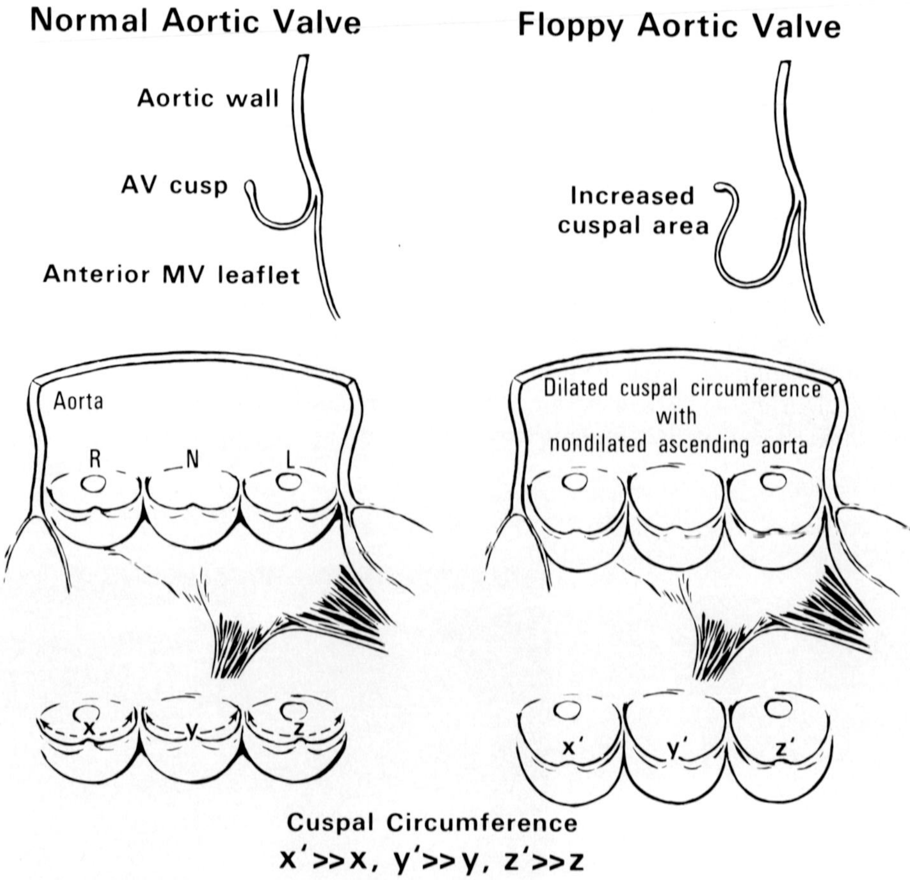

Figure 10–21. Definition of "floppy aortic valve." Floppy aortic valves have dilated cuspal circumferences (X, Y, Z) with nondilated ascending aorta, and the leaflet area of each cusp is increased. AV = aortic valve, L = left coronary ostium, MV = mitral valve, N = noncoronary cusp, R = right coronary ostium.

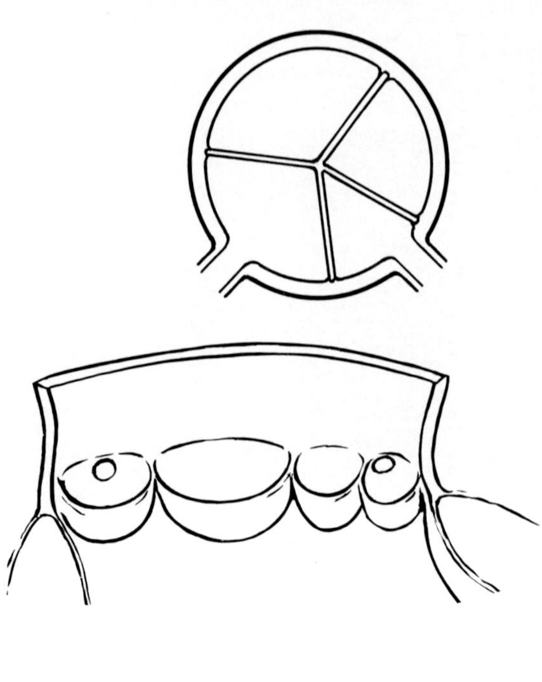

Figure 10–22. Purely regurgitant quadricuspid aortic valve. This variety has four unequal-sized cusps. See specimen in Figure 10–5.

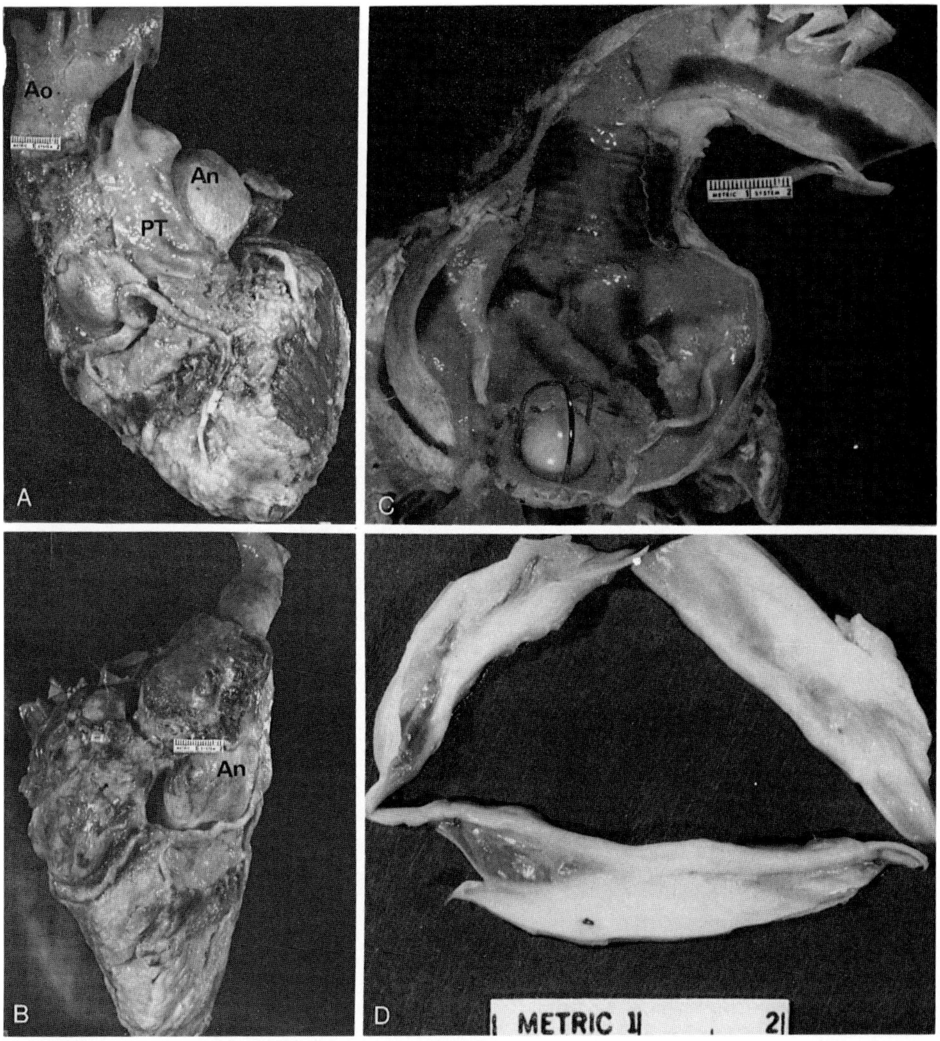

Figure 10–23. Exterior views of heart at necropsy (*A* through *C*) and operatively excised purely regurgitant aortic valve *(D)* from a 69-year-old man with Marfan's cardiovascular disease. The proximal ascending aorta (Ao) has a fusiform aneurysm (An), which produced severe aortic regurgitation requiring aortic valve replacement several years before death. (From Waller et al: Marfan cardiovascular disease without the Marfan syndrome. Chest 77:533, 1980, with permission.)

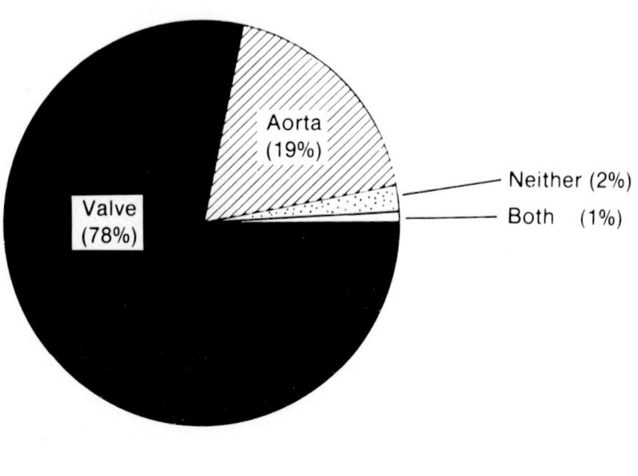

Figure 10–24. Causes of pure aortic regurgitation based on abnormality of the aortic valve, of aorta, of both valve and aorta, or of neither valve nor aorta. (See Table 10–4 for breakdown of etiologies.)

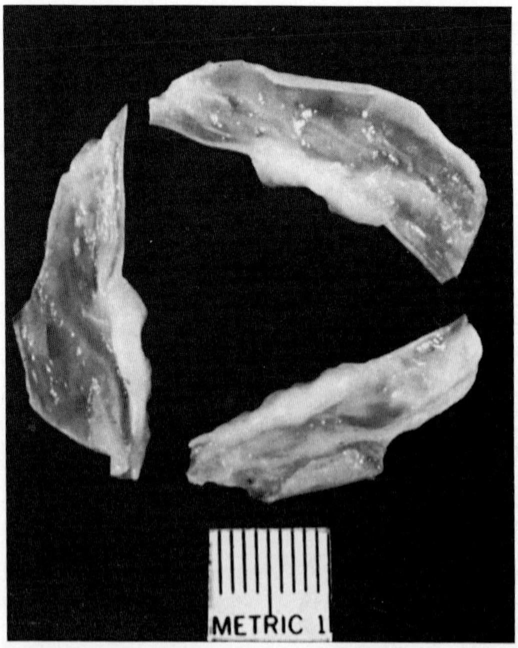

Figure 10–25. Operatively excised three-cuspid aortic valve from a patient with type 1 aortic dissection. The valve is anatomically normal.

percent in 1985. In addition, the frequency of floppy mitral valves increased from 17 percent in 1965 to 44 percent in 1985. Various factors including anatomic recognition, referral practices, and incidence of acute rheumatic fever and sequelae may account for these changes.

Tricuspid Valve

Operatively excised tricuspid valves (isolated or combined) are relatively uncommon (see Table 10–3, Figs. 10–40 through 10–42). Of 1547 patients with one or more operatively excised cardiac valves, pure tricuspid regurgitation occurred in only 21 (1 percent) patients.[10–12] Of the 21 patients, 18 (86 percent) had another stenotic or purely regurgitant valve excised, and only 3 (14 percent) patients had *isolated,* pure tricuspid regurgitation (Tables 10–6, 10–7). Of the 18 patients with tricuspid valve and at least one other valve excised, 16 (90 percent) had associated mitral stenosis, 1 (5 percent) had associated mitral and aortic stenosis, and 1 (5 percent) had pure mitral regurgitation. Other patients with operatively excised aortic valves or mitral valves, or both, may have had pure tricuspid regurgitation, but the tricuspid valve dysfunction was not severe enough to warrant valve replacement or the valve was adequately repaired to prevent or delay replacement.

The etiology for the pure tricuspid regurgitation in the 21 patients with operatively excised tricuspid valves was 9 (43 percent) *rheumatic,* 8 (38 percent) *anatomically normal leaflets with dilated anuli ("functional") tricuspid regurgitation due to pulmonary hypertension from severe mitral stenosis),* 2 (9 percent) *Ebstein's anomaly,* and 1 (5 percent) each, *infective endocarditis* and *floppy valve* (Figs. 10–42 through 10–46). Thus, *rheumatic disease* (primary or secondary effect) was the cause for pure tricuspid regurgitation in 17 (81 percent), whereas *nonrheumatic etiologies* (congenital, floppy, infection) accounted for the remaining 4 (19 percent) patients. This observation contrasts with the causes of pure mitral regurgitation in which nonrheumatic conditions (floppy, infection, papillary muscle dysfunction) accounted for 97 percent of the operatively excised valves, and rheumatic disease was the cause for pure regurgitation in only 3 percent.[24] Tricuspid valve replacement has been reported in other conditions besides those listed in Table 10–5: coronary atherosclerosis,[24] hypereosinophilic syndrome,[25] trauma,[26] Libman-Sacks endocarditis,[27] and carcinoid heart disease.[17] As with pure mitral regurgitation, leaflet area and anular circumference are useful measurements in separating various etiologies of pure tricuspid regurgitation (Figs. 10–46 through 10–54).

Anular *circumferences* of operatively excised tricuspid valves rendered regurgitant by rheumatic disease and infective endocarditis were *normal* (11.4 cm, 10.5 cm, respectively); the anuli of anatomically normal valves associated with pulmonary hypertension due to mitral stenosis were *dilated* (13.4 cm) ($p < 0.05$); and the anular circumferences of the floppy and Ebstein's valves were *markedly dilated* (16.5 cm, 18.3 cm, respectively) compared with those of the other groups ($p < 0.05$) (Figs. 10–48, 10–49). *Thus, measurement of anular circumference was a useful separation*

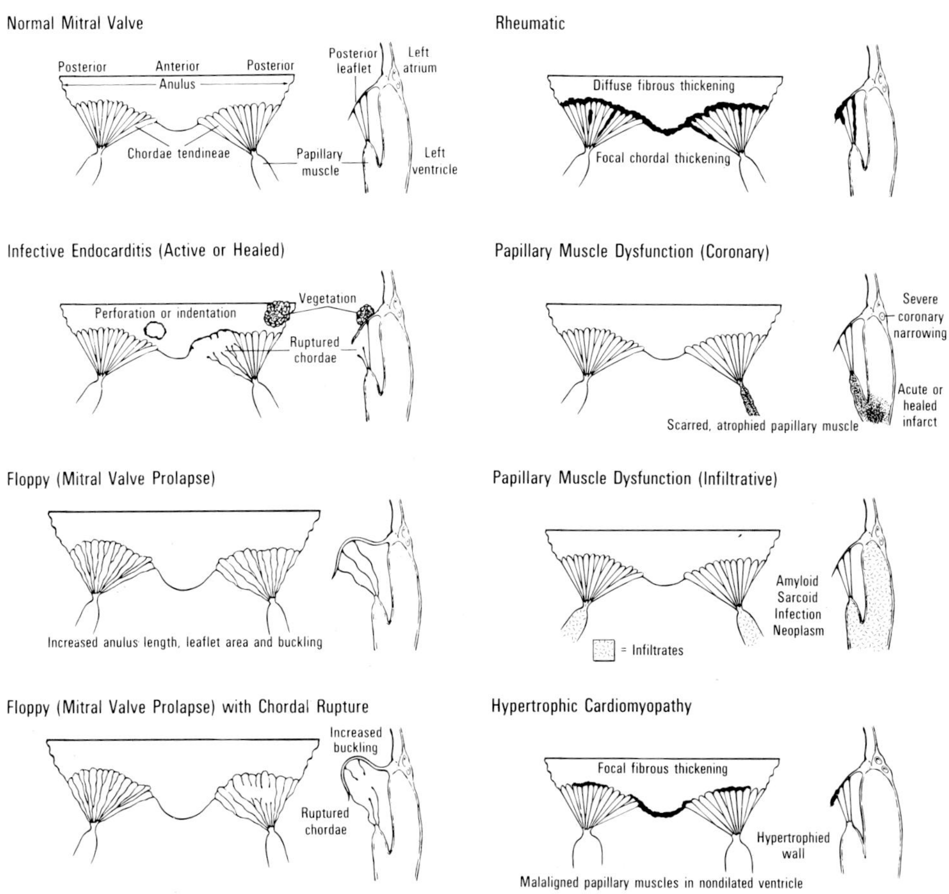

Figure 10–26. Various causes of pure mitral regurgitation.

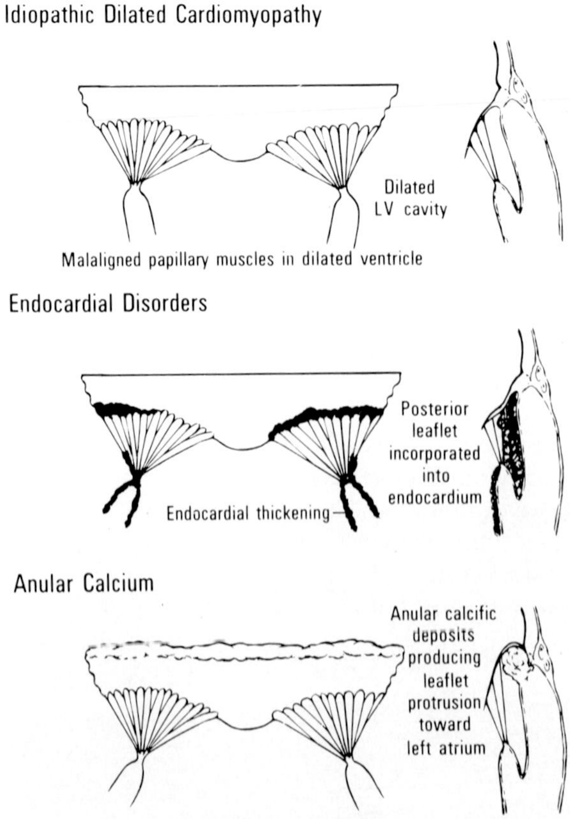

Figure 10–27. Various causes of pure mitral regurgitation (continued).

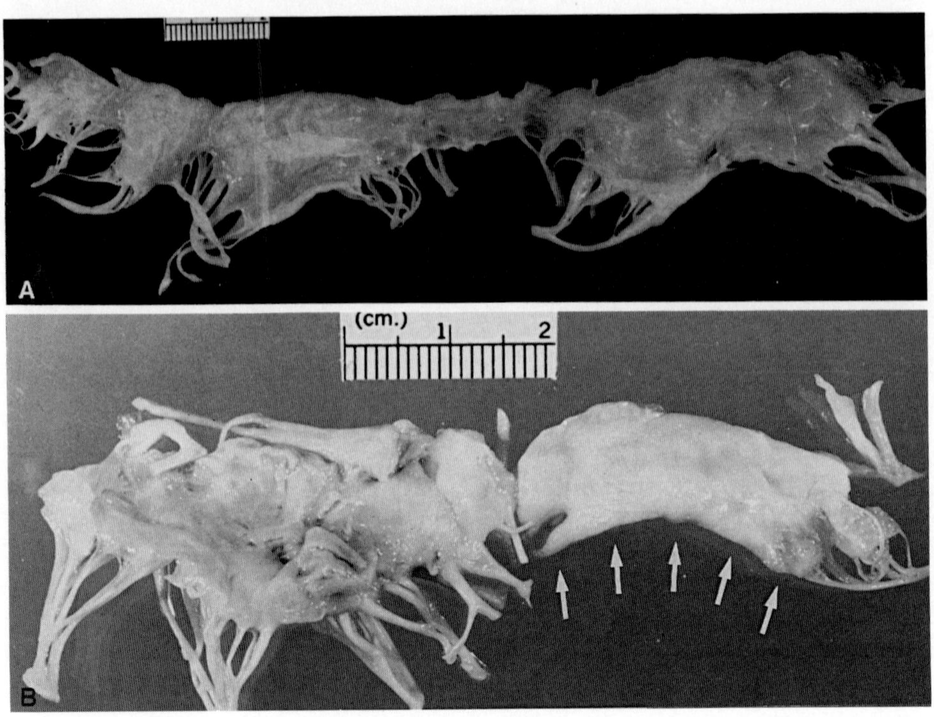

Figure 10–28. Two operatively excised floppy mitral valves producing pure mitral regurgitation. *A*, Mitral valve with increased anular circumference and leaflet area. *B*, Floppy mitral valve with multiple absent chordae tendineae (ruptured) to the posterior leaflet *(arrows)*.

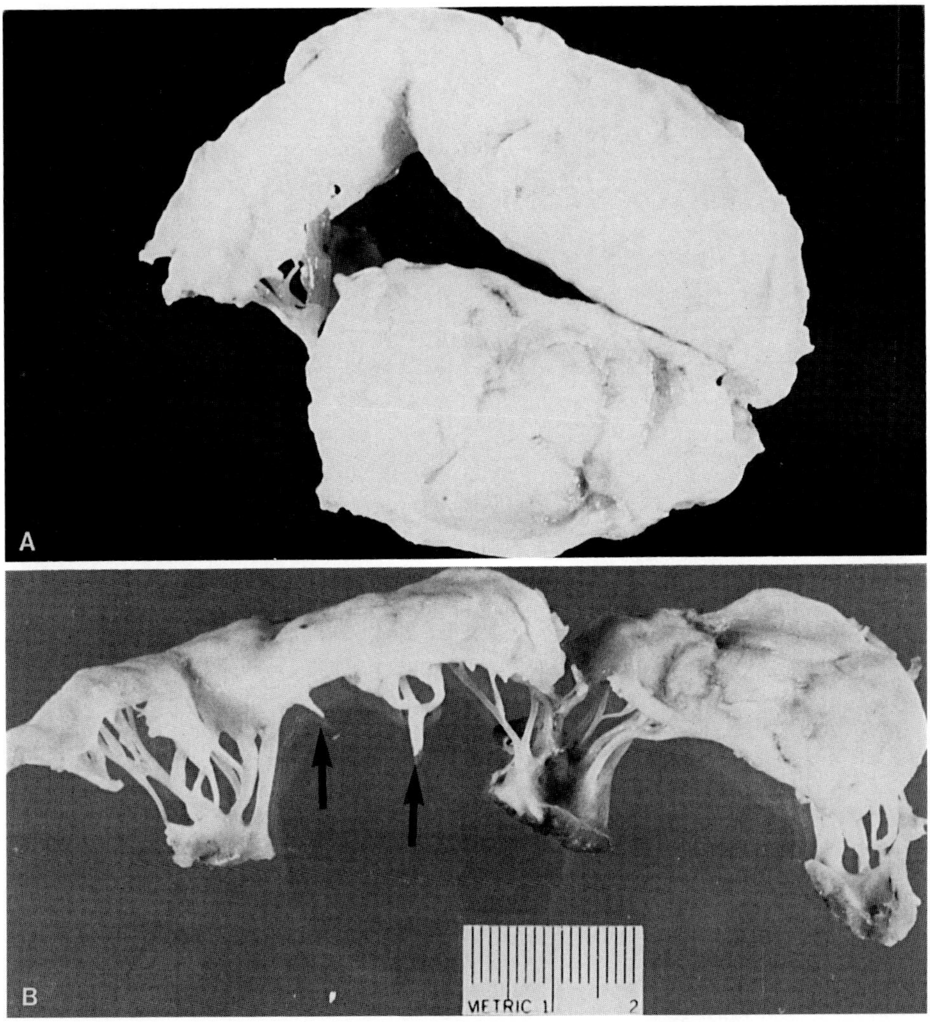

Figure 10-29. Operatively excised floppy mitral valve. *A.* View of valve as seen from left atrium showing increased leaflet area (redundant leaflets). *B,* Opened mitral valve showing ruptured chordae tendineae *(arrows).*

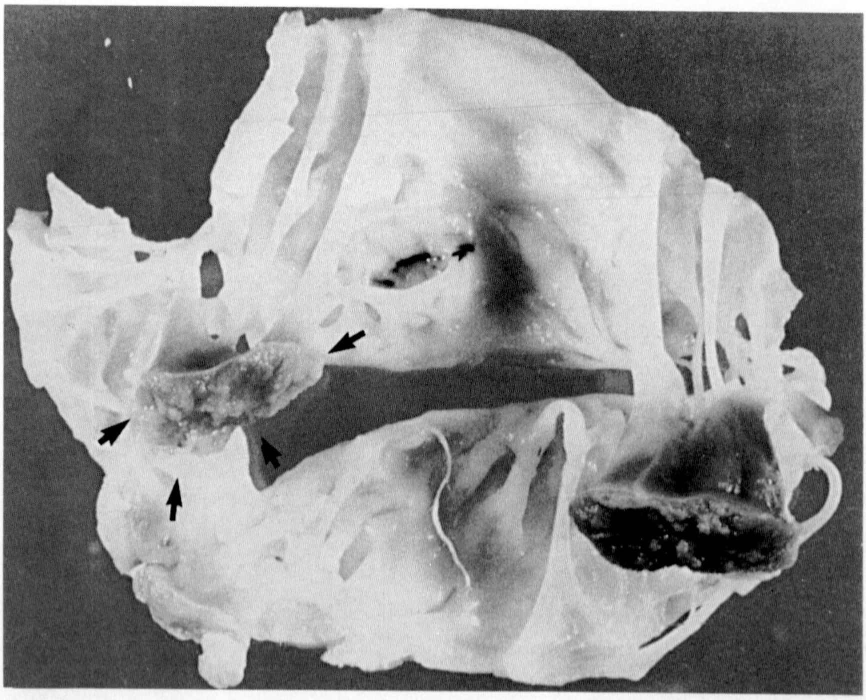

Figure 10–30. Operatively excised purely regurgitant mitral valve secondary to papillary muscle dysfunction from atherosclerotic coronary artery disease. One papillary muscle is scarred and atrophied *(arrows)*.

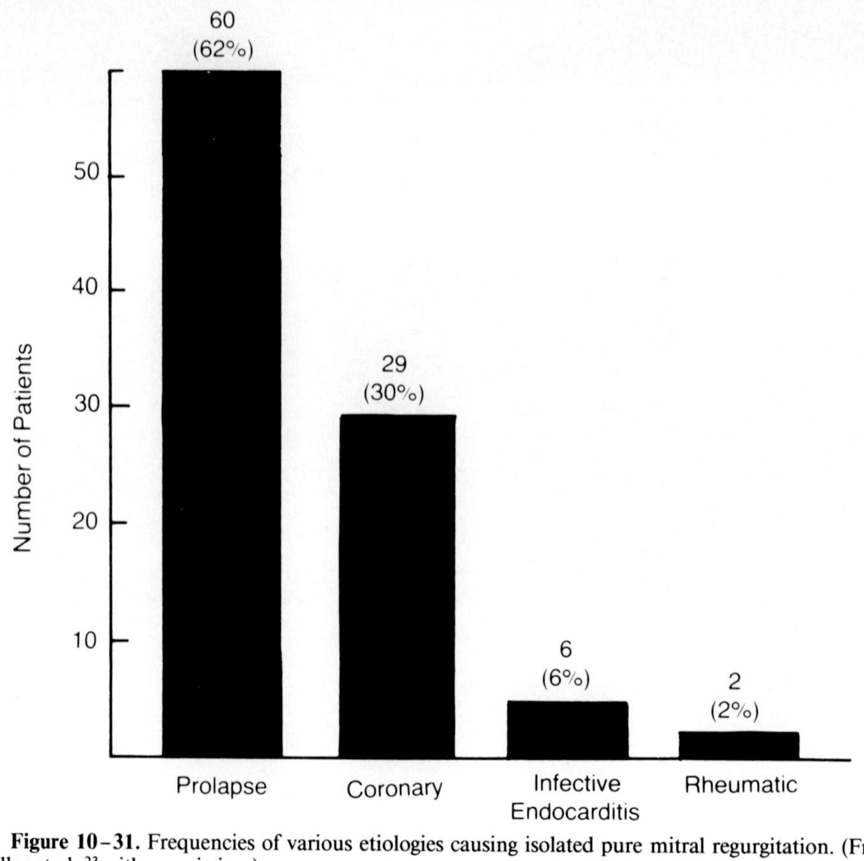

Figure 10–31. Frequencies of various etiologies causing isolated pure mitral regurgitation. (From Waller et al.,[23] with permission.)

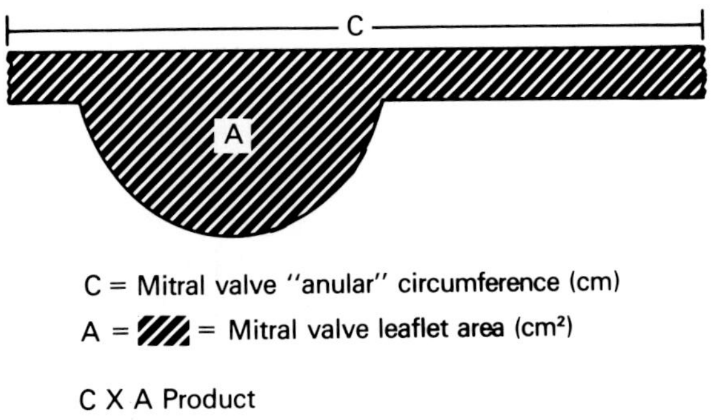

Figure 10–32. Measurements of operatively excised mitral valves. (From Waller et al.,[23] with permission.)

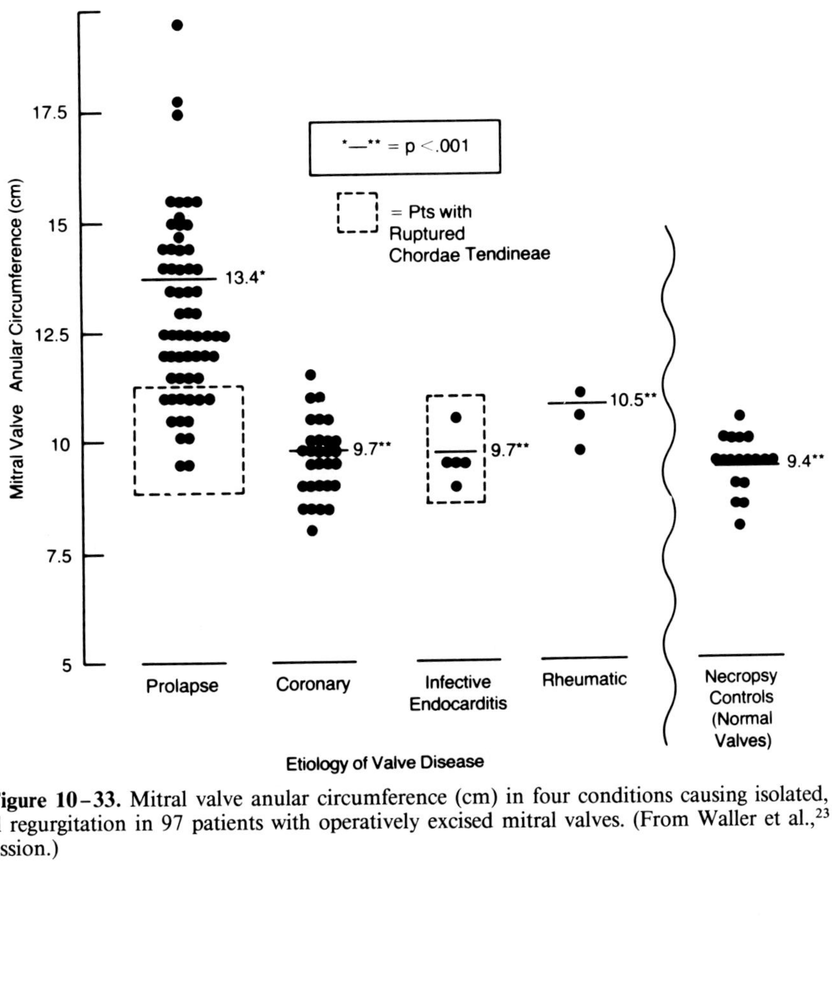

Figure 10–33. Mitral valve anular circumference (cm) in four conditions causing isolated, pure mitral regurgitation in 97 patients with operatively excised mitral valves. (From Waller et al.,[23] with permission.)

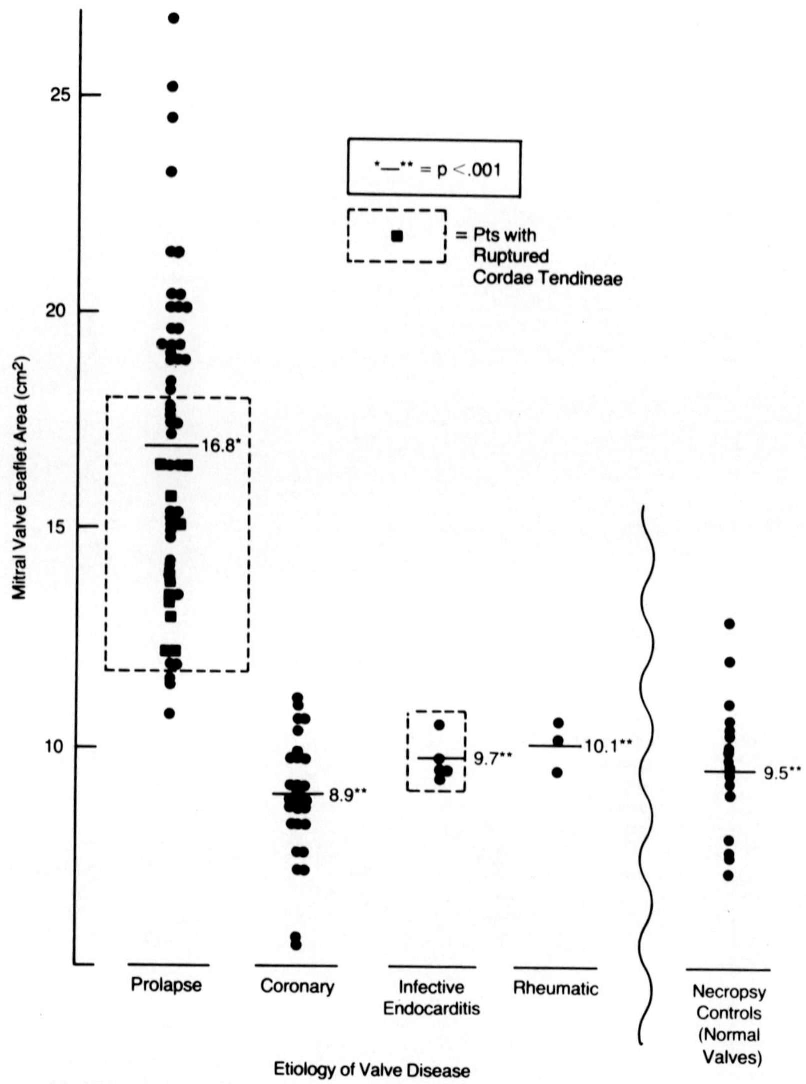

Figure 10–34. Mitral leaflet area (cm^2) in four conditions causing isolated pure mitral regurgitation in 97 patients with operatively excised mitral valves. (From Waller et al.,[23] with permission.)

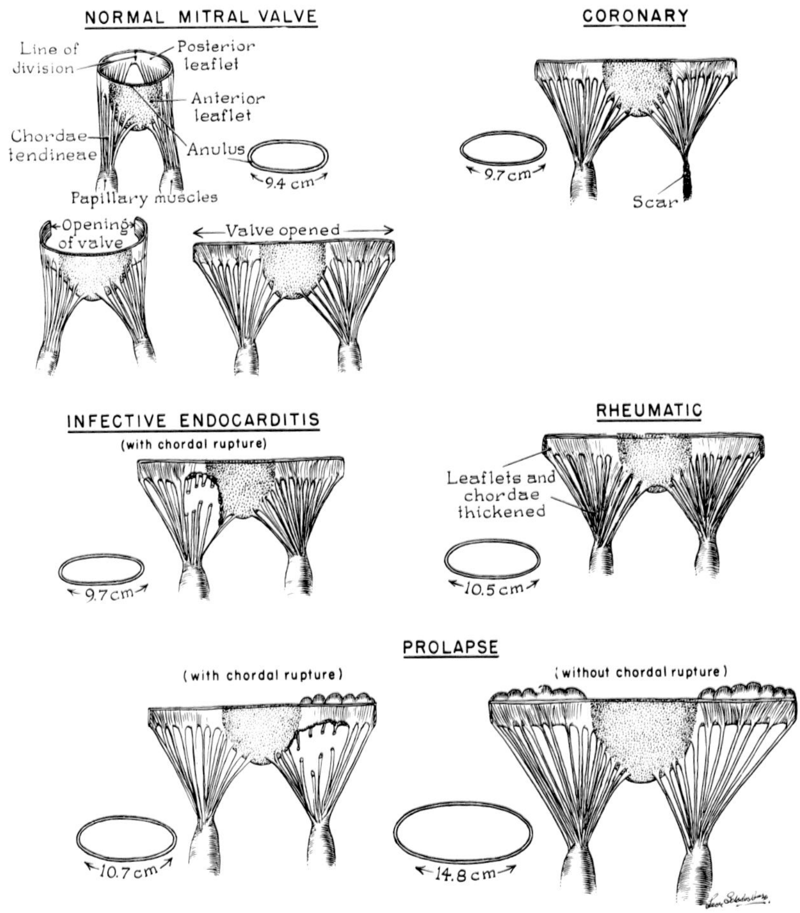

Figure 10–35. Anular circumference and leaflets in four conditions causing isolated pure mitral regurgitation, and comparison with controls. Anular measurements represent averages. (From Waller et al.,[23] with permission.)

Condition	Area	Anular Circumference
1. Floppy	↑	↑
2. Papillary muscle dysfunction	Normal	Normal
3. Rheumatic	↓/Normal	Normal
4. Infective endocarditis	↓/Normal	Normal
5. Dilated cardiomyopathy	Normal	Normal/↑
6. Hypertrophic cardiomyopathy	Normal	Normal

Figure 10–36. Various causes of pure mitral regurgitation, based on measurements of leaflet area and anular circumference.

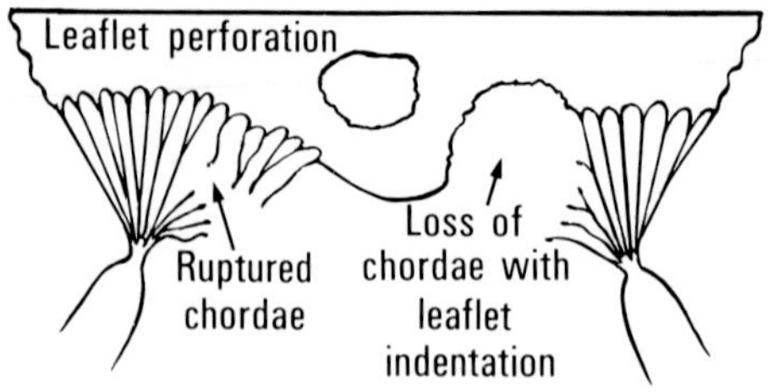

Figure 10–37. Mechanisms of pure mitral regurgitation produced by infective endocarditis.

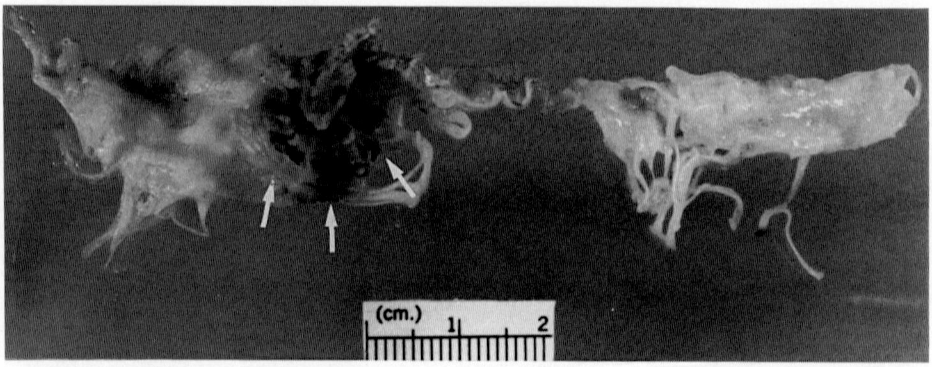

Figure 10–38. Operatively excised mitral valve with active infective endocarditis primarily affecting the anterior mitral leaflet *(arrows).*

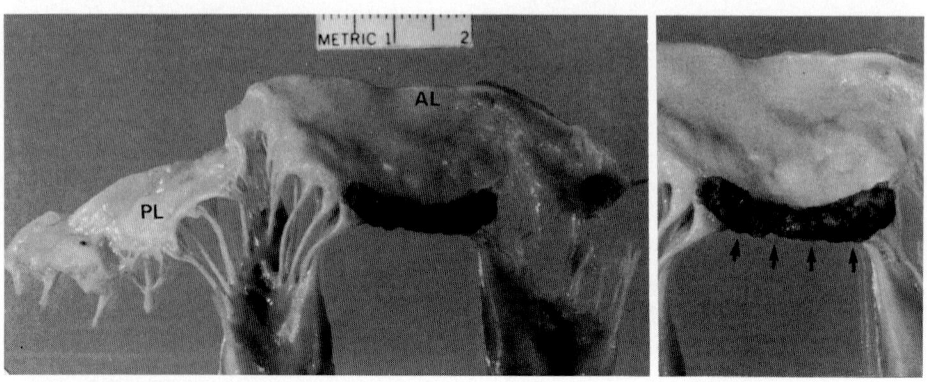

Figure 10–39. Operatively excised mitral valve with active infective endocarditis involving the margins of closure of the anterior leaflet (AL) *(arrows)* and a small segment of posterior leaflet (PL).

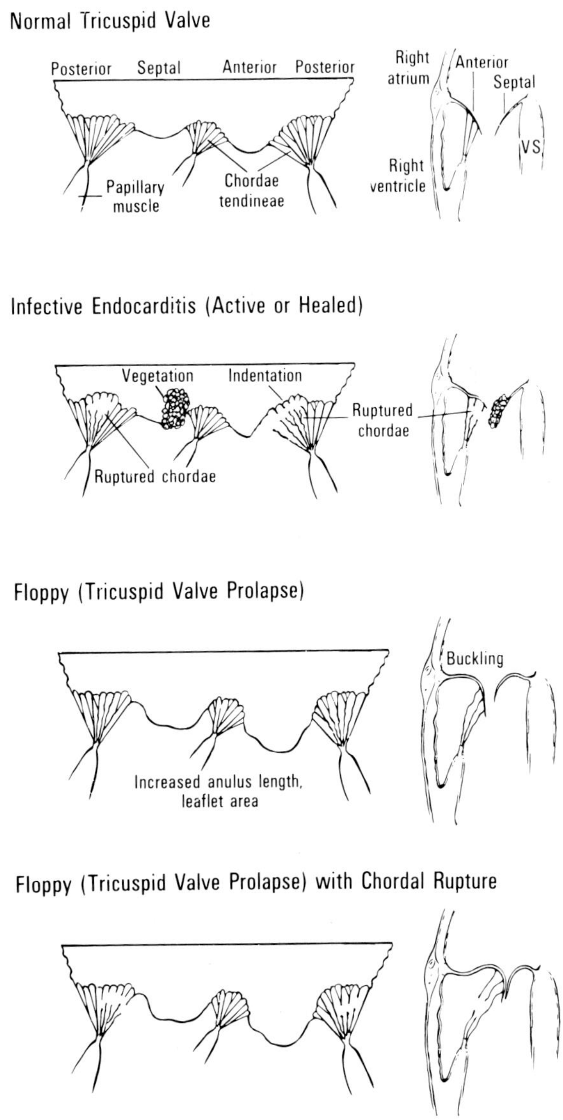

Figure 10–40. Various causes of pure tricuspid regurgitation.

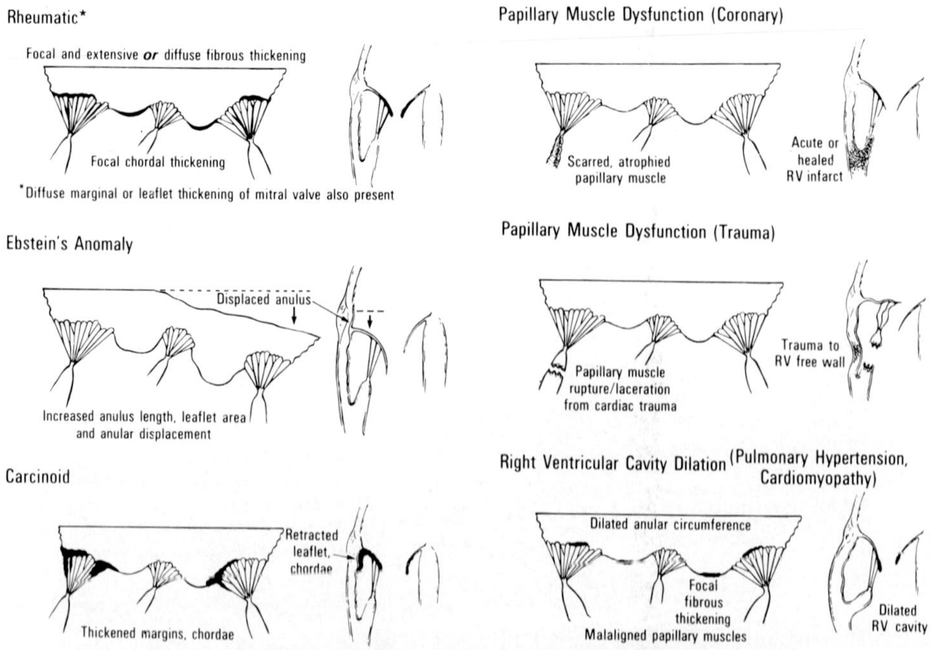

Figure 10–41. Various causes of pure tricuspid regurgitation (continued).

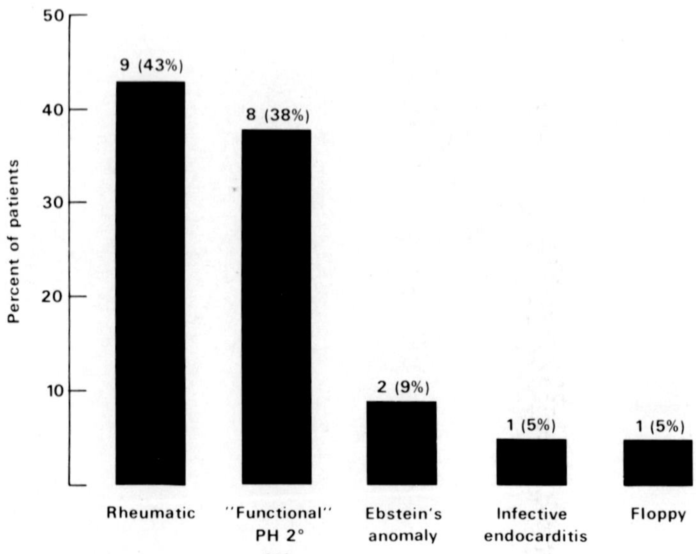

Figure 10–42. Frequency of occurrence of five etiologies of pure tricuspid regurgitation in 21 patients undergoing tricuspid valve replacement.

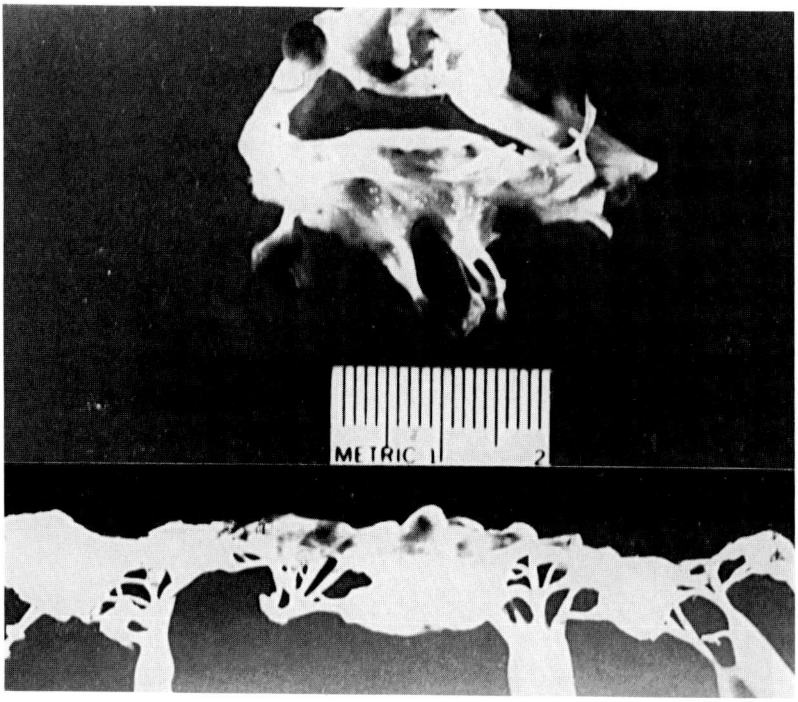

Figure 10–43. Operatively excised purely regurgitant tricuspid valve from a patient with rheumatic heart disease. The valve has diffuse fibrous thickening without calcific deposits and a normal to slightly reduced anular circumference.

of purely regurgitant tricuspid valves into those etiologies with normal anuli (less than 12 cm) (rheumatic, coronary, carcinoid, infective endocarditis), slightly dilated anuli (12 to 14 cm) (various causes of pulmonary hypertension), and those conditions with markedly dilated anuli (more than 14 cm) (Ebstein's anomaly, floppy valves) (Fig. 10–49).[9,10]

In operatively excised purely regurgitant tricuspid valves, floppy and Ebstein valves had significantly larger average *leaflet areas* than tricuspid valves rendered

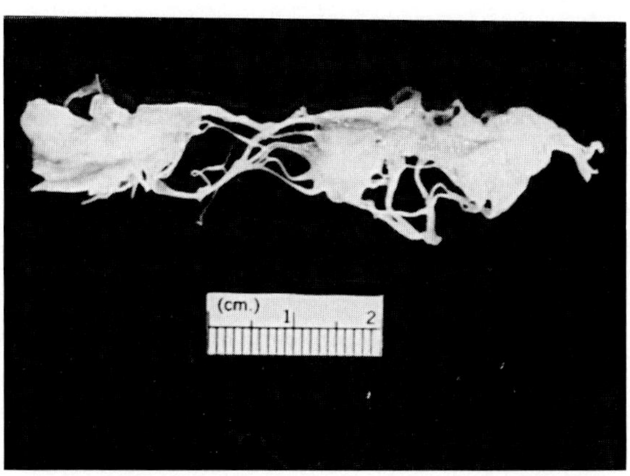

Figure 10–44. Operatively excised purely regurgitant tricuspid valve of primary rheumatic etiology. A stenotic mitral valve was also excised.

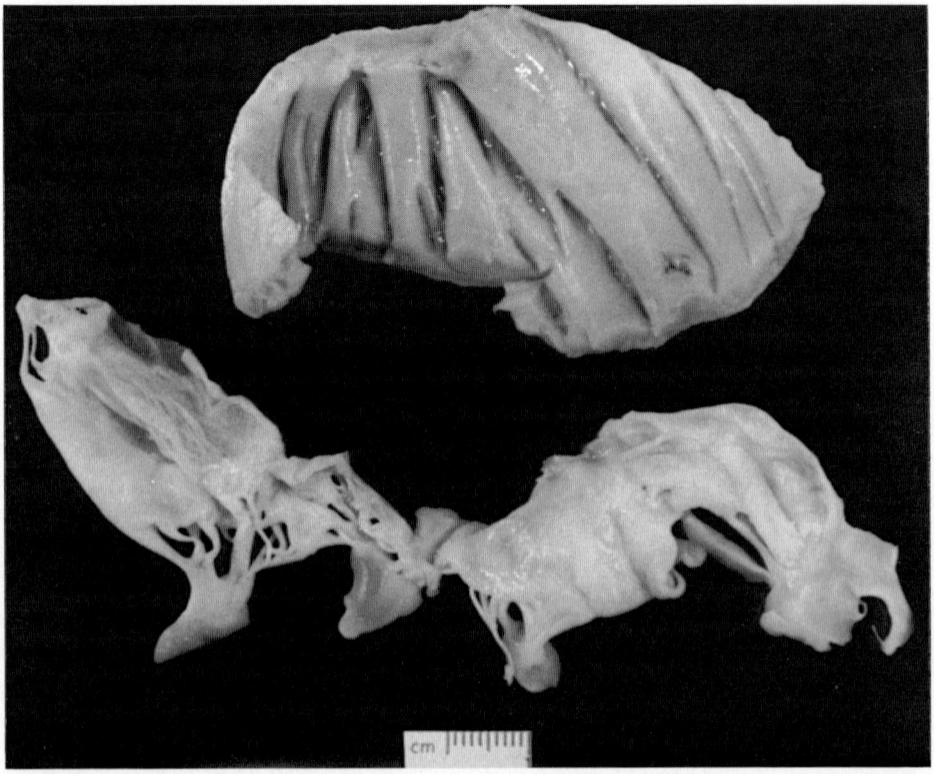

Figure 10–45. Operatively excised purely regurgitant Ebstein's tricuspid valve and portion of massively dilated right atrium.

incompetent by rheumatic disease (primary or secondary effects) or infective endocarditis (27.1 cm^2 and 32 cm^2 versus 13.5 cm^2, 14.0 cm^2, and 11.9 cm^2, respectively) (Fig. 10–50). *Thus, measurement of leaflet areas was useful in separating two conditions (Ebstein's anomaly and floppy valves from remaining causes of purely regurgitant tricuspid valves.* Although anular circumferences of Ebstein valves were slightly larger than those in floppy valves, measurement of leaflet area served to separate further these two etiologies. Tricuspid valves with Ebstein's anomaly have larger leaflet areas compared with floppy tricuspid valves (32.0 cm^2, 27.1 cm^2, respectively) (Fig. 10–51).[9,10]

Thus, the etiology of purely regurgitant operatively excised tricuspid valves can be established by the observation of normal or dilated anular circumferences in conjunction with morphologically normal or abnormal leaflets (Fig. 10–52). Given a purely regurgitant tricuspid valve, if the anulus is normal (less than 12 cm) and the leaflets are normal, papillary muscle dysfunction is the cause of the regurgitation; if the anulus is normal and the leaflets abnormal, rheumatic disease, carcinoid, or infective endocarditis are possible causes; if the tricuspid valve anulus is dilated (12 to 14 cm) and the leaflets normal, various conditions producing pulmonary hypertension and dilated cardiomyopathy are etiologies; and if the anulus is markedly dilated (more than 14 cm) and the leaflets abnormal, Ebstein's anomaly or tricuspid valve prolapse are possible etiologies (Fig. 10–52).

Condition	Anulus	Leaflet Area	Anulus Insertion Site
1. Floppy (prolapsed)	↑	↑	Normal
2. Ebstein's Anomaly	↑	↑	Abnormal
3. Pulmonary Hypertension		Normal	Normal
(a) Cor Pulmonale	↑	Normal	Normal
(b) Mitral Stenosis	↑	Normal	Normal
4. Coronary (Papillary muscle)	Normal	Normal	Normal
5. Carcinoid	Normal/↑	Normal/↑	Normal
6. Rheumatic	Normal	Normal/↑	Normal
7. Infective Endocarditis	Normal	Normal	Normal
8. Dilated Cardiomyopathy	↑	Normal	Normal

Figure 10–46. Various causes of pure tricuspid regurgitation, based on morphometric analysis (leaflet area, anular circumference, and site of leaflet insertion).

A subgroup of patients with pure tricuspid regurgitation are those associated with rheumatic heart disease (Figs. 10–53, 10–54). Each of the patients in this subgroup have abnormal mitral valves (stenotic) in association with the purely regurgitant tricuspid valves. The purely regurgitant tricuspid valves can be divided into those valves that are *anatomically abnormal* ("primary," "organic") and those that are *anatomically normal* ("secondary," "functional"). Anular circumference measurement is a useful tool to distinguish the two conditions. In "organic" (i.e., rheumatic) pure tricuspid regurgitation, the anuli are normal, whereas in the "functional"

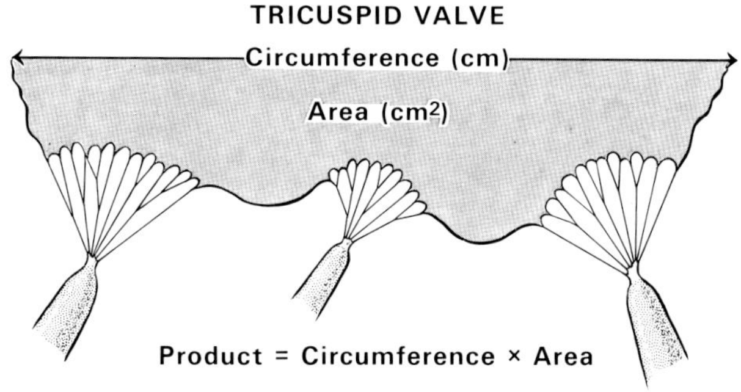

Figure 10–47. Tricuspid valve diagram showing morphologic parameters useful in determining etiology of pure tricuspid regurgitation. (From Waller et al.,[9] with permission.)

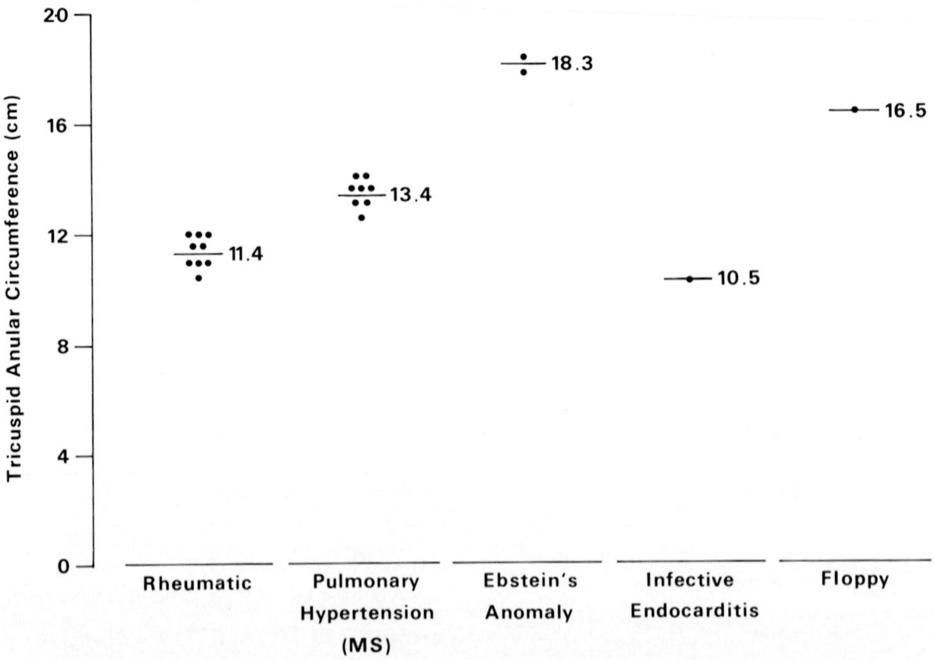

Figure 10–48. Tricuspid anular circumference in five causes of pure tricuspid regurgitation in 21 operatively excised valves.

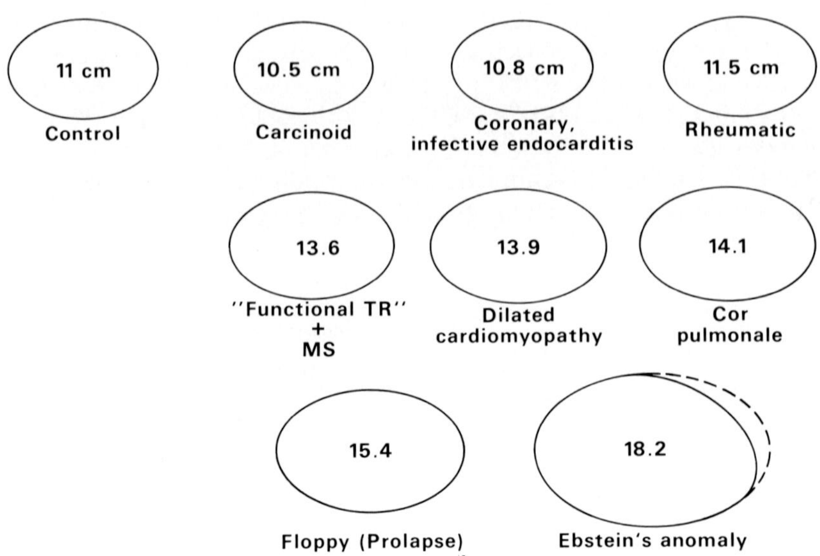

Figure 10–49. Comparison of tricuspid anuli in various causes of pure tricuspid regurgitation. (From Waller.[10])

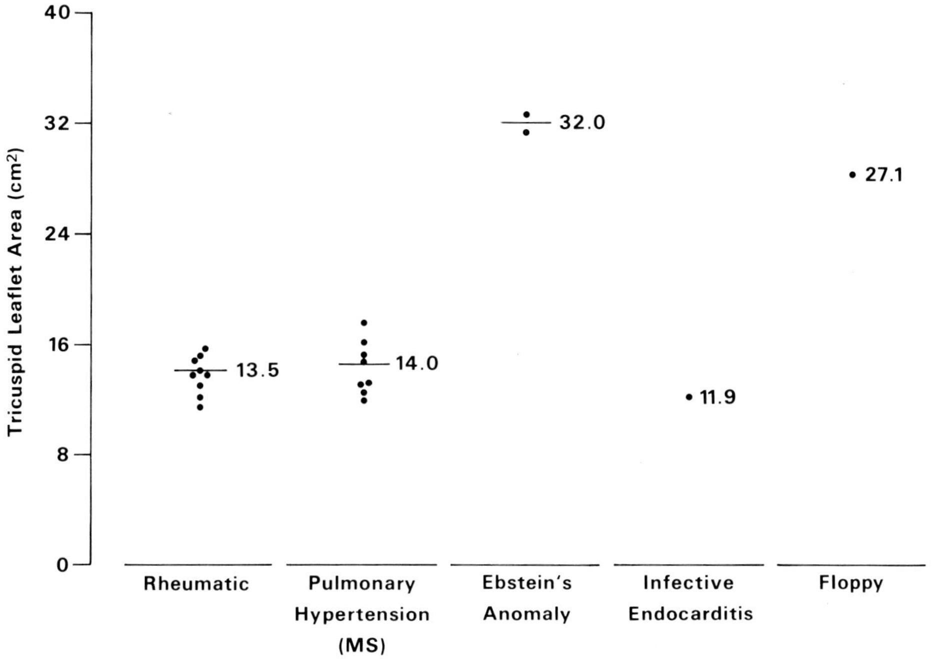

Figure 10–50. Tricuspid leaflet area in five causes of pure tricuspid regurgitation in 21 operatively excised valves.

Figure 10–51. Morphologic approach to etiology of purely regurgitant mitral and tricuspid valves, based on anular circumference and leaflet area measurements.

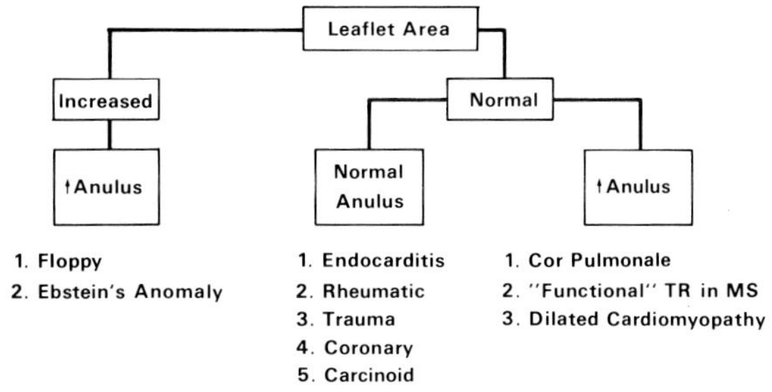

Figure 10–52. Etiology of pure tricuspid regurgitation, based on anular circumference and normal or abnormal tricuspid leaflets. (From Waller et al.,[9] with permission.)

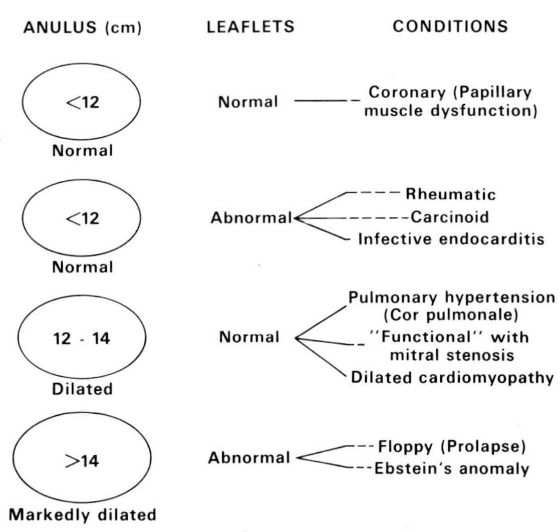

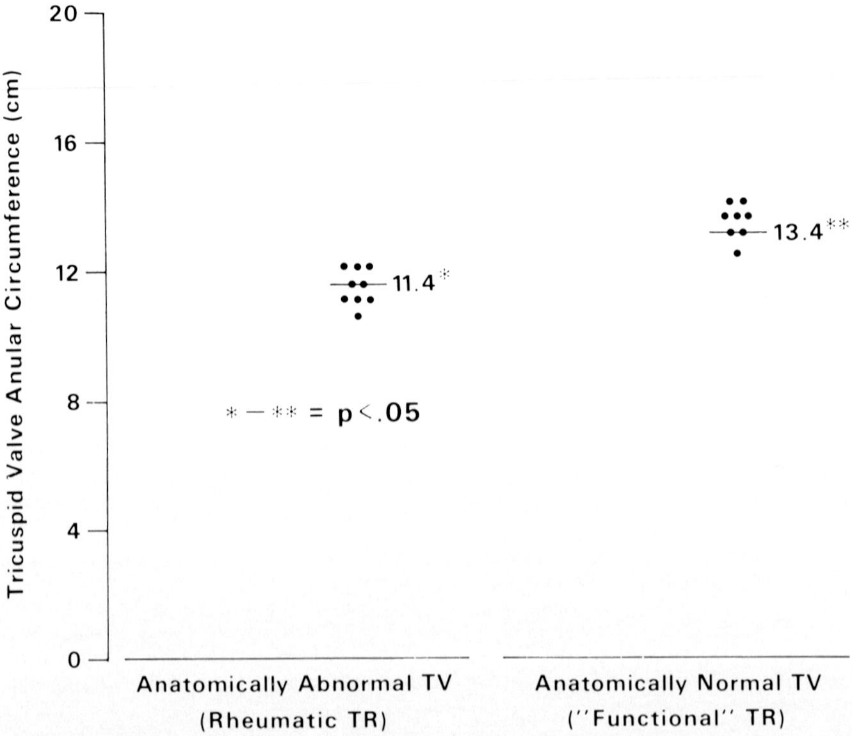

Figure 10–53. Tricuspid anular circumference in primary ("rheumatic") and secondary ("functional") pure tricuspid regurgitation in patients with mitral stenosis. The anatomically abnormal valves have significantly smaller anuli.

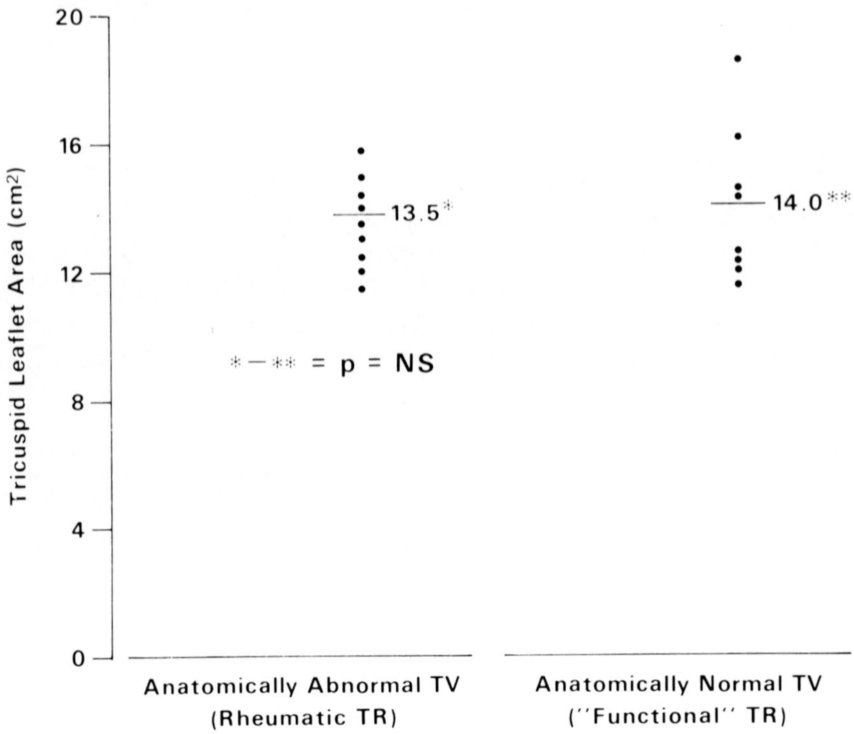

Figure 10–54. Tricuspid leaflet area in primary ("rheumatic") and secondary ("functional") causes of pure tricuspid regurgitation in patients with mitral stenosis. The two groups have similar mean leaflet areas.

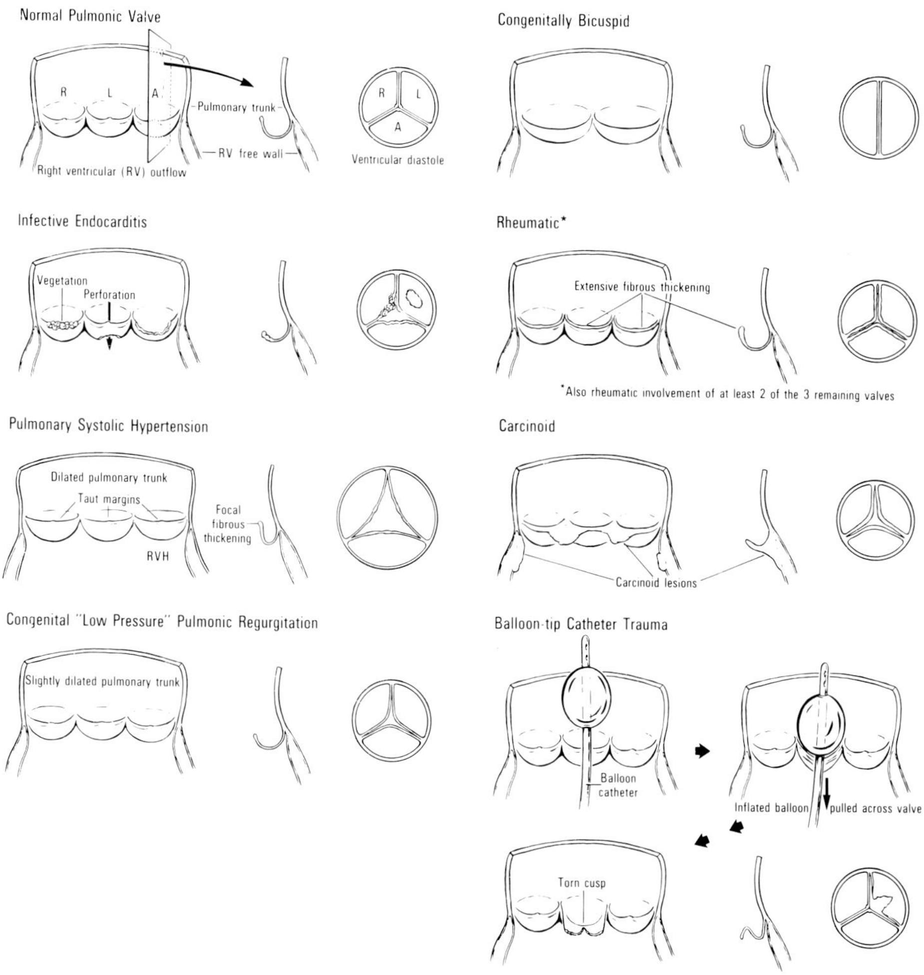

Figure 10–55. Various causes of pure pulmonic regurgitation.

subgroup, the anuli are dilated. Of the 21 operatively excised purely regurgitant tricuspid valves, 17 (81 percent) had associated mitral stenosis. Of these 17, 9 (43 percent) had anatomically abnormal leaflets with normal anuli ("organic"), and 8 (38 percent) had anatomically normal leaflets with dilated anuli ("functional") (Table 10–6).

Pulmonic Valve

Pure pulmonic valve regurgitation may result from anatomically *abnormal* or *normal* valve cusps. Despite occasional patients with pure pulmonic regurgitation, pulmonic valves rarely are excised or replaced with prosthetic valves. Pure pulmonic valve regurgitation may result from congenital or acquired conditions (Fig. 10–55). Of the acquired conditions, infective endocarditis, carcinoid, trauma (from balloon-tipped catheters), and rheumatic etiologies are most common. The most common cause of pure pulmonic valve regurgitation is not intrinsic valve disease, but dilation of the pulmonary trunk and pulmonic valve "anulus" from any of several causes of

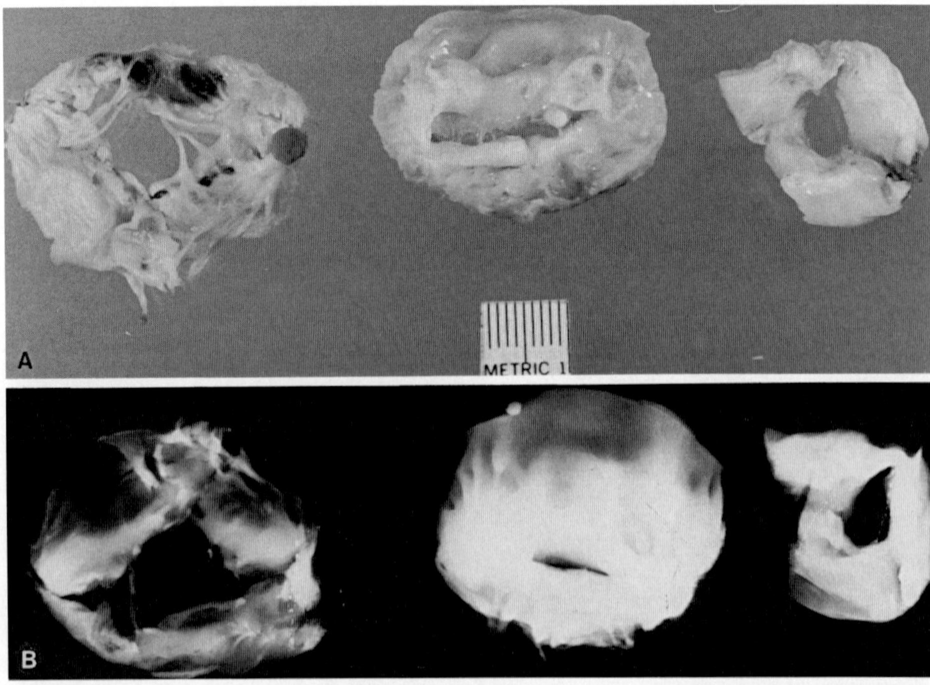

Figure 10–56. *A*, Operatively excised stenotic tricuspid *(left)*, mitral *(middle)*, and aortic *(right)* valves from a patient with rheumatic heart disease. *B*, Radiographs show minimal if any calcific deposits in the three valves.

Table 10–4. Causes of Pure Aortic Regurgitation Based on Site of Abnormality (Valve, Aorta, Neither, Both) in 292 Patients*

Disease Site	Number (%) of Patients
Valve	228 (78)
Rheumatic	120
Infective endocarditis	62
Congenital (bicuspid)	29
Prolapse from VSD	10
Spontaneous tear	2
"Floppy"	2
Subaortic stenosis	2
Trauma	1
Aorta	57 (19)
Noninflammatory	23
Marfan's, Marfan-like	15
Syphilis	9
Aortitis	8
Dissection	2
Neither	
Systemic hypertension	5 (2)
Both	
Ankylosing spondylitis	2 (1)
Combined totals	292 (100)

* Based on data from Davies,[2] Roberts et al.,[21] and Waller et al.[19,22]

Table 10–5. Etiology of Isolated Pure Aortic Regurgitation in 106 Patients Aged ≥ 15 Yr With Operatively Excised Aortic Valves

Etiology	Number (%) of Patients
1. Infective endocarditis	50 (47)
3-cuspid = 29 (58%)	
2-cuspid = 21 (42%)	
2. Congenitally bicuspid	22 (21)
3. Rheumatic	15 (14)
4. Aortic dissection	12 (11)
5. Marfan's syndrome	2 (2)
6. Floppy (prolapse)	2 (2)
7. Syphilis	1 (1)
8. Quadricuspid	1 (1)
9. Radiation	1 (1)
TOTAL	106 (100)

pulmonary arterial systolic hypertension. Pure pulmonic valve regurgitation from intrinsic valve disease or secondary to pulmonary trunk dilation is rarely severe enough to warrant valve replacement.

MULTIPLE VALVE EXCISIONS

Of 1547 patients with one or more operatively excised cardiac valves, 332 (21 percent) had double valve replacement, and 3 (10.2 percent) had triple valve replacement (see Table 10–3). Of the 332 patients with double valve replacement, the

Table 10–6. Certain Morphologic Observations in 21 Patients With Pure Triscupid Regurgitation (TR) Undergoing Triscupid Valve Replacement

Item	Number (%)
1. Etiology of pure TR	
a. Rheumatic*	9 (43)
b. "Functional" (pulmonary hypertension 2° MS)	8 (38)
c. Ebstein's anomaly	2 (9)
d. Infective endocarditis	1 (5)
e. Floppy†	1 (5)
2. Tricuspid valve structure	
a. Abnormal leaflets (thickened, perforated, indented, redundant)	13 (62)
b. Dilated anulus (circumference)	11 (52)
c. Abnormal chordae (ruptured, elongated)	2 (9)
d. Abnormal papillary muscles	0

* Associated mitral stenosis (MS).
† Associated floppy mitral valve.

Table 10–7. Etiology of Isolated, Pure Tricuspid Regurgitation in 3 Patients Aged ≥ 15 Yr With Operatively Excised Tricuspid Valves

Etiology	Number of Patients
1. Ebstein's anomaly	2
2. Infective endocarditis	1
TOTAL	3

etiology was *rheumatic disease* in 318 (96 percent), *infective endocarditis* in 13 (4 percent), and *floppy valve syndrome* in 1 (less than 1 percent). The three patients with triple valve replacement (each aortic plus mitral plus tricuspid) had rheumatic heart disease. Thus, *the vast majority (more than 96 percent) of patients with multiple valve replacements have rheumatic heart disease as the etiology of the valve dysfunction* (Fig. 10–56).

ACKNOWLEDGMENTS

I wish to thank Candice Owens for her invaluable secretarial service, George Buckley for his artistic talents, and Ken Whilhite for his graphics ability.

REFERENCES

1. Roberts, WC and Morrow, AG: Cardiac valves and the surgical pathologist. Arch Pathol 82:309, 1966.
2. Davies, MJ: Pathology of Cardiac Valves. Butterworths, Boston, 1980, p 18.
3. Subramanian, R, Olsen, LJ, and Edwards, WD: Surgical pathology of pure aortic stenosis. A study of 374 cases. Mayo Clin Proc 59:683, 1984.
4. Waller, BF, Bloch, T, Barker, BG, et al: Evaluation of operatively excised cardiac valves: Etiologic determination of valvular heart disease. Cardiol Clin 2(4):687, 1984.
5. Waller, BF: Morphologic assessment of operatively-excised native cardiac valves. Indiana Medicine 4:293, 1985.
6. Roberts, WC, Mason DT, Morrow, AG, et al: Calcific pulmonic stenosis. Circulation 37:973, 1968.
7. Covarrubias, EA, Sheikh, MU, Isner, JI, et al: Calcific pulmonic stenosis in adulthood. Treatment by valve replacement. Chest 75:399, 1979.
8. Roberts, WC: The structural basis of abnormal cardiac function: A look at coronary, hypertensive, valvular, idiopathic myocardial, and pericardial heart diseases. In Levine, HJ (ed): Clinical Cardiovascular Physiology. Grune & Stratton, New York, 1976, p 1.
9. Waller, BF, Moriarty, AT, Eble, JN, et al: Etiology of pure tricuspid regurgitation based upon anular circumference and leaflet area. Analysis of 45 necropsy patients with clinical and morphologic evidence of pure tricuspid regurgitation. J Am Coll Cardiol 7:1063, 1986.
10. Waller, BF: Etiology of pure tricuspid regurgitation. In Fisk, RL (ed): The Right Heart. FA Davis, Philadelphia, 1987.
11. Waller, BF: Morphologic aspects of valvular heart disease—Part I. Curr Probl Cardiol 9(7):1, 1984.
12. Waller, BF: Morphologic aspects of valvular heart disease—Part II. Curr Probl Cardiol 9(8):1, 1984.
13. Rose, AG: Etiology of acquired valvular heart disease in adults. A survey of 18,132 autopsies and 100 consecutive valve-replacement operations. Arch Pathol Lab Med 110:385, 1986.
14. Virmani, R and Roberts, WC: Aschoff bodies in operatively excised atrial appendages and in papillary muscles. Frequency and clinical significance. Circulation 55:559, 1977.
15. Lachman, AS and Roberts, WC: Calcific deposits in stenotic mitral valves. Extent and relation to age, sex, degree of stenosis, cardiac rhythm, previous commissurotomy and left atrial body thrombus from study of 164 operatively excised valves. Circulation 57:808, 1978.

16. Olsen, LJ, Subramanian, R, Ackermann, DM, et al: Surgical pathology of the mitral valve: A study of 712 cases spanning 21 years. Mayo Clin Proc (in press).
17. Miller, BR, Vohr, FH, Christian FV, et al: Cardiac valve replacement in carcinoid heart disease. Am J Med 75:896, 1983.
18. Roberts, WC, Morrow, AG, McIntosh, CL, et al: Congenitally bicuspid aortic valve causing severe, pure aortic regurgitation without superimposed infective endocarditis. Am J Cardiol 47:206, 1981.
19. Waller, BF, Zoltick, JM, Rosen JH, et al: Severe aortic regurgitation from systemic hypertension (without aortic dissection) requiring aortic valve replacement. Am J Cardiol 49:473, 1982.
20. Bulkley, BH and Roberts, WC: Ankylosing spondylitis and aortic regurgitation. Description of the characteristic cardiovascular lesion from study of 8 necropsy patients. Circulation 48:1014, 1973.
21. Roberts, WC, Morrow, AG, McIntosh, CL, et al: Congenitally bicuspid aortic valve causing severe pure aortic regurgitation without superimposed infective endocarditis. Am J Cardiol 47:206, 1981.
22. Waller, BF, Kishel, JC, and Roberts, WC: Severe aortic regurgitation from systemic hypertension. Chest 82:365, 1982.
23. Waller, BF, Morrow, AG, Maron BJ, et al: Etiology of clinically isolated severe, chronic pure mitral regurgitation: An analysis of 97 patients over 30 years of age having mitral valve replacement. Am Heart J 104:276, 1982.
24. Korr, KS, Levinson, H, and Bough, EW: Tricuspid valve replacement for cardiogenic shock after acute myocardial infarction. JAMA 244:1958, 1980.
25. Harley, JB, McIntosh, CL, Kirklin, JJW, et al: Atrioventricular valve replacement in the idiopathic hypereosinophilic syndrome. Am J Med 73:77, 1982.
26. Fracasso, A, Pothen, P, and Gallucci, V: Tricuspid regurgitation caused by blunt chest trauma in association with pericardial agenesis: Surgical correction after 8 years. Thorax 37:75, 1982.
27. Laufer, J, Frand, M, and Milo, S: Valve replacement for severe tricuspid regurgitation caused by Libman-Sacks endocarditis. Br Heart J 48:294, 1982.

CHAPTER 11

Floppy Mitral Valve Syndrome

Jesse E. Edwards, M.D.

Many names are given to the condition that is the subject of this chapter. Among these names are "floppy mitral valve," "myxomatous degeneration of the mitral valve," "ballooning mitral valve," "the redundant cusp syndrome," "mitral valve prolapse," and the "systolic click murmur syndrome." The clinical features of this syndrome were well described nearly 50 years ago by Levine and Thompson,[1] who in turn referred to a paper by Cuffer and Barbillion, who about 100 years earlier described "an extra sound appearing a brief interval following the termination of the first heart sound."[2] Pathologic features of this entity were formally described in 1958 by Fernex and Fernex[3] (mucoid degeneration), in 1961 by Oka and Angrist[4] (billowing sail deformity), and in 1965 and 1966 by Read and associates[5,6] (myxomatous transformation, floppy valve syndrome). A floppy or prolapsed state may involve any of the cardiac valves but is most common in the mitral valve.

This chapter is divided into two major sections. The first section deals with a description of general aspects of floppy mitral valves, including definition of terms, description of primary (basic) and secondary pathologic changes, and discussion of complications and associated conditions. The second section describes an anatomic study of 102 consecutive autopsy cases of floppy mitral valves from a community hospital autopsy population.

GENERAL

Definition of Terms

Gross and Microscopic Anatomy of the Normal Mitral Valve

Ranganathan and associates[7] have defined the gross morphology of the normal human mitral valve. The anterior leaflet is a large, semicircular, or triangular structure. In the great majority of patients, the posterior leaflet is composed of three subdivisions or scallops named according to their position with respect to the mitral valvular commissures: posteromedial, anterolateral, and central scallop. Occasionally, more or fewer of these subdivisions are present. Each leaflet has a rough zone toward the free edge and a central clear zone toward the base. In the normal mitral valve there are interchordal convexities toward the atrium in the rough zone of both leaflets that vary considerably in height. Although the anterior leaflet is *longer* than the posterior leaflet, the posterior mitral leaflet is *wider* by a ratio of nearly 2:1. It is noteworthy that the chordal insertions into the leaflets are focal, so that there are valvular sites receiving chordal attachment and others that lie between these.

There is a tendency for the chordae tendineae to be grouped into three classes, the first order being inserted nearest the free edge of the leaflet and the third order inserted at the basal aspects of the leaflet. The second order occupies a medial position.[8] Normally, the chordae tendineae are thin and delicate structures.

The microscopic appearance of the normal leaflet consists of three elements: the *atrialis,* a thin layer of collagen and elastic tissue forming the atrial aspect of the leaflet and continuous with the endocardium of the left atrium; the *fibrosa,* composed of dense layers of collagen, which forms the basic support of the leaflet; and the *spongiosa,* a central delicate myxomatous (spongy) connective tissue between the atrialis and fibrosa. I consider the ventricularis, a thin layer of collagen and elastic tissue forming the ventricular surface of the mitral leaflet, to be part of the fibrosa.[9,10] Considerable variation exists in the thickness of the atrialis and the spongiosa.

From the foregoing description, it is apparent that the leaflets are relatively thin and flexible structures. Moreover, as the attachments of chordae into the leaflets are focal, pressure applied to the ventricular aspect of the leaflets, as during ventricular systole, will result in "prolapse" or hooding of interchordal aspects of the leaflets toward the atrium. Therein lies a problem in evaluating a mitral valve for the presence of a pathologic state of prolapse. There is a broad "gray" zone between the obvious normal and abnormal for each examiner, whether in the field of pathology,[10] radiology, or echocardiography. For the pathologist the distinction in some aspects depends on degree of "hooding" of leaflet tissue toward the atrium, but more specific signs of abnormality may be apparent by gross and histologic observation of specimens.

Gross and Microscopic Pathology of the Floppy Mitral Valve

I have used the term "floppy mitral valve" to refer to an anatomic condition. The systolic click-murmur is an auscultatory phenomenon. Anatomic floppy mitral valves cause the great majority of systolic click-murmurs. However, systolic click-murmurs are also produced by cardiomyopathies, papillary muscle dysfunction, left ventricular dysfunction, and other mitral valve anomalies. Mitral valve prolapse is defined by echocardiography or angiocardiography. A floppy mitral valve is the usual cause of mitral valve prolapse, but the latter is also produced by dysfunction of papillary muscles, left ventricular myocardial abnormalities, and other mitral valve anomalies. I wish to emphasize that the anatomic condition, the auscultatory events, and the echocardiographic (or angiocardiographic) findings are not synonymous. The clinician has the responsibility to use whichever terms he or she favors for these situations, but the terms must be used precisely and not interchangeably.

Primary (Basic) Changes

A major problem in making an anatomic diagnosis of floppy mitral valve is separating the truly floppy mitral valve from the normal mitral valve with minor degrees of interchordal hooding and increase in spongiosa. On gross examination, most normal mitral valves have interchordal convexities in the rough zone of both leaflets.[10] Moreover, interchordal hooding that involves both the rough and the clear zones of the mitral valve and that is localized to one third or less of the valve leaflet is relatively common.[7,13]

In my opinion, the following *primary* or *basic* features must be present before a gross diagnosis of floppy mitral valve is made:

1. Interchordal hooding involving both the rough and the clear zones of the involved leaflet or leaflets
2. Height of the interchordal hooding 4 mm or greater
3. Interchordal hooding involving at least one half of the anterior leaflet or at least two thirds of the posterior leaflet (it is not known whether patients who have lesser degrees of interchordal hooding represent variations in normal or minor degrees of floppy mitral valve[10])

The feature of interchordal hooding is the most consistent gross sign of the floppy or prolapsed mitral valve. This feature is apparent both in the opened and unopened valve. In the unopened state, the multiple areas of leaflet prolapse tend to obscure the usually simple matter of distinguishing the anterior from the posterior leaflet (Fig. 11–1). In the opened state, it is simple to identify the features of interchordal hooding and also to differentiate the degrees of involvement among the components of the valve (Fig. 11–2). In the classic state, the posterior leaflet is involved either alone or more prominently than the anterior leaflet. When the anterior leaflet is involved, the process is either more localized or involved to a greater degree in its posteromedial half. Features other than interchordal hooding are also part of the basic floppy valve process. In involved segments, the substance of the leaflet tissue on section is translucent or opaque. The chordae tendineae vary considerably. Many chordae are of normal length and noninterfused. In some instances, chordae tendineae are elongated and thin and in others, they are normal. Occasionally, one finds stout chordae that, on histologic examination, are composed of two or more chordae interfused.

A specific feature of the floppy valve syndrome is that commissural fusion, common in rheumatic valvular disease, is absent (Fig. 11–2). This characteristic

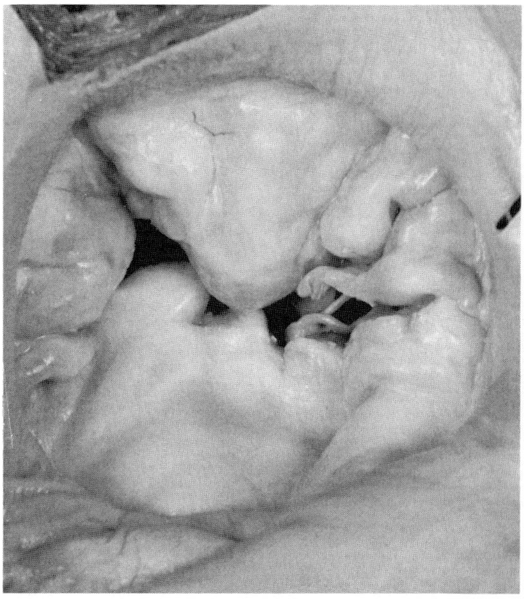

Figure 11–1. Unopened floppy mitral valve, viewed from above. The anterior leaflet is in the upper part of the illustration, the posterior in the lower. Numerous prolapsed units are present.

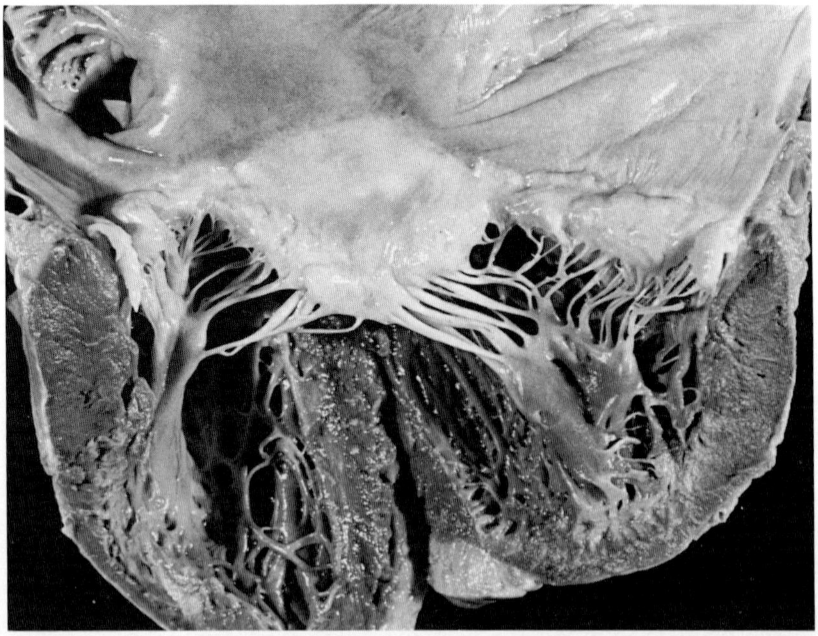

Figure 11–2. Opened mitral valve and left atrium and left ventricle. The anterior leaflet lies in the center of the illustration. The posterior leaflet has been cut in the dissection so that about two thirds of it lie to the right of the anterior leaflet and one third to the left. Prolapsed units are present in both leaflets, particularly the posterior one. In the anterior leaflet, the posteromedial half is more involved than the anterolateral half. Note that the two commissures are normal and not fused, a feature distinguishing this condition from rheumatic disease.

serves grossly to identify the floppy mitral valve in aging persons in whom fibrous thickening and valvular distortion through contracture of connective tissue may be prominent features. The diameter of the mitral orifice or anulus varies from normal to enlarged.[11]

The basic microscopic feature of the floppy mitral valve is significant thickening of the spongiosa, particularly noticeable in the free one third of the leaflet. Moreover, *the spongiosa encroaches on and invades the fibrosa,* causing focal interruption of the fibrosa. It is not known whether patients who have thickened spongiosa layers that do not invade the fibrosa represent a variation of normal or an early state in the myxomatous process. I consider such a state to be a normal variant, and a histologic diagnosis of floppy mitral valve is made when the fibrosa is invaded and disrupted by the spongiosa. Interruption of the fibrosa layer at many foci by extension of elements of the spongiosa into this layer appears to be the element that causes the leaflet to weaken and thus prolapse to abnormal degrees (Fig. 11–3).[9,12]

Quantitation of Severity of the Floppy Mitral Valve

Once the mitral valve has been defined as floppy, a considerable spectrum of severity exists. For this reason, Lucas and Edwards[10] devised a grading system for qualitating severity. This system is based on the magnitude and extent of interchordal hooding and is described as follows:

Grade I —Interchordal hooding involving more than one half of the anterior leaflet *or* more than two thirds of the posterior leaflet (one leaflet involved)

Grade II —Interchordal hooding involving more than one half of the anterior leaflet *and* more than two thirds of the posterior leaflet (both leaflets involved)

Grade III—A significantly greater magnitude of interchordal hooding than that present in Grade II

Secondary manifestations (e.g., friction lesions) were not used in this grading system.

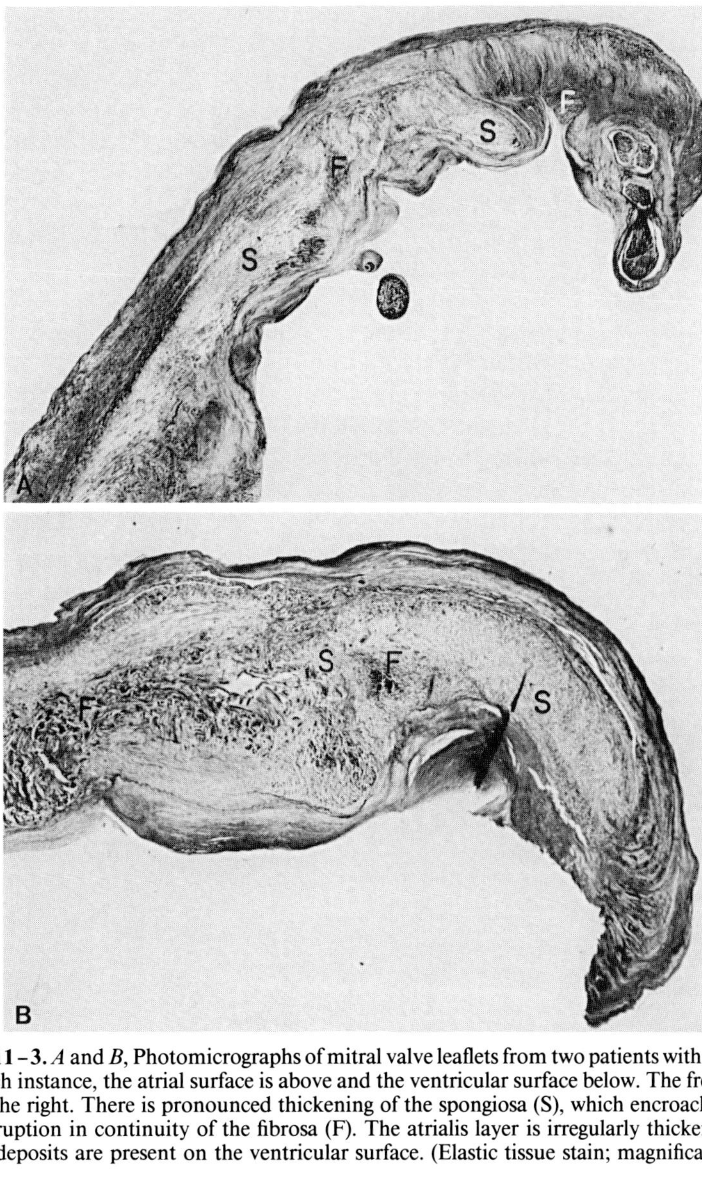

Figure 11-3. *A* and *B*, Photomicrographs of mitral valve leaflets from two patients with floppy mitral valve. In each instance, the atrial surface is above and the ventricular surface below. The free edge of the leaflet is to the right. There is pronounced thickening of the spongiosa (S), which encroaches upon and causes interruption in continuity of the fibrosa (F). The atrialis layer is irregularly thickened. Fibrous, "stuck on" deposits are present on the ventricular surface. (Elastic tissue stain; magnification *A* ×5, *B* ×40.)

Secondary Effects

In addition to the primary or basic features of the floppy mitral valve, other anatomic changes, termed "secondary effects," have been described.[9,13] These secondary lesions appear to represent responses to the stresses on and injury to the prolapsing elements.

Among the secondary effects of the floppy mitral valve are (1) *fibrous thickening of the free aspect of the leaflet;* (2) *fibrous deposits on the ventricular surface of the leaflets* (Figs. 11–3, and 11–4); (3) *friction lesions* involving the mural endocardium of the left ventricle; and (4) *contact thrombosis.*

Fibrous thickening of the free aspect of the leaflet involves thickening of the auricularis layer with collagen and elastic tissue. The fibroelastic thickening at the summit of the atrial aspect of prolapsing units is considered a response of the injury to the prolapsed segment, as during ventricular systole it makes abnormal contact with an opposite element of the valve. In addition to abnormal contact with an opposite element, within a given leaflet, one prolapsed segment may rub abnormally against an adjacent segment, to which a fibroelastic response also occurs. The precursor of this process may at times be observed in the form of endothelial denudation with deposits of fibrin on the denuded surface.[9,12]

Fibrous deposits on the left ventricular surface of involved leaflets is one of the more specific secondary effects in floppy valves. These changes in the noncontact aspect of the leaflets consist of connective tissue aggregates that are composed primarily of collagen with varying numbers of intermixed elastic fibers. This fibrous tissue acts as a "pad-like filler" between inserting chordae tendineae and does not invade the leaflets.[9,12] The pad-like thickening in the concavity produced by the prolapse appears to be a response to the tension and stretching that occurs at the undersurface of the prolapsing units. Occasionally, the fibrous reaction between the inserting chordae tendineae may extend onto related chordae.[9]

The fibrotic changes that occur secondary to the process of prolapse and the underlying element of increased spongiosa do not disturb the identity of the various

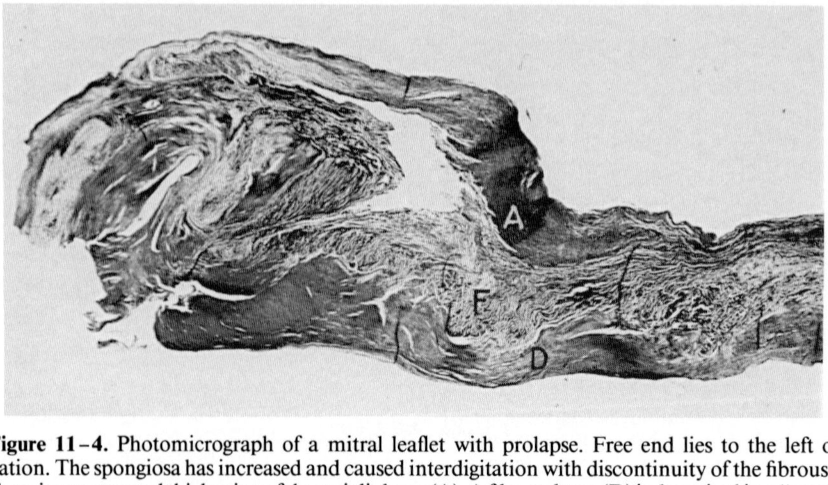

Figure 11–4. Photomicrograph of a mitral leaflet with prolapse. Free end lies to the left of the illustration. The spongiosa has increased and caused interdigitation with discontinuity of the fibrous layer (F). There is pronounced thickening of the atrialis layer (A). A fibrous layer (D) is deposited in a "stuck on" fashion on the ventricular surface of the leaflet. Bulbous thickening of the free aspect leaflet is considered secondary to mitral regurgitation. (Elastic tissue stain; magnification ×10.)

elements of the leaflet. Thus, while the prolapsed mitral valve may become fibrotic, the fibrosis does not affect all layers of the leaflet and cause a loss of distinction between one layer and another, as in chronic deforming rheumatic mitral valve disease. This is an important distinction that should help in avoiding an incorrect pathologic diagnosis of rheumatic disease in those valves involved by the process of prolapse and secondary fibrosis. Another point of distinction is absent commissural fusion in the floppy mitral valve despite marked secondary fibrosis.

Friction lesions as secondary effects of the floppy mitral valve involve the mural endocardium of the left ventricle in relation to chordae that insert into the posterior leaflet of the mitral valve. These lesions, described by Salazar and Edwards,[14] commonly bear the name of Salazar. While the chordae tendineae of the floppy mitral valve initially are long and thin, they may become thickened by aggregation of fibrous tissue on their surfaces.[13] As the posterior mitral leaflet protrudes to abnormal degrees into the left atrium, its chordae tendineae may come in contact with the lining of the related mural endocardium of the left ventricle.

Initially, the Salazar lesion is represented by one or several thin linear thickenings of the left ventricular mural endocardium. The thickenings may become more elaborate so as (1) to result in coalescence of individual lesions (Fig. 11–5), (2) to cause adhesion of the lower aspects of the chordae to the thickened left ventricular endocardium, and (3) to allow the lesion to calcify and be identified echocardiographically (Fig. 11–5*D*). The adhesion of chordae tendineae to the mural endocardium yields a state wherein chordae that initially had been abnormally long become effectively shortened. Related chordae may show surface deposits of new connective tissue (Fig. 11–6). These ultimate responses to friction by chordae tendineae on the left ventricular endocardium yield a complex picture that may be misinterpreted as the end stage of healed infective endocarditis.[9] In addition, in the floppy valve the reaction to friction may cause fusion of chordae tendineae, which is common with rheumatic disease, giving a basis for confusing the floppy valve with one diseased on a rheumatic basis. Distinction between these two states depends to a great extent on the associated nature of the leaflets and of the commissures. Chordal adhesion resulting from rheumatic endocarditis causes simple fusion of chordae, whereas in the floppy valve, interadherent chordae characteristically are interadherent along with fusion to the left ventricular mural endocardium.[9]

Contact thrombosis may occur in two sites of preference; one is on the *atrial surface* of prolapsed units, and the other is in the angle formed by the junction of the left atrial endocardium and the atrial surface of the posterior leaflet (the so-called *angle lesion*) (Fig. 11–7). Contact thrombosis on the atrial surface of the leaflet is less common than the angle lesion. Each is a potential source for systemic embolism including the cerebral vascular tree. Such a phenomenon is suspected of being the cause of transient cerebral ischemic attacks known to occur in patients with floppy mitral valves.[15]

Complications

The uncomplicated floppy mitral valve appears to be a benign condition. On the other hand, complications of the floppy mitral valve, when they occur, carry a significant morbidity and mortality. Among the complications of floppy mitral valve are (1) *mitral insufficiency with intact chordae tendineae,* (2) *infective endocarditis,*

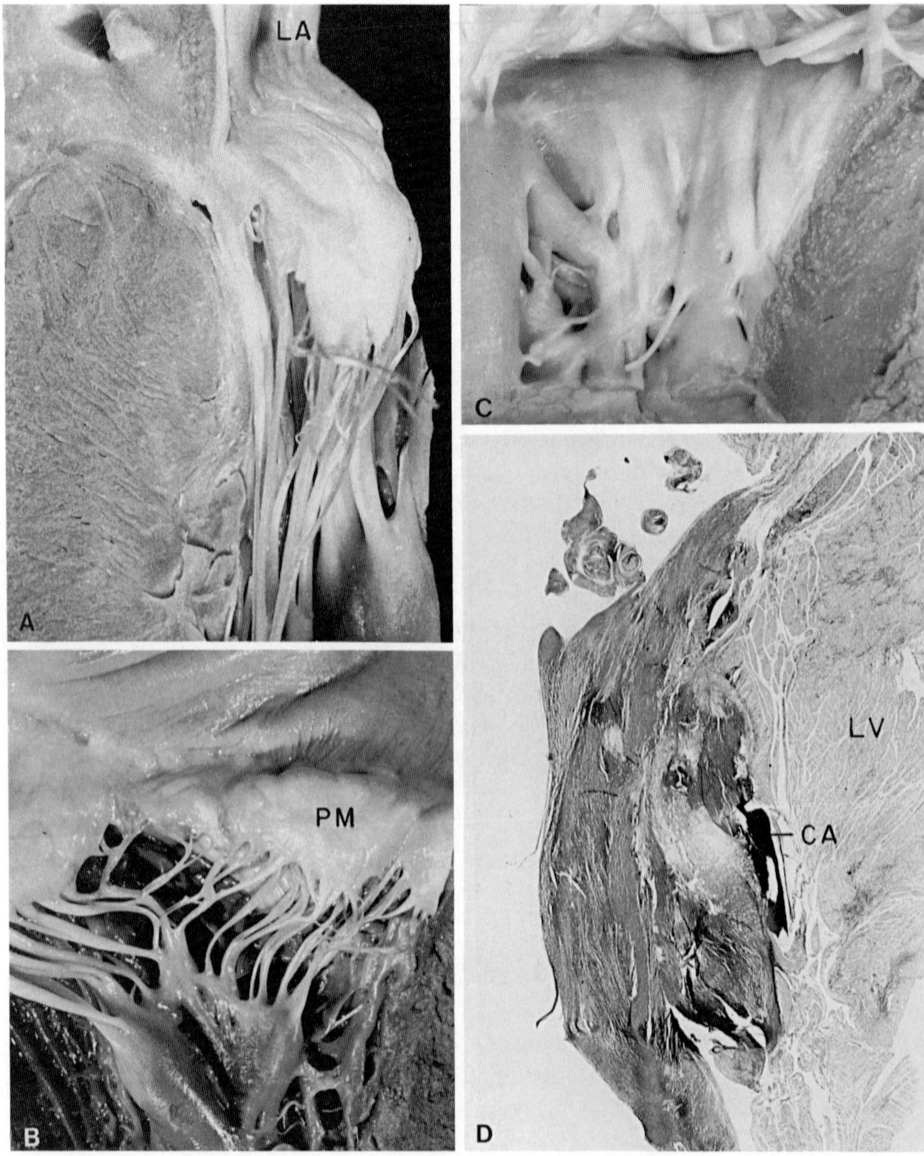

Figure 11–5. Friction lesions of the left ventricular mural endocardium, so-called Salazar lesions. *A,* Close-up view of junction of left atrium (LA) and left ventricle, along with the posterior mitral leaflet. Tertiary cords inserting into the posterior leaflet have made contact with the mural endocardium of the left ventricle causing secondary fibrous (Salazar) lesions. *B,* Opened left atrium and left ventricle. Inferior to the posterior leaflet of the mitral valve (PM) there is endocardial thickening of the mural endocardium of the left ventricle in relation to chordae inserting into the posterior leaflet. *C,* Inferior wall of left ventricle inferior to the mitral valve. The mitral valve has been reflected upward, exposing a series of endocardial thickenings (Salazar lesions) that have tended to coalesce. *D,* Low-power photomicrograph of inferior wall of left ventricle (LV) showing major thickening of the left ventricular endocardium *(dark area).* There is calcification (CA). (Hematoxylin-eosin stain magnification ×5; reduced 13 percent.)

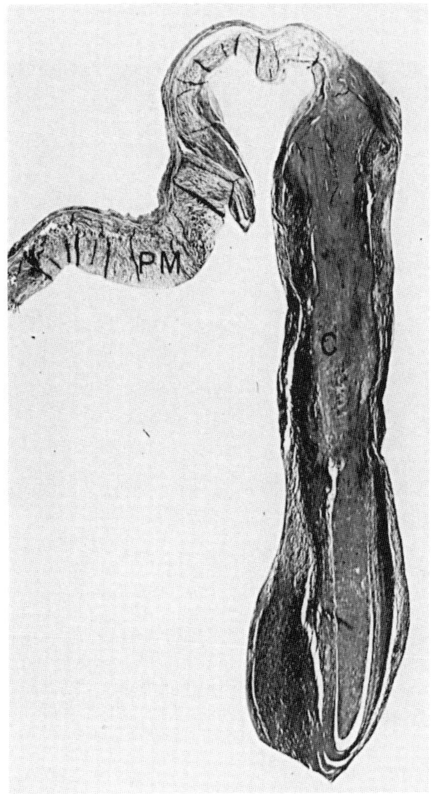

Figure 11-6. Photomicrograph of posterior mitral leaflet (PM) and an inserting cord (C). The cord is encased by fibrous tissue that probably has resulted from friction. (Elastic tissue stain; magnification ×5.)

(3) *ruptured chordae tendineae unassociated with endocarditis,* (4) *sudden death,* (5) *calcification of the posterior mitral leaflet,* and (6) *neuropsychiatric symptoms.*

Mitral Insufficiency With Intact Chordae Tendineae

Various degrees of mitral insufficiency may occur chronically in some subjects with floppy mitral valves with intact chordae tendineae. In such individuals, the mechanism for the valvular malfunction is commonly explained by the enlargement of the mitral orifice ("anulus," "anular circumference") that occurs with the floppy mitral valve. Entrapment of chordae tendineae in left ventricular friction lesions also may produce mitral insufficiency. Anatomic evidence to support a diagnosis of mitral regurgitation includes left atrial "jet lesion," left atrial dilation, and left ventricular dilation. Mitral insufficiency as a cause of death among patients with floppy mitral valve is relatively uncommon (2 percent).[10] Clinically, the progression to mitral regurgitation from an isolated nonejection systolic click is rare, and rapid progression from mild to severe mitral regurgitation is extremely rare.[16] Barlow has observed patients with mitral valve prolapse reflected by a late systolic murmur advancing to a pansystolic murmur during a 10- to 20-year period, but rapid progression is very unusual in the absence of infective endocarditis, idiopathic ruptured chordae tendineae, or Marfan's syndrome.[16]

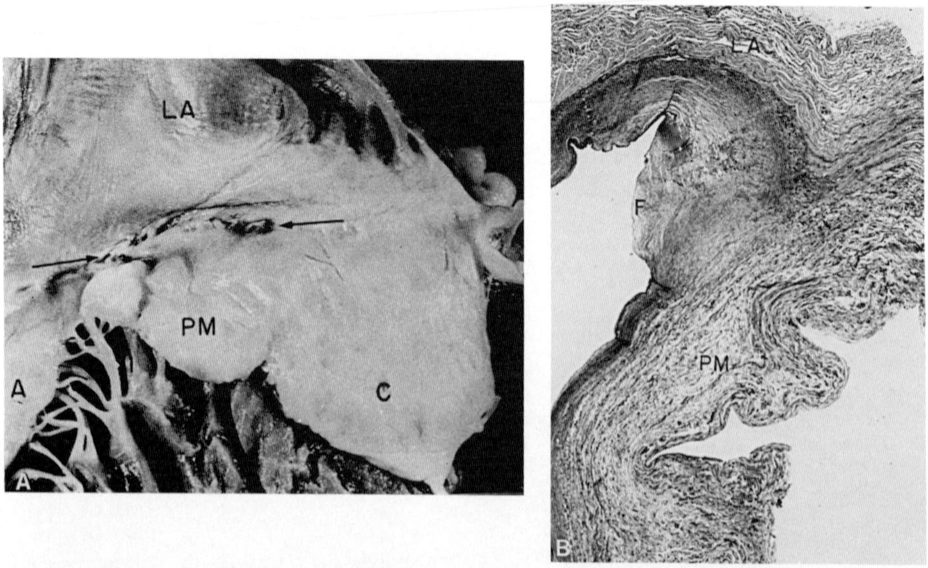

Figure 11–7. Angle contact lesion in floppy mitral valve. *A,* Gross specimen shows a linear deposit of fibrin *(between arrows)* at the junction of the left atrium (LA) and the posteromedial scallop (PM) of the posterior leaflet. C = central scallop of posterior mitral leaflet; A = anterior leaflet. *B,* Low-power photomicrograph of the junction of the left atrium and left ventricle shows a deposit of fibrin (F) in the angle between the left atrium (LA) and the posterior mitral leaflet (PM). The latter shows features of excess in spongiosa. (Elastic tissue stain; magnification ×10, reduced 30 percent.)

Infective Endocarditis

Infective endocarditis is now recognized as a possible complication of the floppy mitral valve.[10,17,18] This complication is probably favored by the trauma of impact of one prolapsed unit against another during ventricular systole. Usually the infection starts in a classic position, on the atrial surface of the valve. It may result in perforation of cuspal tissue or chordal rupture (Fig. 11–8). In a case reported by Kuhn and Weber,[19] infection started at the site of a Salazar lesion.

The incidence of bacterial endocarditis among 102 autopsy patients with floppy mitral valve studied by Lucas and Edwards[10] was 7 percent. This is comparable to the 6 percent incidence reported by Pomerance.[13] Allen and associates[20] reported bacterial endocarditis in 8 percent of 62 patients with late systolic murmur who were followed clinically for 9 to 22 years. In that clinical study, myocardial and ischemic heart diseases were excluded as causes of the late systolic murmur, and thus floppy mitral valve was a statistically reliable diagnosis. These studies suggest that patients with floppy mitral valve have a definite (7 percent) risk of bacterial endocarditis.

When patients with bacterial endocarditis are evaluated, a significant percentage have floppy mitral valve: 30 percent (10 of 33) in the study of Nolan and associates[21] and 36 percent (10 of 28) in that of Corrigall and associates.[22] Since floppy mitral valve is a common condition, even a small risk of bacterial endocarditis will result in a large number of cases of bacterial endocarditis.

Ruptured Chordae Tendineae Unassociated With Endocarditis

Rupture of chordae tendineae in the absence of infection is now generally accepted as a complication of the floppy mitral valve. The autopsy incidence of spontaneous chordal rupture in floppy mitral valves is about 7 percent.[10] To determine the causes of ruptured chordae tendineae and a suspected etiologic role of floppy mitral valve, Jeresaty and associates[23] examined surgically excised mitral valves in 25 consecutive cases of surgically proved chordal rupture. Of the 25 patients, 23 had floppy mitral valves, and in 22 of the 23 cases, mitral valve prolapse was the only underlying morphologic abnormality. Only 1 of 23 patients had infective

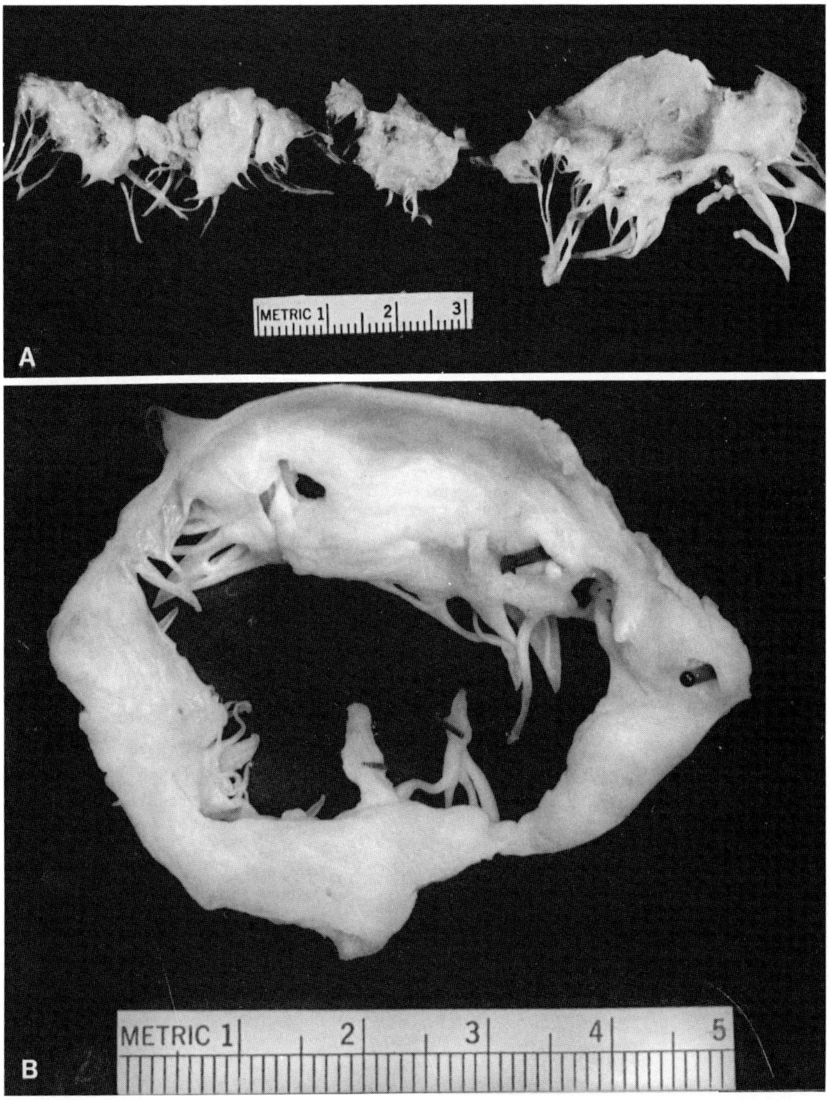

Figure 11-8. *A,* Surgically excised mitral valve showing results of bacterial endocarditis complicating the prolapsed state. In the anterior leaflet, there is a focus involving the posteromedial half with pronounced upward deformity of the leaflet, beneath which is a thickened and ruptured cord. On the posterior leaflet, the atrial surface is corrugated, which is caused by either secondary infection or regurgitation or lesions resulting from regurgitation incident to the ruptured cord of the anterior leaflet. *B,* Surgically excised mitral valve viewed from above in a case of prolapsed mitral valve with old bacterial endocarditis. Evident are four perforations *(black probes).* Chordae attached to the posterior leaflet (lower part of illustration) have ruptured.

endocarditis that was responsible for the chordal rupture. In 4 of the 23 patients, mitral valve prolapse was documented 4 to 11 years earlier. Morphologic and historic evidence from these patients would indicate that floppy mitral valve is probably the most common cause of so-called "spontaneous chordal rupture."[23] Although chordae of any part of the valvular mechanism may rupture, the site of greater predilection for rupture involves the chordae inserting into the central scallop of the posterior leaflet (Fig. 11–9*A*). As a unit of valve loses its chordal support, it hoods to a greater extent than the rest of the valve. This hooding is responsible for the regurgitant stream of blood to be deflected toward the opposite aspect of the left atrium (Figs. 11–9, 11–10). When the central scallop of the posterior leaflet is so involved, the regurgitant stream strikes the atrial septum and yields a systolic murmur at the "aortic area," a phenomenon that may lead to a clinical suspicion of aortic stenosis. Characteristically, jet lesions are identifiable on the septal wall of the left atrium.[24]

Examination of ruptured ends of chordae tendineae yields varying results. The most common change is loss of specific collagenous staining and shredding of elements of chordal substance (Fig. 11–11).

It is of interest that in some cases considered to be examples of spontaneous ruptured chordae tendineae, no stumps of ruptured chordae can be identified. This leads to an alternate explanation for the phenomenon, as follows. As the process of prolapse progresses, the leaflet tissue widens. In so doing, the spaces between the chordal insertions become greater. The ultimate effect may be that the distance between intact chordae is so great that intervening valvular tissue is inadequately supported and prolapses excessively. That unit of leaflet tissue then gives the illusion of having lost chordal support whereas in actuality the chordae tendineae are intact.

Sudden Death

Sudden death[9,26–52] is a feared potential complication among patients with floppy mitral valves. When histories are available, such patients characteristically have shown a *mid-late systolic mitral click, prolapse of the mitral valve* as demonstrated on echocardiography, and *ventricular premature contractions.*[9] Ventricular arrhythmias are commonly observed in subjects with floppy mitral valves.[49,50] It is not clearly established whether or not in general those who suffer sudden death have had prior ventricular premature contractions. In the studies of Shappell and associates,[51] such ectopy need not have been present.

When present, the basis for the premature ventricular contractions is unclear. Some have considered that there is ischemic change in the region of the posteromedial papillary muscle. Because there is evidence of abnormal contact of chordae tendineae with the left ventricular wall, the question arises as to whether such contact may stimulate premature ventricular contractions. A third possibility, suggested by Criley and associates,[25] is that the prolapsing valve creates abnormal tension at the chordal papillary muscle junctions and that this tension stimulates premature ventricular contraction.

Sudden death did not occur in the 102 autopsy cases of floppy mitral valves studied by Lucas and Edwards.[10] In addition, sudden death did not occur in the autopsy series of Pomerance[13] (30 patients) or of Davies and associates[26] (86 patients). It is perhaps not surprising that these hospital series had no sudden deaths, since sudden death usually occurs outside the hospital.

About 39 reported cases of sudden death have been attributed to mitral valve prolapse.[9,26–47] In only 19 of the reported cases were autopsies performed, but even

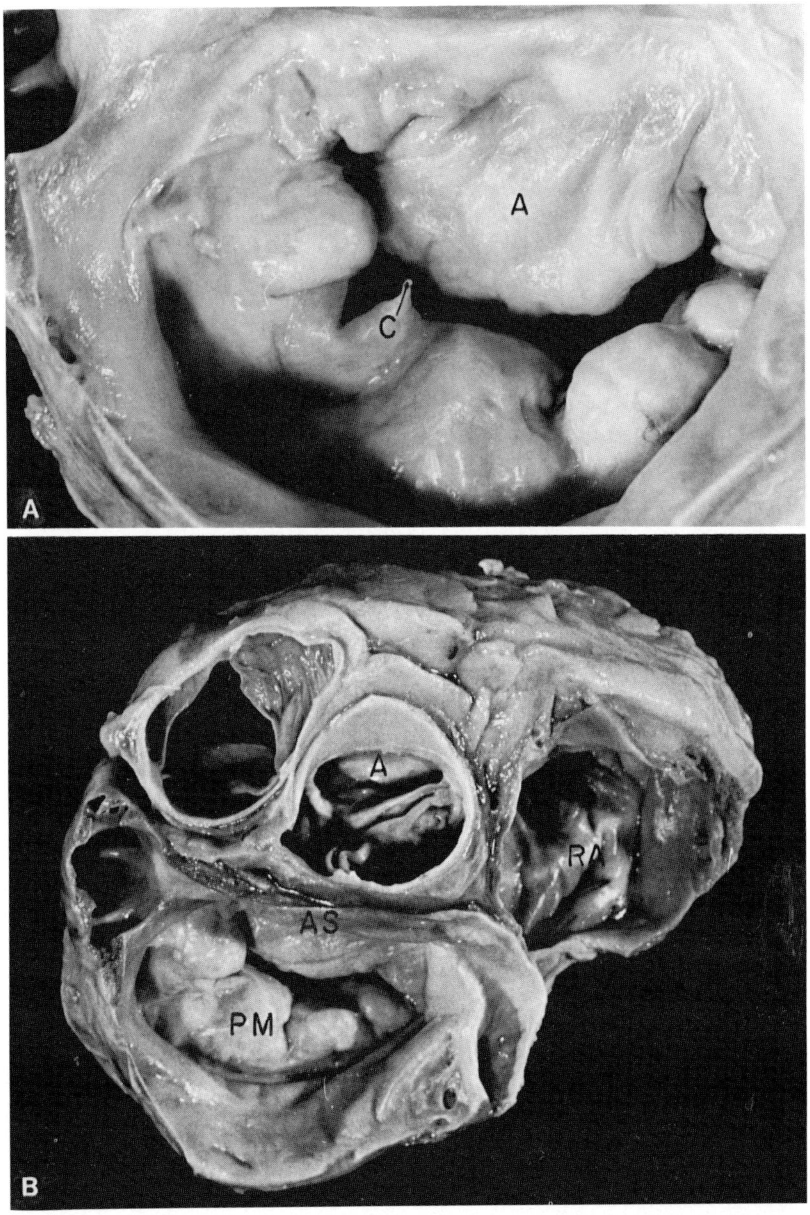

Figure 11–9. *A,* Floppy mitral valve viewed from above. A = anterior leaflet. One of the chordae (C) inserting into the central scallop of the posterior leaflet has ruptured, allowing the involved segment of the valve to prolapse upward so that the end of the ruptured cord is visible from this perspective. *B,* Base of heart in a case of floppy mitral valve with ruptured chordae to the posterior leaflet. As the posterior leaflet (PM) loses support, the stream of blood is directed medially toward the atrial septum (AS); the latter structure lies close to the aortic valve (A) and accounts for the peculiar location of the systolic murmur in such instances. Unlettered vessel = pulmonary trunk; RA = right atrium.

among these cases the information, in many instances, is sparse, so other pathologic conditions cannot be excluded. Recently, Chesler, King, and Edwards[48] reported clinicopathologic features of 14 cases of sudden death in patients with floppy mitral valve. The patients ranged in age from 14 to 59 years (mean 27), and 11 (79 percent) were female. Of seven electrocardiograms available, none showed prolongation of

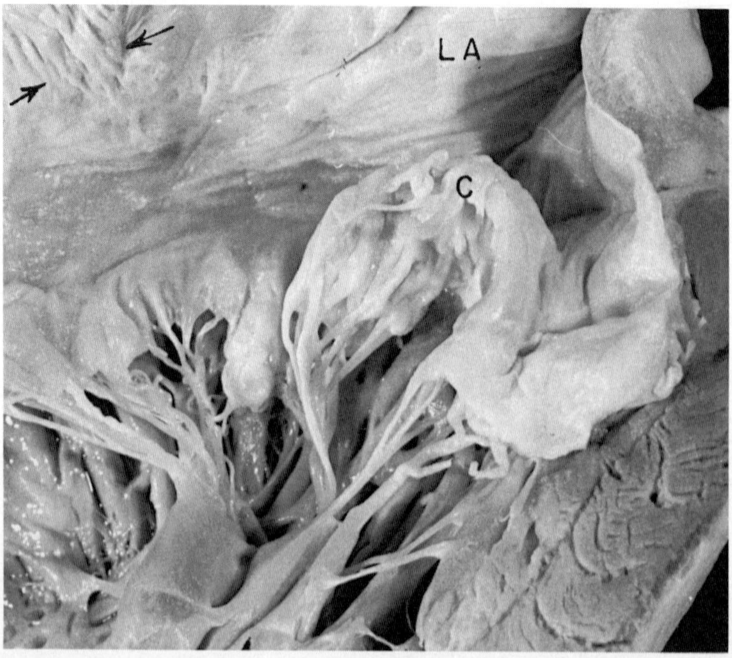

Figure 11-10. A portion of left atrium (LA), left ventricle, and mitral valve. The central scallop (C) of the posterior leaflet has lost chordal support and shows major prolapse toward the atrium. Opposite this location, the atrial septum shows a series of jet lesions *(between arrows)* representing the site of impact of the regurgitant stream from this peculiar type of mitral regurgitation.

the Q-T interval, but two showed repolarization abnormalities. The valves were classified according to the grade of floppiness: grade I, three cases; grade II, eight cases; grade III, three cases. The three cases with minimal prolapse cast some doubt on the hypothesis that traction on the papillary muscles or "diastolic dumping" of the leaflets is implicated in the pathogenesis of ventricular arrhythmias. In one of the cases with minimal prolapse, there was a strong family history of sudden death. Endocardial friction lesions were present in 11 of the 14 cases, including two of the three with minimal prolapse. In five cases a thrombotic lesion of fibrin and platelets was present in the angle between the posterior leaflet and the left atrial wall. These abnormalities may be important in the pathogenesis of the fatal ventricular arrhythmias.

It is my opinion that the risk of sudden death in a patient with floppy mitral valve *and a normal electrocardiogram* is remote. *If electrocardiographic abnormalities are present* in a patient with floppy mitral valve, the patient appears to have a higher, although unknown, risk of sudden death. In his review of 25 cases of sudden death associated with mitral valve prolapse, Jeresaty[52] identified the potential victim as having the following clinical features:

> A 40-year-old woman with a history of syncope who has a late systolic murmur preceded by a click, or a pansystolic murmur with late systolic accentuation. The electrocardiogram shows inferolateral ST-T changes and frequent premature ventricular systoles. Left ventriculography demonstrates obvious mitral valve prolapse and minimal-to-moder-

> ate mitral regurgitation. Patients with "silent" mitral valve prolapse or an isolated click do not appear to be susceptible. A family history of sudden death is an added risk factor.[11]

Our clinical-pathologic features of the 14 cases of sudden death generally confirm these findings.

Histologic evaluation of the cardiac conduction system has been reported in at least five cases.[10,44,45] In two cases studied by Lucas and Edwards,[10] no abnormalities were found. Bharati and colleagues[44,45] performed a detailed study of the conduction system in three cases of mitral valve prolapse and sudden death. In two cases there were premature aging and sclerosis of the cardiac skeleton with involvement of the atrioventricular node and trifascicular conduction system; in one of these cases there was also thrombosis of the sinoatrial node artery.[45] In the third case, there was fatty infiltration in the approaches to the sinoatrial and atrioventricular nodes and atrial preferential pathways.[44] The role of these findings in the pathogenesis of lethal bradyarrhythmias or tachyarrhythmias is uncertain, because their frequency in hearts of patients with floppy mitral valves without sudden death or without floppy valves is unknown. Senges and associates[53] studied three patients electrophysiologically who had mitral valve prolapse, strong family histories of sudden death, and high-grade ventricular ectopy. In these patients, normal intracardiac conduction and refractoriness were demonstrated. These studies provide no evidence for underlying reentrant mechanisms as a potential cause of ventricular ectopy.

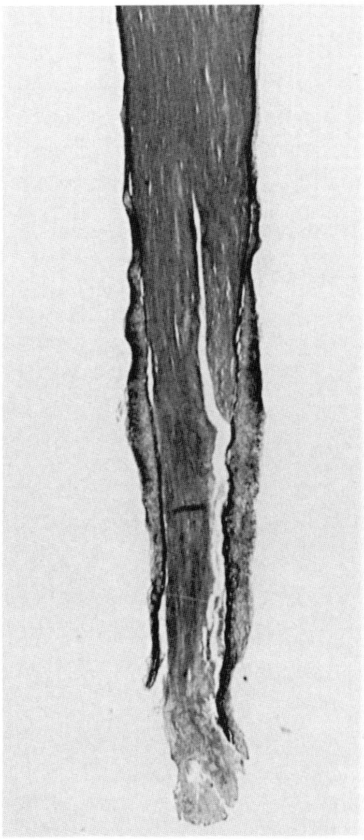

Figure 11–11. Terminal end of ruptured cord. There is loss of density of the collagenous structure of the cord leading to the rupture site (lower part of illustration). In the lowermost half of the photograph, surface deposits of new connective tissue are present on the cord. These may have resulted from friction against adjacent structures. (Elastic tissue stain; magnification ×15.)

Calcification of Posterior Leaflet

The posterior mitral leaflet involved by myxomatous change may show focal calcification beginning at its basal aspect (Fig. 11–12). In such a position the calcification may be confused with or difficult to distinguish from calcification of the mitral ring. Calcification may occur in a large Salazar lesion (see Fig. 11–5), and, uncommonly, chordae tendineae of a floppy valve may calcify.

Neuropsychiatric Symptoms

It has been reported that some patients with floppy mitral valves exhibit "neuropsychiatric" or "psychiatric symptoms."[54] It is not certain whether these phenomena represent manifestations of anxiety in otherwise asymptomatic patients or whether they relate directly to the existence of the mitral valve prolapse. Cerebral embolism from microthrombi that may occur on the contact surfaces or angle lesions of the prolapsed segments is one possible basis for such symptoms or other neurologic events.

Associated Conditions

Certain conditions have a higher than expected frequency in patients with floppy mitral valve. These conditions include floppiness of other valves,[9] connective tissue disorders,[55–57] and secundum atrial septal defect.[58]

Floppiness of Other Valves

In the autopsy study by Lucas and Edwards,[10] the incidence of floppiness of other valves was as follows: tricuspid valve 41 percent, pulmonary valve 11 percent, aortic valve 2 percent. In none of the affected valves was there evidence of abnormal function. It is possible that pulmonary hypertension may result in increased stress on the pulmonary and tricuspid valves, thereby increasing the possibility of valve insufficiency or chordae tendineae rupture.

Connective Tissue Disorders

In some cases of floppy mitral valves, the patient shows the body physique of arachnodactyly (Marfan's syndrome). This has led to the thought that in cases without this condition the myxomatous valve is a forme fruste of Marfan's syndrome. Support for such a concept comes from the fact that when the mitral valve is involved,

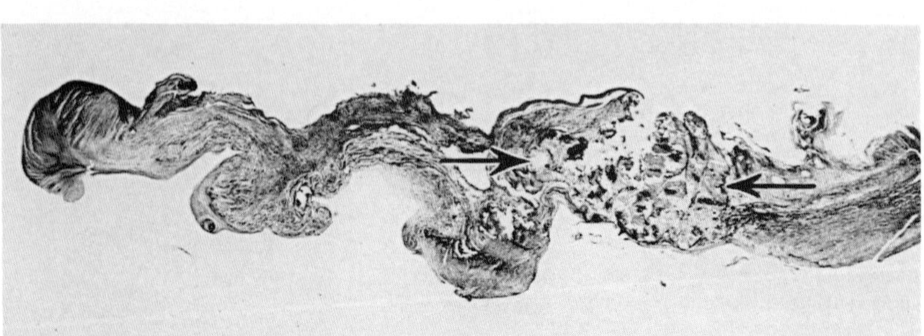

Figure 11–12. Low-power photomicrograph of mitral leaflet with the floppy state in which there is a focus of calcification *(between arrows)*. The free edge of the leaflet (left side of illustration) is bulbous, resulting from fibrous reaction to mitral regurgitation. (Elastic tissue stain; magnification ×20.)

it is common for some degree of myxomatous change to be observed in the other valves and for some degree of cystic medial necrosis of the aorta to occur. McKay and Yacoub[57] reported three nonarachnodactylic patients with myxomatous mitral valve (two with ruptured chordae), in each of whom dissecting aneurysm of the aorta had begun at the site of clamping of the aorta during the operation for replacement of the mitral valve. The identified cystic medial necrosis of the aorta was considered a condition accompanying the myxomatous mitral valve. It is of additional interest that Read and associates[5] found among patients with "floppy" valves certain skeletal deformities that form part of Marfan's syndrome.

Secundum Atrial Septal Defect

The incidence of secundum atrial septal defect in patients with floppy valve is slightly higher than the incidence of secundum atrial septal defect in the general population.[10] There is also a slightly higher incidence of floppy mitral valve among patients with atrial septal defect than in the general population. When the two conditions coexist, the prognosis appears influenced by both. Of 12 patients with atrial septal defect and floppy mitral valve in our study,[10] six died as a result of the atrial septal defect, two as a result of the floppy mitral valve (both with bacterial endocarditis), and one during operation for atrial septal defect closure and mitral valve replacement.

ANATOMIC STUDY OF 102 CONSECUTIVE AUTOPSIES OF FLOPPY MITRAL VALVE CASES FROM A COMMUNITY HOSPITAL

Lucas and Edwards[10] recently studied at autopsy 102 patients who had floppy mitral valves and who died at a community hospital. This section of the chapter provides details from this community hospital series, as well as quantitative data for the previously described primary and secondary pathologic changes, complications, and associated conditions of the floppy mitral valve.

The autopsy records of 1376 consecutive patients who died at the Miller Hospital between January 1, 1969 through December 31, 1980 were reviewed. Miller hospital is a community hospital serving the city of St. Paul, Minnesota, and its environs. The patient population is largely adult. There is no pediatric ward, and only a few older children are admitted. During the period of study, this hospital was not a major referral center for cardiac patients. In 134 cases the mitral valve was considered to be floppy at the time of autopsy. Of these hearts, 109 were available for restudy and 102 met our criteria for the diagnosis of floppy mitral valve. The other seven showed minor degrees of mitral valve floppiness, and on restudy were considered normal. These seven, as well as 25 specimens that were not available for review, were not included in the 102 cases considered to have floppy mitral valves.

Incidence

One hundred two specimens exhibiting a floppy mitral valve from an autopsy population of 1376 represents an incidence of 7.4 percent. This is a minimal incidence; an additional 25 patients had been considered to have floppy mitral valve at autopsy, but these heart specimens were not available for review and are not included as examples of this condition.

Gender Distribution

Among the 102 cases with floppy mitral valve, there were 62 (61 percent) men and 40 (39 percent) women. The 1376 cases of the total autopsy series consisted of 750 (55 percent) men and 626 (45 percent) women. When the male-to-female ratio of the floppy mitral valve group is corrected for that of the total autopsy series, the resultant male-to-female ratio is 1:3.

Age at Death

In women, there was no statistical difference in age at death between the floppy mitral valve group and the control autopsy group (mean 68.2 years, 66.2 years, respectively). On the other hand, the mean age at death of men with floppy mitral valves was 4 years older than the mean age at death of the control autopsy men (mean 69.7 years, 65.6 years, respectively, $p = 0.03$). When men and women were combined, the patients with floppy mitral valve lived longer than the control autopsy group ($p = 0.03$).

Cause of Death

The cause of death in the 102 patients with floppy mitral valves may be compared with the cause of death in the total autopsy series of 1376 patients, respectively, as follows: neoplastic disease—42 percent, 34 percent; cardiovascular disease (floppy mitral valve)—4 percent, 0.3 percent; other cardiovascular disease—30 percent, 37.7 percent; pulmonary disease—14 percent, 6 percent; gastrointestinal disease—6 percent, 7 percent; and miscellaneous—4 percent, 15 percent. Complications of the floppy mitral valve were considered to be the cause of death in four patients. Two patients died of mitral regurgitation following rupture of chordae, and two died of bacterial endocarditis involving the floppy mitral valve. No patient in the community hospital series had a sudden, unexpected, unexplained death.

Severity of Floppy Mitral Valve

The severity of the primary lesion was graded in the 102 floppy mitral valves as follows: grade I, 34 cases (33 percent); grade II, 45 cases (44 percent); and grade III, 23 cases (23 percent). *When the severity of the floppy mitral valve was related to the age at death, older patients did not have more severe mitral valve floppiness. This suggests that the floppy mitral valve is not part of an aging process.* Moreover, the severity grade distribution in patients who had primary rupture of chordae and patients who had bacterial endocarditis was comparable to the severity grade distribution of the total group. When only one leaflet was involved (grade I), the involved leaflet was the posterior one in each of the cases. Moreover, when one leaflet was more hooded than the other, the posterior leaflet consistently was the greater affected.

Secondary Effects

Fibroelastic Lesions of Mitral Valve Leaflets

In all of the hearts with floppy mitral valve, the mitral valvular leaflets had fibrosis involving the atrial or ventricular aspects, or both. Fibrosis of the atrialis surface of the mitral valve seemed to be an accentuation of the normal and was considered to result from abnormal coaptation of one mitral valve unit with its opposite or contiguous member. The ventricular surface of the floppy mitral valve exhibited deposits of fibroelastic tissue involving the hooded interchordal segments.

Abnormalities of Chordae Tendineae

Ninety-one hearts (89 percent) had thin chordae. We did not determine chordal length quantitatively, but on the basis of subjective observations we concluded that chordal length was normal in 75 specimens (74 percent) and elongated in 27 specimens (26 percent).

Left Ventricular Friction Lesions

These lesions, consisting of fibrous patches on the inferobasal aspect of the left ventricular endocardium oriented parallel to contiguous chordae, are considered to result from friction between the chordae and left ventricular wall. Friction lesions of the left ventricular wall were present in 77 of the specimens (75 percent). The chordae that produce the friction lesion typically were covered by collagenous and elastic fibers that did not invade the chordae tendineae.

In three of the specimens (3 percent), the fibroelastic friction lesion resulted in entrapment of the chordae. Even when entrapped, the chordae tendineae were not invaded by the fibroelastic process. The myocardium underlying the friction lesion was normal.

Friction lesions of the inferobasal aspect of the left ventricular endocardium uncommonly occur in conditions other than floppy mitral valve. *Thus, the presence of a friction lesion alone is not sufficient for a diagnosis of floppy mitral valve. Conversely, the absence of a friction lesion does not preclude this diagnosis. However, when a friction lesion accompanies a floppy mitral valve, its presence supports disordered mitral valve function.*

Complications of Floppy Mitral Valve

Primary Rupture of Mitral Valve Chordae

Seven patients had primary rupture of chordae of the mitral valve. All had anatomic evidence of mitral regurgitation. In five, the mitral regurgitation was not severe, and the patients died of other causes. Two patients died of congestive failure from mitral regurgitation. Rupture of chordae serving the central scallop of the posterior leaflet was seen in three specimens. In three other specimens, the ruptured chordae were to other posterior leaflet scallops. In the seventh case, the specific site of rupture could not be identified on reexamination of the heart. Specific chordal abnormalities were not identified at the rupture site in any specimen. The male-to-female ratio in patients with ruptured chordae was 1.3. The mean age at death was 62 years, 7 years less than the mean age of death in the total floppy mitral valve series. The distribution of grade of severity in patients with ruptured chordae was similar to the distribution in the group of 102 patients.

Bacterial Endocarditis

Seven of the 102 floppy valves had anatomic evidence of bacterial endocarditis. In two specimens, the mitral valve endocarditis had healed and mitral valve dysfunction was minimal. These patients died at ages 61 and 71 years of chronic pulmonary disease and myocardial infarction, respectively.

Five patients had active bacterial endocarditis involving the mitral valve. Three of these patients had a far-advanced malignant neoplasm, and the bacterial endocarditis was a clinically unrecognized terminal event. The remaining two patients with active bacterial endocarditis had no apparent predisposing factors. They died at ages

42 and 60 years of complications of bacterial endocarditis, namely, ruptured mycotic aneurysm of the right vertebral artery and perforated mitral valve. Bacterial endocarditis caused ruptured chordae in three patients. In one patient with healed bacterial endocarditis, the ruptured chordae produced minimal mitral valve dysfunction. In the other two patients, significant mitral regurgitation appeared to result from the ruptured chordae, but mitral regurgitation was not the apparent cause of death in either.

The male-to-female ratio for patients with bacterial endocarditis was 1.3. The mean age at death was 58 years, 11 years younger than for the total floppy mitral valve series. The severity grade distribution was comparable to the grade distribution in the total floppy mitral valve group.

Fibrin Deposits at Mitral Leaflet-Left Atrial Angle

Fibrin deposits on the mitral valve or in the left atrial mitral angle were recognized in four hearts. The average age at death of these patients was 73 years. The small size and localized nature of fibrin deposits suggest that they might be missed on initial autopsy examination and would likely be missed on routine sectioning of the valves for microscopic evaluation. Moreover, the fragility of the fibrin deposits suggests they might not survive specimen storage. Thus, autopsy material might underestimate the actual incidence of angle-fibrin deposits.

Associated Conditions

Floppiness of Other Valves in Patients With Floppy Mitral Valve

The normal *tricuspid valve* has a generous amount of valve tissue, and some interchordal hooding is normal. In 41 (40 percent) of 102 hearts with floppy mitral valve, the tricuspid valve had excessive interchordal hooding and was considered to be abnormal. Histologic evaluation of the floppy tricuspid valve revealed changes comparable to those seen in the floppy mitral valve. The spongiosa was increased in volume and had invaded and disrupted the fibrosa. Fibroelastic deposits were present on both the atrial and ventricular aspects of the tricuspid leaflets. Thirty-nine of the 41 specimens had thin tricuspid valve chordae, and 15 of the 41 had friction lesions of the right ventricle. None of these specimens had ruptured chordae of the tricuspid valve, and none showed evidence of tricuspid valve insufficiency or bacterial endocarditis.

A thickened, floppy *pulmonary valve* was noted in 11 specimens; in none of these was there evidence of pulmonary valve regurgitation. A thickened, redundant *aortic valve* was present in two specimens. There was no evidence of aortic valve regurgitation in these hearts.

Connective Tissue Disorders

Marfan's syndrome was present in one of the 102 patients with floppy mitral valve. The male patient had died at age 44 years of complications following operative repair of an aneurysm of the ascending aorta and placement of an aortic valve prosthesis. Cystic medial necrosis of the aorta was present in four of the 102 specimens, two from men, two from women. Three patients had died as a result of dissecting aneurysm of the ascending aorta at ages 68, 71, and 81, respectively. The fourth patient had died of a ruptured abdominal aneurysm at age 76.

Secundum Atrial Septal Defect

The status of the atrial septum was evaluated in each of the 102 specimens. In 73 the foramen ovale was anatomically sealed. In 26 the foramen ovale was patent but guarded. Three (3 percent) had a secundum atrial septal defect. One of these was the heart from a 60-year-old man who had died of active bacterial endocarditis and mitral regurgitation.

Comparison with Other Autopsy Studies

Lucas and Edwards compared their autopsy study[10] with the autopsy studies of Pomerance[13] and of Davies and associates.[26] These latter two studies screened routine adult hospital necropsy specimens for floppy mitral valves and showed the following:

The incidence of floppy mitral valves was 1 percent (30 of 3083) in the study of Pomerance[13] and 4.5 percent (86 of 1984) in the study of Davies and associates.[26] The incidence of floppy mitral valves in our study was 7.4 percent (102 of 1376).[10] This discrepancy of incidence may be partly attributable to the increased awareness of this condition over time, so that it has been recognized more commonly in recent years. Moreover, while our criteria for the diagnosis of floppy mitral valve were comparable to those used by Davies and associates, the criteria of both these studies appeared more inclusive than the criteria of Pomerance.

The male-to-female ratios observed in these autopsy studies were as follows: Pomerance, 1.9;[13] our study, 1.5;[10] and Davies and associates, 1.0.[26] The male preponderance may be partly related to the higher male incidence encountered in routine autopsy studies. This is presumably due to the fact that legal and logistic factors favor obtaining permission for autopsy when the first spouse dies and make it more difficult when the surviving spouse dies. Since husbands more often predecease their wives, it is the men who are more likely to undergo autopsy. This factor also biases routine autopsy series to a younger age at death than that found in the general population. For whatever reason, the female preponderance noted in many clinical studies of prolapsed mitral valves is not confirmed by these three autopsy studies.

In each of the three autopsy studies, the age at death of patients with floppy mitral valve was comparable to the age at death of patients in the control autopsy groups.

The floppy mitral valve was considered to be the cause of death in 17 percent (15 of 86) of the patients studied by Davies and coworkers,[26] in 13 percent (4 of 30) of Pomerance's patients,[13] and in 4 percent (4 of 102) of our patients.[10] Ruptured chordae and bacterial endocarditis accounted for most of the deaths caused by floppy mitral valve in the series of Davies and associates[26] and accounted for all such deaths in the other two studies.[10,13] The relative infrequency of the floppy mitral valve as a cause of death and the normal age at death of patients with floppy mitral valve prompted Pomerance[13] and Davies and colleagues[26] to consider the floppy mitral valve a relatively benign condition. I agree with this view.

We detected no increase in the average severity of the floppy mitral valve as patients grew older. This supports Pomerance's observation that the patients with severe ballooning of the mitral valve showed no progression of this condition with aging.[13] On the other hand, minor degrees of interchordal hooding and minor increases in spongiosa do appear to be more frequent in older patients. It may be that these minor degrees of hooding and spongiosal increase are aging processes, whereas the floppy mitral valve, as defined in these autopsy studies, is not.

REFERENCES

1. Levine, SA and Thompson, WP: Systolic gallop rhythm: A clinical study. N Engl J Med 213:1021, 1935.
2. Harvey, WP, Foreward, IN, Cheitlin, MD, et al: Prolapsed mitral valve: The commonest valve disease? Curr Probl Cardiol 8:1, 1984.
3. Fernex, M and Fernex, C: La degenerescence mucoide des valvules mitrales. Helv Med Acta 25:694, 1958.
4. Oka, M and Angrist, A: Fibrous thickening with billowing sail distortion of the aging heart valve. Proc NY State Assoc Publ Health Lab 46:21, 1961.
5. Read, RC, Thal, AP, and Wendt, VE: Symptomatic valvular myxomatous transformation. Circulation 32:897, 1965.
6. Read, RC and Thal, AP: Surgical experience with symptomatic myxomatous valvular transformation (the floppy valve syndrome). Surgery 59:173, 1966.
7. Ranganathan, N, Lam, JHC, Wigle, ED, et al: Morphology of the human mitral valve: II. The valve leaflets. Circulation 41:459, 1970.
8. Ranganathan, N, Silver, MD, Robinson, TI, et al: Angiographic-morphologic correlation in patients with severe mitral regurgitation due to prolapse of the posterior mitral valve leaflet. Circulation 48:514, 1973.
9. Guthrie, RB and Edwards, JE: Pathology of the myxomatous mitral valve. Nature, secondary changes and complications. Minn Med 59:637, 1976.
10. Lucas, RV, Jr and Edwards, JE: The floppy mitral valve. Curr Probl Cardiol 7:1, 1982.
11. Perloff, JK and Roberts, WC: The mitral apparatus. Functional anatomy of mitral regurgitation. Circulation 46:227, 1972.
12. Shrivastava, S, Guthrie, RB, and Edwards, JE: Prolapse of the mitral valve. Mod Conc Cardiovasc Dis 462:57, 1977.
13. Pomerance, A: Ballooning deformity (mucoid degeneration) of atrioventricular valves. Br Heart J 31:343, 1969.
14. Salazar, AE and Edwards, JE: Friction lesions of ventricular endocardium. Relation to chordae tendineae of mitral valve. Arch Pathol Lab Med 90:364, 1970.
15. Barnett, HMJ: Embolism in mitral valve prolapse. Ann Rev Med 33:489, 1982.
16. Barlow, JB: Perspectives on the Mitral Valve. FA Davis, Philadelphia, 1986, p 98.
17. Corrigal, D, Bolen, J, and Hancock, E: Mitral valve prolapse and infective endocarditis. Am J Med 63:215, 1977.
18. Mills, P, Rose, J, Hollingsworth, BA, et al: Long-term prognosis of mitral-valve prolapse. N Engl J Med 297:13, 1977.
19. Kuhn, D and Weber, N: Mural bacterial endocarditis of a ventricular friction lesion. Arch Pathol Lab Med 95:92, 1973.
20. Allen, H, Harris, A, and Leatham, A: Significance and prognosis of an isolated late systolic murmur: A 9- to 22-year follow-up. Br Heart J 36:525,1974.
21. Nolan, CM, Kane, JJ, and Grunow, WA: Infective endocarditis and mitral prolapse: A comparison with other types of endocarditis. Arch Intern Med 141:447, 1981.
22. Corrigall, D, Bolen, J, Hancock, EW, et al: Mitral valve prolapse and infective endocarditis. Am J Med 63:215, 1977.
23. Jeresaty, RM, Edwards, JE, and Chawla, SK: Mitral valve prolapse and ruptured chordae tendineae. Am J Cardiol 55:138, 1985.
24. Osmundson, PJ, Callahan, JA, and Edwards, JE: Mitral insufficiency from rupture of chordae tendineae simulating aortic stenosis. Mayo Clin Proc 63:215, 1958.
25. Criley, JM, Lewis, KB, Humphries, JO, et al: Prolapse of the mitral valve: Clinical and cine-angiographic findings. Br Heart J 28:488, 1966.
26. Davies, MJ, Moore, BP, and Braimbridge, MV: The floppy mitral valve: Study of incidence, pathology and complications in surgical, necropsy and forensic material. Br Heart J 40:468, 1978.
27. Hancock, EW and Cohn, K: The syndrome associated with midsystolic click and late systolic murmur. Am J Med 41:183, 1966.

28. Barlow, JB, Bosman, CK, Pocock, WA, et al: Late systolic murmurs and non-ejection ("mid-late") systolic clicks: An analysis of 90 patients. Br Heart J 30:203, 1968.
29. Trent, JK, Adelman, AG, Wigle, ED, et al: Morphology of a prolapsed posterior mitral valve leaflet. Am Heart J 79:539, 1970.
30. Shappell, SD, Marshall, CE, Brown, RE, et al: Sudden death and the familial occurrence of mid-systolic click, late systolic murmur syndrome. Circulation 48:1128, 1973.
31. Marshall, CE and Shappell, SD: Sudden death and the ballooning posterior leaflet syndrome. Detailed anatomic and histochemical investigation. Arch Pathol 98:134, 1974.
32. Jeresaty, RM: Mitral valve prolapse-click syndrome. Prog Cardiovasc Dis 15:623, 1973.
33. Jeresaty, RM: Sudden death in the mitral valve prolapse-click syndrome. Am J Cardiol 37:317, 1976.
34. Gulotta, SJ, Gulco, L, Padmanabhan, V, et al: The syndrome of systolic click, murmur, and mitral valve prolapse—a cardiomyopathy? Circulation 49:717, 1974.
35. Appelblatt, NH, Willis, PW, III, Lenhart, JA, et al: Ten to 40 year follow-up of 69 patients with systolic click with or without apical late systolic murmur (abstr). Am J Cardiol 35:119, 1975.
36. Sorenson, HD and Smith RF: Lethal cardiac arrhythmias in the prolapsing valve syndrome (abstr). J Tenn Med Assoc 68:667, 1975.
37. Rakowski, H, Waxman, MB, Wald, RW, et al: Mitral valve prolapse and ventricular fibrillation (abstr). Circulation 52 (Suppl II):II-93, 1975.
38. Belardi, J, Lardani, H, Manubens, S, et al: Idiopathic prolapse of the mitral valve. A follow up study in 137 patients studied by angiography (abstr). Am J Cardiol 37:120, 1976.
39. Koch, FH and Hancock, EW: Ten year follow-up of forty patients with the mid-systolic click/late systolic murmur syndrome (abstr). Am J Cardiol 37:149, 1976.
40. Cobbs, BW, Jr and King, SB, III: Ventricular buckling: A factor in the abnormal ventriculogram and peculiar hemodynamics associated with mitral valve prolapse. Am Heart J 93:741, 1977.
41. Mills, P, Rose, J, Hollingsworth, J, et al: Long-term prognosis of mitral-valve prolapse. N Engl J Med 297:13, 1977.
42. Barnett, HJM, Jones, MW, Boughner, DR, et al: Cerebral ischemic events associated with prolapsing mitral valve. Arch Neurol 33:777, 1976.
43. Mair WJ: Sudden death in young females with floppy mitral valve syndrome. Aust NZ Med 10:221, 1980.
44. Bharati, S, Granston, AS, Liebson, PR, et al: The conduction system in mitral valve prolapse syndrome with sudden death. Am Heart J 101:667, 1981.
45. Bharati, S, Rosen, KM, Miller, LB, et al: Sudden death in three teenagers (abstr). Circulation 64 (Suppl IV):IV-72, 1981.
46. Dupasquier, E and Berney, JL: Le syndrome du prolapsus valvulaire mitral. Deux complications rares: la mort subite, l'embolie cerebrale. Schweiz Med Wochenschr 111:73, 1981.
47. Anderson, RC: Idiopathic mitral valve prolapse and sudden death (letter). Am Heart J 100:941, 1980.
48. Chesler, E, King, RA, and Edwards, JE: The myxomatous mitral valve and sudden death. Circulation 67:632, 1983.
49. Winkle, RA, Lopes, MG, and Fitzgerald, JW: Arrhythmias in patients with mitral valve prolapse. Circulation 52:73, 1975.
50. DeMaria, AN, Amsterdam, EA, Vismara, LA, et al: Arrhythmias in the mitral valve prolapse syndrome. Ann Intern Med 81:656, 1976.
51. Shappell, SD, Marshall, CE, Brown, RE, et al: Sudden death and the familial occurrence of mid-systolic click, late systolic murmur syndrome. Circulation 48:1128, 1973.
52. Jeresaty, R: Mitral valve prolapse. Raven Press, New York, 1979, p 209.
53. Senges, J, Zebe, H, Pelzer, D, et al: Nitrates and ectopic ventricular activity in mitral valve prolapse: Clinical and experimental data. Z Kardiol 68:26, 1979.
54. Malcolm, AD, Boughner, DR, Kostuk, et al: Clinical features and investigative findings in presence of mitral leaflet prolapse: Study of 85 consecutive patients. Br Heart J 38:244, 1976.
55. Murdock, JL, Walker, BA, Halpern, BL, et al: Life expectancy and causes of death in Marfan's syndrome. N Engl J Med 286:804, 1972.
56. Cabeen, WR, Jr, Reza, MJ, Kovick, RB, et al: Mitral valve prolapse and conduction defects in Ehlers-Danlos syndrome. Arch Intern Med 137:1227, 1977.
57. McKay, R and Yacoub MH: Acute aortic dissection and medial degeneration in patients with "floppy" mitral valves. Thorax 31:49, 1976.
58. Leachman, RD, Cokkinos, DV, and Cooley, DA: Association of ostium secundum atrial septal defects with mitral valve prolapse. Am J Cardiol 38:167, 1976.

CHAPTER 12

Complications of Mechanical Heart Valve Prostheses*

Malcolm D. Silver, M.D., Ph.D., F.R.C.P.C., F.R.C.P.A.

J. Butany, M.B.B.S., F.R.C.P.C.

During the past 40 years the management of valvular heart disease has improved remarkably. This change is attributable in part to increasingly sophisticated methods of diagnosis, in part to an enlarging pharmacopoeia that permits better medical management, and in part to improved surgical treatment with new anesthetic, perfusion, and operative techniques. Simple valve commissurotomy and the sophisticated plastic and reconstructive valve surgery practiced today allow palliation. The introduction of the heart valve prosthesis (HVP) more than 25 years ago provided a device that, in theory, allowed both the excision and replacement of a diseased valve and, for the treated patient, an increased life expectancy free of complications. That the insertion of an HVP "relieves a patient's symptoms, reduces the risk caused by the hemodynamic abnormality produced by the valvular disease," [1] and grants the individual a prolonged life is not in doubt; that prostheses do not yet meet full theoretical expectations is not surprising.

The functional parts of an individual prosthesis are composed either of tissue or of nontissue elements, giving rise to two families of HVP. Tissue valves, like native semilunar ones, have three cusps that allow a central flow through their lumens; on the other hand, nontissue or mechanical valves allow either a lateral (caged ball or caged disc valves) or a semicentral flow (tilting disc valves), depending on the location of the valve occluder when the prosthesis is open. The latter difference defines genera within the family of mechanical valves. Explanation of these terms and a description of the components of an artificial heart valve are found in the literature.[2]

To meet design criteria originally defined by Harken and colleagues[3] and to

*Supported in part by grants from the Ontario Heart and Stroke Foundation.

avoid infringing patent claims, HVPs, within the familial and generic categories defined, have a variety of morphologic forms. Recent publications define their gross[4] and radiologic[5] appearances and help both clinician and pathologist to identify them. Many HVPs illustrated in those publications are no longer inserted. Nevertheless, cohorts of patients bearing discontinued models live for many years. They are exposed to the complications associated with the valves, including those that may have caused a valve's withdrawal from the market. The individuals must be monitored closely, to define an optimal time for valve replacement.

Many considerations determine the choice of a prosthesis for a particular patient.[1,6–8] They include such things as the individual's cardiac anatomy, valvular lesion, previous medical history, age, lifestyle, and access to medical care. In addition, perceived advantages or disadvantages of tissue and mechanical valves govern selection. They relate to flow characteristics through, and gradients across, a valve; to the likelihood of its promoting thrombogenesis; and to infection control. The surgeon seeks the best match of patient and prosthesis.

Insertion of an HVP is not without risk. For example, 2 to 5 percent of patients die during the operation or in the immediate postoperative period, usually not from complications directly related to the inserted prosthesis, but to iatrogenic problems.[9] In addition, valve insertion engenders hazards by placing a foreign body in the bloodstream where it may promote thrombogenesis or act as a nidus for infection. Other potential hazards arise from a prosthesis' design, from biochemical degradation of its components, or from an interaction between the prosthesis and body elements. Once inserted, an HVP must open and close 35 to 40 million times a year. This functional demand stresses all components and, with time, some may fatigue or wear, to the detriment of function.

The earliest HVPs were tested by insertion in humans. In some instances, unexpected problems caused disasters. Nowadays, governmental regulations demand that extensive animal and laboratory testing, including accelerated bench tests, be done during valve development. Such tests may identify problems and lead to their correction. Once completed, the tests define a valve that has promising characteristics and performance. Clinical trials are still required because bench tests do not exactly mimic the situation in vivo, where problems not revealed by bench tests may manifest or where those revealed may evolve at a faster rate. Gersh and colleagues[10] have called for guidelines that would clarify procedures used to evaluate valves before market release and standardize initial clinical evaluation. The authors believe that this approach would facilitate the introduction of new models and aid clinicians making comparisons between HVPs.

In this chapter we present a historic perspective of the evolution of mechanical valves. It defines problems associated with prostheses and outlines steps manufacturers have taken to overcome these problems. Then, we discuss complications common to all mechanical valves and emphasize those associated with particular ones because of their design or structure. Most of these problems occur sometime after valve insertion, with many attributable to the valve itself.[8] We do not discuss complications causing "early" morbidity or death (i.e., within a month of valve insertion); rather, we refer the reader to publications that do.[2,11] In a subsequent chapter in this volume, Schoen and colleagues[12] discuss the clinicopathologic features of failure in tissue valves and the pathobiology of their calcification. We make no further reference to complications associated with bioprostheses.

HISTORIC PERSPECTIVE

Caged Ball Valves

The earliest, successful mechanical valves had a ball-shaped occluder or poppet that moved within a naked metal cage. The Starr-Edwards model 1000 prosthesis is an example. In this design, a Silastic ball moving within a metal cage occluded the valve lumen part way between the occluder's equator and pole.

Thrombus developed on these prostheses at sites of relative stasis or at interfaces between different components. Initially, such thrombus is soft and friable but, with time, it can organize to form a tough pannus. Particular sites of thrombus formation were junctions between the cloth sewing ring and the metal ring on both inflow and outflow surfaces and at the base of struts. As complications of this deposition, thrombus could encroach upon the valve lumen and stenose or occlude it; extend along the struts (Fig. 12–1) and interfere with poppet movement or seating; or, rarely, completely encase the cage and freeze poppet movement (poppet entrapment) (Fig. 12–2). If a thrombus formed at the apex of a cage (see Fig. 12–1), it might cause a poppet to stick there. Any thrombus could give rise to emboli or act as a nidus for infection.

Observations on the location of thrombi led initially to a reduction in the amount of metal exposed to the bloodstream at the orifice of Starr-Edwards valves (models 1200, 1260, 6000, and 6120). Subsequently, metal was covered with cloth (Starr-Edwards series 2300 and 6300) or cloth mesh. The Braunwald-Cutter prosthesis was a model for the latter development. The concept was that thrombus would coat the cloth or mesh and, on being organized, provide a nonthrombogenic surface. Regrettably, connective tissue formation, or its coating of cloth- or mesh-covered struts, proved both unpredictable and uncontrollable. Thus, not all of a surface would be coated. Alternatively, the bulk of the coating could interfere with poppet movement. Also, cloth increased hemolysis and obstructed flow through a prosthesis; cloth mesh did this to a lesser extent. In addition, the cloth wore with time and, in

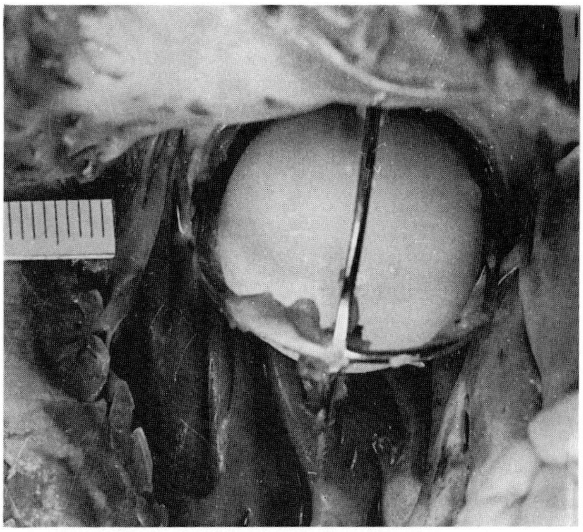

Figure 12–1. Starr-Edwards model 6120 prosthesis in tricuspid area, viewed from its ventricular aspect. Thrombus extends along the struts of the cage from their bases and is attached at the apex of the cage. Thrombus on the struts could interfere with poppet movement; thrombus at the cage's apex causes the ball to stick there. (Scale = 1 cm.)

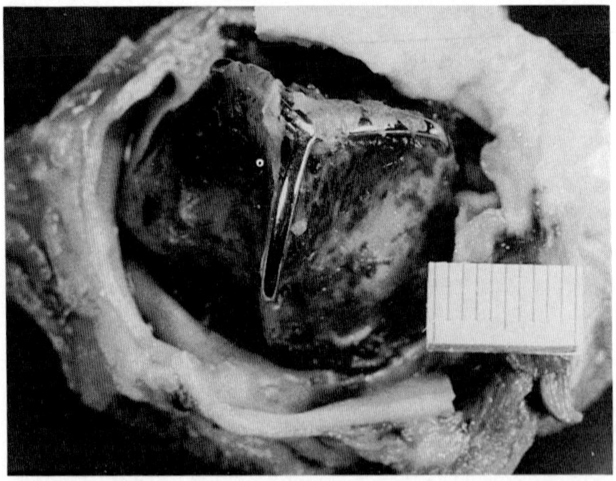

Figure 12–2. Starr-Edwards model 1260 prosthesis in aortic area, viewed from its aortic aspect. Thrombus encased the prosthesis' cage and "froze" poppet movement. (Scale = 1 cm.)

fraying, gave rise to emboli and aggravated hemolysis. Loss of cloth in the Braunwald-Cutter prosthesis allowed poppet escape.[13,14]

A marked reduction in thrombogenesis had to await a better understanding of surface properties. Initially, nonwettable surfaces such as Teflon were used on disc valves. A revolutionary change occurred when pyrolytic carbon was introduced to coat surfaces.[15] It is an extremely hard substance. Smooth, clean, LTI pyrolyte carbon has excellent thromboresistant properties inherent in its physical and chemical structure and does not alter plasma proteins. Its biocompatibility relies on an intermediate, dynamically absorbed, protein layer at its interface. Newer model prostheses are coated with this material.

With time the silicone rubber ball of early valves imbibed lipid with yellowing and softening of its substance (Fig. 12–3). As Schoen[11] comments, this is the only example of a biochemical degradation known to occur in a prosthetic valve component. The resultant changes led to ball "variance." This development interfered with occluder seating, allowed fragments of the ball to embolize distally, or caused the poppet to impact in the valve lumen or escape from its cage. The problem was solved by altering the manner of "curing" the silicone rubber in manufacture.[16] With that change, poppets currently made of this material endure well and rarely show abnormalities.[17]

The introduction of a Stellite ball in the cloth-covered prosthesis (Starr-Edwards 2300 and 6300 series) represented one attempt to overcome poppet variance before the problem with silicone rubber was resolved. In function the metal ball was noisy, a problem not unique to this type of prosthesis. Also, the metal poppet wore cloth coating the struts of the cage. The composite cloth/metal seat (models 2310 and 6310) and track (models 2400 and 6400) followed, so that moving metal was in contact with metal. However, friction caused both metal and cloth to wear[18] (Fig. 12–4).

The high profile of early ball valves could cause disproportion. For example, in the mitral area, a prosthesis might (1) obstruct the left ventricular outflow tract; (2) impinge upon nearby structures, causing endocardial thickening or erosion with mural thrombus formation and the threat of emboli; or (3) become incorporated into the myocardium. If a prosthesis impinged upon the septal wall of the left ventricle and affected conducting system fibers, arrythmias could develop. With aortic valve

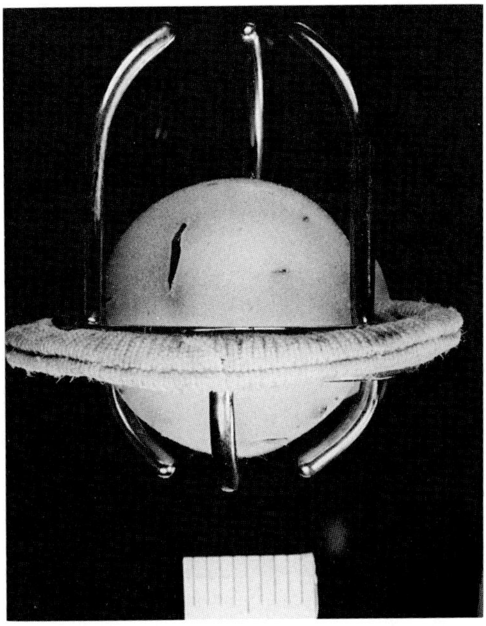

Figure 12–3. Smeloff-Cutter valve showing splits and cracks in silicone rubber occluder caused by lipid imbibition. In the fresh state, the ball was yellow. (Scale = 1 cm.)

replacement, a narrow ascending aorta stretched about the perimeter of the cage could lead to severe hemolysis or prosthesis dysfunction caused by interference with poppet movement. The latter problem is now predicted before, or recognized during, operation and prevented or treated by inserting a cloth gusset in the ascending aorta. Nevertheless, the pathologist sees minor forms of disproportion at necropsy, presenting as areas of endocardial thickening or indentations in the aortic intima, related to the struts of a prosthesis' cage.

The closed cage of early model ball valves was thought to add to turbulence. To overcome this abnormality and enlarge the valve lumen, thereby improving both

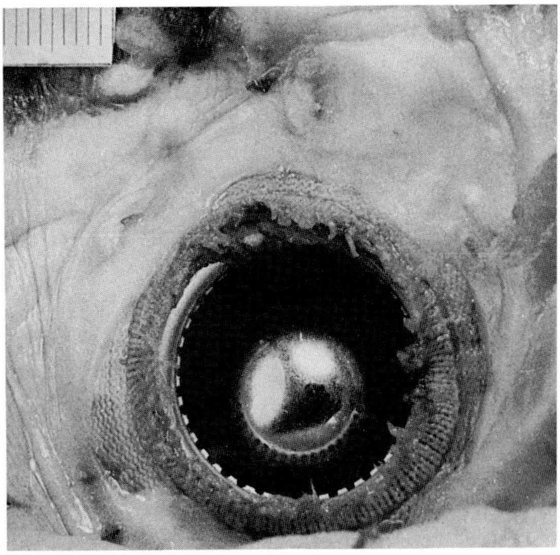

Figure 12–4. Composite seat of cloth covered Starr-Edwards model 6310 prosthesis in mitral area, viewed from its atrial aspect. Note cloth fraying and tearing, wearing of mitral studs in seat characterized by their varying height, and thrombus deposited at cloth-metal interface at 12 o'clock position. (Scale = 1 cm.)

hydraulics and transvalvular gradient, an open-caged prosthesis that had the ball occlude the lumen at its equator was designed. This change lowered valve profile, gave the prosthesis two cages, and permitted modest "back flow" to inhibit thrombogenesis. The Smeloff-Cutter (now Smeloff-Sutter) prosthesis is an example (see Fig. 12–3). Many such prostheses functioned well but, in some, the metal ends of the cage became entangled in pectinate muscles, were incorporated into the myocardium, or affected other cardiac structures (e.g., a coronary artery).[17] This could interfere with prosthesis function.

Caged Disc Valves

The caged disc valve evolved in parallel with the caged ball valve. The Beall model is an example. Its design produced a valve of low profile and larger lumen, because the disc occluded the orifice by covering it. Coating metal surfaces at the ring and in the lumen with Dacron velour reduced thromboembolic complications[19] but made the valve prone to cloth wear where the disc hit it, on occlusion.[19,20] Worn and torn cloth herniated into the valve orifice, obstructed it, and aggravated hemolysis[20] (Figs. 12–5*A*, *B*). In this HVP the disc and struts were coated with Teflon, because of that substance's nonwettable properties. However, the material wore with time (Figs. 12–5*A*, *B*). This development could cause a poppet to tilt, move irregularly, or escape from the cage.[19–22] Nowadays, the metal struts and disc of the Beall valve (model 106) are covered with pyrolytic carbon. This change reduced hemolysis and eliminated poppet wear but not wear of the Dacron velour where the disc strikes it on occluding the valve.[20]

Tilting Disc Valves

Tilting disc valves were the next development. In this design, the disc occluded a valve within its lumen, instead of overlying the orifice. These valves had some of the advantages of a caged disc valve and allowed a semicentral blood flow. The Björk-Shiley prosthesis is such a valve. Its design allowed "backflow" when the disc closed, to inhibit thrombogenesis. Early models had Delrin discs.[23] Subsequently, they were replaced by ones coated with pyrolytic carbon, now used in all disc valves. Thrombi form on disc valves at cloth-metal interfaces (Fig. 12–6) and at or near the disc's pivot point(s) in areas of relative stasis. They could grow to interfere with a disc's movement or completely entrap it (Fig. 12–6). The risk of disc entrapment led to changes in the design of the disc of the Björk-Shiley valve from a flat-topped structure to the current convexoconcave design.[24] Also, the angle of disc opening was increased from 60 to 70 degrees.[24] A problem of metal fatigue affected the minor strut of the 60-degree model at the site where the strut was welded to the ring; strut fracture and disc embolization were the results.[25–29] The defect has been resolved with the current monostrut design.[30]

More recently introduced tilting disc valves permit a wider angle of disc opening and, as a result, more of a central flow through the valve. Lillehei-Kaster,[31] Omniscience,[32,33] and Medtronic-Hall[32,34] prostheses are examples. The St. Jude Medical prosthesis[35,36] has a unique, double-leaflet design. It is made of machined graphite, is coated with pyrolytic carbon, and has neither seams nor welds.

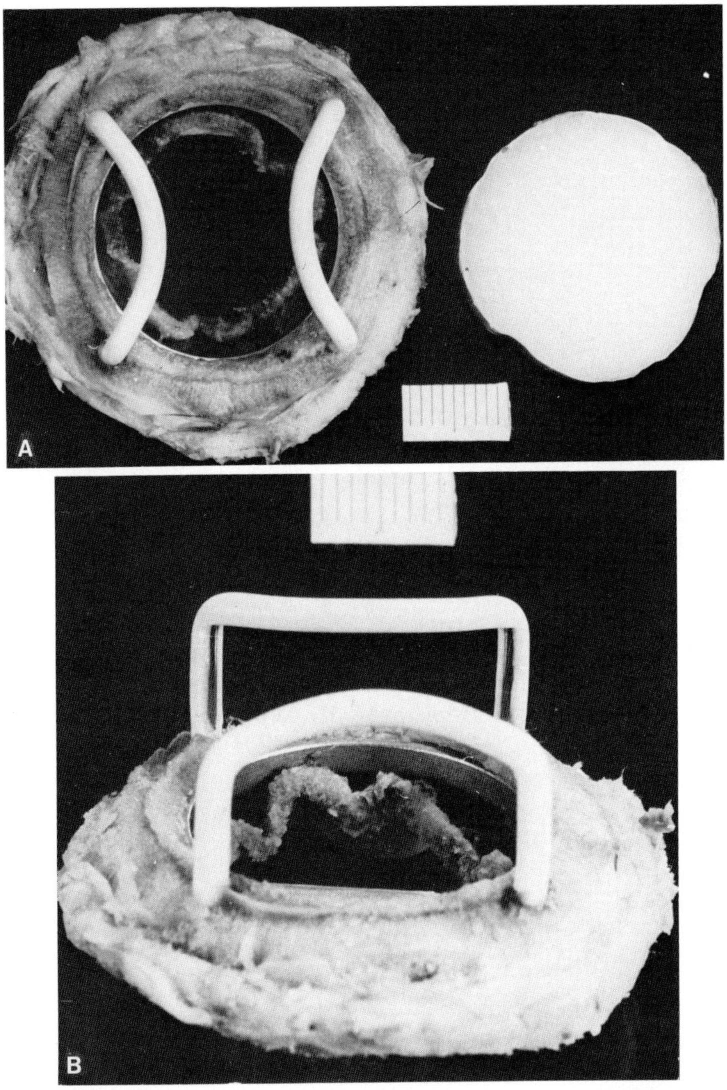

Figure 12–5. Surgically excised model 104 Beall prosthesis from mitral area viewed from its ventricular aspect (*A*). It shows wear at the edge of the Teflon disc caused by friction against the struts of the cage. Note cloth wear, fraying, and tearing where disc hit Dacron velour seat on occluding the valve. Torn cloth has herniated toward inflow surface stenosing the lumen. *B*, Lateral view demonstrates wear of the Teflon on the struts. Note angulated cloth/thrombus surface of the "seat" (to the *left*). Wear at this stage produces distinct shelving of the disc's edge. Once the disc is in contact with metal, wear proceeds at a faster rate. The torn and herniated cloth seat is well seen. (Scale = 1 cm.)

COMPLICATIONS COMMON TO ALL MECHANICAL HEART VALVES

Thrombus Formation/Thromboemboli

When older mechanical valves are examined at necropsy or surgical pathology, they often show minute, if locally inconsequential, thrombi attached to them at the sites previously defined. Histologically, tiny fresh or organized thrombi are also

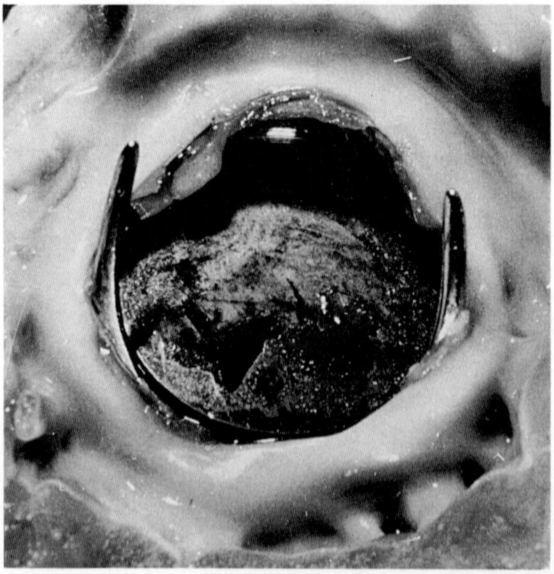

Figure 12–6. Lillehei-Kaster prosthesis in mitral area, viewed from ventricular aspect. Thrombus has entrapped the disc, freezing its movement. Note thrombus at edge of cloth-metal interface.

found on the connective tissue that coats the sewing ring of all mechanical valves. Large thrombi that stenose or occlude a valve lumen or that interfere with poppet movement or seating are found less frequently. When they occur, they are somewhat more prevalent on disc valves. For example, Björk-Shiley prostheses with a flat-topped disc or when placed in the tricuspid area are particularly prone to disc entrapment,[37,38] but this complication is not unique to that type of prosthesis[32,38,39] (Fig. 12–6). A minor degree of stenosis of a valve's orifice, caused by thrombus or pannus, or both, encroaching on it, is also a frequent finding with mechanical HVPs that have been in situ many years (Fig. 12–7).

Thromboembolic complications arising from thrombi are much more frequent than those complications caused by a bulky thrombus affecting a prosthesis' func-

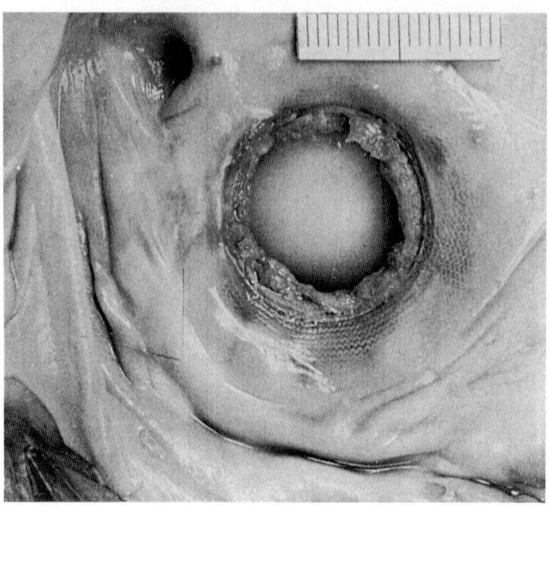

Figure 12–7. Starr-Edwards model 6120 prosthesis that had been in the mitral area for 11 years. Photograph shows the atrial aspect. The cloth sewing ring has been coated with tissue. A combination of thrombus and pannus attached at the cloth-metal interface, encroaches upon the lumen and stenoses it. (Scale = 2 cm.)

tion. Consensus has it that thromboembolic complications diminish in number after a mechanical valve has been in place 12 months.[40] This is attributed to a gradual coating of both surfaces of a cloth sewing ring by connective tissue (Fig. 12–7). However, thromboembolic complications may occur anytime after a mechanical valve is inserted. The tiny thrombi, demonstrable on the valves at necropsy or in surgical pathology, offer a logical explanation for this occurrence. Thus, patients bearing mechanical HVPs require anticoagulant therapy—a dictum not accepted by all.[41] Coating mechanical valves with pyrolytic carbon has reduced the risk of thromboembolic complications[40] but has not eliminated them.[31–36] Factors known to promote thromboemboli include a prosthesis' location in the mitral area, inadequate anticoagulation, a temporary interruption of anticoagulant therapy, and atrial fibrillation.[40,42]

Not all thromboemboli cause clinical symptoms; some symptoms are transient. Edmund[40] has emphasized a need to standardize definitions of thrombotic phenomena and to report the events for valve models and anatomic locations actuarially and in terms of incidence per 100 patient-years of followup. In this respect, comparative studies of such complications made between different valves and at one institution are useful.[33,43,44] Of thromboembolic complications that do cause symptoms, 40 to 50 percent produce severe or fatal effects, with many episodes (about 80 percent) presenting with cerebral symptoms.[40] In general, thromboemboli arise more often from mitral than aortic HVPs (4 per 100 patient-years versus 2 per 100 patient-years).[40]

Coumarin anticoagulants are the usual means of maintaining long-term anticoagulation therapy in patients with mechanical HVPs. The aim is to prolong the prothrombin time 2.0 to 2.5 times over control values. Some authors add antiplatelet drugs to the regimen,[45] while, as indicated, others do not give anticoagulant therapy to children bearing St. Jude Medical prostheses.[41] Of note is the cautionary editorial comment at the end of the latter paper[41] and the opinion of others using the same valve.[35,36]

Anticoagulant treatment promotes the risk of hemorrhage. Trauma and a markedly prolonged prothrombin time are the most frequent precursors of hemorrhage.[40] When it occurs, it is most likely to affect the central nervous system (CNS) or the genitourinary or gastrointestinal tract. Nonfatal hemorrhages have an instance of 0.5 to 6.3 per 100 patient-years, whereas the incidence of fatal bleeding is 0.1 to 0.2 per 100 patient-years. Most fatal episodes are the result of bleeding into the CNS.

Complications caused by thrombi forming on a mechanical HVP or from resultant thromboemboli are recognized by the symptoms and signs that they evince.[37,38,46–48] Valve function can be affected, and valve obstruction may be fatal unless recognized and treated promptly, or symptoms may be referable to distal organs. The latter may be transient or prolonged.

If a valve's function is affected, symptoms may evolve insidiously or rapidly.[46–48] The valve's opening and closing sounds may change or murmurs develop. Fluoroscopy or cineangiography may reveal that the occluder seats improperly, that its excursion is diminished, or that it does not move; echocardiography may show the thrombus if it is large enough or, if there is thrombotic occlusion of the valve, decreased amplitude of valve excursion associated with diminished opening and closing rates or absent disc motion. Doppler techniques may demonstrate valve dysfunction.[49] Cardiac catheterization and angiography may reveal thrombus on the valve, valve incompetence, decreased disc mobility, or excessive pressure gradients across the prosthesis.

A thrombosed valve may be treated by fibrinolytic therapy, if in the tricuspid area,[37,38] by debridement,[47,48] or by valve replacement.[38,46–48] Each form of therapy may be successful. Adequate anticoagulant therapy following lysis or removal of thrombus is essential.

The patient with a thromboembolus is treated symptomatically, and the valve is investigated. The results of the investigation may require any of the aforementioned treatments, but in most instances, no thrombus will be found on the prosthesis. Strict control of anticoagulant therapy is indicated after a thromboembolic event.[40]

Infective Endocarditis

Infective endocarditis may affect a mechanical HVP soon after insertion or have a "late" onset (more than 2 months after valve placement). Unfortunately, the risk of late infection does not diminish with time; Schoen[11] cites a case that occurred after 22 years. The precise incidence of infection is not known because long-term followup studies are often incomplete, but it is estimated at 0.2 to 0.5 percent per annum,[50] affecting up to 3.2 percent of patients with prosthetic valves.[51] Although the disease is infrequent, it is a dreaded complication because of the associated high mortality.[50–52] No type of mechanical valve is less prone to infection than another,[11,32,50] but aortic prostheses are infected approximately twice as often as mitral ones.[50] More than one prosthesis may be infected in a patient, and recurrent infections of a single valve occur.

Prosthetic valve endocarditis is usually preceded by a distinctive event that increases the risk of bacteremia.[52] Usually, the infection begins on the surface coating the sewing ring. Many different organisms may be the cause, but staphylococci and streptococci are still the most frequent; gram-negative and fungal organisms also are infective agents.[50–53]

Infected vegetations attached to an HVP behave in the same manner as a bland thrombus (Fig. 12–8), and give rise to emboli or affect valve function. Damage caused by myocarditis or abscesses and/or areas of myocardial necrosis resulting from emboli may adversely affect the outcome if a patient needs surgical treatment. Mycotic aneurysms are an uncommon complication. If an infection spreads locally to invade adjacent tissues, it may cause an anular abscess.[54] They are more often associated with infections of aortic HVPs and cause dehiscences of a prosthesis, allowing paravalvular leaks (Fig. 12–9). Alternatively, the infection may extend beyond the confines of the anulus, leading to sinuses or fistulas that point toward or enter other cardiac structures.[55] For example, an aortic anular abscess may extend into the aorta proximally. Lateral spread from the aortic area may involve any of the heart chambers, the pulmonary artery, or the pericardium. Distal spread extends into the anterior mitral leaflet or the left ventricle. In the latter instance, an abscess may destroy the atrioventricular node or bundle of His and cause complete heart block or produce a ventricular septal defect. The much less frequent mitral anular abscess can spread proximally into the left atrial wall or interatrial septum, distally into the left ventricle, or laterally to reach the epicardium. The latter is usual. If so, the circumflex coronary artery may develop an arteritis and/or thrombose, with the resultant myocardial infarction adding to the symptom complex.

The signs and symptoms of prosthetic valve endocarditis arise from (1) proliferation of microorganisms in the bloodstream, (2) local or distal complications of the

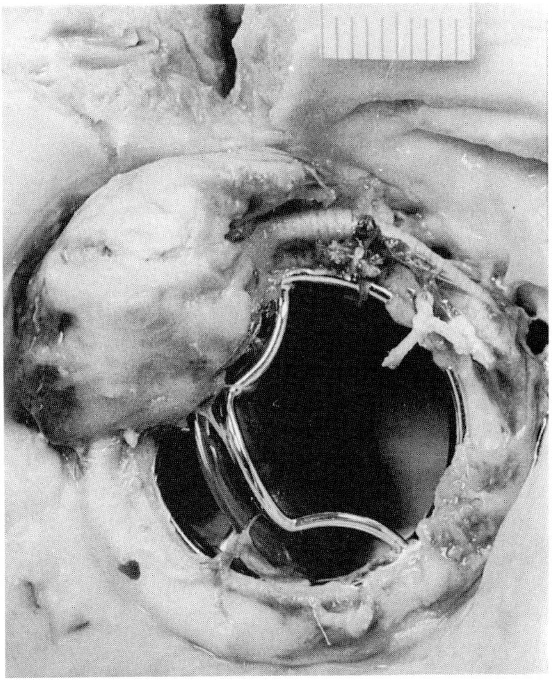

Figure 12-8. Mitral Björk-Shiley prosthesis, viewed from the atrial aspect. The disc is "frozen" in position because of a large infected vegetation (Streptococcus viridans) on the sewing ring and encroaching on the lumen. Note small dehiscences (dark areas) at perimeter of sewing ring at 1 and 2 o'clock positions. (Scale = 1 cm.)

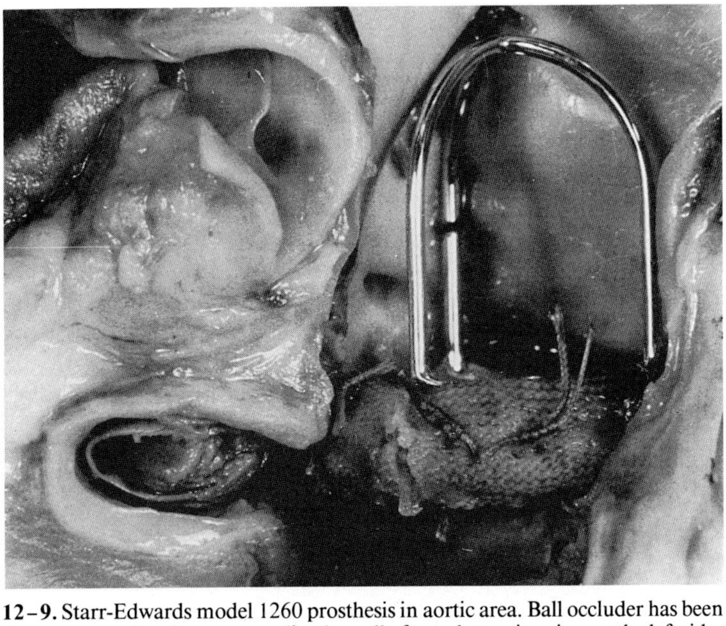

Figure 12-9. Starr-Edwards model 1260 prosthesis in aortic area. Ball occluder has been removed in this lateral view. Note anular abscess extending laterally from the sewing ring on the left side. Sewing ring has infected vegetations (Staphylococcus aureus) on its surface. The prosthesis had dehisced from its anular attachment.

disease, or (3) a loss of valve function. Fever, a new cardiac murmur, or manifestations of neurological complications are the most frequent symptoms.[50–53] Indeed, fever is such a common presenting symptom that it should always raise the suspicion of infective endocarditis.[50] Blood cultures, in patients with symptoms, are usually positive.[50–52] The bacteremia associated with prosthetic valve endocarditis is continuous. Thus, timing blood collection with chills or temperature elevation is not critical.[50] Several separate cultures should be collected. One must remember that bacteremia may occur in a patient with a prosthetic heart valve, without the valve being infected. The recovery of microorganisms from a blood culture should suggest the possibility of infection, but the finding must be related to the patient's history and the likelihood of culture contamination. Isolation of a similar microorganism from two or more separate blood cultures makes contamination less likely.

Echocardiography may define vegetations, but interference by echoes arising from the prosthesis may make interpretation difficult.[50,51,56,57] The technique does help define complications of the infection, such as valve dehiscence or anular abscess.[58] Cinefluoroscopy may reveal valve instability resulting from dehiscence. Cardiac catheterization may be dangerous.

Treatment involves using the appropriate antibiotic in bactericidal doses.[50–53] Medical treatment will cure some cases of prosthetic valve endocarditis but combined medical and surgical treatment is often required. Controversy surrounds some aspects of surgical treatment. Currently, indications for valve replacement during active infective endocarditis include severe heart failure, persistent sepsis, recurrent emboli, or an unstable prosthetic valve.[59,60] Relative indications include early disease and an associated periprosthetic leak.[59] The operative mortality is high.[59,60]

Pathologists must look for signs of healed prosthetic valve endocarditis in patients coming to necropsy.

Turbulent Flow and Hemolysis

Semicentral or central flow prostheses cause less blood turbulence than ones with lateral flow characteristics. The relatively small lumen of high-profile ball valves produces high transvalvular gradients. This is also a problem with small-sized disc valves. These gradients and the turbulence increase shear stress and damage red blood cells, with ensuing hemolysis. Covering the surface of a mechanical prosthesis with cloth aggravated this process as did complications such as ball variance or paravalvular leak. At autopsy, renal tubular hemosiderosis is an almost constant finding in a patient who has borne these types of mechanical valves for many years. Moreover, Harrison and colleagues[61] drew attention to a higher frequency of cholelithiasis in patients with HVPs. Newer, tilting disc models cause far less hemolysis.[34]

Generally, patients compensate for the hemolysis by increasing bone marrow function. A loss of compensation may herald a new complication, for example, a paravalvular leak or degeneration of valve components. Indeed, Schoen[11] suggests that the onset of hemolytic anemia in a patient bearing one of the newer mechanical prostheses should prompt a search for a cause. Few patients with modern prostheses develop anemia. A minority (10 to 15 percent) of those with older prostheses do present with either a hemolytic or an iron-deficiency anemia. The anemia is diagnosed by appropriate hematologic investigation. Treatment with supplementary iron by mouth may suffice, but blood transfusion or valve replacement may be indicated.

Turbulence associated with mechanical HVPs may cause endocardial thickening in the chamber or vessel distal to the prosthesis. To our knowledge, this does not interfere with either valve or cardiac function. Some authors[62,63] have suggested that intimal thickening of the ascending aorta, resulting from turbulence, could cause coronary ostial stenosis.

Paravalvular Leaks and Valve Dehiscence

Small paravalvular defects, found at the edge of a valve's sewing ring and usually no more than 1 to 2 mm in diameter, are the result of tissue retraction on healing. They had been encountered in approximately 10 percent of cases at autopsy, but their frequency has diminished of late. Their presence may be manifest by hemolysis or a murmur and is proven by echocardiographic, Doppler, or hemodynamic studies. If the defect causes a small leak, its effects (e.g., hemolysis) rather than the defect itself may be treated. If it is larger and especially if valve function is compromised, surgical repair may be required. A major dehiscence is usually an indication that the valve is infected.

PARTICULAR PROBLEMS WITH PARTICULAR PROSTHESES

Many of the problems unique to particular prostheses have been mentioned earlier. They reflect a poor design or a poor choice of material for manufacture. Most became obvious as different valves evolved.

The movement of the occluder of a disc valve may be interfered with by long sutures, remnants of chordae tendineae, or adjacent tissue remnants.[64–66] This can interfere with valve function and induce transient cerebral or syncopal symptoms or jam the disc in the closed position and cause sudden death. This problem may affect ball valves, but the effects are less pronounced.[17]

The Beall model 105 valve could be mishandled by a surgeon, stressing the struts and leading to their fracture at their junction with the cross-piece of the cage.[67] This problem usually occurred within the first year of insertion, but it has been overcome. Recently, we have seen Beall model 105 valves in which the pyrolytic carbon coating at the base of struts was cracked. We assume that one fatal case, in which a strut was fractured at that site with disc escape, is a consequence. We are not certain if the morphologic change is principally the result of the "brittleness" of pyrolytic carbon or due to metal fatigue and rupture, promoting secondary changes in the carbon coating.

Rigorous bench testing prior to commercial release and quality control mechanisms during manufacture limit the likelihood of early component failure. Nevertheless, one wonders if reports of catastrophes, such as the loss of a single disc of a St. Jude Medical prosthesis, represent a unique defect in a particular valve, an iatrogenic problem at the time of insertion, or an example of the valve being subject to an unusual stress.[68]

The relentless need for a mechanical valve to function year after year unmasks patterns of wear[18,69] or component fatigue that may cause problems. The experience with the 60-degree Björk-Shiley prosthesis dictates that valves have a monostructure; sites of welding are areas of potential weakness. Fatigue in metal and other components may have future implications. We have described metal wear in the Björk-Shiley[70] and Lillehei-Kaster HVPs.[71] The latter valve presented a corrugated pattern that is probably the result of "stick-slip" wear, related to the layer of protein that exists between stationary metal and the moving disc of that prosthesis. None of the patients in whom metal wear was demonstrated in either prosthesis had clinical abnormalities.

CONCLUSION

Some mechanical valves (e.g., Starr-Edwards models 1260 and 6120) have had a remarkably successful and long life. Indeed, they provide the "gold standard" against which newer models are judged. Newer models, coated with pyrolytic carbon, offer advantages in flow characteristics and reduced thromboembolic complications. However, no available mechanical valve is ideal. Clinicians and pathologists must be vigilant to define yet unknown modes of valve failure.

Arguments as to the value of tissue versus mechanical valves will undoubtedly continue. Protagonists for each type will seek methods of improving models, especially the durability of tissue valves. With the advent of new technologies and materials, one would anticipate that a plastic valve, with semilunar cusps, may not be far off.

REFERENCES

1. Editorial: Which heart valve prosthesis. Lancet 2:756, 1985.
2. Silver, MD and Wilson, GJ: Pathology of cardiovascular prostheses including coronary artery bypass and other vascular grafts. In Silver, MD (ed): Cardiovascular Pathology. Churchill-Livingstone, New York, 1983.
3. Harken, DE, Taylor, WJ, Lefemine, AA, et al: Aortic valve replacement with a caged ball valve. Am J Cardiol 9:292, 1962.
4. Morse, D and Steiner, RM: Cardiac valve identification atlas and guide. In Morse, D, Steiner, RM, and Fernandez, J (eds): Guide to Prosthetic Cardiac Valves. Springer Verlag, New York, 1985.
5. Steiner, RM and Flicker, S: The radiology of prosthetic cardiac valves. In Morse, D, Steiner, RM, and Fernandez, J (eds): Guide to Prosthetic Cardiac Valves. Springer Verlag, New York, 1985.
6. Lefrak, EA and Starr, A: Choice of prostheses. In Cardiac Valve Prostheses. Appleton-Century-Crofts, New York, 1979.
7. Weiland, AP: A review of cardiac valve prostheses and their selection. Heart Lung 12:498, 1983.
8. Selzer, A: Recent status of prosthetic cardiac valves. Arch Intern Med 143:1965, 1983.
9. Schoen, FJ, Titus, JL, and Lawrie, GM: Autopsy-determined causes of death after cardiac valve replacement. JAMA 249:889, 1983.
10. Gersh, BJ, Fisher, LD, Schaff, HV, et al: Issues concerning the clinical evaluation of new prosthetic valves. J Thorac Cardiovasc Surg 91:460, 1986.
11. Schoen, FJ: Pathology of cardiac valve replacement. In Morse, D, Steiner, RM, and Fernandez, J (eds): Guide to Prosthetic Cardiac Valves. Springer Verlag, New York, 1985.
12. Schoen, FJ, Kujovich, JL, Levy, RJ, et al: Bioprosthetic valve failure. In Waller, BF (ed): Contemporary Issues in Cardiovascular Pathology. Vol 18, No 2. FA Davis, Philadelphia, 1987.
13. Schoen, FJ, Goodenough, SH, Ionescu, MI, et al: Implications of late morphology of Braunwald-Cutter mitral heart valve prostheses. J Thorac Cardiovasc Surg 88:208, 1984.
14. Jonas, RA, Barratt-Boyes, BG, Kerr, AR, et al: Late follow-up of the Braunwald-Cutter valve. Ann Thorac Surg 33:554, 1982.
15. Bokros, JC, LaGrange, LD, and Schoen, FJ: Control of structure of carbon for use in bioengineering. In Walker, PL (ed): Chemistry and Physics of Carbon. Marcel Dekker, New York, 1973.
16. Hylen, JC, Hodam, RP, and Kloster, FE: Changes in the durability of silicone rubber in ball-valve protheses. Ann Thorac Surg 13:324, 1972.
17. Harlan, BJ, Smeloff, EA, Miller, GJ, Jr, et al: Performance of the Smeloff aortic valve beyond ten years. J Thorac Cardiovasc Surg. 91:86, 1986.
18. Warnes, CA, McIntosh, CL, and Roberts, WC: Wear of the metallic studs on the component seat of the 2320 Starr-Edwards aortic valve and its clinical consequences. Am J Cardiol 52:1062, 1983.
19. Joob, AW, Kron, IL, Craddock, GB, et al: A decade of experience with the model 103 and 104 Beall valve prosthesis. J Thorac Cardiovasc Surg 89:444, 1985.
20. Fernandez, J, Chang, K, Gooch, A, et al: Anatomic and clinical analysis of 96 Beall prostheses explanted over a 13-year period. Chest 83:632, 1983.
21. Clark, RE, Grubbs, FL, McKnight, RC, et al: Late clinical problems with Beall model 103 and 104 mitral valve protheses: Hemolysis and valve wear. Ann Thorac Surg 21:475, 1976.

22. Silver, MD and Wilson, GJ: The pathology of wear in the Beall model 104 heart valve prostheses. Circulation 56:617, 1977.
23. Montero, CG, Rufilanchas, JJ, Juffe, A, et al: Long-term results of cardiac valve replacement with the Delrin-Disc model of the Björk-Shiley prosthesis. Ann Thorac Surg 37:328, 1984.
24. Björk, VO: The optimal opening angle of the Björk-Shiley tilting disc valve. Scand J Thorac Cardiovasc Surg 15:223, 1982.
25. Sacks, SH, Northeast, AD, and Watkins, J: Late strut fracture in a Björk-Shiley valve prosthesis. Br Heart J 51:578, 1984.
26. Garcia-del-Castillo, H, Larrouse-Pérez, E, Murtra-Férre, et al: Strut fracture and disc embolization of a Björk-Shiley mitral valve prosthesis. Am J Cardiol 55:597, 1985.
27. Khalil, Y, Sethia, B, Quin, RO, et al: Disc and strut embolization after minor strut fracture in a Björk-Shiley mitral valve prosthesis. Thorax 40:158, 1985.
28. Guit, GL, van Voorthuisen, AE, and Steiner, RM: Outlet strut fracture of the Björk-Shiley mitral valve prosthesis. Radiology 154:295, 1985.
29. Sacks, SH, Harrison, M, Bischler, PJE, et al: Metallurgical analysis of failed Björk-Shiley cardiac valve. Thorax 41:142, 1986.
30. Aris, A, Crexelli, C, Augé, JM, et al: Hemodynamic evaluation of the integral monostrut Björk-Shiley prosthesis in the aortic position. Ann Thorac Surg 40:234, 1985.
31. Levang, OW, Levorstad, K, and Haugland, T: Aortic valve replacement. A randomized study comparing the Björk-Shiley and Lillehei-Kaster disc valves. Scand J Thorac Cardiovasc Surg 14:7, 1980.
32. Cortina, JM, Martinell, J, Artiz, V, et al: Comparative clinical results with Omniscience (STM 1), Medtronic-Hall and Björk-Shiley convexo-concave (70 degrees) prostheses in mitral valve replacement. J Thorac Cardiovasc Surg 91:174, 1986.
33. Rábago, G, Martinell, J, Faile, J, et al: Results and complications with the Omniscience prosthesis. J Thorac Cardiovasc Surg 87:136, 1984.
34. Nitter-Hauge, S, Semb, B, Abdelnoor, M, et al: A 5-year experience with the Medtronic-Hall disc valve prosthesis. Circulation 68(Suppl 2):169, 1983.
35. Duveau, D, Michaud, JL, Despins, PL, et al: Mitral valve replacement with St. Jude Medical prosthesis. Incidence of thromboembolic events in 349 patients. Eur Heart J 5(Suppl D):49, 1984.
36. Baudet, IM, Oca, CC, Rogues, XF, et al: A 5 1/2 year experience with the St. Jude Medical cardiac valve prosthesis. J Thorac Cardiovasc Surg 90:137, 1985.
37. Boskovic, D, Elezovic, I, Boskovic, D, et al: Late thrombosis of the Björk-Shiley tilting disc valve in the tricuspid position. J Thorac Cardiovasc Surg vol 91, 1986.
38. Thornburn, CW, Morgan, JJ, Shanahan, MX, et al: Long-term results of tricuspid valve replacement and the problem of prosthetic valve thrombosis. Am J Cardiol 51:1128, 1983.
39. Prabhus, S, Friday, KJ, Reynolds, D, et al: Thrombosis of aortic St. Jude valve. Am Thorac Surg 41:332, 1986.
40. Edmonds, LH: Thromboembolic complications of current cardiac valvular prostheses. Am Thorac Surg 34:96, 1982.
41. Pass, HI, Sade, RM, and Crawford, FA: Cardiac valve prostheses in children without anticoagulation. J Thorac Cardiovasc Surg 87:832, 1984.
42. Acar, J, Enriquez-Sarano, M, Farah, E, et al: Recurrent systemic embolic events with valve prostheses. Europ Heart J 5(Suppl D):33, 1984.
43. Cohn, LH, Allred, EN, Cohn, LA, et al: Early and late risks of mitral valve replacement. J Thorac Cardiovasc Surg 90:872, 1985.
44. Lees, CD, Gill, CC, Cosgrove, DM, III, et al: The St. Jude Medical cardiac valve versus the Björk-Shiley prosthetic valve in the mitral position: A preliminary report. Cleve Clin Q 51:499, 1984.
45. Chesbro, JH, Fuster, V, Elveback, LR, et al: Trial of combined warfarin plus dipyridamole or aspirin therapy in prosthetic heart valve replacement: Danger of aspirin compared with dipyridamole. Am J Cardiol 51:1537, 1983.
46. Kontos, GJ, Jr and Schaff, HV: Thrombotic occlusion of a prosthetic heart valve: Diagnosis and management. Mayo Clin Proc 60:118, 1985.
47. Pavie, A, Bors, V, Baud, F, et al: Surgery of prosthetic valve thrombosis. Eur Heart J 5(Suppl D):39, 1984.
48. Venugopal, P, Kaul, U, Iyer, KS, et al: Fate of thrombectomized Björk-Shiley valves. A long-term cinefluoroscopic, echocardiographic, and hemodynamic evaluation. J Thorac Cardiovasc Surg 91:168, 1986.
49. Veyrat, C, Witchitz, S, Lessana, A, et al: Valvar prosthetic dysfunction. Localization and evaluation of the dysfunction using the Doppler technique. Br Heart J 54:273, 1985.

50. Harris, RL, Wilson, WR, and Williams, TW, Jr: Infections associated with prosthetic heart valves. In Sugarman, B and Young, EJ (eds): Infections Associated With Prosthetic Devices. CRC Press, Boca Raton, FL, 1984.
51. Watanakunakorn, C: Prosthetic valve infective endocarditis. Prog Cardiovasc Dis 22:181, 1979.
52. Leport, C, Vilde, JL, Bricaire, F, et al: Late prosthetic valve endocarditis. Bacteriological findings and prognosis in 29 cases. Eur Heart J 5(Suppl C):139, 1984.
53. Horstkotte, D, Korfer, R, Loogen, F, et al: Prosthetic valve endocarditis: Clinical findings and management. Eur Heart J 5(Suppl C):117, 1984.
54. Arnett, EN and Roberts, WC: Valve ring abscess in active infective endocarditis. Frequency, location and clues to clinical diagnosis from the study of 95 necropsy patients. Circulation 54:140, 1976.
55. Edwards, JE and Burchell, HB: The pathological anatomy of deficiencies between the aortic root and the heart, including aortic sinus aneurysm. Thorax 12:125, 1957.
56. Donaldson, RM, Westgate, C, Bennett, JG, et al: The role of echocardiography in suspected bacterial endocarditis. Eur Heart J 5(Suppl C):53, 1984.
57. Brottier, E, Gin, E, Brottier, L, et al: Prosthetic valve endocarditis: Diagnosis and prognosis. Eur Heart J 5(Suppl C):123, 1984.
58. Neimann, JL, Danchin, N, Godenier, JP, et al: Two-dimensional echocardiographic recognition of aortic valve ring abscesses. Eur Heart J 5(Suppl C):59, 1984.
59. Alsip, SG, Blackstone, EH, Kirklin, JW, et al: Indications for cardiac surgery in patients with active infective endocarditis. Am J Med 78(Suppl 6B):138, 1985.
60. Baumgartner, WA, Miller, DC, Reitz, BA, et al: Surgical treatment of prosthetic valve endocarditis. Ann Thorac Surg 35:87, 1983.
61. Harrison, EC, Roschke, EJ, Meyers, HI, et al: Cholelithiasis: A frequent complication of artificial heart valve replacement. Am Heart J 95:483, 1978.
62. Bjork, VO, Henze, A, and Szamosi, A: Coronary ostial stenosis: A complication of aortic valve replacement of coronary perfusion. Scand J Thorac Cadiovasc Surg 10:1, 1976.
63. Roberts, WC and Morrow, AG: Cause of early postoperative death following cardiac valve replacement. Clinico-pathologic correlations in 64 patients studied at necropsy. J Thorac Cardiovasc Surg 54:422, 1967.
64. Williams, DB, Pluth, JR, and Orszulak, TA: Extrinsic obstruction of the Björk-Shiley valve in the mitral position. Ann Thorac Surg 32:58, 1981.
65. Waller, BF, Jones, M, and Roberts, WC: Postoperative aortic regurgitation from incomplete seating of tilting-disc occluder due to overhanging knots or long sutures. Chest 78:565, 1980.
66. Ziemer, G, Luhmer, I, Oelert, H, et al: Malfunction of a St. Jude Medical heart valve prosthesis in the mitral position. Ann Thorac Surg 33:391, 1981.
67. Gold, H and Hertz, L: Death caused by fracture of Beall mitral valve prosthesis. Report of case. Am J Cardiol 34:371, 1974.
68. Odell, JA, Durandt, J, Shama, DM, et al: Spontaneous embolization of a St. Jude prosthetic mitral valve leaflet. Ann Thorac Surg 39:569, 1985.
69. Sutherland, RD, Guynes, WA, Nichol, CT, et al: Excessive strut wear allowing ball-poppet embolization in a DeBakey-Surgitool aortic valve prosthesis. J Cardiovasc Surg 23:179, 1982.
70. Silver, MD: Wear in Björk-Shiley heart valve prostheses recovered at necropsy or operation. J Thorac Cardiovasc Surg 79:693, 1980.
71. Silver, MD, Koppenhoeffer, H, Heggtviet, HA, et al: Metal wear in Lillehei-Kaster heart valve prostheses. Artif Organs 9:270, 1985.

CHAPTER 13

Bioprosthetic Valve Failure

Frederick J. Schoen, M.D., Ph.D.
Jody L. Kujovich
Robert J. Levy, M.D.
Martin St. John Sutton, M.D.

Valve replacement using mechanical prostheses (composed entirely of synthetic materials) or biologic prostheses (composed largely of human or animal tissues) is a common therapy for patients with severe valvular heart disease. Biologic tissue valves are flexible trileaflet valves that function somewhat similarly to their natural counterparts. Historically, they have included homografts/allografts (human cadaver), heterografts/xenografts (chemically treated porcine aortic valve or bovine pericardial tissue), or autografts (fabricated, for example, from the patient's own pulmonary valve, thigh connective tissue [fascia lata], or pericardium). Various aspects of these valves have been reviewed.[1-5]

Tissue valves have the advantages of pseudoanatomic central flow and low thrombogenicity, usually without anticoagulant therapy. In contrast, because thromboembolic complications are a major cause of mortality and morbidity in patients with mechanical heart valve substitutes, chronic oral anticoagulation is required.[5-10] Thus, tissue valves provide an attractive alternative to mechanical prosthetic valves when anticoagulation is contraindicated or undesirable. However, despite their superficial resemblance to natural valves, contemporary bioprostheses are nonviable, nonrenewing biomaterials that undergo progressive degenerative changes during function. Durability limitations have been the major impediment to their long-term success.[4,5]

This chapter summarizes clinicopathologic issues pertinent to the management of patients in whom bioprosthesis implantation is contemplated or has been done. In particular, we discuss clinical results with contemporary designs, clinicomorphologic correlations in failed valves, clinical characteristics of valve failure, and the pathobiology and potential prevention of bioprosthetic valve degeneration.

VALVES AVAILABLE

According to some investigators, true biologic valves include only cadaveric homografts, obtained fresh, prepared with or without some treatment to ensure sterility, and sewn freehand in the left or right ventricular outflow position, or pulmonary valves autotransplanted to the aortic root.[11] Most other tissue valves are fabricated from chemically altered tissue, subsequently mounted on a flexible stent support. Thus, contemporary "bioprostheses" are hybrids, partly biologic (cuspal tissue) and partly synthetic (the stent supports and fabric sewing ring). The clinical success of specific cardiac valvular bioprostheses depends primarily on the tissue type and source, methods of preservation and preinsertion handling, and the specific manner and method of support. Glutaraldehyde, a dialdehyde ($CHO[CH_2]_3CHO$) that forms complex, degradation-resistant, intermolecular cross links, especially with collagen, has been the most widely used chemical preservative for bioprosthetic tissue treatment.[12]

Currently available bioprostheses (Fig. 13–1) combine the advantages of tissue-derived valves (pseudoanatomic central flow and low thrombogenicity) with the availability and ease of implantation of mechanical heart valve prostheses. Flexible stent-mounted porcine bioprostheses, fabricated from glutaraldehyde-preserved pig aortic valves, have achieved the most extensive clinical application since their introduction in 1971. The most widely used models—Hancock and Carpentier-Edwards bioprostheses—are comparable with respect to durability and overall incidence of

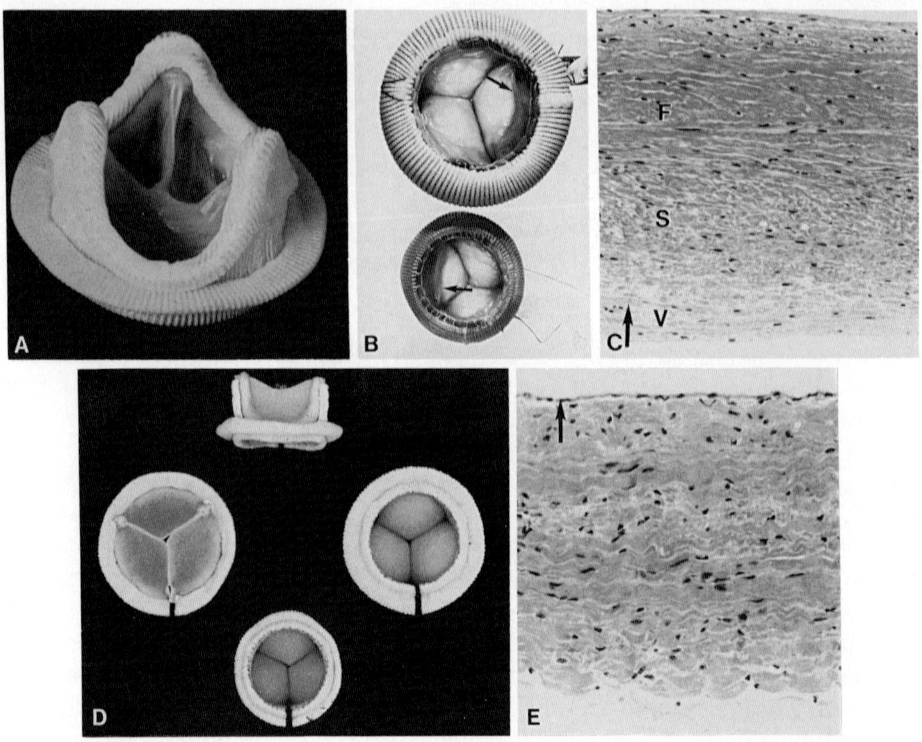

Figure 13–1. Porcine aortic valve and bovine pericardial bioprostheses. *A, B,* Gross photographs of porcine bioprostheses. (Courtesy of Johnson & Johnson Cardiovascular, Inc.) In *B,* with mitral at top and aortic below, *arrows* indicate atrial muscle shelf. *C,* Cross-sectional photomicrograph of porcine aortic valve illustrating layered architecture of porcine aortic valve, with ventricularis (V), spongiosa (S), and fibrosa (F) noted. *Arrow* indicates direction of blood flow. *D,* Gross photograph of pericardial bioprosthesis. (Courtesy of Shiley Laboratories, Inc.) *E,* Cross-sectional photomicrograph of unimplanted pericardium, demonstrating homogeneous, laminated, collagenous structure. Serosal surface is noted *(arrow).* (*C* and *E* hematoxylin-eosin stain; magnifications, *C* ×200, *E* ×260; reduced 42 percent.)

complications. The right coronary cusp of the pig aortic valve is supported by a shelf of interventricular septal muscle, which may prevent full excursion of this cusp of a porcine bioprosthesis. A modified Hancock prosthesis, specifically designed for use in the small aortic root, substitutes a cusp without a muscular ridge from another animal in order to widen the valve orifice.[13] The Carpentier-Edwards design has an asymmetric, contoured orifice that minimizes incorporated septal muscle.

Glutaraldehyde-preserved trileaflet bovine pericardial bioprostheses were first introduced in 1977.[14] Pericardial valves can be tailored efficiently to optimize hemodynamics without the inherent anatomic constraints of porcine valves, and thus novel design configurations are feasible.[15,16] The effective orifice area of pericardial bioprostheses is generally larger than similarly sized porcine aortic valve bioprostheses, especially in small sizes.

Porcine aortic valve and bovine pericardial bioprosthetic cusps have different structures (compare Figure 13–1*C* and *E*). Aortic valve has three well-defined layers: (1) the *ventricularis,* predominantly collagenous with some elastic fibers, facing the inflow surface; (2) the centrally located *spongiosa,* composed of loosely arranged collagen and abundant proteoglycans; and (3) the *fibrosa,* composed of densely packed collagen, facing the outflow surface.[17,18] In contrast, pericardial tissue is a relatively homogenous sheet of laminated collagen with a compact architecture, although not as tightly arranged as porcine valve fibrosa.[19–21] Moreover, although collagen is the most abundant protein in both tissues, the porcine aortic valve contains type I and III collagen,[22] probably in a ratio of approximately 70 percent to 30 percent,[23] whereas bovine pericardial collagen is almost entirely type I.[24] It is unknown whether these structural and biochemical differences are associated with differential surface thrombogenicity, immunoreactivity, or other properties.

CLINICAL RESULTS

Most patients with severe valvular heart disease who undergo valve replacement are functionally improved for extended intervals.[9,14,25–34] The hemodynamic performance of bioprostheses is comparable or superior to that of mechanical prostheses, except in small sizes. Hemolysis is minimal and significant hemolytic anemia generally indicates bioprosthesis dysfunction or paravalvular leak.[35] The overall probability of porcine bioprosthetic valve failure from all causes in adults (defined as death or reoperation owing to periprosthetic leak, thromboembolic complications [including local thrombotic occlusion], infective endocarditis, or degenerative dysfunction),[7] predicted at various institutions by actuarial statistics, is approximately 20 to 30 percent at 7 to 10 years.[5,25,27–29,33,34,36] Risks of specific valve-related complications, reported in recent studies from our institution, are summarized in Table 13–1.

Clinically significant late valve deterioration in the absence of antecedent endocarditis *(primary tissue failure),* with cuspal tears or calcification or both, is frequent, and strongly time-dependent, accounting for an accelerated valve failure rate following 4 to 5 years of function.[5,25,27–29,33,34,36] In a study with maximum 10 years' followup, we found dysfunction owing to degeneration in 5.4 percent of valves implanted in adults for more than 5 years but only 0.7 percent of valves implanted for less than 5 years.[37] Freedom from primary tissue failure is currently reported as 96 to 97 percent at 5 years and 71 percent at 10 years (both mitral and aortic sites),[27] 77 percent at 9.5 years (mitral) and 89 percent at 8 years (aortic),[29] and 83 percent

Table 13–1. Risk of Valve-Related Complications With Bioprostheses and Mechanical Prostheses (Mean %/Pt-Yr)

	Mitral		Aortic	
	Bioprostheses	*Mechanical*	*Bioprostheses*	*Mechanical*
Thrombosis/thromboembolism	2.4	4.6	2.0	2.4
Hemorrhage	0.4	1.7	0.2	1.8
Perivalvular leak	0.7	0.8	0.4	0.2
Endocarditis	0.4	0.2	0.6	0.1
Primary valve dysfunction*	1.2*	0.4	0.8*	0.0
All valve complications	5.2	8.1	3.8	4.2

* 83 ± 4% free at 108 months (mitral); 91 ± 3% free at 108 months (aortic).
Adapted from Cohn, LH, et al.[25,28]

(mitral) and 91 percent (aortic) at 9 years.[25,28] Valve failure owing to calcification is markedly accelerated in children and adolescents with left or right-sided, intracardiac, or conduit-mounted bioprostheses.[27,38–40] Fewer than 60 percent of valves in this population remain intact 3 to 5 years postoperatively. Detailed age-related data suggest that the increased risk may continue to age 35.[27] Thus, primary tissue failure is the predominant late valve-related complication with porcine bioprostheses.

Because the reported clinical experience with bovine pericardial bioprostheses is limited, the long-term fate of these valves remains undetermined. Nevertheless, despite favorable early clinical results from some centers,[14,32] calcific and noncalcific degenerative failures are occurring frequently in both adults and children.[31,33,41–44] Recent data suggest that bovine pericardial bioprostheses may have an even greater propensity to late primary tissue failure than their porcine valve counterparts.[33]

Thromboembolic risk (fatal and nonfatal thromboembolism and local thrombosis) for porcine bioprostheses, without anticoagulation, is less than that for contemporary mechanical valve prostheses in anticoagulated patients.[6,25,27,28,29,36] In recent studies from our institution, freedom from thrombosis or thromboembolism at 9 years for patients with porcine bioprostheses was 85 percent (mitral and aortic), compared with 77 percent (mitral) and 83 percent (aortic) with tilting disc prosthetic valves[25,28]—data almost identical to those of other series.[27,29] Patients with biologic prostheses in normal sinus rhythm have very low thromboembolic risk, but risk increases with atrial fibrillation[25] (Fig. 13–2). Indeed, patients with atrial fibrillation of any etiology have a substantially increased risk of cerebrovascular emboli.[45,46] Therefore, inasmuch as such patients would require chronic anticoagulation irrespective of valve prosthesis type, the major advantage of bioprostheses is negated.

Most studies demonstrate that the lower rates of thromboembolic complications with bioprostheses are balanced by more frequent late reoperations for primary tissue failure; and thus freedom from reoperation and postoperative survival are similar for patients with contemporary mechanical prostheses and bioprostheses (Fig. 13–3).[25,26,28,47,48] Therefore, the probability of late survival primarily reflects preoperative functional classification and associated cardiovascular disease, rather than the specific prosthesis-type implanted. The major consideration in valve selection is the trade-off between risks of thromboembolic complications and anticoagulation hemorrhage (favoring the use of bioprostheses) and limited durability (favoring mechanical prostheses). However, extraordinary clinical circumstances may prevail in selected patients. For example, bioprostheses are recommended for young women

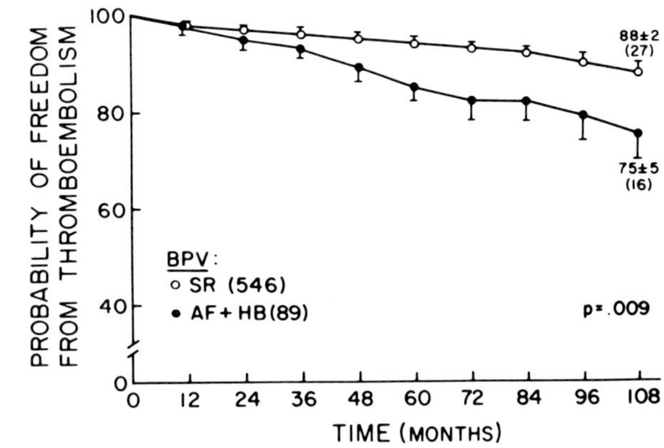

Figure 13–2. Probability of freedom from thromboembolism in patients with porcine bioprostheses (BPV) who were in sinus rhythm (SR) versus atrial fibrillation or heart block (AF + HB). (From Cohn, LH, et al: Early and late risk of aortic valve replacement: A 12 year concomitant comparison of the porcine bioprosthetic and tilting tissue disc prosthetic aortic valve. J Thorac Cardiovasc Surg 88:695, 1984; with permission.)

wishing to become pregnant,[49] in order to avoid anticoagulation, which is not only teratogenic but also associated with increased spontaneous abortion from retroplacental hemorrhage.[50] In contrast, mechanical valves may be preferable in children and young adults, despite the need for anticoagulation, because failure of bioprostheses is accelerated in this population.[27,38–40]

BIOPROSTHETIC HEART VALVE FAILURE: PATHOLOGIC AND CLINICAL CHARACTERISTICS

Tissue preservation procedures and subsequent implantation induce progressive nonspecific microscopic and ultrastructural morphologic changes in porcine aortic valve bioprostheses.[18,51] Glutaraldehyde processing induces loss of surface endothelium, autolytic disruption of porcine connective tissue cells, collagen bundle loosening, and loss of ground substance. Subsequent implantation leads to additional structural alterations including plasma protein insudation, superficial fibrin deposition, inflammatory cell adherence with occasional penetration, generalized architectural homogenization with connective tissue disruption, mineralization, and, in some cases, amyloid deposition.[52] Except for mineralization and collagen structural degeneration, the extent to which these pathologic processes contribute to specific late failure modes has not been determined.

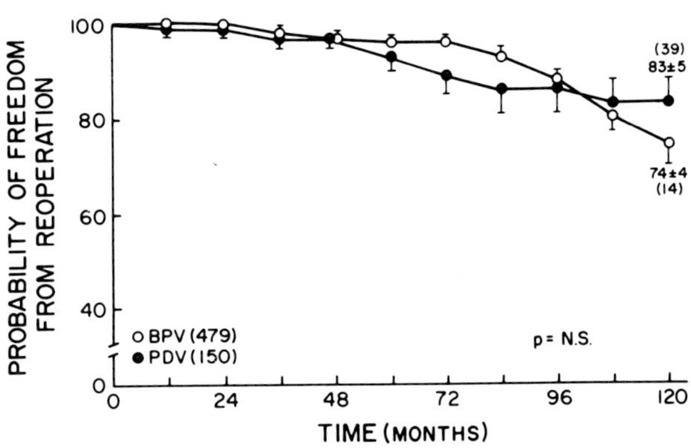

Figure 13–3. Probability of freedom from reoperation after bioprosthetic (BPV) and tilting disc mechanical prosthetic (PDV) valve replacement. (From Cohn, LH, et al: Early and late risk of mitral valve replacement: A 12 year concomitant comparison of the porcine bioprosthetic and prosthetic disc mitral valves. J Thorac Cardiovasc Surg 90:872, 1985, with permission.)

Predominant indications for reoperation or causes of death in patients with mechanical or bioprosthetic valve prostheses include thromboembolic complications, valve-related infective endocarditis, paravalvular leak, and degenerative dysfunction.[5,7–10,25–30,36] Etiologies of dysfunction of 112 consecutive porcine bioprostheses surgically removed at our hospital during a 66-month interval (July 1980 through December 1985) are summarized and compared with those of 45 mechanical valves in Figure 13–4.[53] The most frequent cause of bioprosthesis failure was sterile primary tissue degeneration (74 percent of bioprosthetic valve failures). Bioprosthetic valve removal was necessitated by endocarditis in 11 patients (9 percent) and by thrombosis in four (4 percent). In contrast, thrombosis was a major cause of mechanical valve dysfunction (18 percent of failures). Sterile paravalvular leak and prosthetic infective endocarditis were equally frequent with mechanical and bioprosthetic valves. These results agree with those of other studies.[9,10,25,27–30,34] Pathologic and clinical features of the predominant failure modes are described subsequently.

Bioprosthetic Valve Endocarditis (BVE)

Endocarditis is an infrequent but potentially serious complication of all valve replacements, occurring in 1 to 4 percent of patients.[36,54,55] Rates of infection do not differ consistently among bioprostheses and mechanical valve replacements. Although endocarditis occurs most frequently in the first several months postoperatively, the risk is life-long.[10,36,54–56] Prosthetic valve endocarditis may be complicated (1) by embolization of vegetations; (2) by congestive heart failure secondary to valvular obstruction or regurgitation caused by bulky vegetations; or (3) by paravalvular leaks.[5,10,57–59] Because the synthetic biomaterials used in mechanical prostheses cannot support bacterial or fungal growth, infections are localized to the prosthesis-tissue interface at the sewing ring *(ring abscess).*[59] Damage to contiguous structures, as evidenced by new regurgitant murmurs, atrioventricular conduction disturbances, or valve dehiscence with accelerated hemodynamic deterioration, generally necessitates reoperation.

Although BVE is often localized to the prosthesis sewing ring and complicated by ring abscesses, infections may also involve, and occasionally be limited to, the cuspal tissue (Fig. 13–5).[37,57–59] Histologic examination often demonstrates clumps

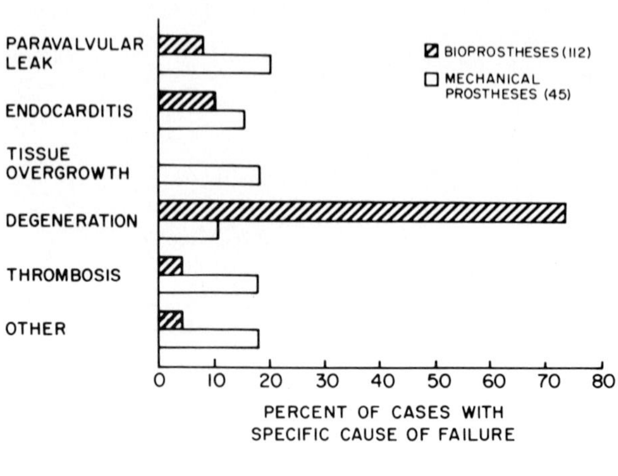

Figure 13–4. Cause of failure of mechanical prosthetic valves (various types) and porcine aortic bioprosthetic heart valves removed at operation, 1980 to 1985. Failure modes of mechanical valves are diverse. In contrast, bioprosthetic valves fail most frequently by degenerative processes. (From Schoen, FJ: Surgical pathology of removed natural and prosthetic heart valves. Hum Pathol 1987 [in press], with permission.)

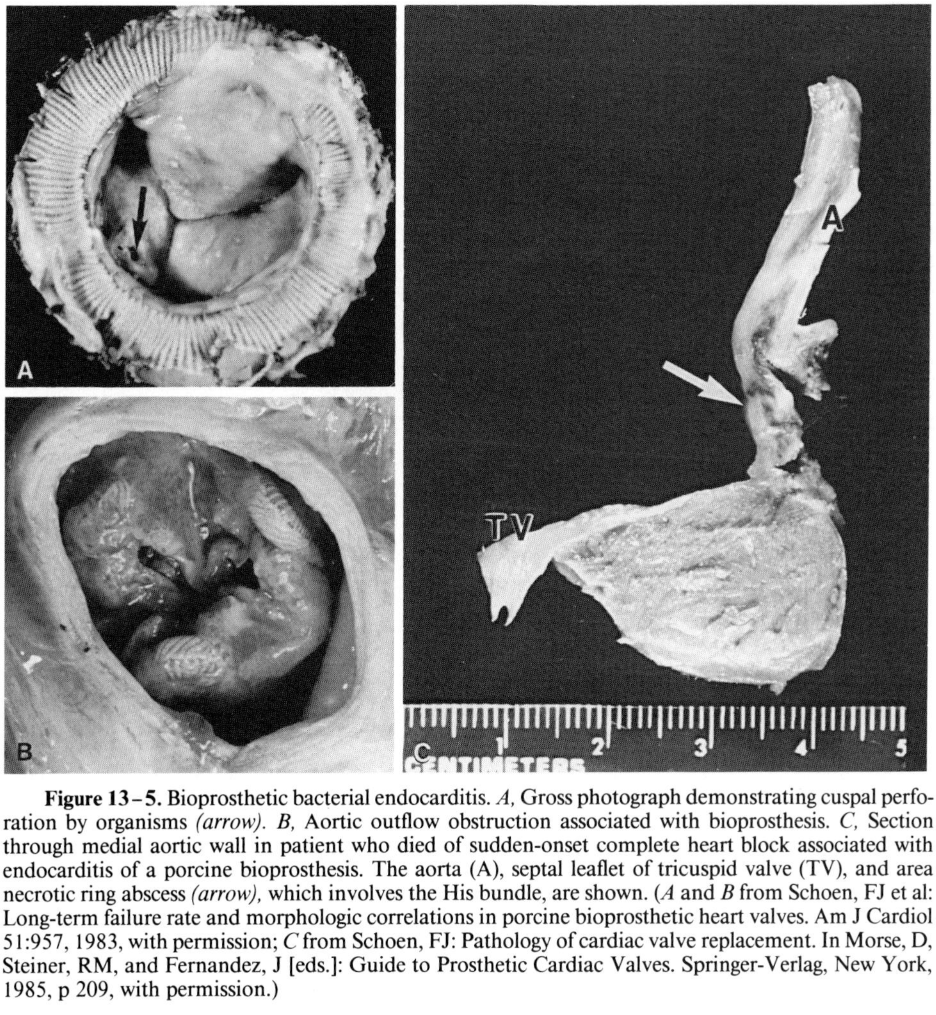

Figure 13-5. Bioprosthetic bacterial endocarditis. *A,* Gross photograph demonstrating cuspal perforation by organisms *(arrow). B,* Aortic outflow obstruction associated with bioprosthesis. *C,* Section through medial aortic wall in patient who died of sudden-onset complete heart block associated with endocarditis of a porcine bioprosthesis. The aorta (A), septal leaflet of tricuspid valve (TV), and area necrotic ring abscess *(arrow),* which involves the His bundle, are shown. (*A* and *B* from Schoen, FJ et al: Long-term failure rate and morphologic correlations in porcine bioprosthetic heart valves. Am J Cardiol 51:957, 1983, with permission; *C* from Schoen, FJ: Pathology of cardiac valve replacement. In Morse, D, Steiner, RM, and Fernandez, J [eds.]: Guide to Prosthetic Cardiac Valves. Springer-Verlag, New York, 1985, p 209, with permission.)

of organisms deep in the cusps. Cuspal vegetations of BVE may mineralize (extrinsic calcification).[37,60] Secondary incompetence may occur owing to tears, perforations, or widespread cuspal destruction; and large vegetations can cause stenosis by obstructing the valve orifice. Medical cure of BVE may be achieved in some cases.[61] Infection limited to the cusps is probably more easily cured by antibiotics.

Irrespective of valve type, prosthetic valve endocarditis is classified as *early,* within 60 days of valve replacement, or *late,* after 60 days, because the etiology, risk factors, causative microorganisms, and treatment are different.[54,55,59] Early infections reflect perioperative contamination, whereas late infections are usually of hematogenous origin. Although the most useful clinical indicator of early infections is unremitting fever, multiple alternative causes of early postoperative fever and leukocytosis, including wound infection, pulmonary atelectasis, and postperfusion and postpericardiotomy syndromes, may confound the diagnosis until positive blood cultures are obtained. Early infection, often accompanied by partial sewing ring dehiscence and resultant paravalvular leaks with regurgitant murmurs, may cause sudden, severe, and rapidly progressive congestive heart failure.

Late prosthetic valve endocarditis usually presents insidiously as low-grade fever with nonspecific symptoms, although a minority of patients have rapidly progressive hemodynamic decompensation. A precipitating cause, such as dental treatment without appropriate antibiotic prophylaxis, is documented in only 50 percent of patients or less.[54,55] The most frequent findings are fever, new cardiac murmurs, splenomegaly, and anemia with elevated white blood cell count; classic cutaneous signs of endocarditis are uncommon. Subtle alterations in prosthetic valve sounds with new murmurs suggest the diagnosis, and Doppler echocardiographic examination of the bioprosthesis often visualizes vegetations and assesses the severity of either prosthetic obstruction or regurgitation.[62–65] Identification of causative microorganisms is critical for specific antibiotic therapy. Nevertheless, the results of medical treatment for early infections are poor, with mortality greater than 80 percent; surgical removal of the infected device is usually required.[54,66] In contrast, half of patients who develop late infections can be cured with appropriate antibiotic therapy. Reoperation is usually indicated for continuing uncontrolled infection, ring abscess, recurrent systemic embolization, or progressive heart failure.

Thromboembolic Complications

Early thrombosis (or thromboembolism) after bioprosthetic valve replacement usually originates at the proximal host tissue-valve interface, reflecting predisposing risk factors of atrial fibrillation, increased atrial size, low cardiac output syndromes, and inadequate anticoagulation therapy, superimposed on a thrombogenic sewing ring. This provides the rationale for early, temporary anticoagulation therapy in patients with bioprosthetic valves. Because growth of tissue into the sewing ring confers thromboresistance, late thrombosis is associated with the cusps themselves, with large thrombotic deposits in the bioprosthetic sinuses of Valsalva (Fig. 13–6).[5,10,67] Pathologic determination of the age of thrombi on bioprosthetic (or mechanical) valves is difficult, because the lack of adjacent vascularity retards histologic progression of organization. The greater frequency of thromboembolism in

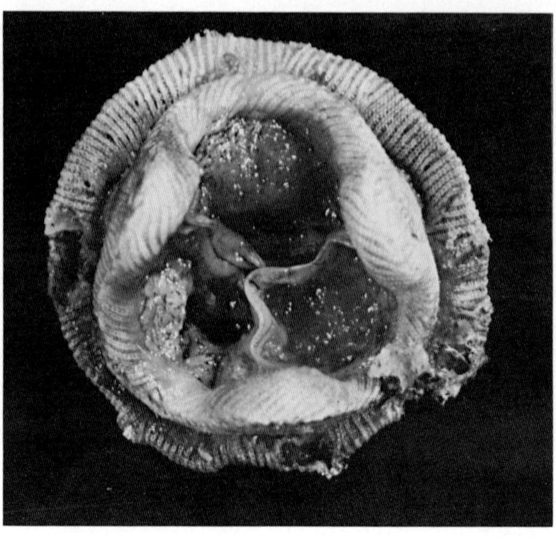

Figure 13–6. Thrombosis of an aortic bioprosthetic heart valve. Thrombotic deposits completely fill the prosthetic sinuses of Valsalva. (From Schoen, FJ and Hobson, CE: Anatomic analysis of removed prosthetic heart valves: Causes of failure of 33 mechanical valves and 58 bioprostheses, 1980–1983. Hum Pathol 16:549, 1985, with permission.)

mitral than in aortic bioprosthetic replacement is probably due to the increased frequency of atrial dysrhythmias and larger atrial size in mitral valve disease.

Thromboembolism frequently presents dramatically with acute neurologic deficits, acute extremity ischemia, or infarction of an abdominal viscus. Many patients have only mild and transitory sequelae, but almost half sustain permanent neurologic damage or death. Every attempt should be made to determine the presence of intracardiac thrombus, the adequacy of prosthetic valve function (often aided by two-dimensional [2-D] echocardiography), the status of anticoagulation, and any change in cardiac rhythm. Two episodes of documented thromboembolism are usually an indication for valve replacement.

Primary Tissue Failure (PTF)

PTF, especially that related to cuspal mineralization, is the major cause of dysfunction of cardiac valve bioprostheses.[5,10,25,27–30,34] Degenerative processes cause cuspal stiffening or structural defects, accounting for the clinical symptoms of stenosis or regurgitation or both (Figs. 13–7, 13–8).[5,10] Our studies demonstrated calcification in 86 percent of valves removed for PTF, and cuspal defects in 79 percent.[10] Regurgitation through tears secondary to calcification characterized 67 percent of valves with PTF, whereas stenosis owing to calcific cuspal stiffening was present in 20 percent. In 13 percent, cuspal tears or perforations were unrelated to either calcification or endocarditis; most bioprostheses with noncalcific tissue defects were mitral replacements.

Degenerative calcific deposits generally predominate at the cuspal commissures and basal attachments,[5,10] the sites of highest dynamic mechanical stress during function.[68] Calcific deposits are grossly visible as nodular grey-white masses that often ulcerate through the cuspal tissue. Microscopically, calcific deposits are most extensive in the porcine valve spongiosa.[60] Ultrastructurally, they are related to cuspal connective tissue cells and collagen.[69] The detailed pathologic features of calcification in clinically failed pericardial bioprostheses have not yet been described.

Bioprosthetic degenerative processes are strongly time-dependent.[25,27–30,36,37] Mineral deposits tend to increase with time of function, but the extent of calcification varies widely among individuals after long-term implantation, and it is not unusual to encounter bioprostheses with minimal or no radiographically demonstrable calcific deposits after extended implantation (6 to 10 years).[10] We encountered intrinsic (sterile, nonthrombotic) bioprosthetic valve calcification with leaflet tears 27 months postoperatively in one patient but only following at least 44 months in others. Mean duration of function of valves with PTF was 73 months (range 8 to 122). Radiographically demonstrable calcific deposits were noted in 84 percent of bioprostheses without endocarditis implanted for at least 44 months.

Although most cuspal tears probably result from the mechanical discontinuity in the tissue associated with focal calcific nodules,[5,10,70] some cuspal tears reflect direct mechanical destruction of collagen architecture.[71,72] Stress-induced collagen deterioration is revealed by scanning electron microscopy as fraying and disruption of collagen fibers.[18,71,72] This pathology may be reproduced using in vitro pulse accelerators (fatigue testers).[73] Although clinical degradative failure modes are generally simulated in mechanical valve prostheses investigated with these methods, whether contemporary testing devices accurately reproduce bioprosthetic failures is controversial, inasmuch as relevant biologic processes occurring in vivo are usually

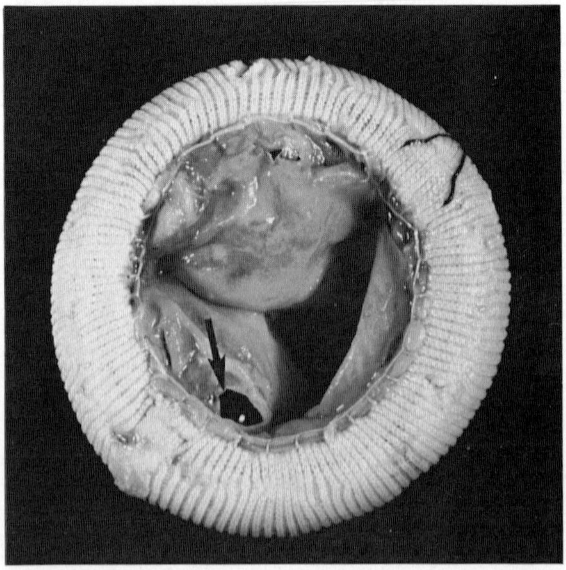

Figure 13–7. Small perforation *(arrow)* at base of cusp of mitral bioprosthesis causing regurgitation. (From Schoen, FJ, et al: Long-term failure rate and morphologic correlations in porcine bioprosthetic heart valves. Am J Cardiol 51:957, 1983, with permission.)

destructive rather than reparative. Therefore, bioengineering durability studies of bioprostheses at best predict only an optimistic upper limit of functional longevity.

The contribution to failure of noncalcific degenerative processes may be more important in clinical pericardial than porcine bioprostheses (Fig. 13–9).[74] Cuspal tears are encountered frequently. Loss of cuspal architectural definition and deep fluid insudation are prominent after clinical function.[41] In addition, stretching of cuspal pericardial tissue associated with considerable collagen bundle loosening is frequently observed in experimental implants and may have clinical significance, especially in designs with larger cusps.[75] Furthermore, implanted pericardium appears to elicit an aggressive host inflammatory response with local tissue disruption.[74–76]

The clinical presentation of primary bioprosthetic valve failure varies from the slow insidious reduction of exercise tolerance that accompanies leaflet calcification and stenosis to the dramatic development of congestive heart failure owing to acute severe prosthetic regurgitation from cuspal tears. Increasing cuspal thickness and transvalvar gradients are noted with extended postoperative intervals.[77,78] The extent to which inward deflection of the stent posts *(stent creep)* of some porcine bioprostheses contributes to progressive stenosis is unknown.[79] The symptomatic expression and physical findings of mitral bioprosthetic stenosis are indistinguishable from those of native rheumatic mitral stenosis, including deterioration of exercise tolerance and congestive heart failure, accompanied by a late apical diastolic murmur. Bioprosthetic mitral stenosis may be more difficult to diagnose in patients in whom mitral valve replacement was delayed or performed after development of pulmonary vascular disease, which itself may contribute to late functional deterioration. Problems of diagnosis also arise in patients with prosthetic stenosis with atrial fibrillation and poor rate control, and in those with multiple prosthetic valves. The clinical suspicion of bioprosthetic stenosis can usually be confirmed by noninvasive techniques. Calcified and immobile mitral prosthetic leaflets can be visualized by 2-D echocardiography in the majority of cases (Fig. 13–10). The severity of orifice compromise can be determined by accurately measuring the increased blood flow velocity across the mitral prosthesis with pulse wave Doppler, and calculating the mitral diastolic gradient and valve area.[64,80,81] Doppler velocity flow spectra of bioprostheses are generally more easily interpreted than those of mechanical valves with central occluders or tilting discs.

Aortic bioprosthetic stenosis presents with symptoms of left ventricular outflow tract obstruction, including syncope, chest pain, and increasing dyspnea. When left ventricular function is preserved, a characteristic harsh ejection systolic murmur and abnormal carotid pulse contour are evident. These findings are accompanied by electrocardiographic evidence of either persistent or developing left ventricular hypertrophy. In aortic bioprosthetic stenosis, the calcified leaflets themselves as well as their reduced motion can be visualized by 2-D echocardiography (Fig. 13–11), and the marked elevation of blood flow velocity measured by Doppler can be used to

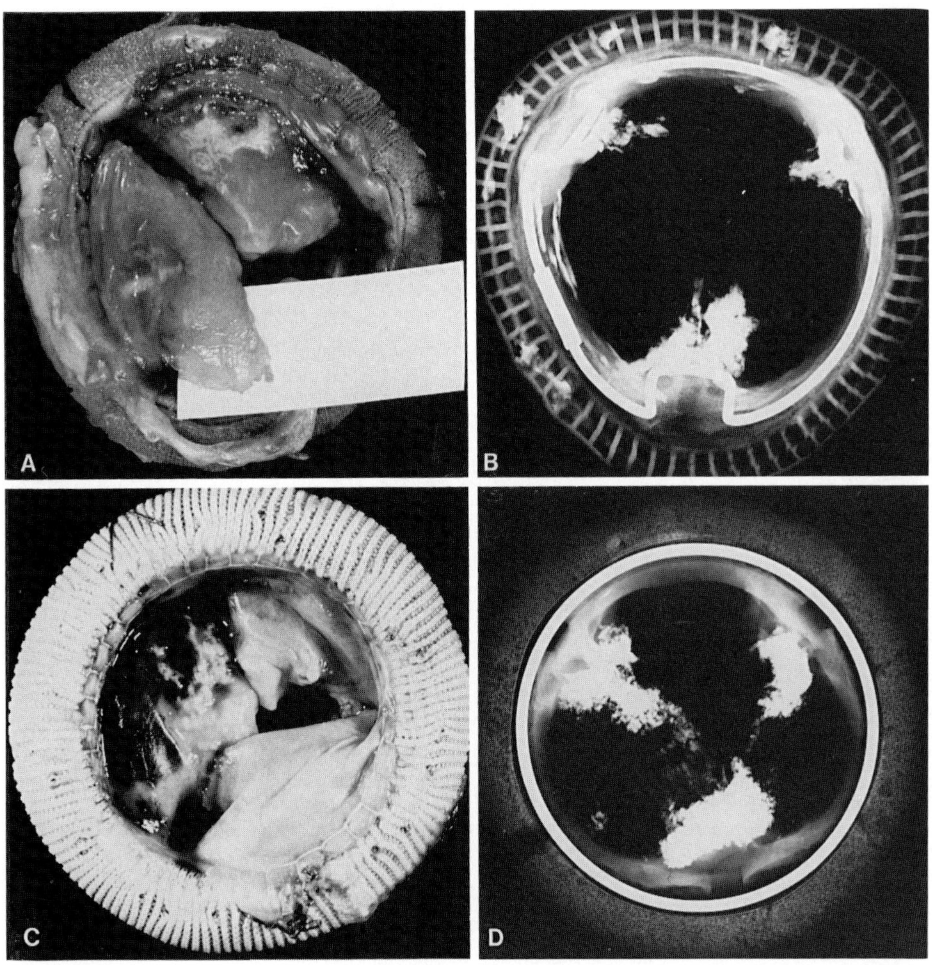

Figure 13–8. Calcification causing primary tissue failure of porcine aortic valve bioprostheses. *A*, Calcification with cuspal tear. B, Radiograph of valve specimen illustrated in *A*. *C*, Valve stenosis due to calcification. *D*, Radiograph of valve illustrated in *C*. (From Schoen, FJ and Hobson, CE: Anatomic analysis of removed prosthetic heart valves. Causes of failure of 33 mechanical valves and 58 bioprostheses, 1980–1983. Hum Pathol 16:549, 1985, with permission.)

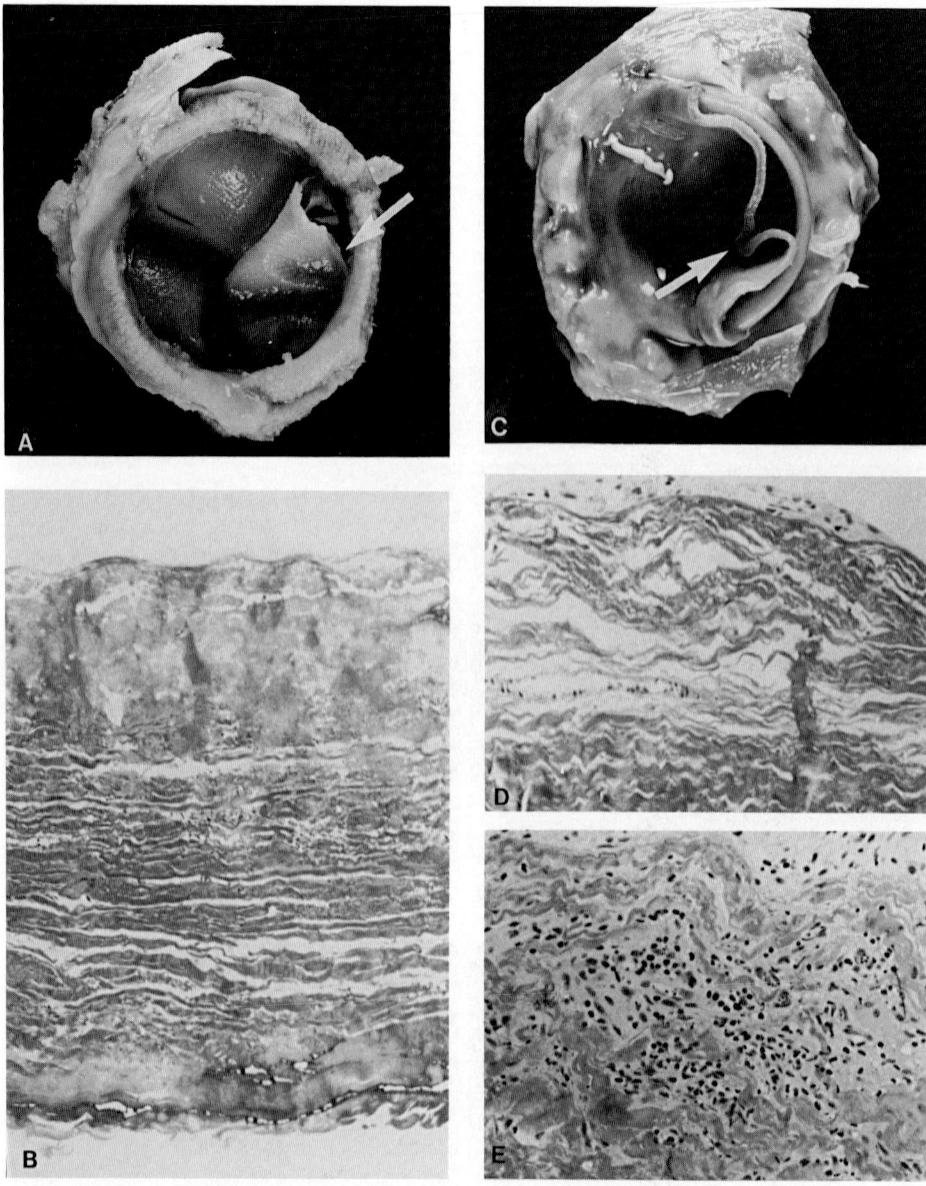

Figure 13–9. Noncalcific degenerative pathologies in clinical and experimental bovine pericardial bioprostheses. *A,* Clinical mitral bovine pericardial bioprosthesis implanted for 35 months. There is an extensive tear of one cusp (arrow) rendering this prosthesis grossly incompetent. *B,* Photomicrograph of cross section of cusp from valve shown in *A.* There is extensive fluid insudation and homogenization of the cuspal structure, with wide separation of collagen bundles. *C,* Experimental unileaflet bioprosthesis implanted as a sheep orthotopic mitral replacement for 3 months. There is severe cuspal stretching with redundancy at the free edge *(arrow). D,* Photomicrograph of cross section of cusp from bioprosthesis shown in *C,* indicating wide separation of collagen bundles. *E,* Photomicrograph of area of experimental bovine pericardial bioprosthesis indicating severe inflammatory disruption of the collagen architecture. *B, D,* and *E,* hematoxylin-eosin stain; *B* and *D* magnification ×200, *E* ×350; reduced 18 percent.) (*A* and *B,* courtesy L. Scotten.)

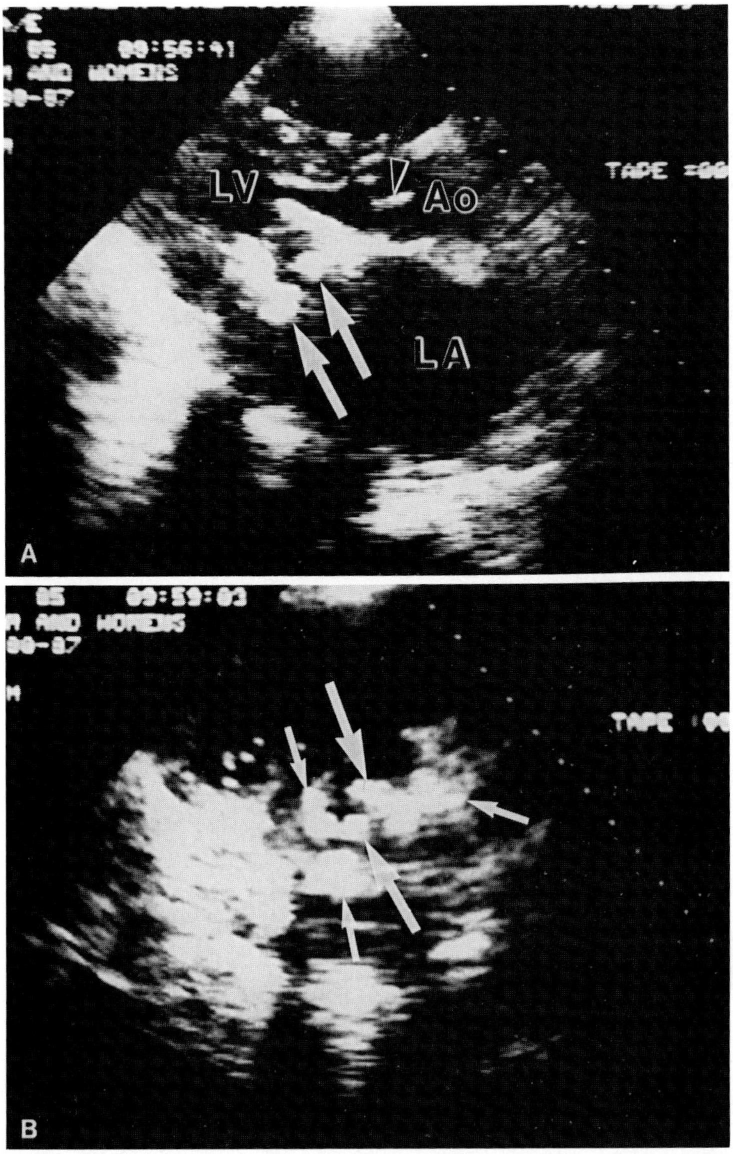

Figure 13–10. Stenotic, calcified porcine bioprosthesis in the mitral site. *A,* 2-D echocardiographic long-axis view of the left ventricle in diastole, showing a bioprosthesis in the mitral position with heavily calcified, fixed, and partially closed cusps. *B,* 2-D echocardiographic short axis view of the left ventricle showing three mitral bioprosthetic stents and heavy calcification and stenosis of the bioprosthetic leaflets. Cuspal calcific nodules indicated by *large arrows,* bioprosthetic valve stents by *small arrows,* and aortic valve cusps by *arrowhead.*

calculate the severity of stenosis.[80] Diagnostic difficulties arise, however, in patients with severely impaired left ventricular function; often they derive little or no symptomatic benefit or objective functional improvement from operation and may have continuing symptoms of dyspnea and chest pain. In this group, 2-D echocardiography demonstrates normal leaflet motion and Doppler demonstrates no aortic systolic gradient.

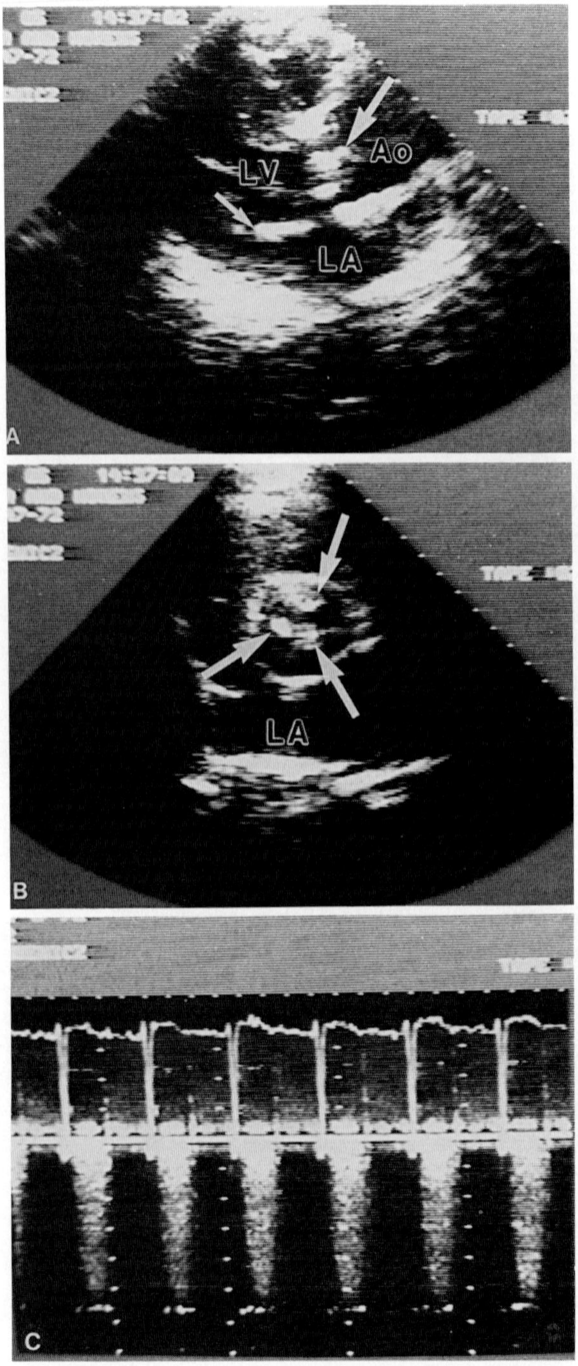

Figure 13–11. Stenotic, calcified porcine bioprosthesis in the aortic position. *A,* 2-D echocardiographic long-axis view of the left ventricle demonstrating heavy calcification and limited mobility of the bioprosthetic valve cusps, and a small hypertrophied left ventricle. *B,* 2-D echocardiographic short-axis view of the aorta showing three calcified aortic bioprosthetic cusps. Calcific nodules demonstrated by *large arrows* in *A* and *B*. In *A,* anterior mitral leaflet marked by *small arrow*. *C,* Doppler velocity spectra recorded across the calcific stenotic aortic bioprosthesis with peak velocity of 5 m/sec, corresponding to a bioprosthetic gradient of 100 mmHg.

The degree of valvular regurgitation owing to cuspal tears correlates with the extent of anatomic valvular disruption. Bioprosthetic regurgitation may occasionally be detected on auscultation at routine followup of a completely asymptomatic patient. The degree of regurgitation may remain stable or progress only very slowly. Elective reoperation can be performed when symptoms develop or there is noninvasive evidence by Doppler echocardiography of increasing left ventricular size or deteriorating function.

In other patients, bioprosthetic cuspal tears result in acute severe regurgitation with rapid decompensation, resting tachycardia, free regurgitation, low-volume pulse, and congestive heart failure. Characteristic auscultatory findings may be absent or equivocal. Thus, when sudden cardiac decompensation occurs in patients with prosthetic valves, whether biologic or mechanical, prosthetic malfunction should be anticipated and immediately investigated noninvasively with Doppler echocardiography. The abnormal, low-frequency chaotic motion of the torn bioprosthetic leaflet is usually identifiable by 2-D echocardiography (Fig. 13–12, 13–13) and the regurgitant signal detected unequivocally by Doppler. Severity of regurgitation can be assessed by flow mapping of the left atrium or ventricle and by calculation of the regurgitant fraction by echocardiography.[82]

PATHOBIOLOGY OF BIOPROSTHETIC VALVE MINERALIZATION

Experimental models used to investigate the pathophysiology of bioprosthetic tissue calcification include orthotopic tricuspid or mitral replacements or conduit-mounted valves in sheep[83] or calves,[67,84–86] and heterotopic tissue samples implanted in and around the heart[87] and subcutaneously in mice,[88] rabbits,[89] or rats.[24,88,90,91] In both circulatory and subcutaneous models, bioprosthetic tissue calcifies progressively with a morphology similar to that observed in clinical specimens, but with accelerated kinetics. Orthotopic valve replacements in sheep or calves calcify extensively in 3 to 6 months (Fig. 13–14), compared with the several years normally required for calcification of adult clinical bioprostheses. The process is even more dramatically accelerated in subcutaneous implants of bioprosthetic tissue in young rats, with maximal accumulation of mineral within 8 weeks, to levels comparable to those of failed clinical explants (200 to 225 μg calcium/mg tissue) (Fig. 13–15).[5,24,85]

The similar morphologic progression of calcification in the different experimental models and clinical bioprostheses suggests a common pathophysiology, independent of implant site. Calcification appears to depend only on exposure of a susceptible substrate to extracellular fluid;[24] this concept, however, does not rule out a possible regulatory role for circulating bloodborne substances. The subcutaneous model is a technically convenient and economically advantageous vehicle for investigating host and implant determinants and mechanisms of mineralization, as well as for screening potential strategies for its inhibition. Promising approaches may be investigated further in a large animal valve implant model. Orthotopic implants may be used not only to elucidate further the processes accounting for clinical failures but also to evaluate the performance of design and biomaterials modifications in valve development studies, and to assess the importance of blood/surface interactions and sewing ring healing on performance. Our current state of understanding of bioprosthetic tissue calcification, largely derived from subcutaneous implantation experiments, is summarized subsequently.

Determinants of Mineralization (Table 13–2)

Clinical and experimental studies strongly suggest that dynamic mechanical stress and strain promote calcification.[5,68] Macroscopic calcification of bioprosthetic valves begins in areas of leaflet flexion where deformations are maximal, especially

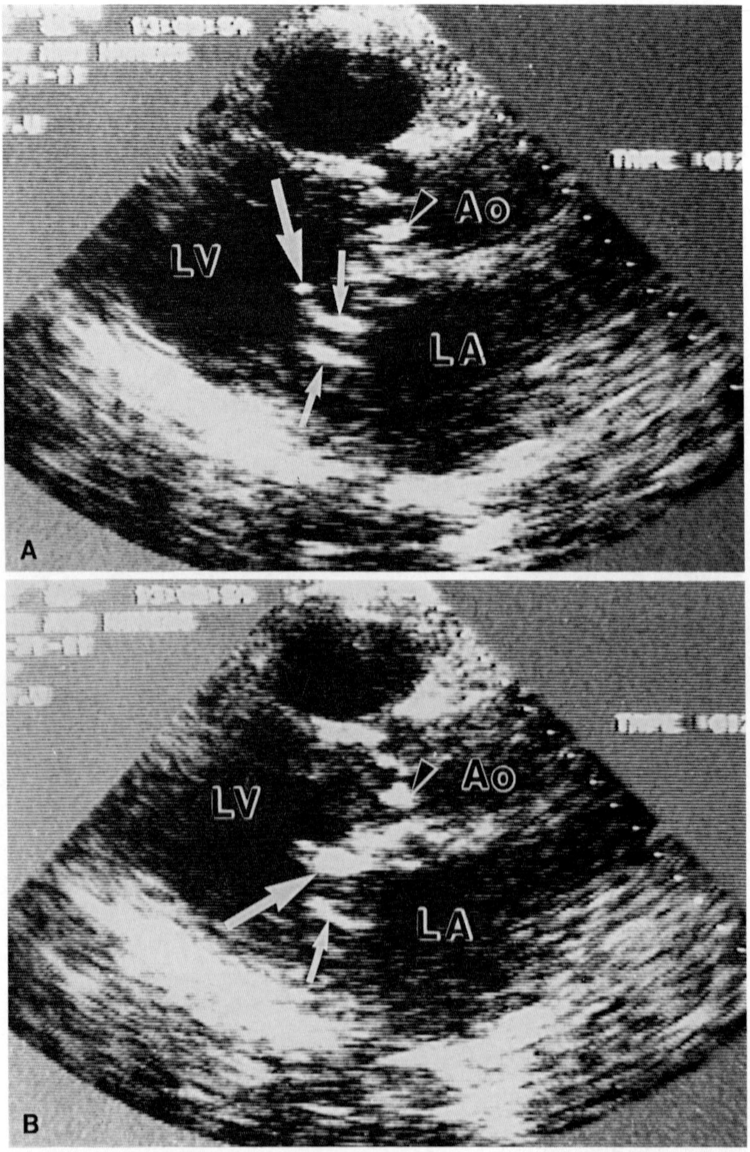

Figure 13–12. Calcified mitral porcine bioprosthesis with secondary tear demonstrated in 2-D echocardiographic long-axis view. In systole *(A)*, torn and flail cusp *(large arrow)* is visualized within the left ventricle. In diastole *(B)*, cuspal calcific nodule is indicated by *large arrow*. Mitral bioprosthetic valve stents are marked by *small arrows*, aortic valve cusp by *arrowhead*.

the cuspal commissures and bases (see Fig. 13–14).[5,68,85] The morphology and extent of calcification in subcutaneous implants is analogous to that observed in clinical and experimental circulatory implants, despite the lack of dynamic mechanical activity characteristic of the circulatory environment.[24,85,90] This suggests that dynamic stress promotes but is not a prerequisite for calcification of bioprosthetic tissue, and that metabolic and implant factors alone are required. Nevertheless, in the subcutaneous model, enhanced calcification is noted in areas of tissue folds and bends,[90] suggesting that static mechanical deformation also potentiates mineralization. The mechanisms by which stress enhances calcification are unknown but could include stress-generated crystal nucleation sites, structural disruption of the collagen architecture creating internal spaces that facilitate crystal growth, piezoelectric crystal growth augmentation, or increased fluid insudation deep into bioprosthetic valve cusps.

The rate of bioprosthetic tissue calcification is dependent on host metabolic factors. For example, renal failure and young age potentiate mineralization. The age-dependence of calcification rate is simulated in the rat subcutaneous model, in which the amount of calcium accumulated in bioprosthetic tissue implanted in

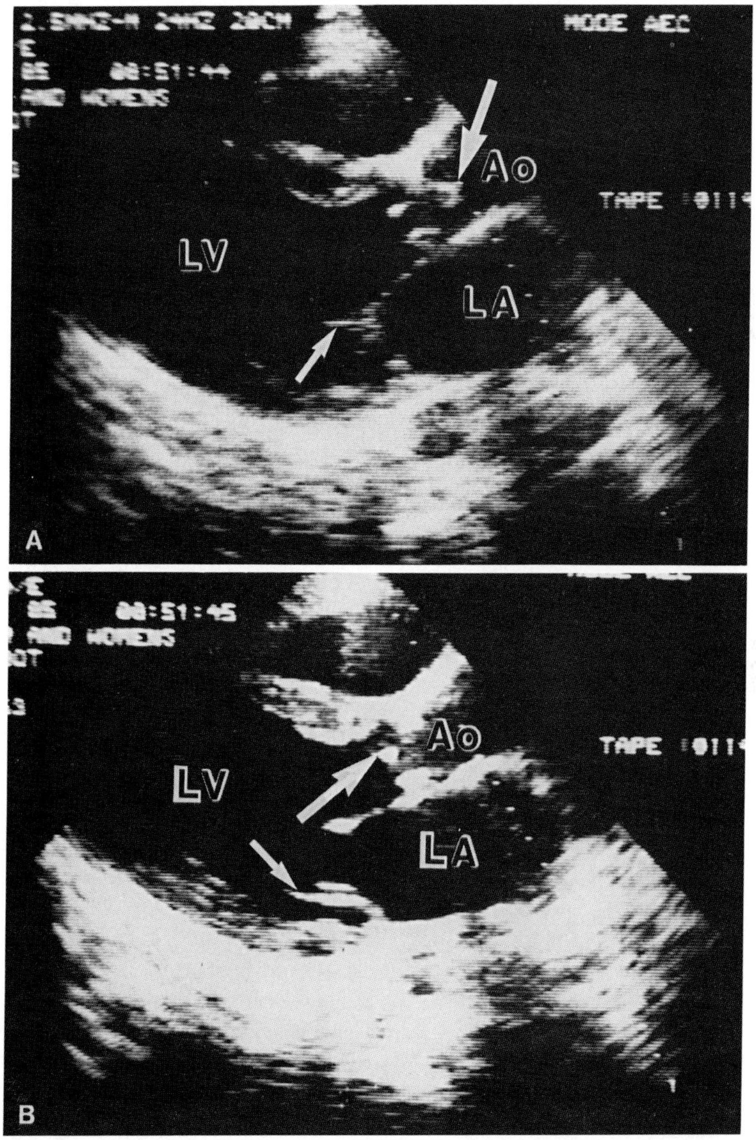

Figure 13–13. Calcified aortic porcine bioprosthesis with tear shown by 2-D echocardiographic long-axis view of the left ventricle. In systole *(A)*, calcified torn aortic bioprosthetic leaflet is visualized in the aorta *(large arrow)*. During diastole *(B)*, this cusp is in the left ventricular outflow tract. *Small arrow* indicates mitral valve leaflet.

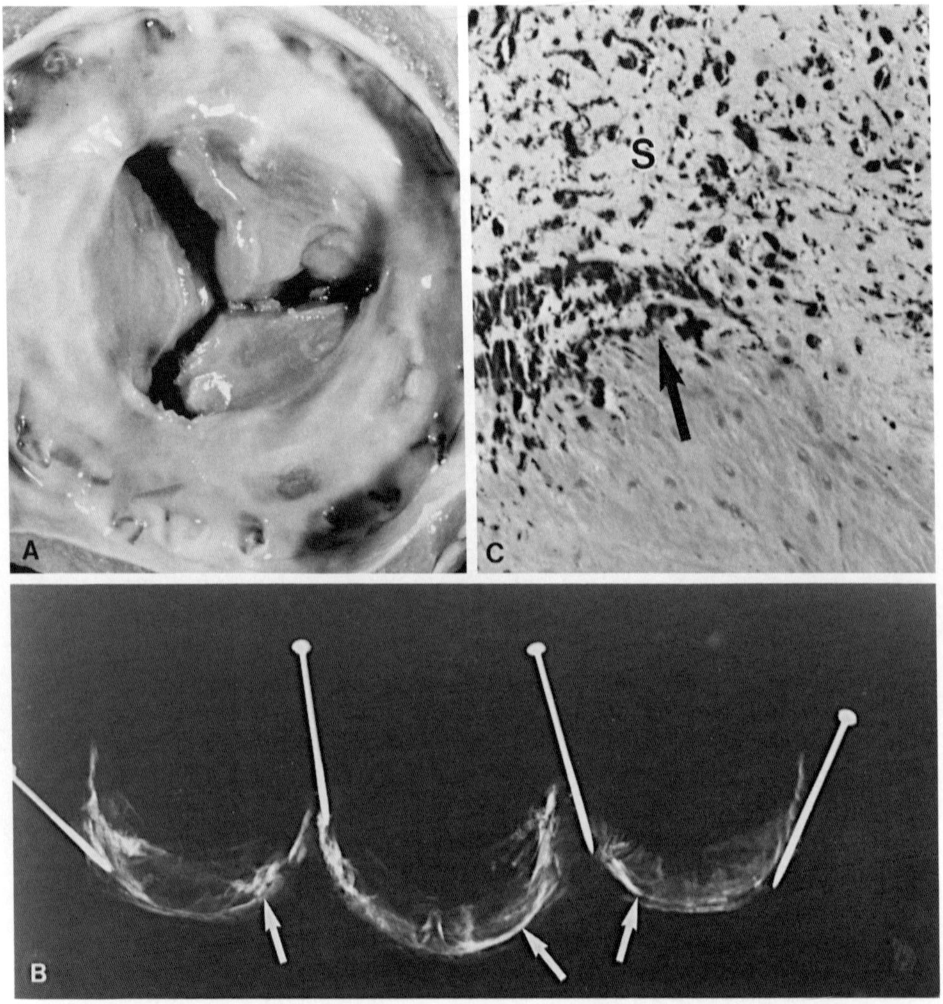

Figure 13-14. Morphology of porcine aortic valve implanted into the mitral position of calf for 92 days. *A,* Gross photograph. *B,* Radiograph of specimen shown in *A* demonstrating predominant calcification at cuspal attachment sites *(arrows)*. *C,* Light photomicrograph demonstrating diffuse calcific deposits predominantly in the spongiosa (S), with early nodule formation at the spongiosa/fibrosa junction *(arrow)*. (From Schoen, FJ, et al: Onset and progression of experimental bioprosthetic heart valve calcification. Lab Invest 52:523, 1985, with permission.)

8-month-old rats is less than 15 percent of that accumulated in implants in 3-week-old rats.[90] The basis for this differential rate of calcification is likely due to poorly understood age-related differences in calcium and phosphorus metabolism.

Neither nonspecific inflammation nor specific immunologic responses appear to mediate bioprosthetic tissue calcification.[88,90] Inflammation induces neither mineral deposition nor resorption. Morphologic examination of both circulatory and subcutaneous porcine valve implants reveals a classic "foreign body reaction," primarily composed of nonlymphocytic mononuclear cells.[90] Furthermore, inflammatory cell penetration into this tissue and host cell reaction to mineral deposits are minimal and inconsistent.[5,85,90] Enclosure of valve cusps in chambers that prevent

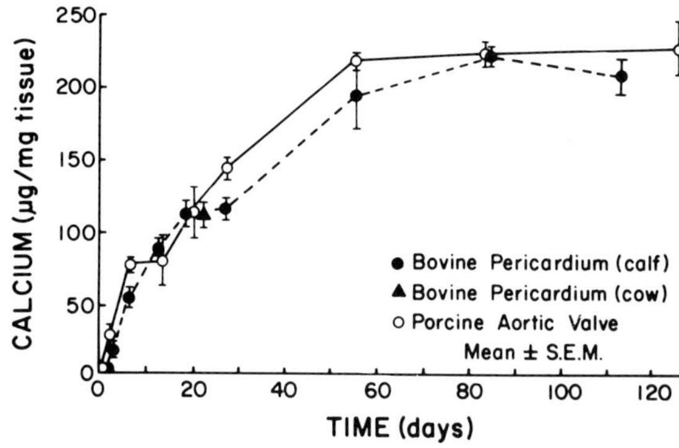

Figure 13-15. Progression of calcification (calcium assay by atomic absorption spectroscopy) in glutaraldehyde-pretreated porcine aortic valve and bovine pericardium implanted subcutaneously in rats. (From Schoen, FJ and Levy, RJ: Pathophysiology of bioprosthetic heart valve calcification. In Bodnar, E and Yacoub, MH (eds): Biological and Bioprosthetic Valves. Yorke, New York, 1986, p 418; with permission.)

host cell contact with tissue but allow free diffusion of extracellular fluid alters neither the extent nor morphology of mineralization in rat subcutaneous implants.[90] Moreover, valve tissue implanted in congenitally athymic ("nude") mice, who have essentially no T-cell function, calcifies to the same extent as implants in immunologically competent hosts.[88] These experimental findings are consistent with clinical data that show that second bioprosthetic valve replacements fail no sooner than initial replacements.[91] Previous clinical and experimental data detecting antibodies to valve tissue after failure probably reflect a secondary response to valve damage and resultant exposure of new antigenic determinants, rather than a cause of failure.[92]

Whether anticoagulation retards bioprosthetic valve and other pathologic calcifications remains a controversial and unsettled issue. It has been hypothesized that warfarin therapy might limit calcification of bioprosthetic heart valves by inhibiting vitamin K-dependent synthesis of γ-carboxyglutamic acid-containing calcium-binding proteins, which are associated with normal and pathologic calcification.[93] Nevertheless, several studies from our laboratories have failed to demonstrate an effect of warfarin on calcification of porcine aortic valves implanted in the calf

Table 13-2. Calcification of Subcutaneously Implanted Bioprosthetic Tissue (21-Day Implants)

	Calcium Content (μg/mg tissue)	Reference
Unimplanted PAV cusp	3 ± 1	90
3-wk-old recipient rat		
Untreated (fresh) PAV cusp	6 ± 1	90
Glutaraldehyde-treated PAV cusp	108 ± 16	90
Glutaraldehyde-treated bovine pericardium	114 ± 8	24
Millipore chamber-enclosed PAV cusp*	92 ± 18	90
Purified type I collagen*	57 ± 6	99
6-8-mo-old recipient rat	13 ± 4	90
3-wk-old recipient mouse		
PAV* in control (BALBc) mouse	102 ± 5	88
PAV* in nude (thymus-deficient)	96 ± 25	88

Mean ± SEM.
PAV = porcine aortic valve.
* Highly glutaraldehyde cross-linked.

circulatory system[86] or rat subcutaneous space,[90] or on calcification of functioning cardiac assist device bladders.[85] In contrast, an inhibitory effect of sodium warfarin on mineralization was suggested by a retrospective study of patients with clinical bioprosthetic valves[94] and an experimental investigation of elastomeric cardiac assist pump sacs.[95]

The most important determinant of the propensity of bioprosthetic tissue to calcify is probably the tissue preparation method. Pretreatment of tissue with an aldehyde cross-linking agent is a prerequisite for calcification in a nonflexing experimental environment.[90] Nonpreserved cusps implanted subcutaneously in rats do not mineralize. However, a recent report suggests that prolonged incubation of bioprosthetic valve tissue in glutaraldehyde inhibits mineralization.[96] Considerable additional work will be necessary before the relative roles of specific tissue preparation variables are understood. Despite differences in composition and structure, glutaraldehyde-treated porcine aortic valve and bovine pericardium calcify comparably with respect to kinetics, extent, and morphology.[24, 85] This not only suggests fundamental mechanisms of bioprosthetic tissue mineralization that depend on specific biochemical modifications of implant microstructural components induced by aldehyde pretreatment, but also predicts that calcification will critically limit the late durability of clinical pericardial bioprostheses.

Mechanisms of Calcification

Descriptive morphology of experimental bioprosthetic valve calcification is illustrated in Figures 13–16 and 13–17. Calcific deposits in either porcine valve or bovine pericardial tissue are evident morphologically and chemically within 48 hours following subcutaneous implantation.[24,85] Ultrastructural examination shows that initial deposits are localized to transplanted connective tissue cells but do not involve extracellular collagen fibers.[24,85] With increasing duration of implantation, cell-associated deposits increase in size and number, obliterating cells and dissecting among the collagen bundles. Direct collagen involvement occurs later. Proliferation of nucleation sites and crystal growth result in progressive confluence of diffusely distributed microcrystals into macroscopic nodules, which focally obliterate implant architecture and ulcerate through the cuspal surface. These gross nodules are analogous to those responsible for clinical valve failures. This sequence is summarized schematically in Figure 13–18.

The specific mechanisms by which glutaraldehyde fixation facilitates mineralization are not understood. Initial calcification of transplanted connective tissue cells could result from glutaraldehyde-induced cellular "devitalization" and the resulting disruption of cellular calcium regulation.[24] The concentration of ionic calcium is only approximately 10^{-7} M inside living animal cells, but approximately 10^{-3} M in the extracellular fluid. Thus, there is normally a steep, inwardly directed electrochemical gradient across the plasma membrane. Calcium entry into cells is passive, but the intracellular calcium concentration is kept low, in part by mechanisms that require the energy of ATP hydrolysis in order to pump calcium out of the cell. Intracellular phosphate levels, in contrast, are normally relatively high. Phosphate is incorporated in many proteins, lipids, and the nucleus and is especially prevalent within plasma and organellar membranes in the form of phospholipids and proteolipids. Using a newly available technique called electron energy loss spectrometry (EELS), we have recently demonstrated focally high concentrations of intracellular phosphorus in unimplanted, glutaraldehyde-preserved porcine aortic valve and bovine pericardium.[97]

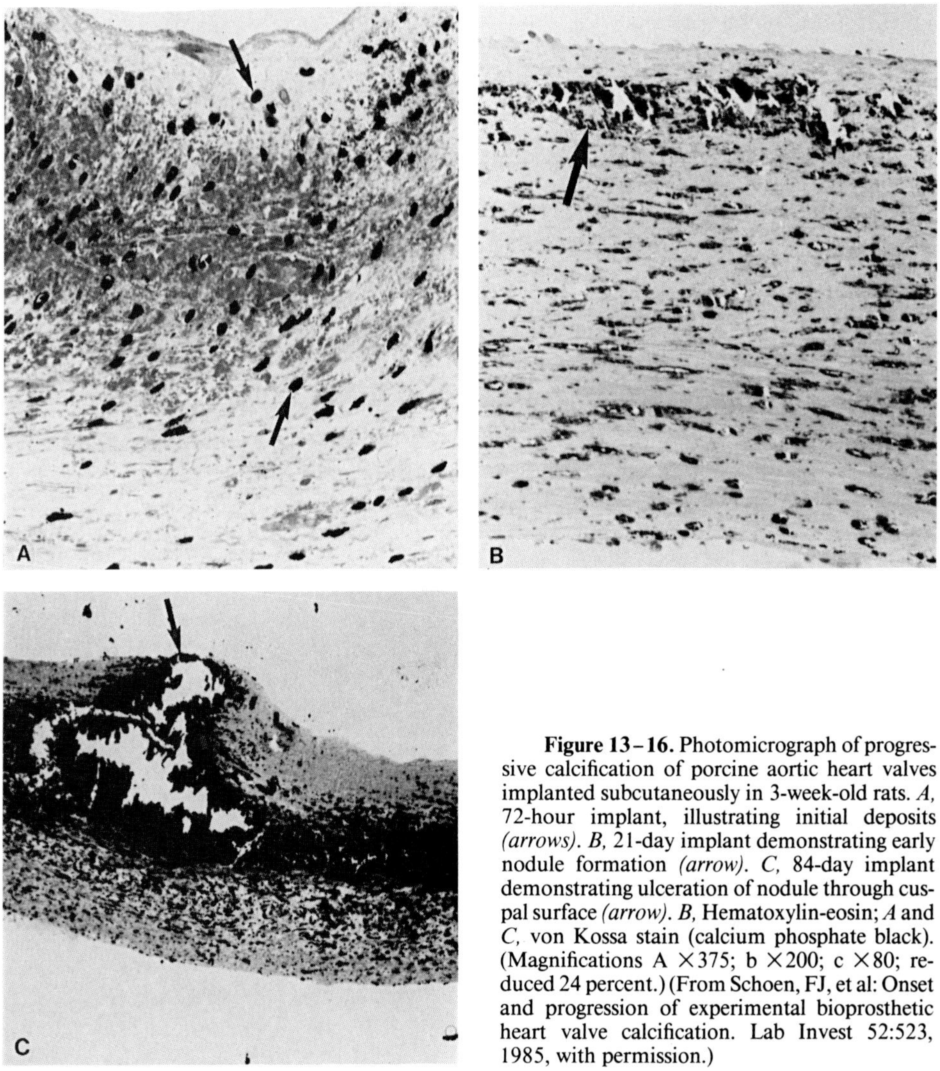

Figure 13–16. Photomicrograph of progressive calcification of porcine aortic heart valves implanted subcutaneously in 3-week-old rats. *A,* 72-hour implant, illustrating initial deposits *(arrows)*. *B,* 21-day implant demonstrating early nodule formation *(arrow)*. *C,* 84-day implant demonstrating ulceration of nodule through cuspal surface *(arrow)*. *B,* Hematoxylin-eosin; *A* and *C,* von Kossa stain (calcium phosphate black). (Magnifications A ×375; b ×200; c ×80; reduced 24 percent.) (From Schoen, FJ, et al: Onset and progression of experimental bioprosthetic heart valve calcification. Lab Invest 52:523, 1985, with permission.)

The effects of glutaraldehyde fixation and other aspects of tissue preparation on the cellular components of bioprosthetic tissue include paralysis of ATP-generating metabolic activity and disruption of the structural integrity of cell membranes and organelles. Both effects probably contribute to the initiation and progression of cell-associated calcification. When bioprosthetic tissue is bathed in either blood or extracellular fluid, substantial amounts of calcium are available. Depletion of cellular ATP stores reduces the activity of all energy-dependent transport mechanisms, thereby impairing calcium efflux from the cell. The net effect is a dramatic increase in intracellular calcium concentrations. Increased permeability owing to loss of membrane integrity exacerbates the inward ion flow. The imbalance between influx and efflux induced by loss of cell vitality is analogous to the mitochondrial calcification that occurs when cardiac myocytes are irreversibly damaged by severe ischemia and exposed to plasma during reperfusion.[98] The plasma membranes of necrotic myocytes, similar to connective tissue cells devitalized by glutaraldehyde, are incapable of

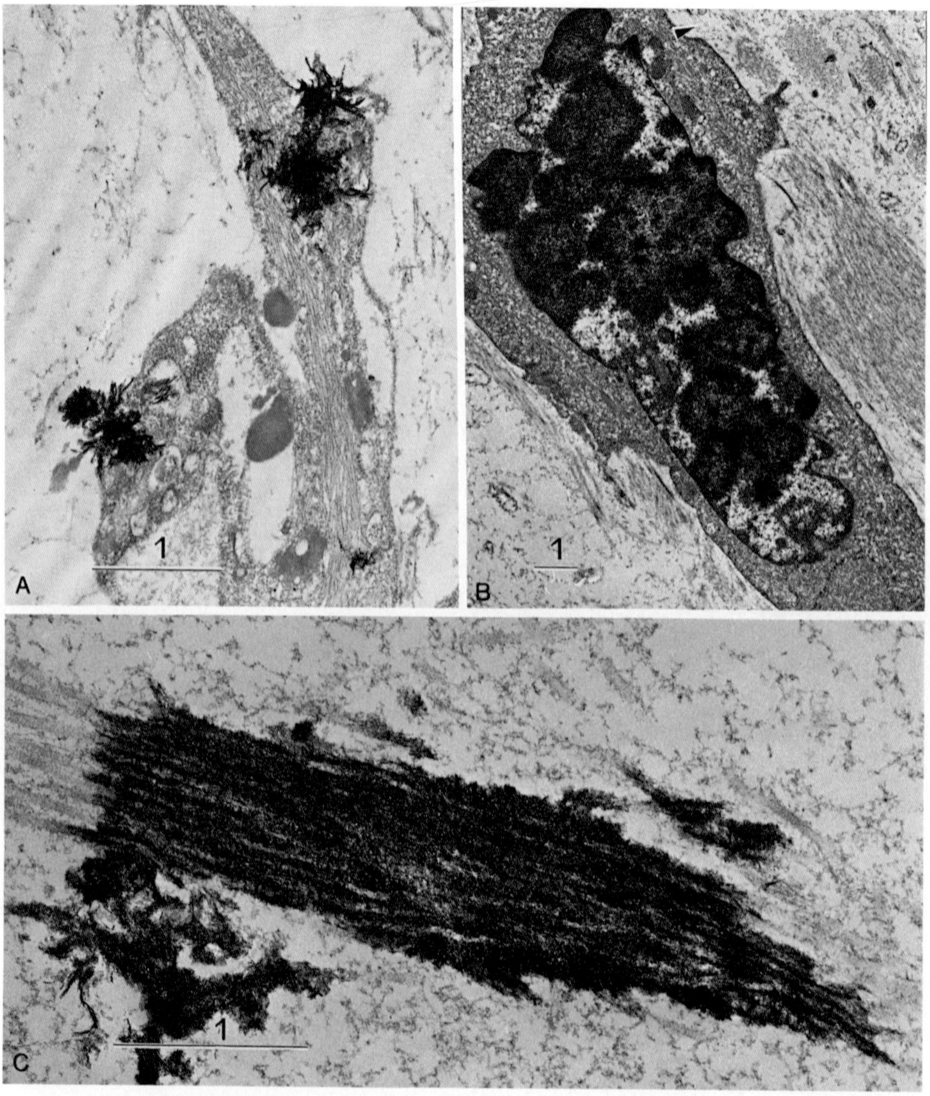

Figure 13–17. Ultrastructure of porcine connective tissue cell and collagen-associated calcific deposits in subcutaneous implants. *A*, Focal deposits at cell surface and cytoplasm. *B*, Extensive intranuclear calcification. *C*, Collagen calcification. *A*, 48 hours; *B*, 72 hours; *C*, 21 days. Bar = 1 μm. Sections stained with uranyl acetate and lead citrate. (*B* and *C* from Schoen, FJ, et al: Onset and progression of experimental bioprosthetic heart valve calcification. Lab Invest 52:523, 1985, with permission.)

excluding massive quantities of calcium ions, in the presence of transport systems that are no longer functional.

Although calcification of bioprosthetic tissue collagen occurs subsequently to cell and membrane involvement, experimental observations suggest that mineralization of the two components may represent independent processes. Implanted aldehyde-treated purified type I collagen sponges calcify without associated cell-oriented mineral deposition. Therefore, bioprosthetic tissue calcification may be mediated in part by direct interaction of glutaraldehyde with cuspal collagen.[99]

The extent to which mechanisms of bioprosthetic tissue calcification resemble those of physiologic and other forms of pathologic mineralization is not clear.[99-101] The pathologic calcification that occurs in bioprosthetic valves, degenerative senile native aortic valve sclerosis,[102] and nonfixed tissue valve implants (such as homografts[103] and fascia lata[104] valves), may be similar to the extent that, in each case, cell injury secondary to mechanical flexion probably renders the tissue susceptible to mineralization. Moreover, cell injury may be enhanced by local hypoxia in each of these poorly vascularized tissues. The typical molar ratio of Ca:P in calcified bioprosthetic tissue (approximately 1.6)[85] and crystal structure determined by x-ray diffraction[90] are consistent with those of hydroxyapatite, the predominant mineral phase in bone, and most instances of pathologic calcification.[100,105]

Prevention of Bioprosthetic Valve Calcification

An ultimate goal of investigations of the mechanisms of bioprosthetic tissue calcification is the development of preventive therapies. Since calcification has both host and implant determinants, strategies of prevention involve modifications of valve preparation and the local host environment of the implant. Experimental evidence suggests that the most promising approaches are cuspal pretreatment with detergents or diphosphonate compounds, or systemic or local therapy of the host with diphosphonates (Table 13–3).[106-109] Diphosphonates are synthetic pyrophosphate analogues, used to treat some types of metabolic bone disease, which probably inhibit calcification by binding to developing hydroxyapatite crystals, thereby restricting crystal growth.[110] Cuspal pretreatment by covalent linkage of aminopropane diphosphonate (APDP) to residual aldehyde groups in the glutaraldehyde-pretreated bioprosthetic tissue results in significant inhibition of calcification without any adverse effects.[106,107] Recent experiments indicate that a near-complete inhibition of mineralization may be achieved by optimization of APDP treatment conditions.[111] Pretreatment for 24 hours in 5 percent sodium dodecyl sulfate (SDS) also significantly inhibits calcification of porcine aortic valve tissue implanted subcutaneously in rats.[106] However, results with SDS-treated valves as orthotopic implants in large animal experimental models have been inconsistent. Some reports indicate that SDS pretreatment inhibits calcification of porcine valves in sheep and calves,[112,113] whereas other studies suggest that pretreated valves in the circulatory position calcify comparably to untreated controls.[114,115] One study[113] suggested that SDS inhibited calcification of orthotopic porcine valvular but not bovine pericardial implants in sheep. SDS pretreatment is currently used in the preparation of some clinical porcine aortic valves.[13]

Administration of diphosphonate compounds to the host consistently inhibits bioprosthetic tissue calcification. Daily subcutaneous injections of ethanehydroxy diphosphonate (EHDP) nearly completely inhibit calcification of subcutaneous bioprosthetic tissue implants but cause retardation of somatic growth and disruption of bone development in the recipient.[107] However, local controlled-release administra-

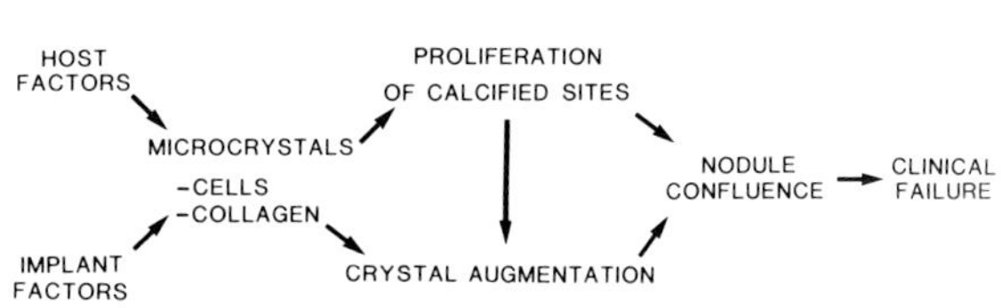

Figure 13–18. Schematic model for critical events in bioprosthetic heart valve calcification. (From Schoen, FJ, et al: Onset and progression of experimental bioprosthetic heart valve calcification. Lab Invest 52:523, 1985, with permission.)

Table 13–3. Inhibition of Calcification of Subcutaneously Implanted Porcine Aortic Valves by Host and Implant Modification

Group	Duration (d)	Calcium (μg/mg)	% Inhibition	Reference
Control	14	135 ± 6	—	107
Control	21	155 ± 4	—	107
Control	84	219 ± 14	—	108
EHDP, systemic	21	4 ± 1	97	107
EHDP, local	14	4 ± 1	97	107
EHDP, controlled release polymer	84	16 ± 6	93	108
APDP, cuspal pretreatment	21	24 ± 7	84	107
EHDP, cuspal pretreatment	21	114 ± 10	24	107
SDS, cuspal pretreatment	21	19 ± 4	84	106

Mean ± SEM.
EHDP = ethanehydroxy diphosphonate; APDP = aminopropane diphosphonate; SDS = sodium dodecyl sulfate.

tion of EHDP by osmotic mini-pump implanted in direct contact with the tissue prevents calcification without adverse systemic effects. More recently, controlled drug-release matrices containing EHDP dispersed in a copolymer of ethylene vinyl acetate, implanted adjacent to bioprosthetic tissue, also inhibited calcification without adverse effects (Fig. 13–19).[108] Because ethylene vinyl acetate–containing EHDP matrices can be formed in any shape, one attractive possibility is the direct incorporation of the diphosphonate-containing copolymer into the bioprosthesis, perhaps as part of the sewing ring. Studies directed toward further development of this concept are in progress.[76]

CONCLUSIONS

The overwhelming majority of patients who undergo valve replacement with either bioprosthetic or mechanical prosthetic valves have increased survival and enhanced functional status for extended intervals. Nevertheless, reoperation necessitated by or death caused by prosthesis-associated complications is common. Although thromboembolic complications are a frequent source of mortality and morbidity with mechanical prostheses, despite chronic anticoagulation, thromboembolic sequelae are infrequent in patients with bioprostheses, especially those in sinus rhythm. However, primary degenerative failure, predominantly due to cuspal mineralization, causing stenosis or regurgitation with or without cuspal tears, is a frequent cause of bioprosthetic valve dysfunction. Reoperation, largely owing to primary tissue failure, is required in approximately 20 to 30 percent of bioprosthetic valve recipients by 10 years postoperatively. Diagnosis of primary bioprosthetic valve dysfunction is enhanced substantially by 2-D Doppler echocardiography.

Experimental models, using either circulatory implants in large animals or subcutaneous implants in rodents, have contributed substantially to our understanding of the pathophysiology of bioprosthetic valve mineralization and its determinants. A complex interplay of host factors (particularly those influencing calcium and phosphorus metabolism) and implant factors (particularly those concerned with tissue source and preservation) mediate bioprosthetic valve calcification. Mechanical

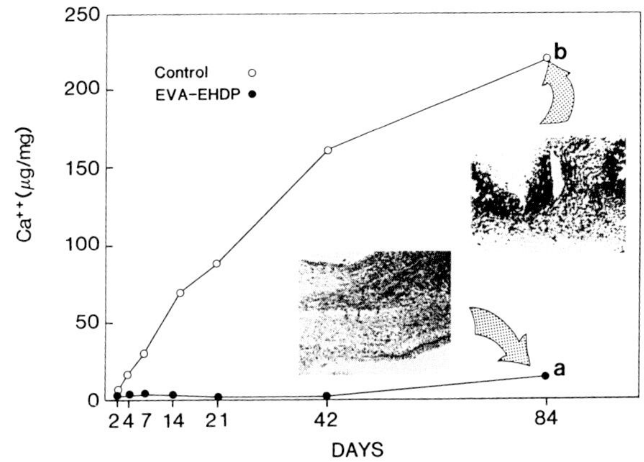

Figure 13–19. Inhibition of calcification in subcutaneously implanted porcine aortic valve by localized controlled release diphosphonate. *a,* Controlled-release implant. *b,* Untreated implant. Insets show photomicrographs of retrieved implants stained with the von Kossa technique (calcium phosphates—*black*). Extensive intrinsic calcification was noted at 84 days in control specimen, but no visible deposits were noted in implants treated with ethylene vinyl acetate–containing ethanehydroxydiphosphonate (EHDP). (From Levy, RJ, et al: Inhibition of calcification of bioprosthetic heart valves by local controlled release diphosphonate. Science 227:190, 1985, with permission.)

stress accelerates but is not a prerequisite for mineralization. Immunologic and other inflammatory reactions appear to be noncontributory. Bovine pericardium calcifies equivalently to porcine aortic valve in experimental models, and recent clinical data suggest that rates of failure of pericardial valves will be less favorable than those of porcine valves. Current investigation is directed toward elucidation of the pathophysiology of mineralization, development of specific pharmacological modifications of host and implant in order to inhibit it, and design modifications that could reduce degeneration and thus valve failure.

REFERENCES

1. Ionescu, MI (ed): Tissue Heart Valves. Butterworths, Boston, 1979, pp 1–373.
2. Cohn, LH and Gallucci, V (eds): Cardiac Bioprostheses. Yorke Medical Books, New York, 1982, pp 1–591.
3. Bodnar, E and Yacoub, MH (eds): Biological and Bioprosthetic Valves. Yorke Medical Books, New York, 1986, pp 1–874.
4. Titus, JL: Pathology of grafted heart valves. Adv Cardiol 7:149, 1972.
5. Schoen, FJ and Levy, RJ: Bioprosthetic heart valve failure: Pathology and pathogenesis. Cardiol Clin 2:717, 1984.
6. Edmunds, LH: Thromboembolic complications of current cardiac valvular prostheses. Ann Thorac Surg 34:96, 1982.
7. Miller, DC, Oyer, PE, Stinson, EB, et al: Ten to fifteen year reassessment of the performance characteristics of the Starr-Edwards model 6120 mitral valve prosthesis. J Thorac Cardiovasc Surg 85:1, 1983.
8. Schoen, FJ, Titus, JL, and Lawrie, GM: Autopsy-determined causes of death after cardiac valve replacement. JAMA 249:899, 1983.
9. Rahimtoola, SH: Valvular heart disease: A perspective. J Am Coll Cardiol 1:199, 1983.
10. Schoen, FJ and Hobson, CE: Anatomic analysis of removed prosthetic heart valves: Causes of failure of 33 mechanical valves and 58 bioprostheses, 1980–1983. Hum Pathol 16:549, 1985.
11. Ross, DN, Martelli, V, and Wain, WH: Allograft and autograft valves used for aortic valve replacement. In Ionescu, MI (ed): Tissue Heart Valves. London, Butterworths, 1979, p 127.
12. Carpentier, A, Lemaigre, G, Robert, L, et al: Biological factors affecting long-term results of valvular heterografts. J Thorac Cardiovasc Surg 58:467, 1969.
13. Wright, JT, Eberhardt, CE, Gibbs, ML, et al: Hancock II: An improved bioprosthesis. In Cohn LH and Gallucci V (eds): Cardiac Bioprostheses. New York, Yorke Medical Books, 1982, p 425.
14. Ionescu, MI, Smith, DR, Hasen, SS, et al: Clinical durability of the pericardial xenograft valve: Ten years' experience with mitral replacement. Ann Thorac Surg 34:265, 1982.

15. Bodnar, E, Bowden, NLR, Drury, PJ, et al: Bicuspid mitral bioprosthesis. Thorax 36:45, 1981.
16. Gabbay, S, Bortolotti, U, Cipolletti, G, et al: The Meadox unicusp pericardial bioprosthetic heart valve: New concept. Ann Thorac Surg 37:448, 1984.
17. Gross, L and Kugel, MA: Topographic anatomy and histology of the valves in the human heart. Am J Pathol 7:445, 1931.
18. Ferrans, VJ, Spray, VJ, Billingham, ME, et al: Structural changes in glutaraldehyde-treated porcine heterografts used as substitute cardiac valves: Transmission and scanning electron microscopy observations in 12 patients. Am J Cardiol 41:1159, 1978.
19. Ishihara, T, Ferrans, VJ, Jones, M, et al: Structure of bovine parietal pericardium and of unimplanted Ionescu-Shiley pericardial valvular bioprostheses. J Thorac Cardiovasc Surg 81:747, 1981.
20. Ishihara, T, Ferrans, VJ, Jones, M, et al: Histologic and ultrastructural features of normal human parietal pericardium. Am J Cardiol 46:744, 1980.
21. Allen, DJ, Didio, LJ, Zacharias, A, et al: Microscopic study of normal parietal pericardium and unimplanted Puig-Zerbini pericardial valvular heterografts. J Thorac Cardiovasc Surg 87:845, 1984.
22. Mannschott, P, Herbage, D, Weiss, M, et al: Collagen heterogeneity in pig heart valves. Biochem Biophys Acta 434:177, 1976.
23. Eyre, DR: Personal communication, 1983.
24. Schoen, FJ, Tsao, JW, and Levy, RJ: Calcification of bovine pericardium used in cardiac valve bioprostheses: Implications for the mechanisms of bioprosthetic tissue mineralization. Am J Pathol 123:134, 1986.
25. Cohn, LH, Allred, EN, DiSesa, VJ, et al: Early and late risk of aortic valve replacement: A 12 year concomitant comparison of the porcine bioprosthetic and tilting disc prosthetic aortic valves. J Thorac Cardiovasc Surg 88:695, 1984.
26. Starr, A and Grunkemeier, GL: Selection of a prosthetic heart valve. JAMA 251:1739, 1984.
27. Magilligan, DJ, Lewis, JW, Tilley, B, et al: The porcine bioprosthetic valve: Twelve years later. J Thorac Cardiovasc Surg 89:499, 1985.
28. Cohn, LH, Allred, EN, Cohn, LA, et al: Early and late risk of mitral valve replacement: A 12 year concomitant comparison of the porcine bioprosthetic and prosthetic disc mitral valves. J Thorac Cardiovasc Surg 90:872, 1985.
29. Oyer, PE, Stinson, EB, Miller, DC, et al: Thromboembolic risk and durability of the Hancock bioprosthetic cardiac valve. Eur Heart J 5(Suppl D):81, 1984.
30. Bosch, X, Pomar, JL, and Pelletier, LC: Early and late prognosis after reoperation for prosthetic valve replacement. J Thorac Cardiovasc Surg 88:567, 1984.
31. Reul, GJ, Cooley, DA, Duncan, JM, et al: Valve failure with the Ionescu-Shiley bovine pericardial bioprostheses: Analysis of 2680 patients. J Vasc Surg 2:192, 1985.
32. Brais, MP, Bedard, JP, Goldstein, W, et al: Ionescu-Shiley pericardial xenografts: Follow-up of up to 6 years. Ann Thorac Surg 39:105, 1985.
33. Nistal, F, Garcia-Satue, E, Artinano, E, et al: Comparative study of primary tissue valve failure between Ionescu-Shiley pericardial and Hancock porcine valves in the aortic position. Am J Cardiol 57:161, 1986.
34. Bortolotti, U, Milano, A, Mazzucco, A, et al: Results of reoperation for primary tissue failure of porcine bioprostheses. J Thorac Cardiovasc Surg 90:564, 1985.
35. Lader, E, Kronzon, I, Trehan, N, et al: Severe hemolytic anemia in patients with a porcine aortic valve prosthesis. J Am Coll Cardiol 1:1174, 1983.
36. Blackstone, EH and Kirklin, JW: Death and other time-related events after valve replacement. Circulation 72:753, 1985.
37. Schoen, FJ, Collins, JJ, and Cohn, LH: Long-term failure rate and morphologic correlations in porcine bioprosthetic heart valves. Am J Cardiol 51:957, 1983.
38. Sanders, SP, Levy, RJ, Freed, MD, et al: Use of Hancock porcine xenografts in children and adolescents. Am J Cardiol 46:429, 1980.
39. Dunn, JM: Porcine valve durability in children. Ann Thorac Surg 32:354, 1981.
40. Miller, DC, Stinson, EB, Oyer, PE, et al: The durability of porcine xenograft valves and conduits in children. Circulation 66(Suppl I):I-172, 1982.
41. Gabbay, S, Bortolotti, U, Wasserman, F, et al: Long-term follow-up of the Ionescu-Shiley mitral pericardial xenograft. J Thorac Cardiovasc Surg 88:758, 1984.
42. Ionescu, MI, Tandon, AP, Silverton, NP, et al: Long-term durability of the pericardial valve. In Bodnar, E and Yacoub, M (eds): Biologic and Bioprosthetic Valves. Yorke Medical Books, New York, 1986, p 165.

43. Cooley, DA, Ott, DA, Reul, GJ, et al: Ionescu-Shiley bovine pericardial bioprostheses: Clinical results in 2,701 patients. In Bodnar, E and Yacoub, M (eds): Biologic and Bioprosthetic Valves. Yorke Medical Books, New York, 1986, p 177.
44. Gonzalez-Lavin, L, Chi, S, Lewis, B, et al: An 8-year experience with the standard Ionescu-Shiley pericardial valve in the aortic position. In Bodnar, E and Yacoub, M (eds): Biologic and Bioprosthetic Valves. Yorke Medical Books, New York, 1986, p 199.
45. Wolf, PA, Dawber, TR, Thomas, HE, et al: Epidemiologic assessment of chronic atrial fibrillation and risk of stroke: The Framingham Study. Neurology 28:973, 1978.
46. Gajewski, J and Singer, RB: Mortality in an insured population with atrial fibrillation. JAMA 245:1540, 1981.
47. Magilligan, DJ, Oyama, C, and Alam, M: Comparison of dysfunction with mechanical and porcine mitral valve prostheses. Circulation 72(Suppl II):II-129, 1985.
48. Douglas, PS, Hirshfeld, JW, Edi, RN, et al: Clinical comparison of St. Jude and porcine aortic valve prostheses. Circulation 72(Suppl II):II-135, 1985.
49. Bortolotti, U, Milano, A, Mazzucco, A, et al: Pregnancy in patients with a porcine valve bioprosthesis. Am J Cardiol 50:1051, 1982.
50. Salazar, E, Zajarias, A, Gutierrez, N, et al: The problem of cardiac valve prostheses, anticoagulants, and pregnancy. Circulation 70(Suppl I):I-169, 1984.
51. Fishbein, MC, Gissen, SA, Collins, JJ, et al: Pathologic findings after cardiac valve replacement with glutaraldehyde-fixed porcine valves. Am J Cardiol 40:331, 1977.
52. Goffin, YA, Gruys, E, Sorenson, GD, et al: Amyloid deposits in bioprosthetic cardiac valves after long-term implantation in man: A new localization of amyloidosis. Am J Pathol 114:431, 1984.
53. Schoen, FJ: Surgical pathology of removed natural and prosthetic heart valves. Hum Pathol 1987 (in press).
54. Wilson, WR, Danielson, GK, Giuliani, ER, et al: Prosthetic valve endocarditis. Mayo Clin Proc 57:155, 1982.
55. Calderwood, SB, Swinski, LA, Waternaux, CM, et al: Risk factors for the development of prosthetic valve endocarditis. Circulation 72:31, 1985.
56. Muller, WA, Cohn, LH, and Schoen, FJ: Infection with a degenerated Starr-Edwards silicone rubber poppet in the aortic valve position. Am J Cardiol 54:1146, 1984.
57. Bortolotti, U, Thiene, G, Milano, A, et al: Pathological study of infective endocarditis on Hancock porcine bioprosthesis. J Thorac Cardiovasc Surg 81:934, 1981.
58. Ferrans, VJ, Ishihara, T, Jones, M, et al: Pathogenesis and stages of bioprosthetic infection. In Cohn, LH and Gallucci, V (eds): Cardiac Bioprostheses. New York, Yorke Medical Books, 1982, p 346.
59. Schoen, FJ: Pathology of cardiac valve replacement. In Morse, D, Steiner, RM, and Fernandez, J (eds): Guide to Prosthetic Cardiac Valves. Springer-Verlag, New York, 1985, p 209.
60. Ferrans, VJ, Boyce, SW, Billingham, ME, et al: Calcific deposits in porcine bioprostheses: Structure and pathogenesis. Am J Cardiol 46:721, 1980.
61. Rossiter, SJ, Stinson, EB, Oyer, PE, et al: Prosthetic valve endocarditis. Comparison of heterograft tissue valves and mechanical valves. J Thorac Cardiovasc Surg 76:795, 1978.
62. Alam, M, Lakier, JB, Pichard, SD, et al: Echocardiographic evolution of porcine bioprosthetic valves: Experience with 309 normals and 59 dysfunctional valves. Am J Cardiol 35:309, 1983.
63. Kotler, MN, Mintz, GS, Panidis, I, et al: Non-invasive evaluation of normal and abnormal prosthetic valve function. J Am Coll Cardiol 2:151, 1983.
64. Effron, MK and Popp, RL: Two-dimensional echocardiographic assessment of bioprosthetic valve dysfunction and infective endocarditis. J Am Coll Cardiol 2:597, 1983.
65. Hatle, L and Angelsen, B: Doppler Ultrasound in Cardiology—Physical Principles and Clinical Applications, ed 2. Lea & Febiger, Philadelphia, 1985, pp 188–205.
66. Kloster, FE: Diagnosis and management of complications of prosthetic heart valves. Am J Cardiol 35:372, 1975.
67. Thiene, G, Bortolotti, U, Panizzon, G, et al: Pathological substrates of thrombus formation after heart valve replacement with the Hancock bioprosthetic valves. J Thorac Cardiovasc Surg 80:414, 1980.
68. Thubrikar, MJ, Deck, JD, Aouad, J, et al: Role of mechanical stress in calcification of aortic bioprosthetic valves. J Thorac Cardiovasc Surg 86:115, 1983.
69. Valente, M, Bortolotti, U, and Thiene, G: Ultrastructural substrates of dystrophic calcification in porcine bioprosthetic valve failure. Am J Pathol 119:12, 1985.
70. Stein, PD, Kemp, SR, Riddle, JM, et al: Relation of calcification to torn leaflets of spontaneously degenerated porcine bioprosthetic valves. Ann Thorac Surg 40:175, 1985.

71. Ishihara, T, Ferrans, VJ, Boyce, SW, et al: Structure and classification of cuspal tears and perforations in porcine bioprosthetic cardiac valves implanted in patients. Am J Cardiol 48:665, 1981.
72. Riddle, JM, Magilligan, DJ, and Stein, PD: Surface morphology of degenerated porcine bioprosthetic valves four to seven years following implantation. J Thorac Cardiovasc Surg 81:279, 1981.
73. Gabbay, S and Kresh, J: Bioengineering of mechanical and biologic heart valve substitutes. In Morse, D, Steiner, RM, and Fernandez, J (eds): Guide to Prosthetic Cardiac Valves. Springer-Verlag, New York, 1985, p 239.
74. Schoen, FJ: Causes of failure and pathological findings in surgically removed Ionescu-Shiley standard bovine pericardial heart valve bioprostheses: Emphasis on progressive structural deterioration. Circulation (in press).
75. Schoen, FJ, Shemin, RJ, and Cohn, LH: Pathologic evaluation of a unileaflet pericardial bioprosthesis after implantation as tricuspid and mitral valve replacements in sheep. In Transactions, Society for Biomaterials 9:76, 1986.
76. Levy, RJ, Schoen, FJ, and Golumb, G: Bioprosthetic heart valve calcification: Clinical features, pathobiology, and prospects for prevention. CRC Critical Reviews in Biocompatibility 2:147, 1986.
77. Alam, M, Goldstein, S, and Lakier, JB: Echocardiographic changes in the thickness of porcine valves with time. Chest 79:309, 1985.
78. Lipson, LC, Kent, KM, Rosing, DR, et al: Long-term hemodynamic assessment of the porcine heterograft in the mitral position. Late development of valvular stenosis. Circulation 64:397, 1981.
79. Schoen, FJ, Schulman, LJ, and Cohn, LH: Quantitative anatomic analysis of "stent creep" of explanted Hancock standard porcine bioprostheses used for cardiac valve replacement. Am J Cardiol 56:110, 1985.
80. Williams, GA and Labovitz, AJ: Doppler hemodynamic evaluation of prosthetic (Starr-Edwards and Bjork-Shiley) and bioprosthetic (Hancock and Carpentier-Edwards) cardiac valves. Am J Cardiol 56:325, 1985.
81. Ryan, T, Armstrong, WF, Dillon, JC, et al: Doppler echocardiographic evaluation of patients with porcine mitral valves. Am Heart J 111:237, 1986.
82. Abbasi, AS, Allen, MW, Decristofaro, D, et al: Detection and estimation of the degree of mitral regurgitation by range-gated pulse Doppler echocardiography. Circulation 61:143, 1980.
83. Barnhart, GR, Jones, M, Ishihara, T, et al: Bioprosthetic valvular failure. Clinical and pathological observations in an experimental animal model. J Thorac Cardiovasc Surg 83:618, 1982.
84. Levy, RJ, Zenker, JA, and Bernhard, WF: Porcine bioprosthetic valve calcification in bovine left ventricle-aorta shunts: Studies of the deposition of vitamin K-dependent proteins. Ann Thorac Surg 36:187, 1983.
85. Schoen, FJ, Levy, RJ, Nelson, AC, et al: Onset and progression of experimental bioprosthetic heart valve calcification. Lab Invest 52:523, 1985.
86. Lian, JB, Levy, RJ, Bernhard, W, et al: LVAD mineralization of gammacarboxyglutamic acid containing proteins in normal and pathologically mineralized tissue. Trans Am Soc Artif Intern Organs 27:683, 1981.
87. Gabbay, S, Bortolotti, U, Factor, S, et al: Calcification of implanted xenograft pericardium: Influence of site and function. J Thorac Cardiovasc Surg 87:782, 1984.
88. Levy, RJ, Schoen, FJ, and Howard, SL: Mechanism of calcification of porcine bioprosthetic aortic valve cusps: Role of T-lymphocytes. Am J Cardiol 52:629, 1983.
89. Fishbein, MC, Levy, RJ, Ferrans, VJ, et al: Calcification of cardiac valve bioprostheses: Biochemical, histologic and ultrastructural observations in a subcutaneous implantation model system. J Thorac Cardiovasc Surg 83:602, 1982.
90. Levy, RJ, Schoen, FJ, Levy, JT, et al: Biologic determinants of dystrophic calcification and osteocalcin deposition in glutaraldehyde-preserved porcine aortic valve leaflets implanted subcutaneously in rats. Am J Pathol 113:143, 1983.
91. Magilligan, DJ, Lewis, JW, Heinzerling, RH, et al: Fate of a second porcine bioprosthetic valve. J Thorac Cardiovasc Surg 85:362, 1983.
92. Rocchini, AP, Weesner, KM, Heidelberger, K, et al: Porcine xenograft valve failure in children: An immunologic response. Circulation 64(Suppl II):II-162, 1981.
93. Gallop, PM, Lian, JB, and Hauschka, PV: Carboxylated calcium-binding proteins and vitamin K. N Engl J Med 302:1460, 1980.
94. Stein, PD, Riddle, JM, Kemp, SR, et al: Effect of warfarin on calcification of spontaneously degenerated porcine bioprosthetic valves. J Thorac Cardiovasc Surg 90:119, 1985.
95. Pierce, WS, Donachy, JH, Rosenberg, G, et al: Calcification inside artificial hearts: Inhibition by warfarin sodium. Science 208:601, 1980.

96. Schryer, PJ, Tomasek, ER, Starr, JA, et al: Anticalcification effect of glutaraldehyde-preserved valve tissue stored for increasing time in glutaraldehyde. In Bodnar, E and Yacoub, M (eds.): Biologic and Bioprosthetic Valves. Yorke Medical Books, New York, 1986, p 471.
97. Schoen, FJ and Levy, RJ: Unpublished results.
98. Hagler, HK, Lopez, LE, Murphy, ME, et al: Quantitative x-ray microanalysis of mitochondrial calcification in damaged myocardium. Lab Invest 45:241, 1981.
99. Levy, RJ, Schoen, FJ, Sherman, FS, et al: Calcification of subcutaneously implanted Type I collagen sponges: Effects of glutaraldehyde and formaldehyde pretreatments. Am J Pathol 122:71, 1986.
100. Anderson, HC: Calcific diseases: A concept. Arch Pathol Lab Med 107:341, 1983.
101. Glimcher, MJ: On the form and function of bone: From molecules to organs. Wolff's law revisited. In Veis, A (ed): The Chemistry and Biology of Mineralized Connective Tissues. North Holland, Elsevier, 1981, p 617.
102. Kim, KM, Valigorsky, JM, Mergner, WJ, et al: Aging changes in the human aortic valve in relation to dystrophic calcification. Hum Pathol 7:47, 1976.
103. Wallace, RB, Londe, SP, and Titus, JL: Aortic valve replacement with preserved aortic valve homografts. J Thorac Cardiovasc Surg 67:44, 1974.
104. Silver, MD, Hudson, REB, and Trimble, AS: Morphologic observations on heart valve prostheses made of fascia lata. J Thorac Cardiovasc Surg 70:360, 1975.
105. Posner, AS: The mineral of bone. Clin Orthop Rel Res 200:87, 1985.
106. Levy, RJ, Levy, JT, Schoen, FJ, et al: Prevention of bioprosthetic heart valve calcification. Circulation 68(Suppl 3):III-395, 1983.
107. Levy, RJ, Hawley, MA, Schoen, FJ, et al: Inhibition by diphosphonate compounds of calcification of porcine bioprosthetic heart valve cusps implanted subcutaneously in rats. Circulation 71:349, 1985.
108. Levy, RJ, Wolfrum, J, Schoen, FJ, et al: Inhibition of calcification of bioprosthetic heart valves by local controlled-release diphosphonate. Science 228:190, 1985.
109. Golumb, G, Langer, R, Schoen, FJ, et al: Controlled-release of diphosphonate to inhibit bioprosthetic heart valve calcification: Dose-response and mechanistic studies. J Control Release 4:181, 1986.
110. Russell, RGG and Smith, R: Diphosphonates: Experimental and clinical aspects. J Bone Joint Surg 55:66, 1973.
111. Webb, C, Benedict, J, Schoen, FJ, et al: Inhibition of bioprosthetic (BHV) calcification (CALC) with covalently bound aminopropanehydroxydiphosphonate (APD). Trans Am Soc Artif Intern Organs (in press).
112. Lentz, DJ, Pollock, EM, Olsen, DB, et al: Prevention of intrinsic calcification in porcine and bovine xenograft materials. Trans Am Soc Artif Intern Organs 28:494, 1982.
113. Arbustini, E, Jones, M, Moses, RD, et al: Modification by the Hancock T6 process of calcification of bioprosthetic cardiac valves implanted in sheep. Am J Cardiol 53:1388, 1984.
114. Thubrikar, MJ, Nolan, SP, Deck, JD, et al: Intrinsic calcification of T6-processed and control porcine and bovine bioprostheses in calves. Trans Am Soc Artif Intern Organs 29:245, 1983.
115. Thiene, G, Laborde, F, Valente, M, et al: Experimental evaluation of porcine-valved conduits processed with a calcium-retarding agent (T6). J Thorac Cardiovasc Surg 91:215, 1986.

PART 4

Special Topics

CHAPTER 14

Pathology of Pulmonary Hypertension

William D. Edwards, M.D.

Pulmonary hypertension denotes elevated blood pressure in the pulmonary circulation and is defined clinically as pulmonary arterial pressure of more than 30/15 mmHg (or a mean of more than 25 mmHg).[1] It may be *primary* (idiopathic) or *secondary* to a known underlying disorder such as a ventricular septal defect or recurrent pulmonary thromboembolization. *Acute* pulmonary hypertension (associated with the adult respiratory distress syndrome, for example) usually exhibits few, if any, hypertensive lesions on light microscopy. Alternatively, *chronic* cases exhibit widespread pulmonary vascular abnormalities that typically include medial hypertrophy, obstructive intimal lesions, and thrombosis. In patients with *precapillary* obstructions, only the pulmonary arteries tend to be involved. In contrast, *postcapillary* obstructions are also associated with venous, capillary, and lymphatic alterations.

Consequently, pulmonary hypertension may be categorized according to cause (primary or secondary), duration (acute or chronic), or location (precapillary or postcapillary). More commonly, however, it is classified according to *histopathologic patterns,* as discussed in detail in several texts.[1-3] An understanding of the hypertensive patterns is facilitated by familiarity with normal pulmonary vascular histology.

NORMAL PULMONARY VASCULATURE

In contrast to the systemic circulation, the pulmonary vascular bed is a low-pressure and low-resistance system, and its structure reflects these hemodynamic features (Table 14–1). Both the pulmonary arteries (Fig. 14–1) and the pulmonary veins (Fig. 14–2) are normally thin-walled.[1-3]

In human lungs, pulmonary arteries travel with their respective bronchi. Elastic pulmonary arteries extend from the level of the pulmonary valve to the small (1 mm) subsegmental bronchi, and they function as compliant conduits for blood flow. Normally, the diameter of the pulmonary trunk is similar to that of the ascending aorta, and the diameters of intrapulmonary elastic arteries are similar to those of adjacent bronchi.

Muscular pulmonary arteries accompany airways from the level of subsegmental bronchi to respiratory bronchioles (Table 14–2; see Fig. 14–1), and their diame-

Table 14–1. Comparison of Pulmonary and Systemic Circulations

	Circulation	
Feature	*Pulmonary*	*Systemic*
Arterial pressure, mmHg	22/10 (mean, 13)	120/80 (mean, 90)
Capillary pressure, mmHg	6–9 (mean, 7)	10–30 (mean, 17)
Venous pressure, mmHg	1–4 (mean, 2)	0–10 (mean, 6)
Arterial M/D ratio, %*	3–8 (mean, 5)	15–25 (mean, 20)
Venous M/D ratio, %*	2–5 (mean, 3)	3–6 (mean, 4)
Vascular resistance, $U \cdot m^2$	1–4 (mean, 3)	10–25 (mean, 15)
Blood flow, liters/min	5	5

* M/D ratio = ratio of thickness of media to external diameter of vessel.

ters are somewhat smaller than those of the adjacent airways. They primarily control pulmonary vascular resistance. In humans, the muscular pulmonary arteries show great individual variability in response to oxygen and other vasoactive substances. Therefore, vascular reactivity, as well as vascular obstruction, may contribute to the development of some forms of pulmonary hypertension.[1,2]

Pulmonary arterioles are intra-acinar and, accordingly, travel either beside respiratory bronchioles and alveolar ducts or within alveolar walls. As they taper, they

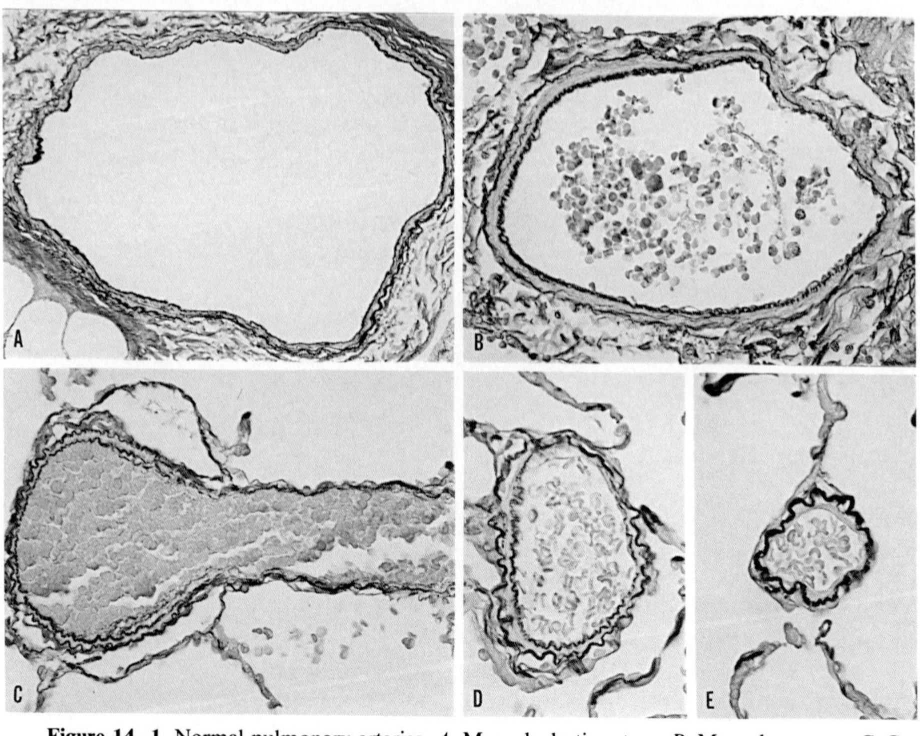

Figure 14–1. Normal pulmonary arteries. *A,* Musculoelastic artery. *B,* Muscular artery. *C,* Cross section of small artery and longitudinal section of its arteriolar branch demonstrates loss of smooth muscle in arteriole. *D, E,* Cross sections of small artery *(D)* and arteriole *(E)* show muscular and nonmuscular medias, respectively. (Elastic–van Gieson stain; magnification *A,* ×90; *B* and *C,* ×360; *D* and *E,* ×450; reduced 38 percent.)

Table 14–2. Diameters of Histologic Types of Pulmonary Arteries

Histologic Type	Diameter, μ	Adjacent Airways
Elastic	>1000 (1mm)	Lobar, segmental, and subsegmental bronchi
Musculoelastic	500–1500	Subsegmental bronchus
Muscular	50–1000	Subsegmental bronchus, terminal bronchiole
Arteriole	15–150	Respiratory bronchiole, alveolar duct, and alveolar wall

gradually lose their medial smooth muscle and internal elastic membrane (see Fig. 14–1).[1–4] Because the arterioles contribute little to pulmonary vascular resistance in the normal lung, the clinical term "arteriolar resistance" is anatomically misleading.

The pulmonary capillaries form a vascular network within alveolar walls and are primarily concerned with gas exchange and various metabolic functions (such as angiotensin-converting activity). Normally, most capillary beds in the lung are only partially open. However, if pulmonary blood flow increases (as with exercise), capillary beds open to accommodate the increased flow. In this manner, pulmonary blood flow may increase without an appreciable increase in pulmonary vascular resistance. Extensive loss of intra-acinar vessels, however, may contribute to the development of some forms of pulmonary hypertension.[4]

Small pulmonary venules course between alveolar walls and are similar in both location and structure to normal arterioles. Larger venules are located at the periphery of the acinus, and pulmonary veins travel within the interlobular septa.[1] Pulmonary veins have an indistinct external elastic membrane and thereby differ from pulmonary arteries not only in location but also in structure (Fig. 14–2). They function as compliant conduits for blood flow, and their obstruction may lead to the development of pulmonary hypertension.

Lymphatics also course within the interlobular septa, as well as the pleurae, and are distinguished from veins by the presence of valves and the absence of luminal erythrocytes. Their role is to drain excess interstitial fluid and thereby maintain dry alveoli.

Bronchial vessels nourish the tracheobronchial tree and the vasa vasora of the pulmonary vessels. Bronchial arteries usually arise from the descending thoracic aorta at the level of the carina, and pulmonary veins normally drain into the left atrium or the azygos and hemiazygos veins.[5] Arterial bronchopulmonary anastomoses occur in the lung but are less frequent than their venous counterpart.[1–3,5] Pulmonary and bronchial arteriovenous anastomoses are rare in the normal lung.

With increasing age, the mediastinal pulmonary arteries dilate and may harbor a few shallow nonobstructive atheromas. Elastic arteries within the lungs may also develop occasional atheromas, and muscular arteries frequently develop shallow eccentric intimal fibrotic patches (Fig. 14–3).[3,6] With age, capillaries become slightly thicker, and veins may show patchy or circumferential intimal hyalinization (Fig. 14–3).

PHYSIOLOGIC FETAL PULMONARY HYPERTENSION

During fetal life, the ductus arteriosus allows free communication between the pulmonary and systemic circulations. Moreover, the relative hypoxemia of fetal

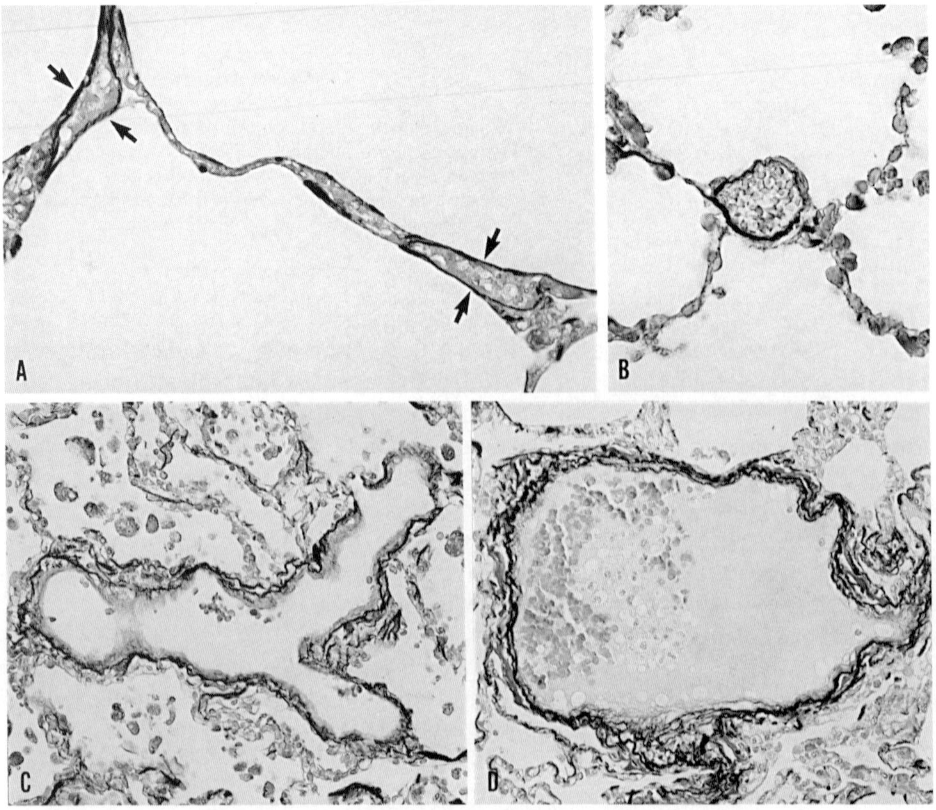

Figure 14–2. Normal pulmonary microcirculation and veins. *A,* Alveolar capillaries *(between arrows). B, C,* Venules. *D,* Vein. (Elastic–van Gieson stain; magnification *A,* ×360; *B,* ×450; *C* and *D,* ×225; reduced 28 percent.)

blood and the collapsed state of the lungs promote further vasoconstriction. The relatively high pressure and high resistance that occur as a result in the pulmonary vascular bed are manifested morphologically by medial hypertrophy of muscular and elastic pulmonary arteries (Fig. 14–4) and by physiologic right ventricular hypertrophy (Fig. 14–5).

At birth, hemodynamic changes take place that transform the pulmonary vascular bed into a low-pressure and low-resistance circulation. Closure of the ductus arteriosus occurs functionally during the first day of postnatal life and anatomically within 2 or 3 months. Furthermore, as the lungs expand and arterial oxygen saturation increases, pulmonary vasoconstriction abates.

As a result, the relative thicknesses of the pulmonary arterial media and the right ventricular free wall gradually diminish during the first few months after birth (see Figs. 14–4, 14–5).[1,2,4,7] By the age of 6 months, the anatomic hallmarks of physiologic fetal pulmonary hypertension have regressed completely. Some investigators[8,9] have observed that during childhood and adolescence there is a progressive extension of smooth muscle into the peripheral small arterial branches within acini, whereas others[10] have reported an age-related loss of medial smooth muscle in small (less than 100 μm) pulmonary arteries.

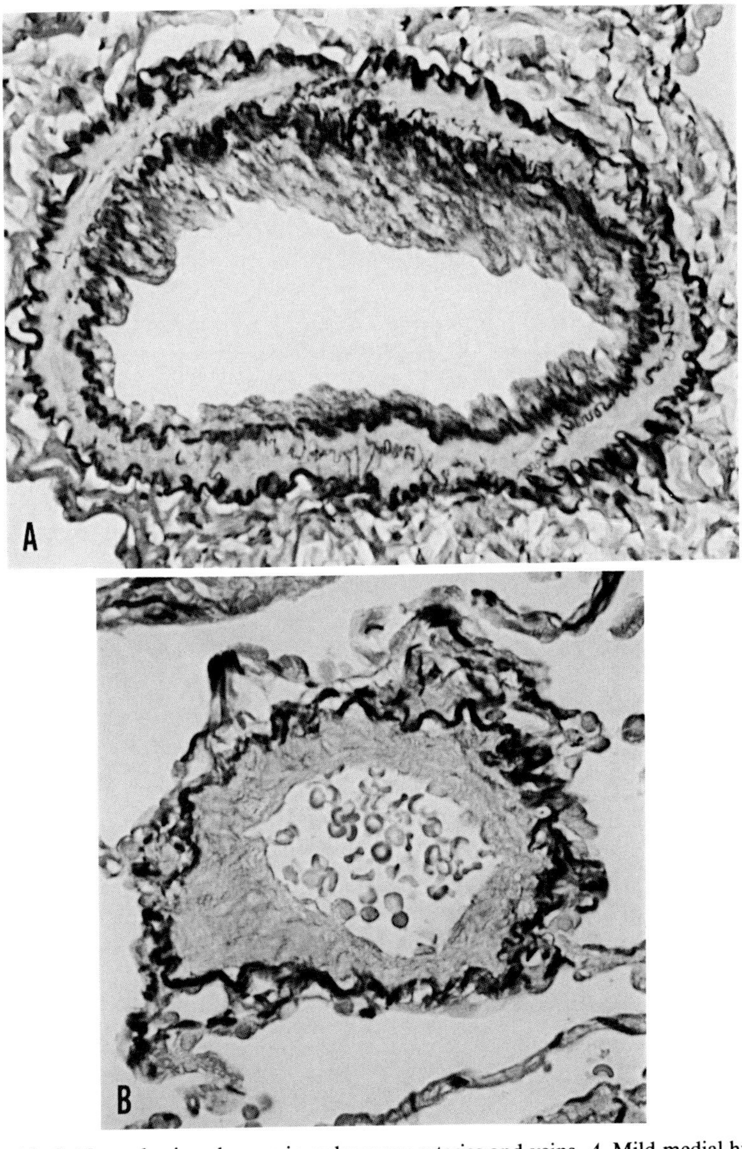

Figure 14-3. Normal aging changes in pulmonary arteries and veins. *A,* Mild medial hypertrophy and mild focal eccentric intimal fibrosis of small artery. *B,* Concentric intimal hyalinization of small vein. (Elastic-van Gieson stain; magnification ×450.)

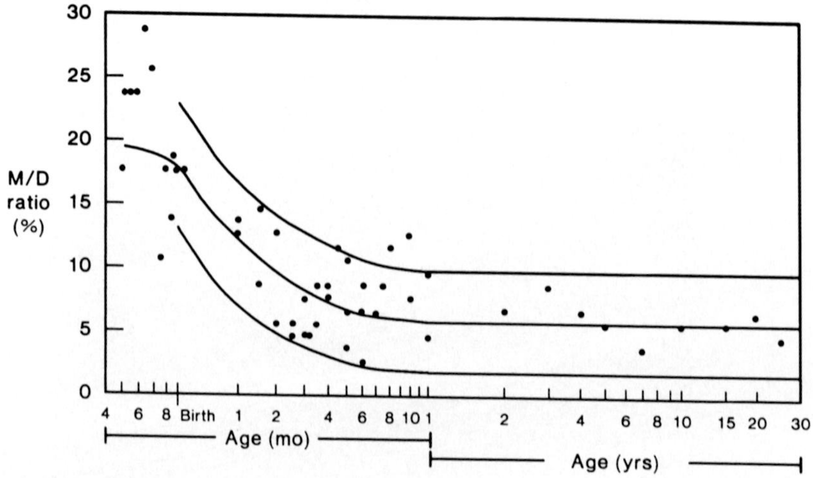

A

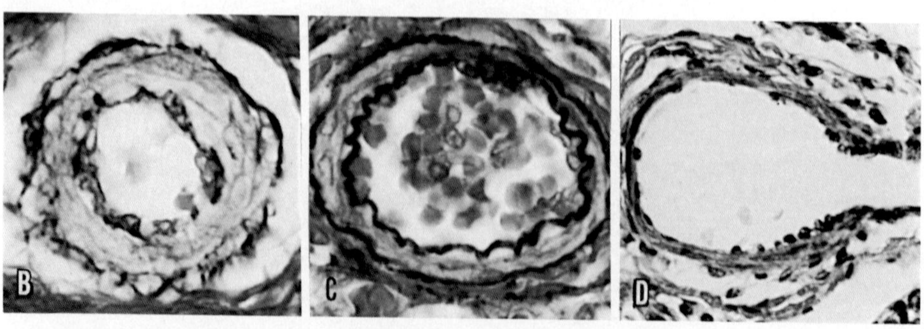

Figure 14-4. Changes in pulmonary arteries after birth. *A,* Ratio of medial thickness to external arterial diameter (M/D), in 50 normal heart-lung specimens, diminishes from prenatal value of approximately 20 percent, when physiologic fetal pulmonary hypertension exists, to approximately 5 percent by 6 months of age. *B* through *D,* Comparison of relative medial thicknesses at birth *(B),* at age 2 months *(C),* and at age 7 months *(D).* (*B* through *D,* Elastic–van Gieson stain; magnification ×360; reduced 17 percent.) (*A* from Petersen, RC and Edwards, WD: Pulmonary vascular disease in 57 necropsy cases of total anomalous pulmonary venous connection. Histopathology 7:487, 1983, with permission of Blackwell Scientific Publications.)

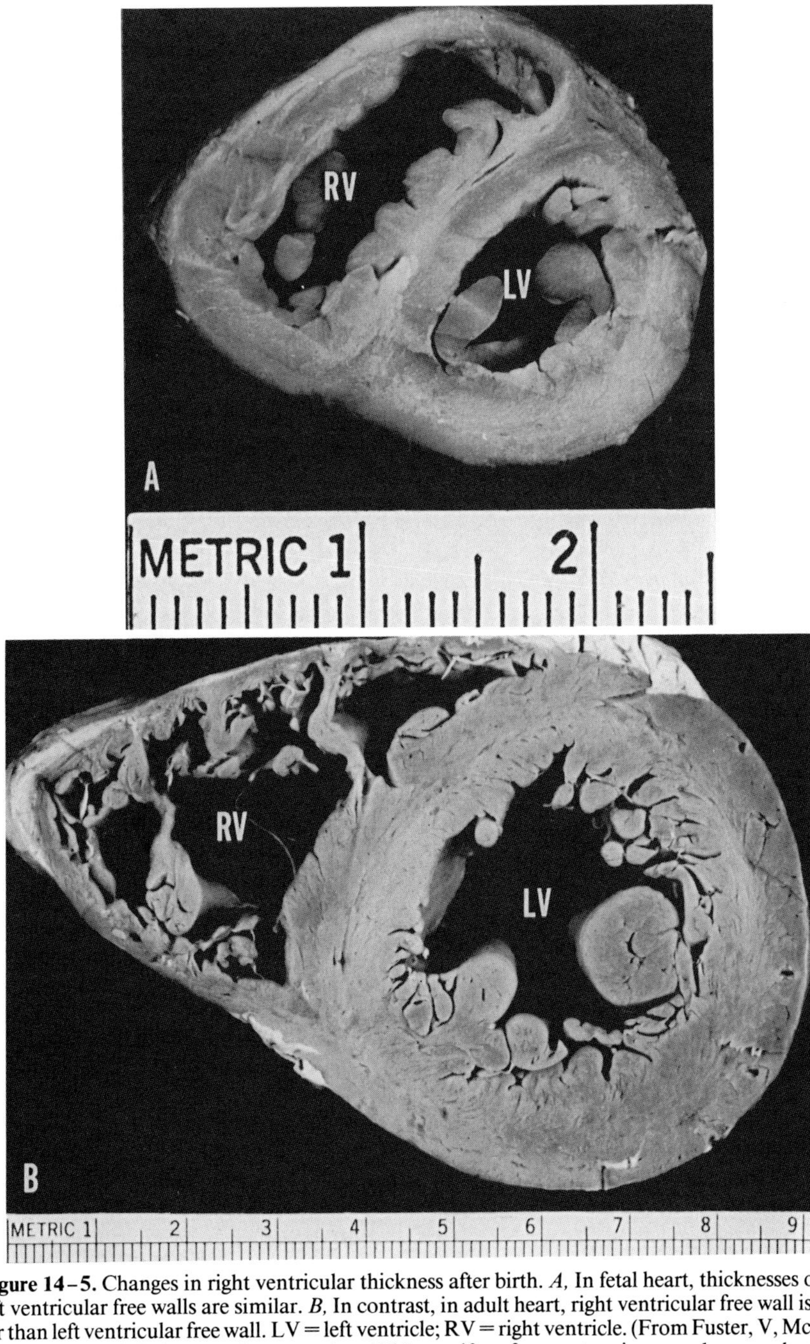

Figure 14-5. Changes in right ventricular thickness after birth. *A,* In fetal heart, thicknesses of right and left ventricular free walls are similar. *B,* In contrast, in adult heart, right ventricular free wall is much thinner than left ventricular free wall. LV = left ventricle; RV = right ventricle. (From Fuster, V, McGoon, MD, Dines, DE, et al: Pulmonary hypertension: With specific reference to primary pulmonary hypertension. In Brandenburg, RO, Fuster, V, Giuliani, ER, et al [eds]: Cardiology: Fundamentals and Practice. Year Book Medical Publishers, Chicago, 1987, with permission of Mayo Foundation.)

PERSISTENT PULMONARY HYPERTENSION OF THE NEWBORN

In some full-term or post-term infants, pulmonary vascular resistance and pressure do not decrease after birth.[11,12] The ductus arteriosus maintains its patency, and right-to-left shunts exist at the levels of the ductus arteriosus and the foramen ovale. This hemodynamic pattern apparently results from hypoxemia and acidosis and is usually related to intrauterine or perinatal asphyxia, aspiration of meconium, or shock. Respiratory symptoms develop during the first few postnatal days and generally resolve within 2 weeks. However, chronic and fatal cases may occur.

Histologically, the pulmonary vasculature exhibits the expected findings in normal neonates (that is, medial hypertrophy of muscular and elastic pulmonary arteries) and may also be involved by platelet-fibrin thrombosis. The pulmonary parenchyma may appear normal or may be damaged by aspiration pneumonia.

GENERAL FEATURES OF CHRONIC PULMONARY HYPERTENSION

In all forms of chronic pulmonary hypertension, the following morphologic features are present to varying degrees: (1) medial hypertrophy of muscular and elastic pulmonary arteries, (2) dilatation and shallow intimal atheromas of elastic pulmonary arteries, and (3) right ventricular hypertrophy, with or without dilatation (Fig. 14–6).[1,13,14] Clinically, right ventricular hypertrophy due to pulmonary hypertension is termed "cor pulmonale."

Straightening of the ventricular septum may appreciably alter the shape and function of *both* ventricles (Fig. 14–7).[15] Moreover, dilatation of the pulmonary and tricuspid anuli commonly produces valvular regurgitation (Fig. 14–8). Chronic pulmonary hypertension may also be associated with dilatation of the right atrium and coronary sinus, right-to-left shunting across a patent foramen ovale, and chronic passive congestion of systemic viscera. In some patients, the dilated and hypertensive mediastinal pulmonary arteries cause tracheobronchial indentation and may produce hoarseness by compression of the left recurrent laryngeal nerve.

HISTOPATHOLOGY OF CHRONIC PULMONARY HYPERTENSION

In addition to the aforementioned features of chronic pulmonary hypertension, certain histopathologic lesions typically involve the arteries, and others are characteristically observed in the microcirculation and veins.[14]

Arterial Lesions

Medial Lesions

Medial hypertrophy accompanies all forms of chronic pulmonary hypertension (Fig. 14–9) and is presumably the result of chronic vasoconstriction in most cases.[1,2,14] Its severity, which may be masked by arterial dilatation, often varies from vessel to vessel and tends to be less in thromboembolic disease than in other forms of pulmonary hypertension.[1] Furthermore, among patients with plexogenic arteriopathy, appreciable medial hypertrophy may delay the development of the more omi-

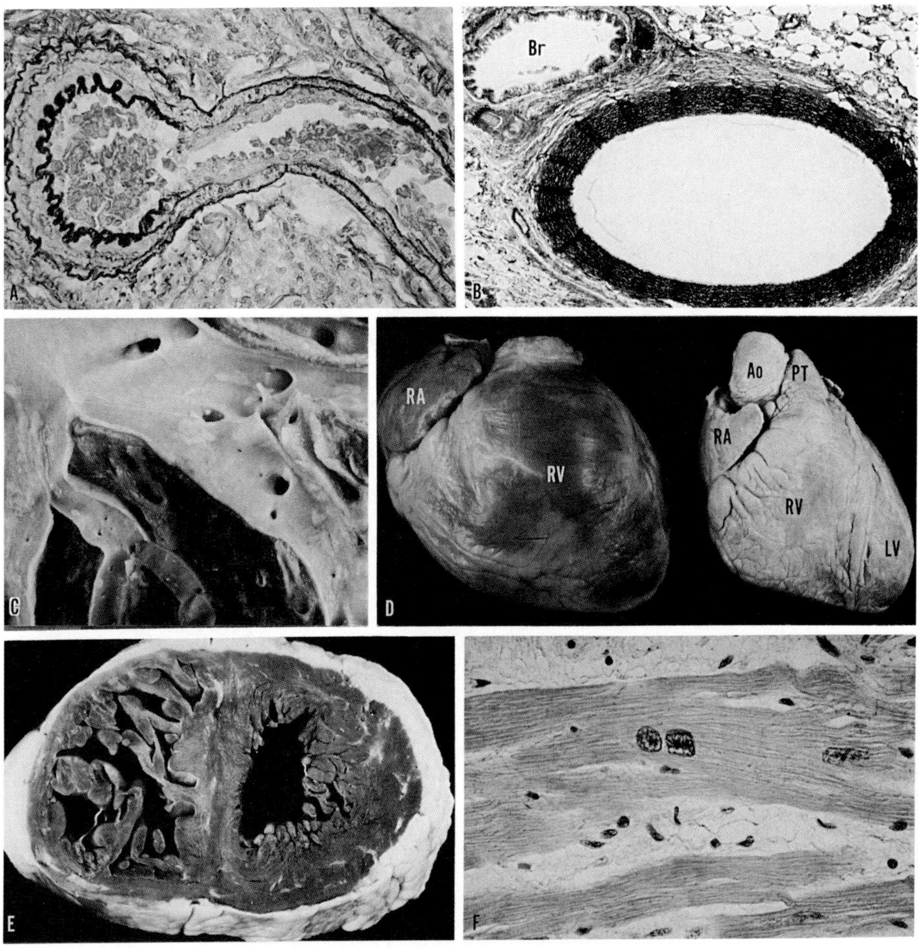

Figure 14–6. General features of chronic pulmonary hypertension. *A,* Medial hypertrophy of muscular pulmonary artery and muscularization of arteriole. *B,* Dilatation and medial hypertrophy of elastic pulmonary artery. Diameter of normal artery should be similar to that of adjacent bronchus (Br). *C,* Shallow atheromas of large elastic pulmonary arteries. *D,* Right ventricular (RV) hypertrophy and dilatation and right atrial (RA) dilatation. Normal heart at right is for comparison. Ao, aorta; LV, left ventricle; PT, pulmonary trunk. *E,* Marked hypertrophy of right ventricular free wall and trabeculae carneae. *F,* Hypertrophy of right ventricular myocardial cells and pericellular interstitial fibrosis. (*A* and *B,* Elastic–van Gieson stain; magnification ×360 and ×36, respectively, reduced 45 percent; *F,* hematoxylin-eosin stain; magnification ×360, reduced 45 percent.) (*A* to *C* from Fuster, V, McGoon, MD, Dines, DE, et al: Pulmonary hypertension: With specific reference to primary pulmonary hypertension. In Brandenburg, RO, Fuster, V, Giuliani, ER, et al [eds]: Cardiology: Fundamentals and Practice. Year Book Medical Publishers, Chicago, 1987, with permission of Mayo Foundation.)

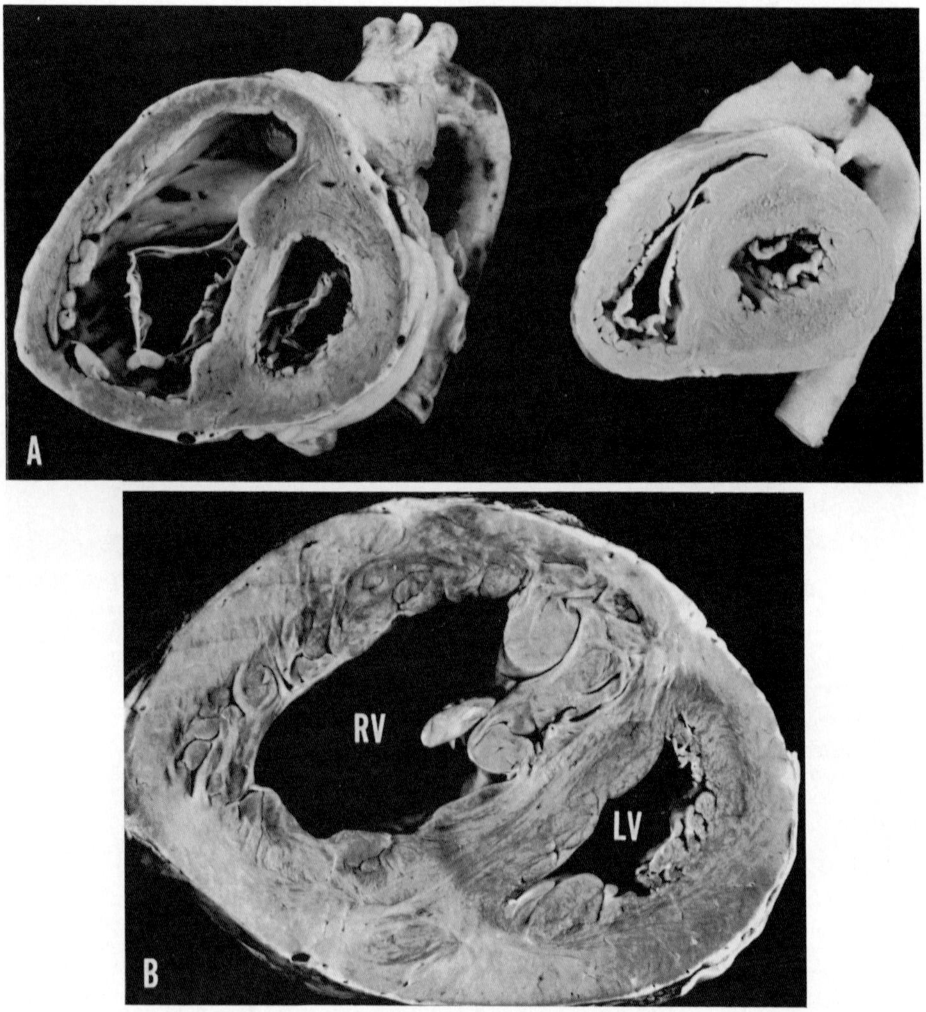

Figure 14–7. Right ventricular hypertrophy and dilatation in chronic pulmonary hypertension. *A,* Straightening of ventricular septum results in D-shaped chambers. Normal heart at right is for comparison. *B,* Leftward bowing of ventricular septum produces circular right ventricular (RV) and crescentic left ventricular (LV) chambers (that is, a reversal in cross-sectional ventricular shapes. (*A* from Edwards, WD: Applied anatomy of the heart. In Brandenburg, RO, Fuster, V, Giuliani, ER, et al [eds]: Cardiology: Fundamentals and Practice. Year Book Medical Publishers, Chicago, 1987, with permission of Mayo Foundation.)

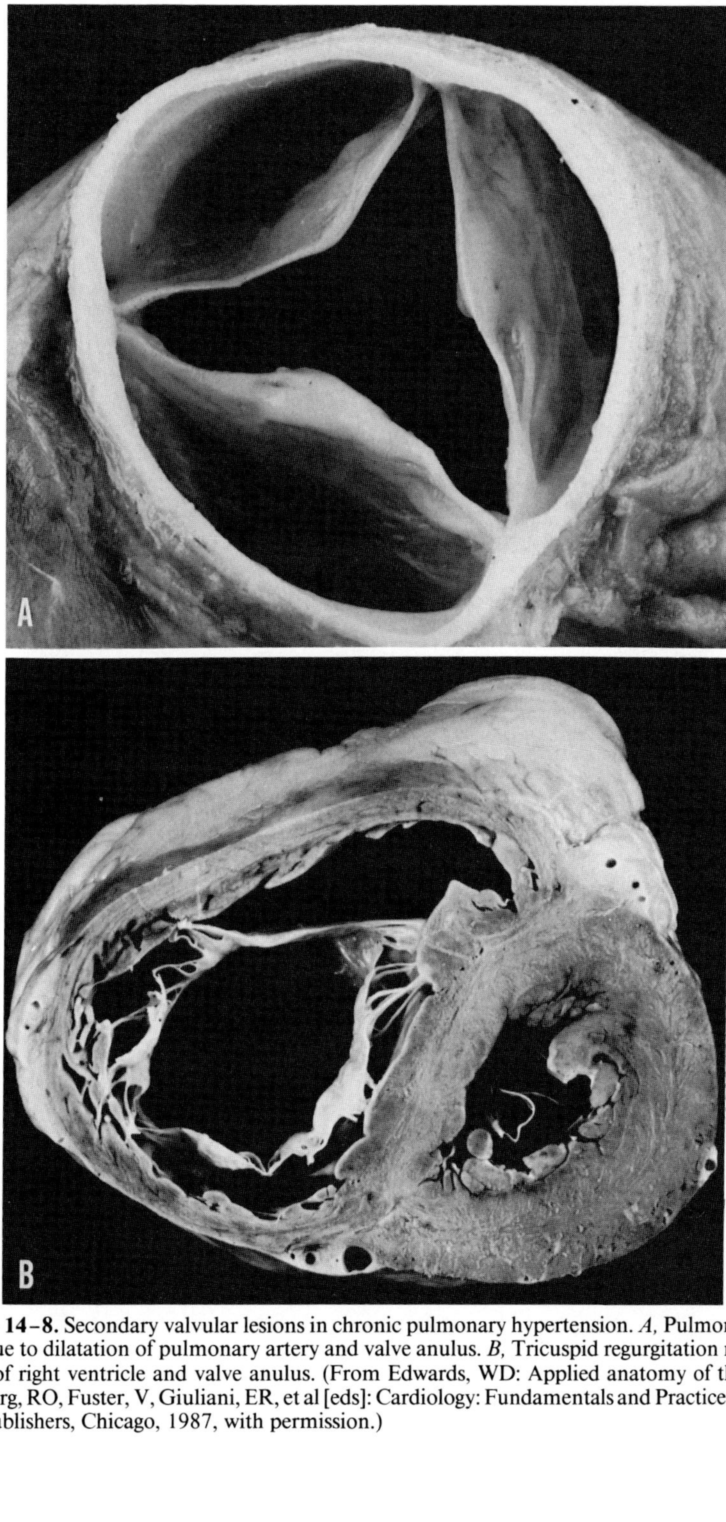

Figure 14-8. Secondary valvular lesions in chronic pulmonary hypertension. *A,* Pulmonary insufficiency is due to dilatation of pulmonary artery and valve anulus. *B,* Tricuspid regurgitation results from dilatation of right ventricle and valve anulus. (From Edwards, WD: Applied anatomy of the heart. In Brandenburg, RO, Fuster, V, Giuliani, ER, et al [eds]: Cardiology: Fundamentals and Practice. Year Book Medical Publishers, Chicago, 1987, with permission.)

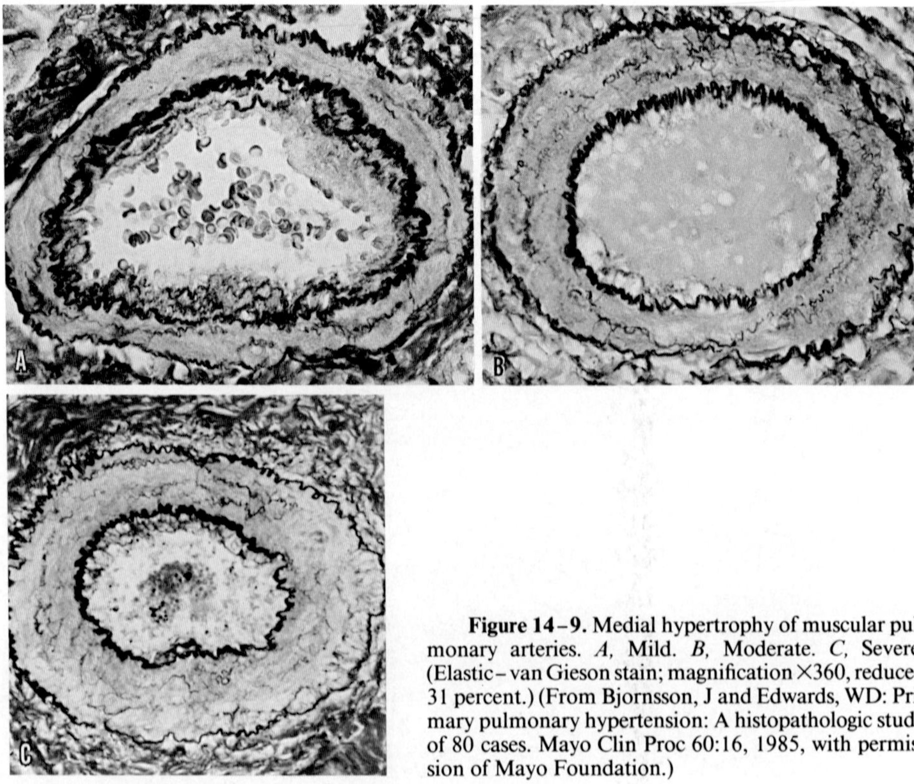

Figure 14–9. Medial hypertrophy of muscular pulmonary arteries. *A,* Mild. *B,* Moderate. *C,* Severe. (Elastic–van Gieson stain; magnification ×360, reduced 31 percent.) (From Bjornsson, J and Edwards, WD: Primary pulmonary hypertension: A histopathologic study of 80 cases. Mayo Clin Proc 60:16, 1985, with permission of Mayo Foundation.)

nous intimal lesions and, thereby, may impart an element of protection to the pulmonary circulation.[16] Regardless of its severity, however, medial hypertrophy is considered a potentially reversible lesion if the cause of pulmonary hypertension is removed (for example, repair or replacement of a stenotic mitral valve or patch closure of a ventricular septal defect).[17,18]

Peripheral extension of medial smooth muscle into the intra-acinar arterioles also commonly occurs and is termed "muscularization of arterioles" (Fig. 14–10).[1,2] Neomuscularization seems to be associated with increased pulmonary blood *flow* and medial hypertrophy with increased *pressure.*[4]

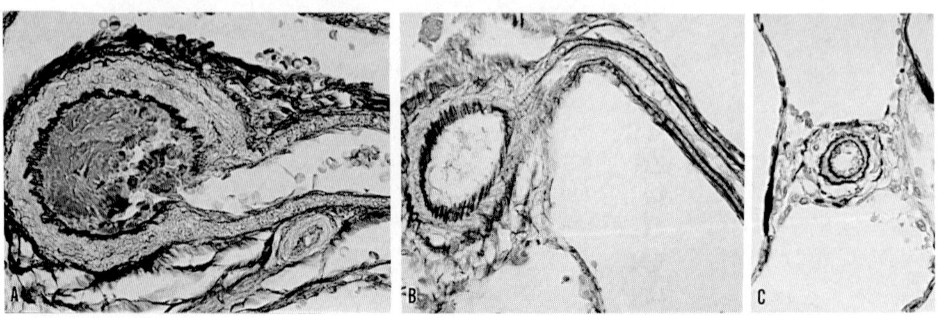

Figure 14–10. Muscularization of intra-acinar arterioles. *A, B,* Longitudinal sections of arteriolar branches. *C,* Cross section of muscularized arteriole. (Elastic–van Gieson stain; magnification ×360, reduced 46 percent.)

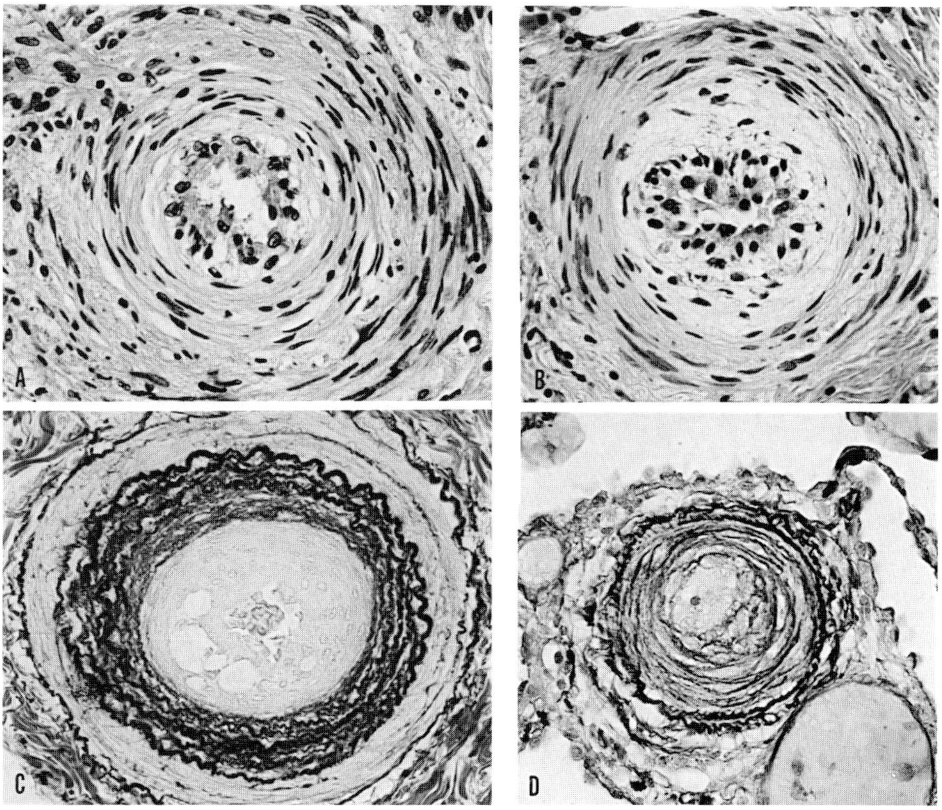

Figure 14–11. Concentric arterial intimal lesions. *A, B,* Concentric intimal proliferation. *C,* Concentric intimal proliferation (centrally) and fibroelastosis (peripherally). *D,* Concentric intimal fibrosis (fibroelastosis). (*A* and *B,* Hematoxylin-eosin stain, magnification ×360, reduced 29 percent; *C* and *D,* elastic–van Gieson stain, magnification ×360, reduced 29 percent.) (*B* from Fuster, V, McGoon, MD, Dines, DE, et al: Pulmonary hypertension: With specific reference to primary pulmonary hypertension. In Brandenburg, R, Fuster, V, Giuliani, ER, et al [eds]: Cardiology: Fundamentals and Practice. Year Book Medical Publishers, Chicago, 1987, with permission. *D* from Bjornsson, J and Edwards, WD: Primary pulmonary hypertension: A histopathologic study of 80 cases. Mayo Clin Proc 60:16, 1985, with permission of Mayo Foundation.)

Intimal Lesions

The most commonly observed intimal lesions are proliferation and fibrosis, and the resulting obstruction may be severe (Figs. 14–11 through 14–13).[1,2,14] Intimal proliferation is considered a potentially reversible process, as are eccentric fibrosis and concentric *non*laminar fibrosis.[18] Wagenvoort and colleagues[18] reported that in contrast, the onion-skin lesions of severe concentric laminar fibrosis are not reversible and may have a tendency to progress, even if the cause of pulmonary hypertension is alleviated. It is unclear whether the eccentric and nonlaminar processes represent organized thrombi or nonthrombotic proliferations. However, regardless of the type of the intimal lesion, the cellular elements are almost exclusively smooth muscle cells and myofibroblasts, and they are presumably derived from the media.[19,20]

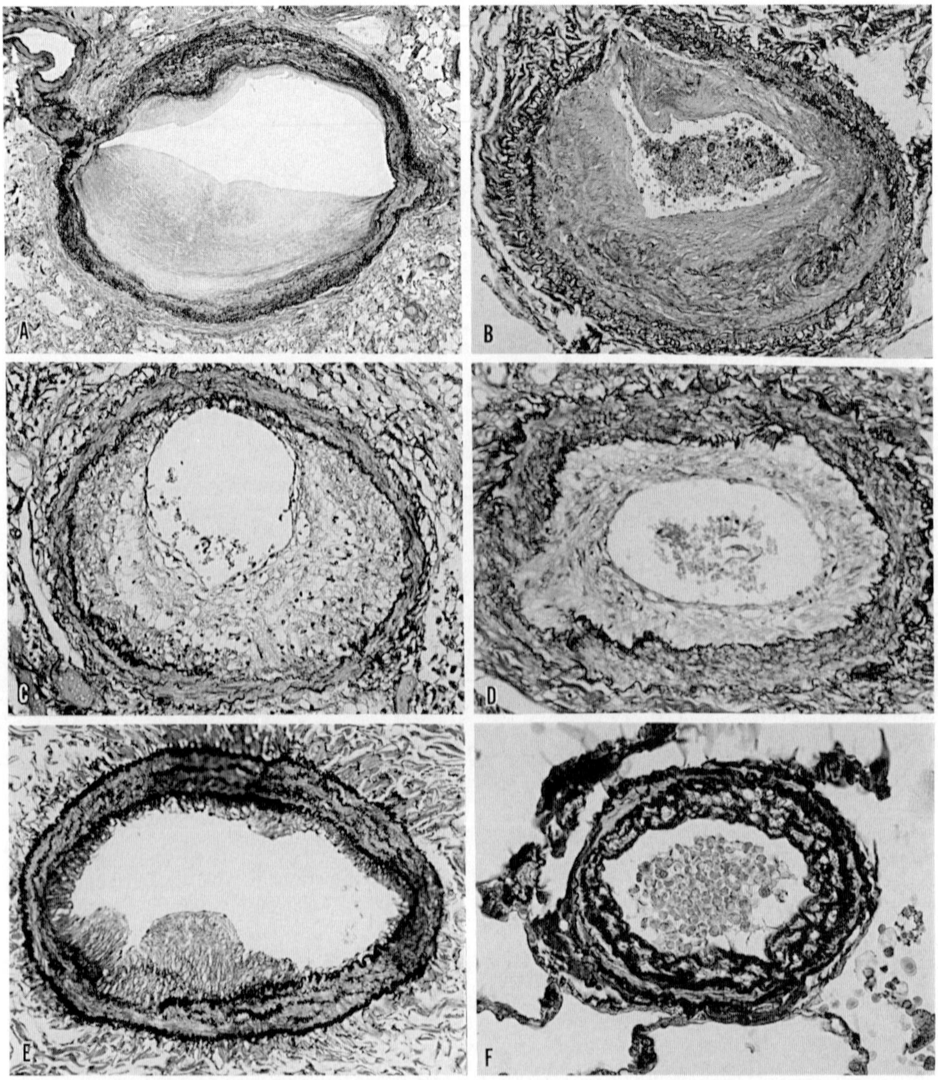

Figure 14–12. Eccentric arterial intimal lesions. *A* and *B*, Eccentric intimal fibrosis in elastic *(A)* and muscular *(B)* pulmonary arteries. *C* and *D*, Eccentric *(C)* and nonlaminar concentric *(D)* intimal proliferation. *E*, Eccentric intimal fibrous pads. *F*, Intimal longitudinal smooth muscle bundles. (Elastic–van Gieson stain; magnifications *A*, ×18; *B*, ×90; *C* through *E*, ×180; *F*, ×360; all reduced 37 percent.) (*B* from Bjornsson, J and Edwards, WD: Primary pulmonary hypertension: A histopathologic study of 80 cases. Mayo Clin Proc 60:16, 1985, with permission. *C*, *D*, and *F* from Fuster, V, McGoon, MD, Dines, DE, et al: Pulmonary hypertension: With specific reference to primary pulmonary hypertension. In Brandenburg, RO, Fuster, V, Giuliani, ER, et al [eds]: Cardiology: Fundamentals and Practice. Year Book Medical Publishers, Chicago, 1987, with permission of Mayo Foundation.)

Complex Intimal-Medial Lesions

Several pulmonary arterial lesions tend to involve both the intima and the media. Fibrinoid degeneration (Fig. 14–14) and necrotizing arteritis (Figs. 14–15, 14–16) are two such lesions. They may be associated with the formation of microaneurysms and are thereby considered by some authors to be the precursors of plexiform and dilatation lesions.[1]

Plexiform lesions (Fig. 14–17) characteristically involve small muscular pulmonary arteries near their origins from larger parent vessels. They are associated with focal medial disruption and aneurysmal dilatation, within which forms a complex proliferative tuft of intimal cells and capillary channels (hence, the older designation as glomeruloid lesions).[1,2,14] The proliferative intimal cells are smooth muscle cells, myofibroblasts, and fibrillary cells that resemble vasoformative reserve cells.[20] Proximal to the plexiform lesion, obstructive fibroelastic intimal mounds are commonly observed, and distally, the artery is usually very thin-walled and dilated. Within the plexiform lesion, thrombotic elements, particularly platelets and fibrin, frequently adhere and may be phagocytosed by the fibrillary cells.[20] Although the typical plexiform lesion is quite cellular, older lesions may become less cellular and even fibrotic.

In some cases, the distinction between plexiform lesions and organized thrombi may be difficult (Fig. 14–18). However, in contrast to plexiform lesions, organized thrombi tend to involve arteries of various sizes and to be unassociated with medial disruption or aneurysm formation.

Dilatation, or angiomatoid, lesions are clusters of dilated and tortuous arterial channels (Fig. 14–19).[1,2] They may be associated with fibrinoid degeneration or may be poststenotic dilatations.

The aforementioned lesions (fibrinoid degeneration, necrotizing arteritis, plexiform lesions, and dilatation lesions) are considered irreversible processes and generally are associated with severe pulmonary hypertension.[1,3,18]

In some forms of pulmonary hypertension, there may be an actual loss of distal pulmonary arteries and arterioles, as evidenced by a decreased numerical density of arteries relative to alveoli.[8,9] However, this is controversial, and some investigators consider it to be an artifactual change.[21,22]

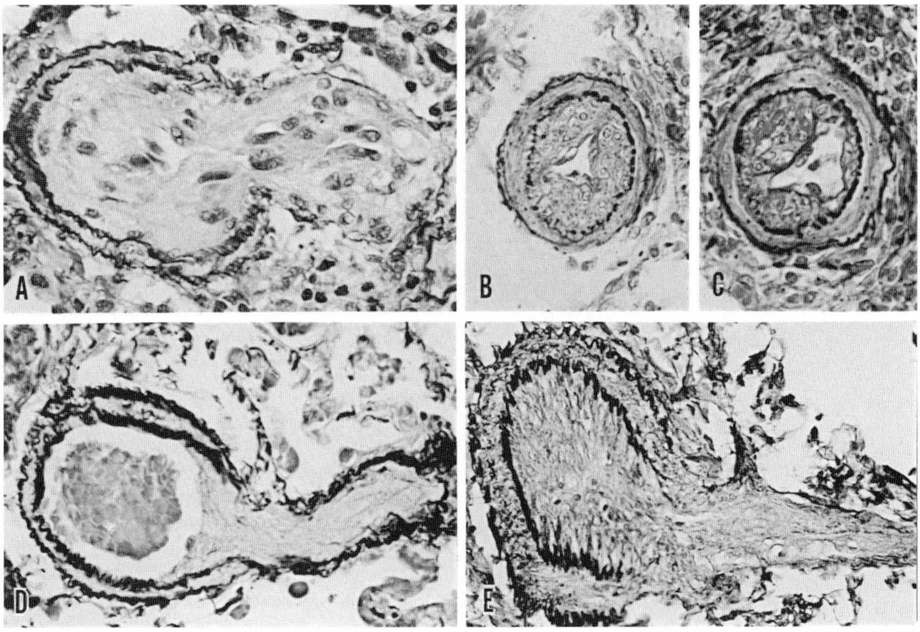

Figure 14–13. Arteriolar intimal lesions. *A* through *C*, Obstructive intimal proliferation. *D, E*, Occlusive intimal fibrosis. (Elastic–van Gieson stain; magnification *A* through *D*, ×360; *E*, ×180; reduced 17 percent.)

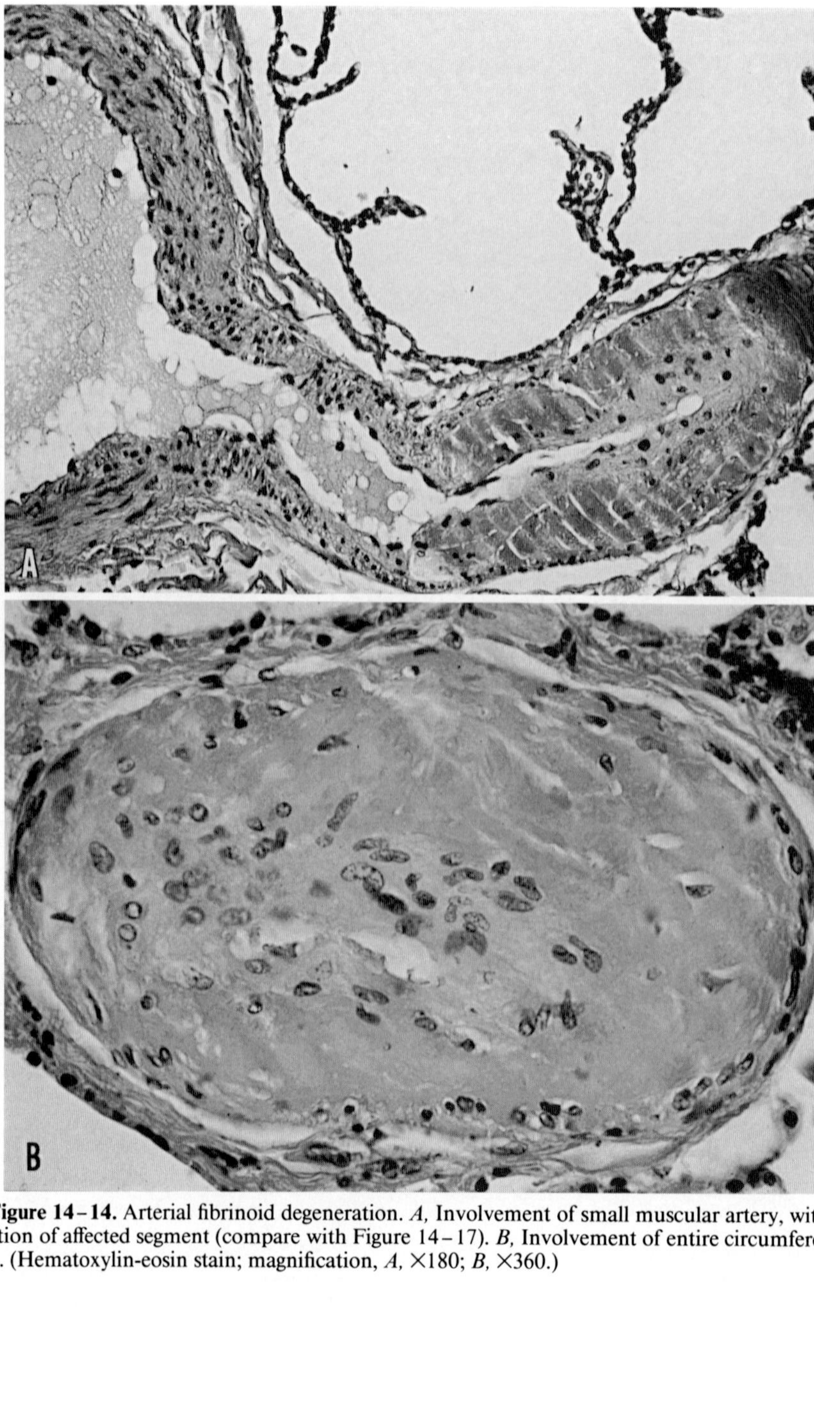

Figure 14–14. Arterial fibrinoid degeneration. *A,* Involvement of small muscular artery, with mild dilatation of affected segment (compare with Figure 14–17). *B,* Involvement of entire circumference of artery. (Hematoxylin-eosin stain; magnification, *A,* ×180; *B,* ×360.)

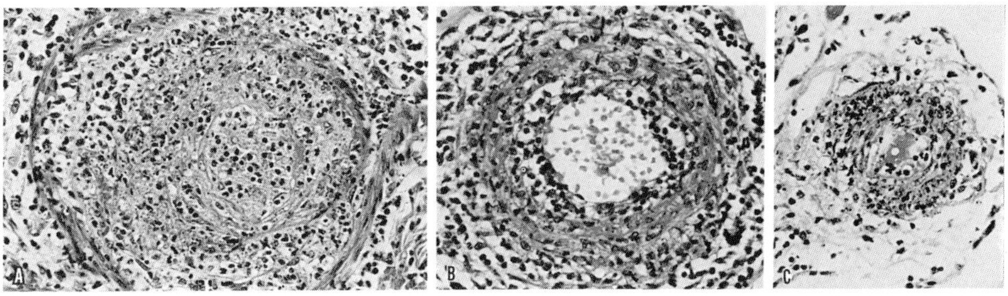

Figure 14–15. Active arteritis. *A* through *C,* Involvement of muscular pulmonary arteries of various sizes. (Hematoxylin-eosin stain; magnification ×360, reduced 52 percent.) (*A* from Bjornsson, J, and Edwards, WD: Primary pulmonary hypertension: A histopathologic study of 80 cases. Mayo Clin Proc 60:16, 1985, with permission of Mayo Foundation.)

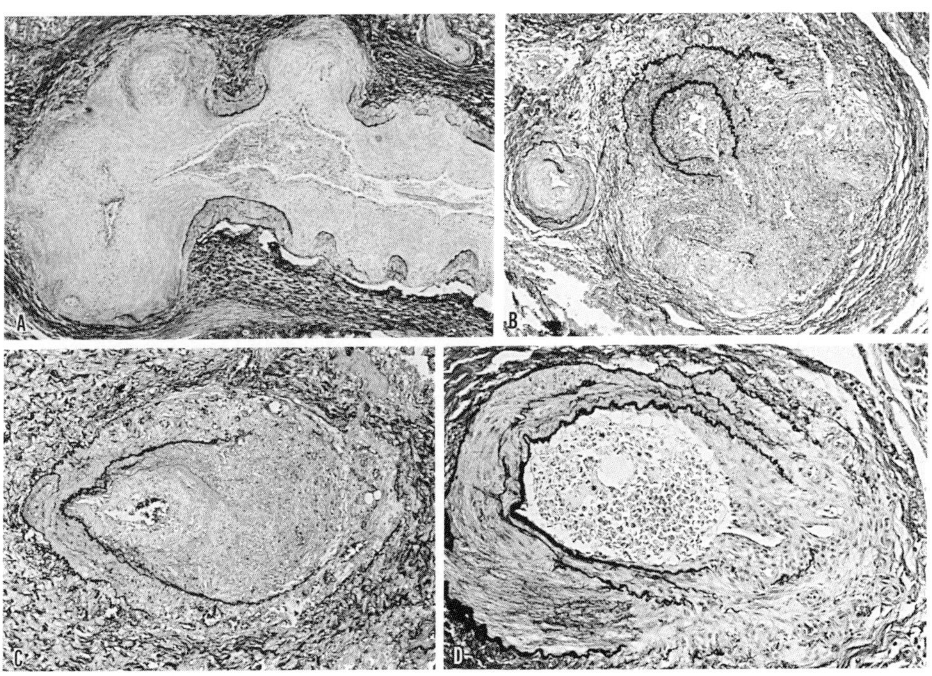

Figure 14–16. Healed arteritis. *A,* Focal disruption of media, with secondary aneurysm formation and intimal proliferation and fibrosis. *B,* Postarteritis microaneurysm with extensive cellular proliferation (compare with Figure 14–17). *C,* Focal medial damage, with secondary medial neovascularization and severely obstructive intimal fibrosis. *D,* Focal arterial disruption, with proliferative fibrovascular granulation tissue. (Elastic–van Gieson stain; magnifications *A,* ×36; *B* and *C,* ×90; *D,* ×180; all reduced 41 percent.) (*B* and *D* from Bjornsson, J and Edwards, WD: Primary pulmonary hypertension: A histopathologic study of 80 cases. Mayo Clin Proc 60:16, 1985, with permission of Mayo Foundation.)

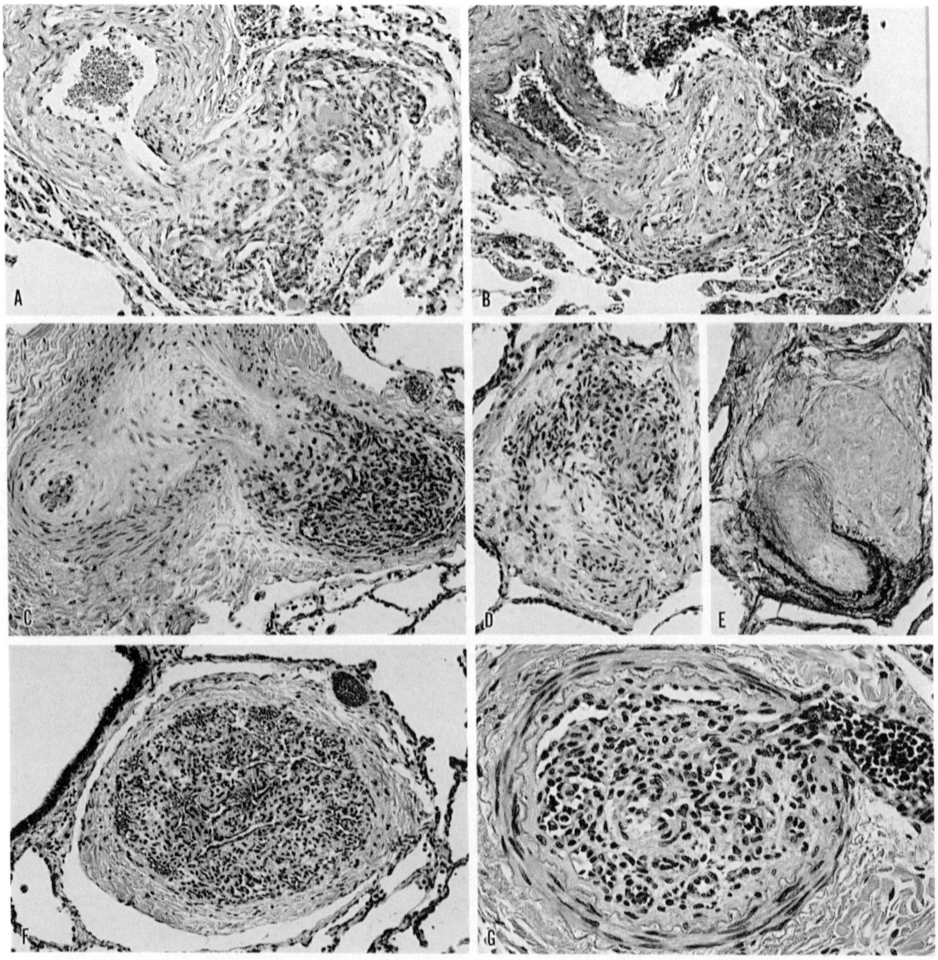

Figure 14–17. Arterial plexiform lesions. *A,* Highly cellular lesion in aneurysmal branch of parent artery. *B,* Fibrotic and poorly cellular lesion (compare with *A*). *C,* Highly cellular lesion *(right),* with obstructive intimal proliferation in parent artery *(left). D* and *E,* Origin of plexiform lesion within postarteritis microaneurysm is better demonstrated with elastic–van Gieson stain *(E)* than with hematoxylin-eosin stain *(D). F, G,* Highly cellular nature of lesions, cut in cross section (compare with Figures 14–18 and 14–21). (*A* through *D, F* and *G,* Elastic–van Gieson stain; *E,* hematoxylin-eosin stain; magnifications *A* through *F,* ×180; *G,* ×360; reduced 44 percent.) (*A* from Fuster, V, McGoon, MD, Dines, DE, et al: Pulmonary hypertension: With specific reference to primary pulmonary hypertension. In Brandenburg, RO, Fuster, V, Giuliani, ER, et al [eds]: Cardiology: Fundamentals and Practice. Year Book Medical Publishers, Chicago, 1987, with permission of Mayo Foundation.)

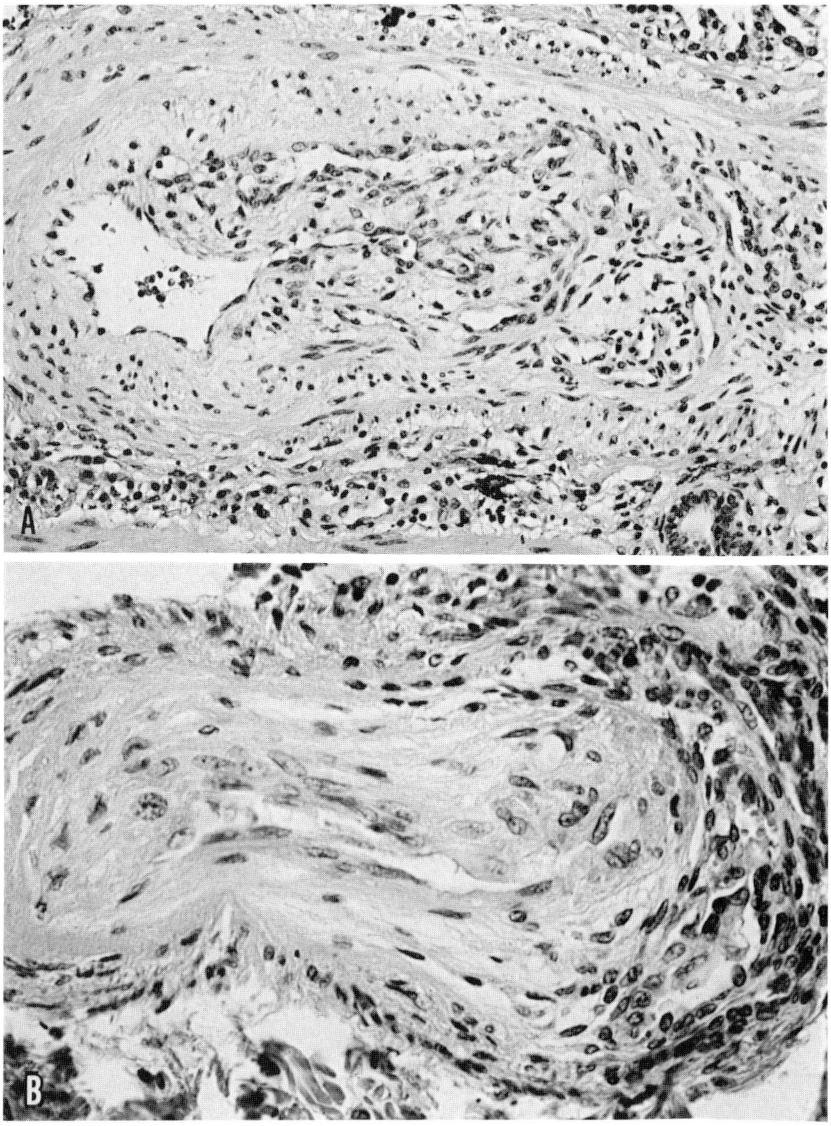

Figure 14–18. Arterial lesions simulating plexiform lesions. *A* and *B*, Oblique sections through muscular pulmonary arteries involved by cellular organization of thrombi. (Hematoxylin-eosin stain; magnifications *A*, ×180; *B*, ×360.)

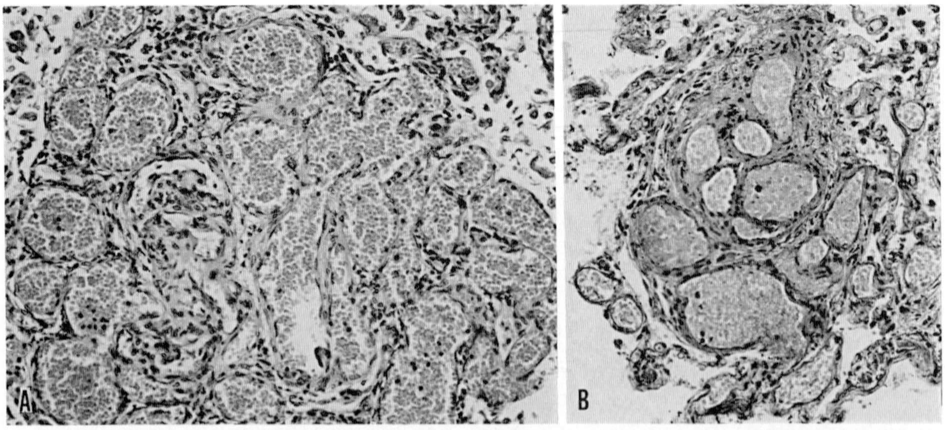

Figure 14–19. Arterial dilatation (angiomatoid) lesions. *A, B,* Focal clusters of tortuous and dilated arterial channels. (Hematoxylin-eosin stain; magnification ×180, reduced 25 percent.) (*B* from Bjornsson, J and Edwards, WD: Primary pulmonary hypertension: A histopathologic study of 80 cases. Mayo Clin Proc 60:16, 1985, with permission of Mayo Foundation.)

Luminal Lesions

Thrombosis is the most commonly encountered obstructive process within the pulmonary arterial lumen. In some instances, it is unclear whether thrombi are embolic in origin or have developed in situ. The thrombi may be fresh or may be in various stages of lysis, organization, or recanalization (so-called colander lesions), and they tend to involve arteries of various sizes.[1,2,14] Old organized lesions in the elastic arteries are manifested grossly as fibrous luminal webs or cords, and larger lesions may become calcified (Fig. 14–20).

Organized thrombi in small muscular pulmonary arteries are generally recanalized (Fig. 14–21) but may appear quite myxoid and usually contain no iron. In small arteries and arterioles, organized thrombi may be recanalized or may form occlusive and retracted fibrotic cords. The hemodynamic effect of thrombi depends on their degree of obstruction and the number of vessels involved. Although areas of nonlaminar intimal fibrosis are commonly believed to represent organized thrombi, such lesions, in some instances, may represent nonthrombotic intimal proliferations.

Fresh thrombi, organizing thrombi, and nonlaminar intimal fibrosis are potentially reversible lesions.[18] However, densely fibrotic luminal webs and occlusive luminal plugs are probably irreversible.

Rarely, neoplastic emboli may occlude a sufficient portion of the pulmonary arterial bed to produce elevated vascular resistance (Fig. 14–22). This most commonly occurs in the setting of carcinoma of the breast or lung, although other neoplasms have been reported.[1,23–26]

Other causes of arterial luminal obstruction in cases of pulmonary hypertension include ova in pulmonary schistosomiasis and talc in intravenous drug abuse (Fig. 14–22).[1,27–32] Hydatid embolism in echinococcosis has also been described.[33]

Adventitial Lesions

In most cases of chronic pulmonary hypertension, the adventitia remains uninvolved.[1] Occasionally, it may be fibrotic or the site of an inflammatory infiltrate.

Adventitial periarterial (and peribronchial) lymphatics may be dilated in severe forms of postcapillary obstruction.

MICROCIRCULATORY LESIONS

The microcirculation is relatively normal in cases of *pre*capillary pulmonary hypertension but is distinctly abnormal in cases of chronic *post*capillary obstruction (Fig. 14–23).[1,2,34,35] In the latter, the alveolar capillaries are distended and engorged with blood, and alveolar hemosiderin-laden macrophages mark the sites of previous intra-alveolar hemorrhages. In the setting of increased venous and capillary pressure, edema fluid accumulates in the pleurae and interstitial spaces, and the lymphatics become dilated. Hemorrhagic alveolar edema may also develop. All microcirculatory lesions are considered reversible if the cause of the postcapillary obstruction can be relieved (for example, repair or replacement of a stenotic mitral valve).[1,17]

VENOUS LESIONS

In cases of postcapillary obstruction, the most common venous lesions are medial hypertrophy and dilatation (Fig. 14–24).[1,2,14,36,37] The formation of a distinct external elastic membrane often accompanies medial hypertrophy and represents so-called arterialization of veins. Such veins may be distinguished from arteries by their location in the interlobular septa rather than adjacent to bronchi.

Eccentric intimal pads may develop and are interpreted by some investigators as organized in situ mural thrombi.[1] However, only the appearance of recanalized

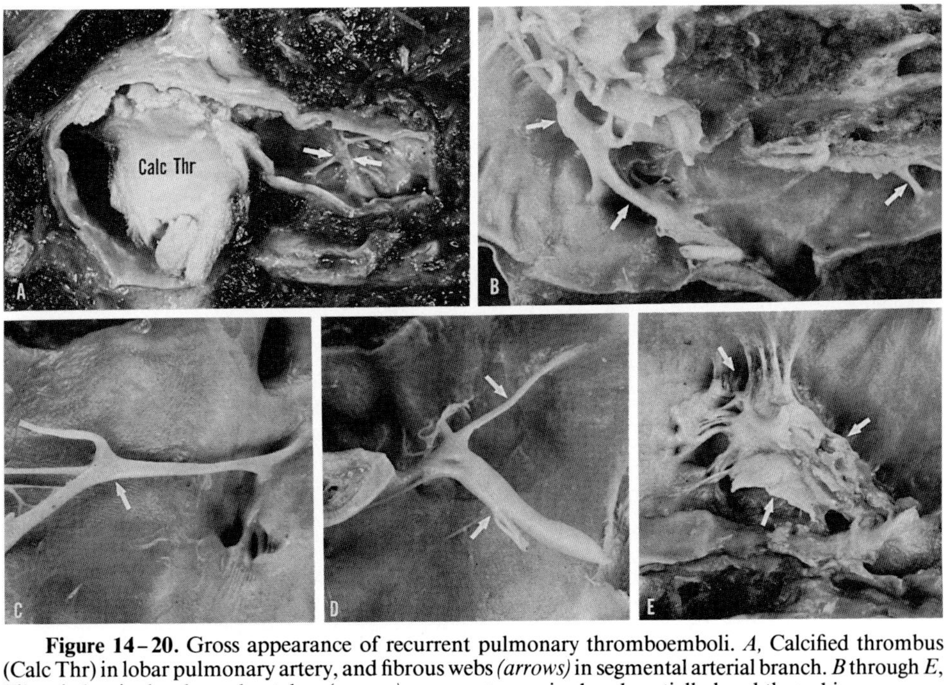

Figure 14–20. Gross appearance of recurrent pulmonary thromboemboli. *A,* Calcified thrombus (Calc Thr) in lobar pulmonary artery, and fibrous webs *(arrows)* in segmental arterial branch. *B* through *E,* Fibrotic luminal webs and patches *(arrows)* represent organized and partially lysed thrombi.

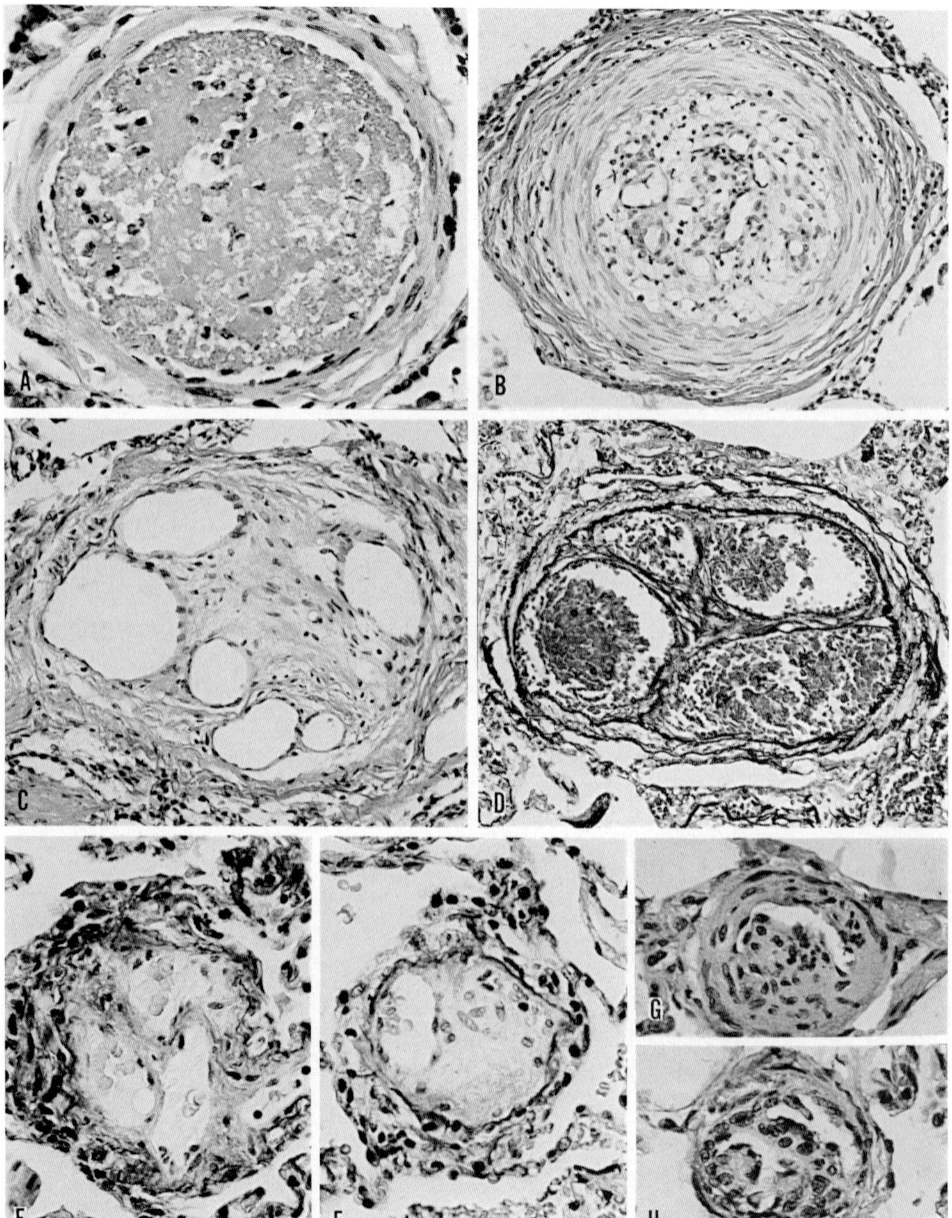

Figure 14–21. Thrombotic arterial lesions. *A,* Fresh thrombus. *B,* Cellular organizing thrombus (compare with Figures 14–16 to 14–18). *C* through *H,* Organized and recanalized thrombi in muscular arteries (*C* and *D*) and in arterioles (*E* through *H*). (*A* through *C, G* and *H,* Hematoxylin-eosin stain; *D* through *F,* elastic–van Gieson stain; magnifications *B* through *D,* ×180; *A* and *E* through *H,* ×360; reduced 27 percent.) (*C, E,* and *F* from Bjornsson, J, and Edwards, WD: Primary pulmonary hypertension: A histopathologic study of 80 cases. Mayo Clin Proc 60:16, 1985, with permission of Mayo Foundation.)

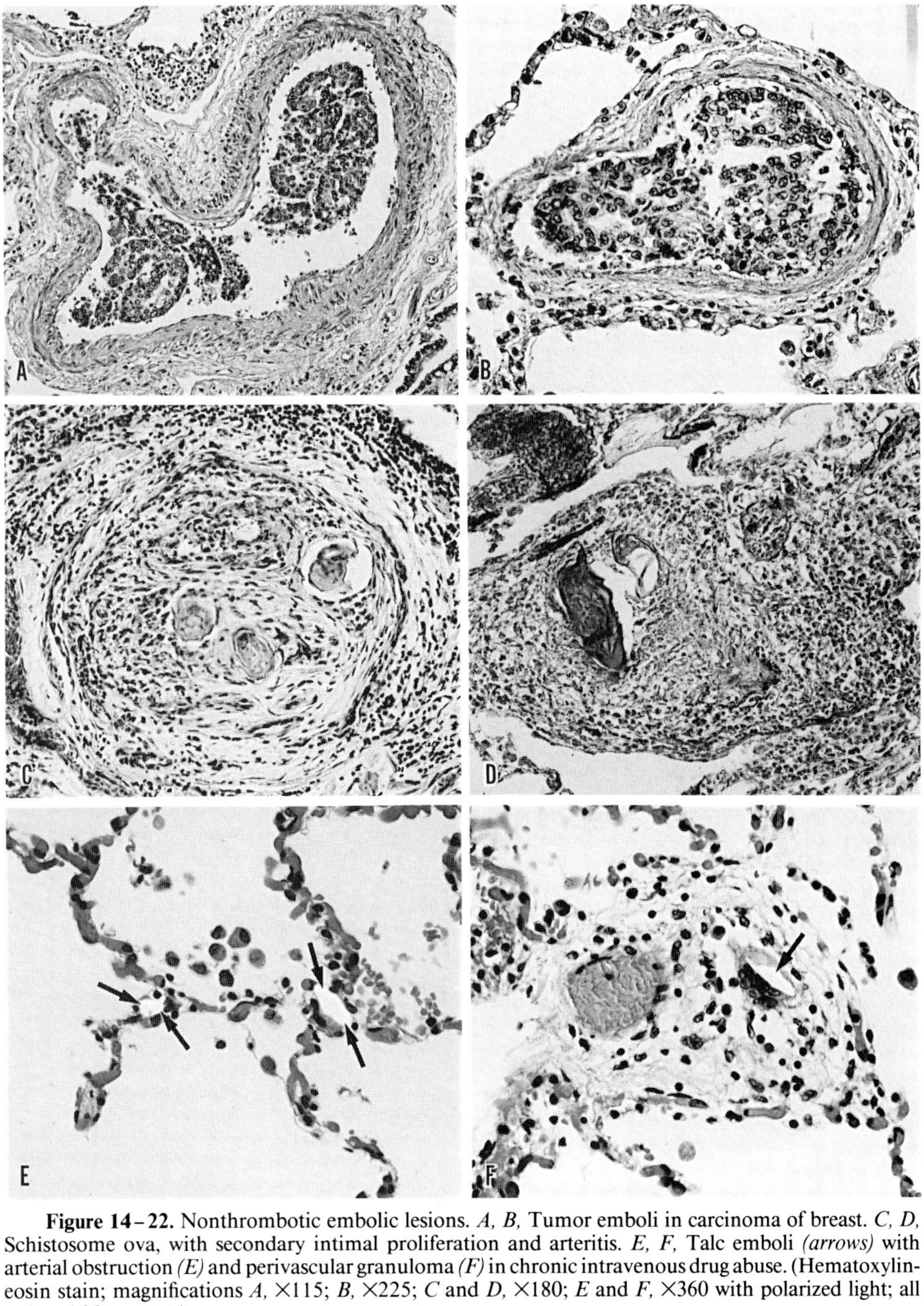

Figure 14–22. Nonthrombotic embolic lesions. *A, B,* Tumor emboli in carcinoma of breast. *C, D,* Schistosome ova, with secondary intimal proliferation and arteritis. *E, F,* Talc emboli *(arrows)* with arterial obstruction *(E)* and perivascular granuloma *(F)* in chronic intravenous drug abuse. (Hematoxylin-eosin stain; magnifications *A,* ×115; *B,* ×225; *C* and *D,* ×180; *E* and *F,* ×360 with polarized light; all reduced 28 percent.)

channels is considered truly pathognomonic of previous thrombotic obstruction (Fig. 14–25). Pulmonary phlebitis and fresh venous thrombosis are exceedingly rare.

Venous medial hypertrophy and mild intimal fibrosis are potentially reversible processes.[1,17] However, densely fibrotic luminal webs and luminal plugs are probably irreversible lesions.

Histopathologic Patterns

Pulmonary hypertension due to precapillary obstruction tends to affect the arteries alone, whereas that due to postcapillary obstruction involves not only the

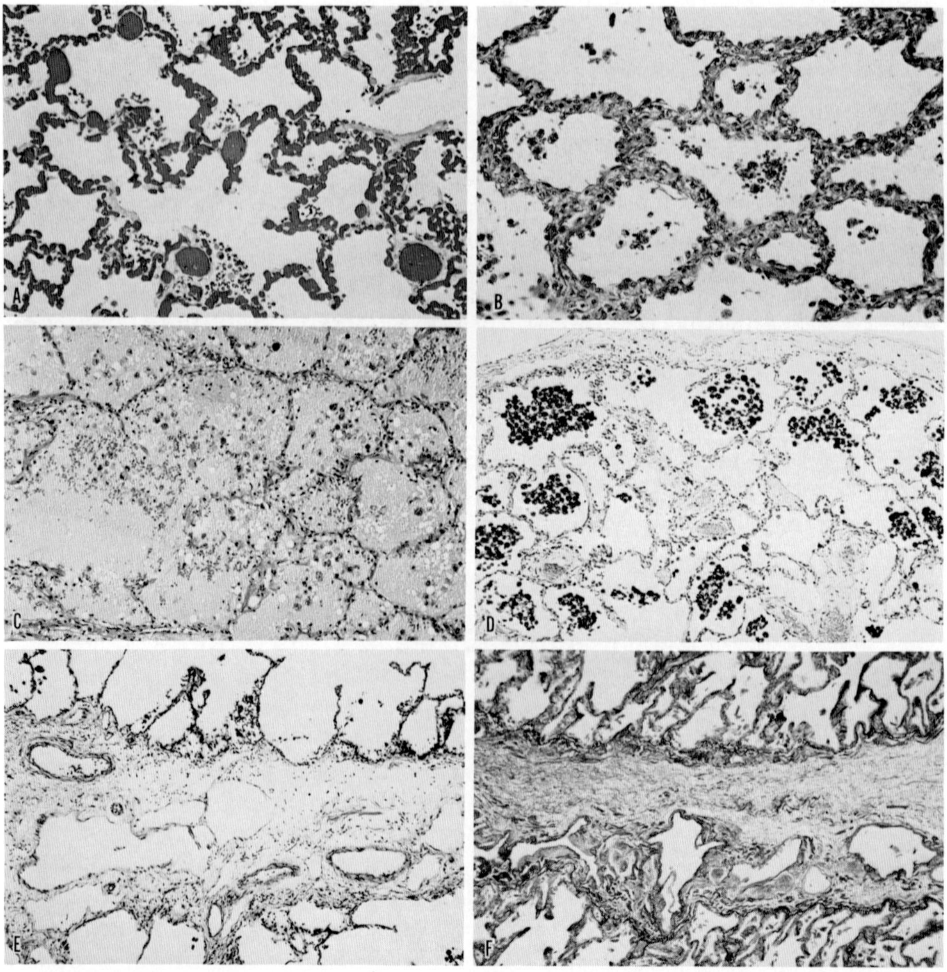

Figure 14–23. Microcirculatory lesions. *A,* Dilatation and engorgement of alveolar capillaries. *B,* Fibrotic thickening of alveolar walls. *C,* Hemorrhagic alveolar edema. *D,* Alveolar clusters of hemosiderin-laden macrophages. *E* and *F,* Dilatation of septal lymphatics, and edema *(E)* and fibrosis *(F)* of interlobular septa. (*A* through *D,* hematoxylin-eosin stain; *E* and *F,* elastic–van Gieson stain; magnifications *A* and *B,* ×180; *C* through *F,* ×90; reduced 44 percent.) (*D* from Fuster, V, McGoon, MD, Dines, DE, et al: Pulmonary hypertension: With specific reference to primary pulmonary hypertension. In Brandenburg, RO, Fuster, V, Giuliani, ER (eds): Cardiology: Fundamentals and Practice. Year Book Medical Publishers, Chicago, 1987, with permission of Mayo Foundation.)

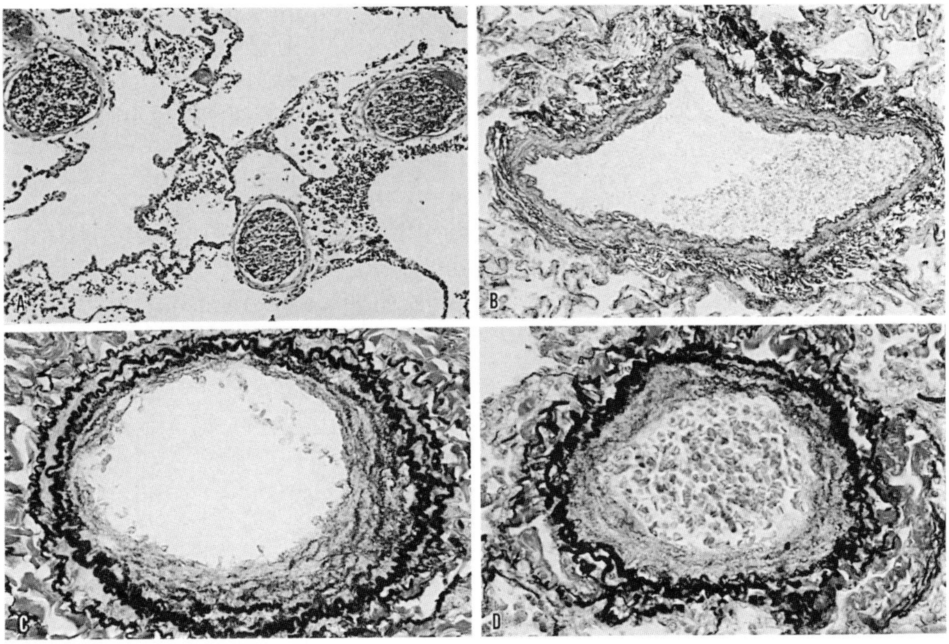

Figure 14-24. Nonthrombotic venous lesions. *A,* Dilated and engorged venules. *B,* Arterialization and medial hypertrophy of vein. *C,* Arterialization and eccentric intimal fibrosis. *D,* Concentric intimal fibrosis. (*A,* Hematoxylin-eosin stain; magnification ×90, reduced 44 percent. *B* through *D,* elastic-van Gieson stain; magnifications *B,* ×90; *C* and *D,* ×360; all reduced 44 percent.)

arteries but also the microcirculation and veins.[1,2,14] Furthermore, within these two broad categories, certain etiologic settings are associated with relatively specific constellations of histopathologic lesions. Some overlap occurs, however, particularly among cases of idiopathic, or primary, pulmonary hypertension.

PULMONARY HYPERTENSION DUE TO PRECAPILLARY OBSTRUCTION

Plexogenic Pulmonary Arteriopathy

This form of pulmonary hypertension may exist as a primary disorder or may be associated with congenital cardiac left-to-right shunts, portal hypertension, pulmonary schistosomiasis, or the drug aminorex fumarate.[1-3] However, regardless of the clinical setting, the spectrum of arterial lesions is similar. These include medial hypertrophy, muscularization of arterioles, concentric intimal proliferation, concentric laminar intimal fibrosis, fibrinoid degeneration, necrotizing arteritis, dilatation lesions, and plexiform lesions (see Figs. 14-9 to 14-11, 14-14 to 14-19). In addition, fresh and organized thrombi and, in particular, eccentric intimal fibrosis may coexist to various degrees (see Figs. 4-12, 4-13, 4-21). The microcirculation and veins are relatively uninvolved, although focal areas of alveolar hemosiderosis may be observed. Because of the variety of lesions encountered in this form of pulmonary hypertension, some investigators consider the term "plexogenic arteriopathy" to be too restrictive and misleading.

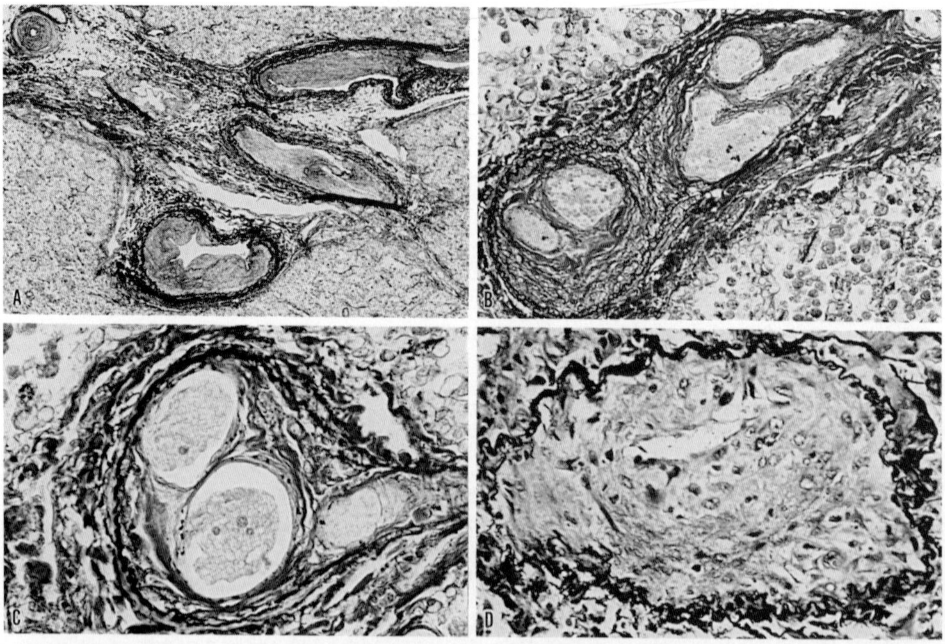

Figure 14–25. Thrombotic venous lesions. *A*, Highly obstructive eccentric intimal fibrosis with focal luminal fibrous bands. *B, C*, Organized and recanalized thrombi. *D*, Highly obstructive intimal proliferation with early recanalization channels. (Elastic–van Gieson stain; magnifications *A*, ×45; *B*, ×180; *C* and *D*, ×360; all reduced 44 percent.) (*C* from Edwards, WD and Edwards, JE: Recent advances in the pathology of the pulmonary vasculature. Monogr Pathol 19:235, 1978, with permission of the International Academy of Pathology.)

Primary Plexogenic Pulmonary Arteriopathy

The idiopathic form affects women twice as frequently as men, tends to occur in young adults, and is associated with sudden death in more than 40 percent of cases.[38–42] Although the cause of the primary form is unknown, the basic lesion is considered to be chronic severe vasoconstriction by some investigators[38] and endothelial proliferation and loss of arterioles by others.[39] However, because biopsy or autopsy tissue from the lungs is generally available only late in the course of the disease, the various pulmonary arterial lesions are usually advanced and highly obstructive. Hence, the basic primary lesion may be masked, and its identification is currently speculative.

Congenital Cardiac Left-to-Right Shunts

The shunts associated with plexogenic pulmonary arteriopathy include ventricular septal defect (without pulmonary stenosis), patent ductus arteriosus, and, rarely, atrial septal defect.[43–46] Patients with transposition of the great arteries, with or without a ventricular septal defect, are also prone to develop plexogenic pulmonary arteriopathy[47–50] or thrombotic obstructions.[51]

Among such patients, investigators have documented a tendency to develop arterial lesions in a typical order, as described by Heath and Edwards[52] and later modified by Wagenwoort:[1,53] medial hypertrophy and muscularization of arterioles (grade 1), concentric intimal proliferation (grade 2), concentric laminar intimal fibrosis (grade 3), fibrinoid degeneration or necrotizing arteritis (grade 6), plexiform lesions (grade 4), and dilatation lesions (grade 5). More recently, investigators have subdivided the grade 1 lesions into peripheral extension of smooth muscle (grade A) and medial hypertrophy (grade B) and have emphasized the importance of the loss of distal small arteries and arterioles (grade C).[54-57] The observance of fewer vessels, however, does not necessarily imply a *congenital* underdevelopment of the pulmonary arterial tree,[58] and may in fact represent an artifact related to the method of perfusion.[21,22]

The complexity of the coexisting lesions suggests the need for a semiquantitative descriptive diagnosis, rather than the use of a single grade.[59] In general, however, grade 1 and 2 lesions are potentially reversible, grade 3 lesions are borderline, and grade 4 through 6 lesions indicate a severely and irreversibly obstructed pulmonary arterial bed with a high fixed pulmonary vascular resistance.[1-3,60] The extent to which the small peripheral arteries are lost tends to increase with the higher Heath-Edwards grades.[58] However, in some cases, irreversible pulmonary hypertension may be associated with only medial hypertrophy, muscularized arterioles, and, possibly, appreciable loss of the distal arterial bed.[54] The *numerical* Heath-Edwards grades, if used at all, should be reserved *only* for the evaluation of hypertensive pulmonary vascular disease associated with congenital cardiac left-to-right shunts.

Other Causes

Pulmonary hypertension associated with portal hypertension (cirrhosis or portal vein thrombosis) or with pulmonary schistosomiasis tends to be characterized by a mixed histopathologic pattern of plexogenic, thrombotic, and fibrotic lesions.[27,28,61] Plexogenic pulmonary arteriopathy associated with the use of the appetite suppressant aminorex fumarate is discussed later with dietary pulmonary hypertension.

Embolic Pulmonary Hypertension

In this category, the vast majority of cases are related to chronic recurrent thromboembolism from the veins of the legs or from the pelvic venous plexus.[1-3,62,63] Rarely, emboli may originate from right atrial thrombi, from ventriculoatrial shunt catheters for hydrocephalus, or from nonthrombotic sources, such as neoplasms, talc, or parasites.[23-33,64,65] The obstructive emboli cause an increase in pulmonary vascular resistance and subsequent elevation of pulmonary arterial pressure.

Thromboembolic pulmonary hypertension tends to occur in adults and affects women more frequently than men.[1,2,38-40] Sudden death occurs in some patients, and the remainder usually die of right heart failure.[1,2,40,42] The clinical course may be characterized by episodes of obvious pulmonary embolism, with acute dyspnea, chest pain, and even hemorrhagic pulmonary infarction, or it may present as progressive dyspnea, without obvious embolic events.[1,2,66] In the latter setting, the emboli are presumably small and affect only the muscular pulmonary arteries, and even pulmonary ventilation-perfusion scans may be unable to detect the embolic nature of the disease. Accordingly, some cases of thromboembolic disease may present clinically as idiopathic (primary) pulmonary hypertension.[38,40] Mediastinal fibrosis or adenopathy may result in pulmonary arterial and venous compression and, thereby, mimic thromboembolic pulmonary hypertension.[67-70]

Grossly, the elastic pulmonary arteries may contain fibrous webs or bands that represent organized and partially lysed thromboemboli (see Fig. 14–20). Microscopically, the muscular and elastic pulmonary arteries harbor thromboemboli of various ages (see Fig. 14–21). Medial hypertrophy is present and is considered to represent a secondary response to elevated arterial resistance and pressure (see Fig. 14–9); however, it is usually less severe than in other forms of pulmonary hypertension.[1] The pulmonary microcirculation and veins are not appreciably involved.

Hypoxic Pulmonary Hypertension

In humans, chronic alveolar hypoxia is a very potent pulmonary vasoconstrictor, and its causes are numerous (Table 14–3).[1,3,71–74] Polycythemia accompanies most cases and contributes to elevated pulmonary vascular resistance,[74] as may acidosis.[75]

Microscopically, the small muscular arteries are the site of mild to moderate medial hypertrophy and muscularization of arterioles, which were shown in Figures 14–9 and 14–10.[1–3,75–78] In addition, some arteries are involved by eccentric intimal fibrosis or by longitudinal muscle bundles in the intima, media, or adventitia (see Fig. 14–12). The small pulmonary veins may also exhibit medial hypertrophy and longitudinal smooth muscle bundles (see Fig. 14–24).[77,79] In destructive disorders such as pulmonary emphysema, capillary beds may be lost. The bronchial arteries and veins commonly become dilated and tortuous, and arterial bronchopulmonary anastomoses become enlarged, particularly in patients with bronchiectasis.[1]

Pulmonary Hypertension and Pulmonary Parenchymal Disease

Various chronic fibrosing disorders of the lung may be associated with the development of pulmonary hypertension (Table 14–4). Fibrosis, hypoxia, and thrombosis are considered responsible for the vascular alterations.[1–3] In fibrotic areas, capillary beds are lost, and small pulmonary arteries and veins are commonly involved by medial hypertrophy and by eccentric intimal proliferation and fibrosis (see Figs. 14–12, 14–24).[80] In some vessels, recanalized and organized thrombi (presumably in situ in origin) and occlusive fibrotic plugs are observed (see Fig.

Table 14–3. Causes of Chronic Alveolar Hypoxia

Residence at high altitude
Chronic upper airway obstruction
Congenital webs
Enlarged tonsils
Impaired thoracic excursion
Extreme obesity (pickwickian)
Kyphoscoliosis
Thoracic ankylosing spondylitis
Chronic poliomyelitis
Progressive muscular dystrophy
Pulmonary parenchymal diseases
Pulmonary emphysema
Chronic bronchitis
Asthmatic bronchitis
Bronchiectasis

Table 14–4. Pulmonary Fibrosing Disorders Associated With Pulmonary Hypertension

Pulmonary interstitial fibrosis
Pneumoconioses
Sarcoidosis
Collagen vascular diseases
Scleroderma (progressive systemic sclerosis)
Dermatomyositis
Systemic lupus erythematosus
Rheumatoid arthritis

14–21). Bronchial vessels may be dilated and tortuous, and arterial bronchopulmonary anastomoses are often enlarged.

Dietary Pulmonary Hypertension

An epidemic of pulmonary hypertension in Switzerland, West Germany, and Austria was associated with the use of the appetite suppressant aminorex fumarate during the years 1967 to 1972. The histopathologic lesions were identical to those of plexogenic pulmonary arteriopathy.[1,3,81] However, in experimental animals, aminorex has not produced similar hypertensive pulmonary vascular lesions.

An unusual form of pulmonary hypertension in Spain has been linked to the illegal use of denatured rapeseed oil as a cooking substitute for olive oil during the years 1981 and 1982.[82–84] This late manifestation of the toxic oil syndrome occurs more commonly in women than in men. Muscular pulmonary arteries are characterized by medial hypertrophy, eccentric and often highly obstructive intimal proliferation, focal medial degeneration or destruction, and adventitial lymphoplasmacytic cuffing. Arterioles are commonly muscularized, and veins are occasionally the site of eccentric intimal proliferation or fibrosis.

Pyrrolizidine alkaloids, such as monocrotaline and fulvine, cause pulmonary hypertension in various laboratory animals but not in humans.[1,85] Jamaican bush-tea, which contains pyrrolizidine alkaloids, may produce *hepatic* veno-occlusive disease and cirrhosis in humans but has not been associated with pulmonary hypertension.

PULMONARY HYPERTENSION DUE TO POSTCAPILLARY OBSTRUCTION

Pulmonary Veno-occlusive Disease

Pulmonary veno-occlusive disease is an obstructive thrombotic disorder of the pulmonary venules and veins.[1–3,86–90] The cause is unknown, but it is *not* related to *hepatic* veno-occlusive disease. Because venous and capillary pressures are elevated, pulmonary congestion and edema are commonly observed roentgenographically.

This is a rare disease that usually affects children, adolescents, and young adults. A few cases involve infants and middle-aged or elderly adults, and familial cases have been reported.[91–94] The sex distribution is equal. Clinically, the disease is characterized by progressive dyspnea and, thereby, may present as primary pulmonary hypertension.[38,40,84] The pulmonary artery pressure is elevated, and the pulmonary wedge pressure may be elevated or may appear normal. The disease is usually fatal within 2 or 3 years after diagnosis, and death may be sudden or associated with pulmonary or right heart failure.

The histopathologic hallmark of this disease is the presence of organized and recanalized thrombi in the pulmonary venules and veins (see Fig. 14–25).[1–3] Eccentric fibrous pads are commonly observed and may represent organized mural thrombi. Veins are also involved by medial hypertrophy and arterialization (see Fig. 14–24). Only rarely is fresh thrombus or pulmonary phlebitis encountered.[95,96] Because of the postcapillary obstruction, the following microcirculatory lesions are also present: capillary congestion, interstitial and pleural edema, dilatation of interstitial and pleural lymphatics, and alveolar clusters of hemosiderin-laden macrophages (see Fig. 14–23). Pulmonary arteries exhibit medial hypertrophy (see Fig. 14–9), and the small muscular arteries occasionally show eccentric intimal fibrosis or organized thrombi (see Figs. 14–12, 14–13, 14–21), similar to those observed in the veins.[97,98]

Pulmonary Venous Hypertension

Pulmonary venous hypertension results from obstruction distal to the small pulmonary veins (Table 14–5) and involves all portions of the pulmonary vasculature.[1–3,34–36,99–110] It is the most common form of pulmonary hypertension and is considered reversible if the cause of the obstruction can be eliminated.[17,111–113] However, regression of the secondary pulmonary vascular lesions may take months to years.

The extent of the vascular lesions depends on both the severity and the duration of the postcapillary obstruction. In general, the entire pulmonary vascular bed is engorged with blood, and this may affect pulmonary function.[114] The pulmonary venules and veins are involved by medial hypertrophy, arterialization, dilatation, and eccentric intimal fibrosis (see Fig. 14–24). The microcirculation is characterized by capillary congestion, edema of interlobular septa and pleurae, dilatation of interstitial and pleural lymphatics, and alveolar hemosiderosis (see Fig. 14–23). Arterioles are often muscularized (see Fig. 14–10). Secondary medial hypertrophy of muscular arteries may be quite striking (see Fig. 14–9), and eccentric or nonlaminar

Table 14–5. Causes of Chronic Pulmonary Venous Hypertension

Pulmonary veins	Left ventricle
Mediastinitis	Chronic heart failure
Mediastinal neoplasm	Constrictive pericarditis
Mediastinal fibrosis	Restrictive cardiomyopathy
Congenital pulmonary vein stenosis	Hypertrophic cardiomyopathy
Left atrium	Congenital subaortic stenosis
Cardiac myxoma	Aortic valve
Ball-valve thrombus	Aortic stenosis
Cor triatriatum	Aortic regurgitation
Mitral valve	Thoracic aorta
Mitral stenosis	Supravalvular aortic stenosis
Mitral regurgitation	Coarctation of aorta

concentric fibrosis is commonly observed and considered to represent in situ stasis thrombosis (see Fig. 14–12). Muscular and elastic arteries may be quite dilated.

COEXISTENT FORMS OF PULMONARY HYPERTENSION

In some instances, the characteristic lesions of two different histopathologic forms of pulmonary hypertension may be observed in the same patient. For example, if a patient with a ventricular septal defect and severe pulmonary hypertension develops chronic heart failure, then the vascular lesions of chronic pulmonary venous hypertension may coexist with those of plexogenic pulmonary arteriopathy. As another example, a patient with mitral stenosis and chronic pulmonary venous hypertension may, by virtue of limited activity and sluggish blood flow, develop systemic venous thrombosis, recurrent pulmonary embolization, and thromboembolic pulmonary hypertension.

PRIMARY PULMONARY HYPERTENSION

Among patients with pulmonary hypertension, a group exists in whom no underlying cardiopulmonary disorder can be clinically identified to account for the hypertensive state. Such patients are considered to have primary, or idiopathic, pulmonary hypertension. It is important to recognize, however, that this single clinical entity encompasses several histopathologic forms (Table 14–6).[1–3,38,40,84,115,116] Thrombotic and plexogenic patterns are the most commonly observed types of primary pulmonary hypertension, but considerable overlap of lesions commonly occurs in individual cases.

Women are affected twice as frequently as men, and the disorder most commonly occurs in young and middle-aged adults.[38,40] Familial cases have been reported.[1,117] Survival is generally 2 to 5 years; sudden death occurs in 25 percent of patients, but it is observed twice as often in patients with plexogenic disease as in those with other histopathologic patterns.[38,40] Right heart failure is the usual cause of death in the remainder. Rarely, the disease regresses spontaneously.[118,119]

NOMENCLATURE

The World Health Organization has designated three histopathologic forms of primary pulmonary hypertension: plexogenic pulmonary arteriopathy, thromboembolic pulmonary hypertension, and pulmonary veno-occlusive disease.[120]

According to this recommendation, cases characterized only by medial hypertrophy or concentric laminar intimal fibrosis are categorized by most investigators as plexogenic pulmonary arteriopathy.[1,115] This is based on the assumption that these cases, like those associated with congenital cardiac left-to-right shunts, will later develop arteritis and plexiform and dilatation lesions.[121] However, this temporal sequence of events has not been demonstrated by serial lung biopsies among individual patients with primary pulmonary hypertension. Accordingly, it is difficult to be confident of the diagnosis of primary plexogenic pulmonary arteriopathy in cases without plexiform lesions.[40]

Moreover, some investigators have been reluctant to accept small-vessel thromboembolic disease as a legitimate category.[39] However, the concept that plexogenic disease represents the only true form of primary pulmonary hypertension is contro-

Table 14-6. Histopathologic Forms of Primary Pulmonary Hypertension

Terminology of World Health Organization	Descriptive Diagnosis
	Primary pulmonary hypertension, with:
Plexogenic pulmonary arteriopathy	Plexiform lesions
	Plexiform lesions and thrombosis
	Isolated medial hypertrophy
	Isolated concentric laminar intimal fibrosis
	Isolated (primary) pulmonary arteritis
Thromboembolic pulmonary hypertension	Arterial thrombosis
	Arterial thrombosis and fibrosis
	Arterial eccentric fibrosis
Pulmonary veno-occlusive disease	Venous thrombosis
	Venous thrombosis and fibrosis
None	Pulmonary capillary hemangiomatosis

versial, because, by definition, the cause of arterial and venous thrombosis is not known in the nonplexogenic cases. Therefore, it seems premature to remove either thromboembolic pulmonary hypertension or pulmonary veno-occlusive disease from the category of idiopathic disorders.

Recently, investigators have questioned the embolic nature of thromboembolic disease and have suggested that in situ thrombosis seems more likely in some cases.[40] Moreover, mixed plexogenic and thrombotic patterns occur frequently, and primary patterns other than plexogenic, thromboembolic, and veno-occlusive have been described.[40]

For these reasons, I favor a more descriptive system of nomenclature that emphasizes the spectrum of histopathologic features in individual cases (for example, primary pulmonary hypertension with mixed plexogenic and thrombotic features, or primary pulmonary hypertension with concentric laminar intimal fibrosis) (see Table 14-6).

Histopathologic Patterns

The thrombotic form is identical to cases of thromboembolic pulmonary hypertension that involve only the muscular and small elastic pulmonary arteries (see Fig. 14-21). Clinically, there is no apparent thrombotic obstruction of the mediastinal, lobar, or segmental arteries.[38,40,84,115,116] To establish the diagnosis of primary pulmonary hypertension with thrombotic features, organized and recanalized lesions must be observed. However, in some cases, eccentric intimal fibrosis, without recanalization, is the dominant lesion (see Figs. 14-12, 14-13). In this setting, the histopathologic pattern may be designated as primary pulmonary hypertension with fibrotic and thrombotic features.

Lesions associated with primary plexogenic disease are identical to those observed in secondary forms of plexogenic pulmonary arteriopathy (see Figs. 14-11, 14-14 to 14-17, 14-19).[1-3,38,40,84,115] To establish the diagnosis of primary pulmonary hypertension with plexogenic pattern, unequivocal plexiform lesions must be present. In some cases, fresh and organized thrombi may be present and may even represent the dominant lesions. Such mixed forms may be termed "primary pulmonary hypertension with plexogenic and thrombotic features."

Cases characterized by the lesions of plexogenic arteriopathy, but without plexiform lesions, may be designated according to the highest grade lesion observed. Examples include primary pulmonary hypertension with medial hypertrophy only (or primary medial hypertrophy)[40,122,123] and primary pulmonary hypertension with concentric laminar intimal fibrosis.[124]

Primary nongranulomatous pulmonary arteritis is a rare disorder of children and young adults that is associated with arterial destruction and secondary thrombosis (see Fig. 14–16*A*).[40,125] It produces a clinical picture of primary pulmonary hypertension and appears to differ from the thrombotic and plexogenic forms. It may be designated primary pulmonary hypertension with nongranulomatous arteritis.

Pulmonary veno-occlusive disease often presents clinically as an idiopathic process and may thereby represent primary pulmonary hypertension with venous thrombotic features.[1–3,38,40,84,115] The characteristic lesions were discussed earlier in this chapter (see Figs. 14–23 to 14–25).

Pulmonary capillary hemangiomatosis is characterized by an aggressive infiltration of the pleura and pulmonary interstitium by sheets of thin-walled vessels.[126,127] It may present clinically as primary pulmonary hypertension.[84] Involvement of arteries and bronchi may be associated with hemosiderin-laden macrophages or hemorrhages (parenchymal, hemothorax, or hemoptysis). Venous involvement may be associated with intimal fibrosis and obstruction and with secondary arterialization of veins, muscularization of arterioles, and medial hypertrophy of muscular arteries.

Pulmonary venous hypertension and pulmonary parenchymal or hypoxic disorders may mimic primary pulmonary hypertension and, therefore, may occasionally be observed in tissue from open lung biopsy in patients whose pulmonary hypertension appears idiopathic clinically.[128]

Rationale for Therapy

Medial hypertrophy is present in all histopathologic forms of primary pulmonary hypertension and presumably represents the morphologic counterpart of chronic vasoconstriction.[1] Accordingly, the rationale exists for treatment with pulmonary vasodilators.[122] However, adverse effects on the systemic circulation and the coexistence of irreversible obstructive pulmonary vascular lesions, among other factors, seriously hinder the efficacy of pulmonary vasodilators in most cases.[129–131]

Furthermore, it is doubtful that vasodilators can appreciably alter vessels that harbor intimal fibrotic lesions. However, because platelet-derived smooth muscle growth factor may promote the intimal proliferative lesions,[132] platelet inhibitors may be useful in some patients with primary pulmonary hypertension.

Plexiform lesions, dilatation lesions, fibrinoid degeneration, and necrotizing arteritis are each considered irreversible lesions and are probably unaffected by vasodilators. However, because they may also be the sites of ongoing thrombosis,[40] anticoagulants and platelet inhibitors may be useful.

Pulmonary thrombosis represents either an in situ or an embolic process. The composition of fresh thrombi may reflect the normal proportion of blood elements or may be rich in platelets. Therefore, in some patients, the rationale is provided for anticoagulant and platelet-inhibitor therapy.[116] Successful treatment is reported.[133]

Among patients with primary pulmonary hypertension, the most commonly observed processes are medial hypertrophy, intimal proliferation and fibrosis, and luminal thrombosis. Treatment with pulmonary vasodilators, platelet inhibitors, and anticoagulants is directed toward the alleviation of these obstructive lesions. Currently, however, the high rate of unsuccessful treatment probably reflects the advanced and perhaps irreversible nature of the pulmonary vascular lesions at the time of diagnosis. Accordingly, therapeutic success may depend primarily on earlier detection of the hypertensive state.[40]

End-stage pulmonary hypertension, either primary or secondary, may also be treated by heart-lung transplantation.[134]

OPEN LUNG BIOPSY

For the evaluation of pulmonary hypertension with open lung biopsy, the specimen should be at least 2 cm in greatest dimension.[84] If the disease process is not uniform in distribution, biopsies of both lungs or of upper and lower lobes may be performed. Biopsy tissue should be fixed in a distended state with transbronchial or transalveolar infiltration of formalin under low manual pressure from a syringe with a 25-gauge or 27-gauge needle.[135] After fixation, the tissue should be sectioned so that the arteries and their adjacent bronchi are cut in cross section rather than obliquely or longitudinally. Slides should be prepared from several levels in the paraffin block and stained with both hematoxylin-eosin and elastic–van Gieson stains.

The pathologist should know the patient's age, sex, history of cardiopulmonary and systemic disorders, pulmonary artery and wedge pressures, results of pulmonary ventilation-perfusion studies, if performed, and the lobe from which the biopsy tissue was taken. In the setting of underlying congenital heart disease, the pathologist should also know the previous cardiac operations and the planned future operations.

Open lung biopsy is generally performed in two settings: primary pulmonary hypertension and congenital heart disease.[128,136–141] In primary disease, a description of the types and extent of the obstructive lesions should be provided, in addition to the histopathologic category.

In the setting of congenital cardiac left-to-right shunts without obstructed pulmonary blood flow, secondary plexogenic pulmonary arteriopathy may develop. If congestive heart failure or left-sided valvular stenosis or regurgitation coexists, then the lesions of pulmonary venous hypertension may also be present. Although use of the Heath-Edwards grading system is appropriate for describing the plexogenic arteriopathy, it is *not* used for venous hypertensive lesions.

In the Fontan operation, the right atrium functions as the pumping chamber for the pulmonary circulation. Consequently, even moderate degrees of medial hypertrophy or intimal fibrosis may produce pulmonary arterial resistance too high for the right atrium to pump against. In this setting, a descriptive semiquantitative evaluation is more useful than the Heath-Edwards classification.[142]

REFERENCES

1. Wagenvoort, CA and Wagenvoort, N: Pathology of Pulmonary Hypertension. John Wiley & Sons, New York, 1977, pp 1–290.
2. Harris, PC and Heath, D: The Human Pulmonary Circulation: Its Form and Function in Health and Disease, ed 2. Churchill Livingstone, New York, 1977, pp 22–42, 211–273, 332–351, 398–451, 487–521, 547–566, 595–615, 626–634.
3. Wagenvoort, CA and Wagenvoort, N: Diseases of the pulmonary circulation. In Silver, MD (ed): Cardiovascular Pathology, Vol 2. Churchill Livingstone, New York, 1983, pp 683–705.
4. Meyrick, B and Reid, L: Pulmonary hypertension: Anatomic and physiologic correlates. Clin Chest Med 4:199, 1983.

5. Cudkowicz, L: Bronchial arterial circulation in man: Normal anatomy and responses to disease. Lung Biol Health Dis 14:111, 1979.
6. Warnock, ML and Kunzmann, A: Changes with age in muscular pulmonary arteries. Arch Pathol Lab Med 101:175, 1977.
7. Wagenvoort, CA, Neufeld, HN, and Edwards, JE: The structure of the pulmonary arterial tree in fetal and early postnatal life. Lab Invest 10:751, 1961.
8. Reid, LM: The pulmonary circulation: Remodeling in growth and disease. The 1978 J Burns Amberson Lecture. Am Rev Respir Dis 119:531, 1979.
9. Haworth, SG and Hislop, AA: Pulmonary vascular development: Normal values of peripheral vascular structure. Am J Cardiol 52:578, 1983.
10. Takahashi, T, Wagenvoort, N, and Wagenvoort, CA: The density of muscularized pulmonary arteries in normal lungs: A morphometric study. Arch Pathol Lab Med 107:19, 1983.
11. Lock, JE, Fuhrman, BP, Epstein, ML, et al: Pulmonary hypertension following neonatal shock. Pediatr Cardiol 1:109, 1979/1980.
12. Tiefenbrunn, LJ and Riemenschneider, TA: Persistent pulmonary hypertension of the newborn. Am Heart J 111:564, 1986.
13. Bove, KE and Scott, RC: The anatomy of chronic cor pulmonale secondary to intrinsic lung disease. Prog Cardiovasc Dis 9:227, 1966.
14. Edwards, JE: Pathology of chronic pulmonary hypertension. Pathol Annu 9:1, 1974.
15. Kieffer, RW, Hutchins, GM, Moore, GW, et al: Reversed septal curvature: Association with primary pulmonary hypertension and Shone syndrome. Am J Med 66:831, 1979.
16. Yamaki, S and Wagenvoort, CA: Plexogenic pulmonary arteriopathy: Significance of medial thickness with respect to advanced pulmonary vascular lesions. Am J Pathol 105:70, 1981.
17. Edwards, WD and Edwards, JE: Recent advances in the pathology of the pulmonary vasculature. Monogr Pathol 19:235, 1978.
18. Wagenvoort, CA, Wagenvoort, N, and Draulans-Noë, Y: Reversibility of plexogenic pulmonary arteriopathy following banding of the pulmonary artery. J Thorac Cardiovasc Surg 87:876, 1984.
19. Balk, AG, Dingemans, KP, and Wagenvoort, CA: The ultrastructure of the various forms of pulmonary arterial intimal fibrosis. Virchows Arch [A] 382:139, 1979.
20. Smith, P and Heath, D: Electron microscopy of the plexiform lesion. Thorax 34:177, 1979.
21. Kay, JM, Suyama, KL, and Keane, PM: Failure to show decrease in small pulmonary blood vessels in rats with experimental pulmonary hypertension. Thorax 37:927, 1982.
22. Mooi, W and Wagenvoort, CA: Decreased numbers of pulmonary blood vessels: Reality or artifact? J Pathol 141:441, 1983.
23. Gonzalez-Vitale, JC and Garcia-Bunuel, R: Pulmonary tumor emboli and cor pulmonale in primary carcinoma of the lung. Cancer 38:2105, 1976.
24. Fanta, CH and Compton, CC: Microscopic tumour emboli to the lungs: A hidden cause of dyspnoea and pulmonary hypertension. Thorax 35:794, 1980.
25. Brisbane, JU, Howell, DA, and Bonkowsky, HL: Pulmonary hypertension as a presentation of hepatocarcinoma: Report of a case and brief review of the literature. Am J Med 68:466, 1980.
26. Heath, D and Mackinnon, J: Pulmonary hypertension due to myxoma of the right atrium: With special reference to the behavior of emboli of myxoma in the lung. Am Heart J 68:227, 1964.
27. Naeye, RL: Advanced pulmonary vascular changes in schistosomal cor pulmonale. Am J Trop Med Hyg 10:191, 1961.
28. Chaves, E: The pathology of the arterial pulmonary vasculature in Manson's schistosomiasis. Dis Chest 50:72, 1966.
29. Tomashefski, JF, Jr and Hirsch, CS: The pulmonary vascular lesions of intravenous drug abuse. Hum Pathol 11:133, 1980.
30. Robertson, CH, Jr, Reynolds, RC, and Wilson JE, III: Pulmonary hypertension and foreign body granulomas in intravenous drug abusers: Documentation by cardiac catheterization and lung biopsy. Am J Med 61:657, 1976.
31. Arnett, EN, Battle, WE, Russo, JV, et al: Intravenous injection of talc-containing drugs intended for oral use: A cause of pulmonary granulomatosis and pulmonary hypertension. Am J Med 60:711, 1976.
32. Rajs, J, Härm, T, and Ormstad, K: Postmortem findings of pulmonary lesions of older datum in intravenous drug addicts: A forensic-pathologic study. Virchows Arch [A] 402:405, 1984.
33. Gilsanz, V, Campo, C, Cue, R, et al: Recurrent pulmonary embolism due to hydatid disease of heart: Study of 3 cases, one with intermittent tricuspid valve obstruction (atrial pseudomyxoma). Br Heart J 39:553, 1977.

34. Heath, D and Edwards, JE: Histological changes in the lung in diseases associated with pulmonary venous hypertension. Br J Dis Chest 53:8, 1959.
35. Wagenvoort, CA: Pathology of congestive pulmonary hypertension. Prog Respir Res 9:195, 1975.
36. Hutchins, GM and Ostrow, PT: The pathogenesis of the two forms of hypertensive pulmonary vascular disease. Am Heart J 92:797, 1976.
37. Wagenvoort, CA: Morphologic changes in intrapulmonary veins. Hum Pathol 1:205, 1970.
38. Wagenvoort, CA and Wagenvoort, N: Primary pulmonary hypertension: A pathologic study of the lung vessels in 156 clinically diagnosed cases. Circulation 42:1163, 1970.
39. Anderson, EG, Simon, G, and Reid, L: Primary and thrombo-embolic pulmonary hypertension: A quantitative pathological study. J Pathol 110:273, 1973.
40. Bjornsson, J and Edwards, WD: Primary pulmonary hypertension: A histopathologic study of 80 cases. Mayo Clin Proc 60:16, 1985.
41. Brown, DL, Wetli, CV, and Davis, JH: Sudden unexpected death from primary pulmonary hypertension. J Forensic Sci 26:381, 1981.
42. Ackermann, DM and Edwards, WD: Sudden death as the initial manifestation of primary pulmonary hypertension: Report of four cases. Am J Forens Med Pathol 9:2, 1987.
43. Edwards, JE: Functional pathology of the pulmonary vascular tree in congenital cardiac disease. Circulation 15:164, 1957.
44. Wagenvoort, CA, Neufeld, HN, DuShane, JW, et al: The pulmonary arterial tree in ventricular septal defect: A quantitative study of anatomic features in fetuses, infants, and children. Circulation 23:740, 1961.
45. Wagenvoort, CA and Wagenvoort, N: Pathology of the Eisenmenger syndrome and primary pulmonary hypertension. Adv Cardiol 11:123, 1974.
46. Wagenvoort, CA, Neufeld, HN, DuShane, JW, et al: The pulmonary arterial tree in atrial septal defect: A quantitative study of anatomic features in fetuses, infants, and children. Circulation 23:733, 1961.
47. Viles, PH, Ongley, PA, and Titus, JL: The spectrum of pulmonary vascular disease in transposition of the great arteries. Circulation 40:31, 1969.
48. Newfeld, EA, Paul, MH, Muster, AJ, et al: Pulmonary vascular disease in complete transposition of the great arteries: A study of 200 patients. Am J Cardiol 34:75, 1974.
49. Edwards, WD and Edwards, JE: Hypertensive pulmonary vascular disease in d-transposition of the great arteries. Am J Cardiol 41:921, 1978.
50. Rosengart, R, Fishbein, M, and Emmanouilides, GC: Progressive pulmonary vascular disease after surgical correction (Mustard procedure) of transposition of great arteries with intact ventricular septum. Am J Cardiol 35:107, 1975.
51. Newfeld, EA, Paul, MH, Muster, AJ, et al: Pulmonary vascular disease in transposition of the great vessels and intact ventricular septum. Circulation 59:525, 1979.
52. Heath, D and Edwards, JE: The pathology of hypertensive pulmonary vascular disease: A description of six grades of structural changes in the pulmonary arteries with special reference to congenital cardiac septal defects. Circulation 18:533, 1958.
53. Wagenvoort, CA: Hypertensive pulmonary vascular disease complicating congenital heart disease: A review. Cardiovasc Clin 5:43, 1973.
54. Rabinovitch, M and Reid, LM: Quantitative structural analysis of the pulmonary vascular bed in congenital heart defects. Cardiovasc Clin 11(2):149, 1980.
55. Hislop, A, Haworth, SG, Shinebourne, EA, et al: Quantitative structural analysis of pulmonary vessels in isolated ventricular septal defect in infancy. Br Heart J 37:1014, 1975.
56. Haworth, SG, Sauer, U, Bühlmeyer, K, et al: Development of the pulmonary circulation in ventricular septal defect: A quantitative structural study. Am J Cardiol 40:781, 1977.
57. Haworth, SG: Pulmonary vascular disease in secundum atrial septal defect in childhood. Am J Cardiol 51:265, 1983.
58. Takahashi, T and Wagenvoort, CA: Density of muscularized arteries in the lung: Its role in congenital heart disease and its clinical significance. Arch Pathol Lab Med 107:23, 1983.
59. Wagenvoort, CA: Grading of pulmonary vascular lesions—a reappraisal. Histopathology 5:595, 1981.
60. Wagenvoort, CA: Hypertensive pulmonary vascular disease: The point of no return. Minn Med 68:45, 1985.
61. Edwards, BS, Weir, EK, Edwards, WD, et al: The pathology of pulmonary hypertension complicating portal hypertension (unpublished data).

62. Beckering, RE, Jr and Titus, JL: Temporal-popliteal venous thrombosis and pulmonary embolism. Am J Clin Pathol 52:530, 1969.
63. Freilich, JK and Szatkowski, J: Pelvic vein thrombosis with pulmonary vascular lesions simulating primary pulmonary hypertension. Am J Cardiol 7:297, 1961.
64. James, TN: Thrombi in antrum atrii dextri of human heart as clinically important source for chronic microembolisation to lungs. Br Heart J 49:122, 1983.
65. McMahon, DP and Aterman, K: Pulmonary hypertension due to multiple emboli. J Pediatr 92:841, 1978.
66. Goodwin, JF, Harrison, CV, and Wilcken, DEL: Obliterative pulmonary hypertension and thrombo-embolism. Br Med J 1:701; 777, 1963.
67. Arnett, EN, Bacos, JM, Macher, AM, et al: Fibrosing mediastinitis causing pulmonary arterial hypertension without pulmonary venous hypertension: Clinical and necropsy observations. Am J Med 63:634, 1977.
68. Sobrinho-Simões, MA, Vaz Saleiro, J, Wagenvoort, CA: Mediastinal and hilar fibrosis. Histopathology 5:53, 1981.
69. Berry, DF, Buccigrossi, D, Peabody, J, et al: Pulmonary vascular occlusion and fibrosing mediastinitis. Chest 89:296, 1986.
70. Hietala, S-O, Stinnett, RG, Faunce, HF, III, et al: Pulmonary artery narrowing in sarcoidosis. JAMA 237:572, 1977.
71. Fishman, AP: Chronic cor pulmonale. Am Rev Respir Dis 114:775, 1976.
72. Fishman, AP: Hypoxia on the pulmonary circulation: How and where it acts. Circ Res 38:221, 1976.
73. Bohr, DF: The pulmonary hypoxic response: State of the field. Chest 71:244, 1977.
74. Reid, LM: Structure and function in pulmonary hypertension: New perceptions. Chest 89:279, 1986.
75. Wagenvoort, CA and Wagenvoort, N: Hypoxic pulmonary vascular lesions in man at high altitude and in patients with chronic respiratory disease. Path Microbiol 39:276, 1973.
76. Warnock, ML and Kunzmann, A: Muscular pulmonary arteries in chronic obstructive lung disease. Arch Pathol Lab Med 101:180, 1977.
77. Shelton, DM, Keal, E, and Reid, L: The pulmonary circulation in chronic bronchitis and emphysema. Chest 71(Suppl):303S, 1977.
78. Hale, KA, Niewoehner, DE, and Cosio, MG: Morphologic changes in the muscular pulmonary arteries: Relationship to cigarette smoking, airway disease, and emphysema. Am Rev Respir Dis 122:273, 1980.
79. Wagenvoort, CA and Wagenvoort, N: Pulmonary venous changes in chronic hypoxia. Virchows Arch [A] 372:51, 1976.
80. Young, RH and Mark, GJ: Pulmonary vascular changes in scleroderma. Am J Med 64:998, 1978.
81. Kay, JM, Smith, P, and Heath, D: Aminorex and the pulmonary circulation. Thorax 26:262, 1971.
82. Fernández-Segoviano, P, Esteban, A, and Martínez-Cabruja, R: Pulmonary vascular lesions in the toxic oil syndrome in Spain. Thorax 38:724, 1983.
83. Garcia-Dorado, D, Miller, DD, Garcia, EJ, et al: An epidemic of pulmonary hypertension after toxic rapeseed oil ingestion in Spain. J Am Coll Cardiol 1:1216, 1983.
84. Kay, JM and Heath, D: Pathology study of unexplained pulmonary hypertension. Semin Respir Med 7:180, 1985.
85. Heath, D and Kay, JM: Diet, drugs, and pulmonary hypertension. Prog Cardiol 7:125, 1978.
86. Wagenvoort, CA and Wagenvoort, N: The pathology of pulmonary veno-occlusive disease. Virchows Arch [A] 364:69, 1974.
87. Thadani, U, Burrow, C, Whitaker, W, et al: Pulmonary veno-occlusive disease. Q J Med 44:133, 1975.
88. Wagenvoort, CA: Pulmonary veno-occlusive disease: Entity or syndrome? Chest 69:82, 1976.
89. Dail, DH, Liebow, AA, Gmelich, J, et al: A study of 43 cases of pulmonary veno-occlusive (PVO) disease (abstr). Lab Invest 38:340, 1978.
90. Kay, JM, De Sa, DJ, and Mancer, JFK: Ultrastructure of lung in pulmonary veno-occlusive disease. Hum Pathol 14:451, 1983.
91. Wagenvoort, CA, Losekoot, G, and Mulder, E: Pulmonary veno-occlusive disease of presumably intrauterine origin. Thorax 26:429, 1971.
92. Cagle, P and Langston, C: Pulmonary veno-occlusive disease as a cause of sudden infant death. Arch Pathol Lab Med 108:338, 1984.

93. Joselson, R and Warnock, M: Pulmonary veno-occlusive disease after chemotherapy. Hum Pathol 14:88, 1983.
94. Voordes, CG, Kuipers, JRG, and Elema, JD: Familial pulmonary veno-occlusive disease: A case report. Thorax 32:763, 1977.
95. Braun, A, Greenberg, SD, Malik, S, et al: Pulmonary veno-occlusive disease associated with pulmonary phlebitis. Arch Pathol 95:67, 1973.
96. Crissman, JD, Koss, M, and Carson, RP: Pulmonary veno-occlusive disease secondary to granulomatous venulitis. Am J Surg Pathol 4:93, 1980.
97. Pääkkö, P, Sutinen, S, Remes, M, et al: A case of pulmonary vascular occlusive disease: Comparison of post-mortem radiography and histology. Histopathology 9:253, 1985.
98. Wagenvoort, CA, Wagenvoort, N, and Takahashi, T: Pulmonary veno-occlusive disease: Involvement of pulmonary arteries and review of the literature. Hum Pathol 16:1033, 1985.
99. Becker, DL, Burchell, HB, and Edwards, JE: Pathology of the pulmonary vascular tree. II. The occurrence in mitral insufficiency of occlusive pulmonary vascular lesions. Circulation 3:230, 1951.
100. Smith, RC, Burchell, HB, and Edwards, JE: Pathology of the pulmonary vascular tree. IV. Structural changes in the pulmonary vessels in chronic left ventricular failure. Circulation 10:801, 1954.
101. Ferencz, C and Dammann, JF, Jr: Significance of the pulmonary vascular bed in congenital heart disease. V. Lesions of the left side of the heart causing obstruction of the pulmonary venous return. Circulation 16:1046, 1957.
102. Lucas, RV, Jr, Anderson, RC, Amplatz, K, et al: Congenital causes of pulmonary venous obstruction. Pediatr Clin North Am 10:781, Aug 1963.
103. Beckman, CB, Moller, JH, and Edwards, JE: Alternate pathways to pulmonary venous flow in left-sided obstructive anomalies. Circulation 52:509, 1975.
104. Tandon, HD and Kasturi, J: Pulmonary vascular changes associated with isolated mitral stenosis in India. Br Heart J 37:26, 1975.
105. Haworth, SG and Reid, L: Structural study of pulmonary circulation and of heart in total anomalous pulmonary venous return in early infancy. Br Heart J 39:80, 1977.
106. Dye, TE, Saab, SB, Almond, CH, et al: Sclerosing mediastinitis with occlusion of pulmonary veins: Manifestations and management. J Thorac Cardiovasc Surg 74:137, 1977.
107. Basu, B, Cherian, G, Krishnaswami, S, et al: Severe pulmonary hypertension in advanced aortic valve disease. Br Heart J 40:1310, 1978.
108. Shida, T, Ohashi, H, Nakamura, K, et al: Pulmonary varices associated with mitral valve disease: A case report and survey of the literature. Ann Thorac Surg 34:452, 1982.
109. Wagenvoort, CA and Wagenvoort, N: Smooth muscle content of pulmonary arterial media in pulmonary venous hypertension compared with other forms of pulmonary hypertension. Chest 81:581, 1982.
110. Petersen, RC and Edwards, WD: Pulmonary vascular disease in 57 necropsy cases of total anomalous pulmonary venous connection. Histopathology 7:487, 1983.
111. Reeve, R, Selzer, A, Popper, RW, et al: Reversibility of pulmonary hypertension following cardiac surgery. Circulation 33,34(Suppl 1):I-107, 1966.
112. Ramírez, A, Grimes, ET, and Abelmann, WH: Regression of pulmonary vascular changes following mitral valvuloplasty: An anatomic and physiologic case study. Am J Med 45:975, 1968.
113. Zener, JC, Hancock, EW, Shumway, NE, et al: Regression of extreme pulmonary hypertension after mitral valve surgery. Am J Cardiol 30:820, 1972.
114. Cortese, DA: Pulmonary function in mitral stenosis. Mayo Clin Proc 53:321, 1978.
115. Edwards, WD and Edwards, JE: Clinical primary pulmonary hypertension: Three pathologic types. Circulation 56:884, 1977.
116. Fuster, V, Steele, PM, Edwards, WD, et al: Primary pulmonary hypertension: Natural history and the importance of thrombosis. Circulation 70:580, 1984.
117. Loyd, JE, Primm, RK, and Newman, JH: Familial primary pulmonary hypertension: Clinical patterns. Am Rev Respir Dis 129:194, 1984.
118. Bourdillon, PDV and Oakley, CM: Regression of primary pulmonary hypertension. Br Heart J 38:264, 1976.
119. Fujii, A, Rabinovitch, M, and Matthews, EC: A case of spontaneous resolution of idiopathic pulmonary hypertension. Br Heart J 46:574, 1981.
120. Hatano, S and Strasser, T (eds): Primary pulmonary hypertension. Report on a World Health Organization meeting, Geneva, 15–17 October 1973. Geneva, WHO, 1975.
121. Yamaki, S and Wagenvoort, CA: Comparison of primary plexogenic arteriopathy in adults and children: A morphometric study in 40 patients. Br Heart J 54:428, 1985.

122. Rao, BNS, Moller, JH, and Edwards, JE: Primary pulmonary hypertension in a child: Response to pharmacologic agents. Circulation 40:583, 1969.
123. Robertson, B: Idiopathic pulmonary hypertension in infancy and childhood: Microangiographic and histological observations in five cases. Acta Pathol Microbiol Scand [A] 79:217, 1971.
124. Juaneda, E, Watson, H, and Haworth, SG: An unusual case of rapidly progressive primary pulmonary hypertension in childhood. Int J Cardiol 7:306, 1985.
125. Clausen, KP and Geer, JC: Hypertensive pulmonary arteritis. Am J Dis Child 118:718, 1969.
126. Wagenvoort, CA, Beestra, A, and Spijker, J: Capillary haemangiomatosis of the lungs. Histopathology 2:401, 1978.
127. Whittaker, JS, Pickering, CA, Heath, D, et al: Pulmonary capillary haemangiomatosis. Diagn Histopathol 6:77, 1983.
128. Wagenvoort, CA: Lung biopsy specimens in the evaluation of pulmonary vascular disease. Chest 77:614, 1980.
129. Rich, S and Brundage, BH: Primary pulmonary hypertension: Current update. JAMA 251:2252, 1984.
130. McGoon, MD and Vlietstra, RE: Vasodilator therapy for primary pulmonary hypertension. Mayo Clin Proc 59:672, 1984.
131. Packer, M: Vasodilator therapy for primary pulmonary hypertension: Limitations and hazards. Ann Intern Med 103:258, 1985.
132. Haworth, SG: Primary pulmonary hypertension. Br Heart J 49:517, 1983.
133. Cohen, M, Edwards, WD, and Fuster, V: Regression in thromboembolic type of primary pulmonary hypertension during 2½ years of antithrombotic therapy. J Am Coll Cardiol 7:172, 1986.
134. Jamieson, SW, Stinson, EB, Oyer, PE, et al: Heart-lung transplantation for irreversible pulmonary hypertension. Ann Thorac Surg 38:554, 1984.
135. Churg, A: An inflation procedure for open lung biopsies. Am J Surg Pathol 7:69, 1983.
136. Wagenvoort, CA, Nauta, J, van der Schaar, PJ, et al: The pulmonary vasculature in complete transposition of the great vessels, judged from lung biopsies. Circulation 38:746, 1968.
137. Rabinovitch, M, Haworth, SG, Castaneda, AR, et al: Lung biopsy in congenital heart disease: A morphometric approach to pulmonary vascular disease. Circulation 58:1107, 1978.
138. Rabinovitch, M, Castaneda, AR, and Reid, L: Lung biopsy with frozen section as a diagnostic aid in patients with congenital heart defects. Am J Cardiol 47:77, 1981.
139. Rabinovitch, M, Keane, JF, Norwood, WI, et al: Vascular structure in lung tissue obtained at biopsy correlated with pulmonary hemodynamic findings after repair of congenital heart defects. Circulation 69:655, 1984.
140. Haworth, SG: Pulmonary vascular disease in different types of congenital heart disease: Implications for interpretation of lung biopsy findings in early childhood. Br Heart J 52:557, 1984.
141. Wagenvoort, CA: Open lung biopsies in congenital heart disease for evaluation of pulmonary vascular disease: Predictive value with regard to corrective operability. Histopathology 9:417, 1985.
142. Edwards, WD and Wold, LE: Cardiovascular system. In Coulson, WF (ed): Surgical Pathology, ed 2. JB Lippincott, Philadelphia (in press).

CHAPTER 15

The Very Elderly Heart

Bruce F. Waller, M.D.
Randy Morgan, B.S.

Forty is the old-age of youth
Fifty is the youth of old-age. (Victor Hugo)

"Old age" has become an increasingly prominent subject in the medical and nonmedical media. There are books on longevity and life extension, and numerous products (nutrient supplements, minerals, skin creams, and so on) have been promoted to delay aging and prolong life. Whereas the average *length of life* has risen from 47 to 73 years in this century, the maximum *lifespan* has not apparently increased.[1] Data on the number of centenarians have been available in England since the early 19th century, and over this time, despite a great change in mean life expectancy, there has been no appreciable change in the number of people living longer than 100 years nor in the maximum age of persons dying in a given year.[1,2] The 1986 edition of the *Guinness Book of World Records* notes that the greatest authenticated age in the world is recorded in Japan—120 years.[2] In Sweden, where careful investigations of centenarians are carried out, apparently no one has yet exceeded 110 years of age.[1,2] About 1 in 10,000 persons in developed countries lives beyond the age of 100. The 1982 Chinese census, reported in February 1984, revealed only 3765 centenarians (0.04 percent), of whom two thirds were women.[2] In the United States, the mid-1983 figure of centenarians was 32,000 (0.01 percent).[2] Although reports of persons living longer than 130 years have been published,[3,4] there has been no satisfactory documentation of exceptional longevity in these societies.

Although the maximum lifespan may not be increasing, the number of persons surviving into the 70s, 80s, and 90s is increasing. In the United States, the population segment aged 85 years and older is about 2.6 million (1 percent), and it is projected that this segment of our population will be the fastest growing in the next 10 years, doubling by the year 2000 and rising five-fold by the year 2050.[5,6]

With an increasingly large segment of the population surviving into the "old-age" category, knowledge of "normal" or "expected" aging changes in the cardiovascular system has practical importance. In addition, knowledge of the relative incidence of various types of cardiovascular disease and causes of death in this age group has value in terms of treatment. Despite an increasing percentage of individuals surviving 90 years or more, little information is available on morphologic (normal or abnormal) changes in the old-age heart.[7–22] Previous publications reporting necropsy observations have been confined for the most part to patients aged 65 to 85 years, and only a limited number of studies have reported observations in necropsy patients aged 90 years and older.[5,13,15–17] The paucity of information in this very elderly age group is related in part to the limited number of necropsies performed on patients aged 90 years or older.[6] The percentage of deaths for which necropsies are performed drops off markedly with increasing age, such that only about 5 percent of those dying at age 85 years or older and about 4 percent of those dying at age 90 years or older undergo necropsy examination.[6]

AGING

Aging processes are usually considered to be "normal," in that they occur in all members of a population.[23] They are usually progressive and physiologically irreversible processes that are inevitable, occurring in spite of optimal nutrition and environment. Changes in the cardiovascular system appear to be central to the general concept of aging, in that aging of the cardiovascular system per se may promote the generalized debilitation of many organ systems characterizing the aging syndromes.[24] This concept was proposed centuries ago by Leonardo da Vinci, who described the cause of aging as:

> veins which by the thickening of their tunics on the old restrict the passage of blood, and by this lack of nourishment destroy the life of the aged without fever, the old coming to fail little by little in slow death.[25]

The aging heart represents the sum of anatomic, biochemical, and physiologic changes that have accrued over the years as a result of normal growth and development, the aging process, and age-related diseases.[26] Separation and identification of changes that are due to age alone, however, is a difficult task. The *effects of aging* per se ("genetically programmed") may not always be distinguishable from the *effects of pathology* ("acquired or initiated from external events").[27] Additional views on the normal aging-disease relationship are expressed subsequently:

> We shall never have a science of medicine as long as we separate the explanation of the pathologic from the explanation of normal vital phenomena. (Bernard, 1865)[28]
>
> The textural changes which old age induce in the organism sometimes attain such a point that the physiological and pathological states seem to mingle by an imperceptible transition, and to be no longer sharply distinguishable. (Charcot, 1881)[29]
>
> Can the effects of aging per se be distinguished from those of pathology?. . . . Time alone causing nothing. (Kleemeier, 1965)[30]
>
> Autopsy studies indicate that the concept of pure 'physiological aging' as a cause of death is observed rarely. . . . (McKeown, 1975)[31]
>
> Aging is not a disease, and it is a fact that the physiological decrements that occur with age simply allow for one expression of disease to occur at higher rates. But one must separate the two concepts, and this is the critical point. (Hayflick, 1976)[32]

Morphologic cardiac changes observed in the very elderly heart (90 years of age or older) may be divided into two major subgroups: (1) *changes ("disease processes") beginning at a younger age and continuing on or progressing into the old-age category* (for example, hypertensive, atherosclerotic coronary, and rheumatic heart diseases); and (2) *changes ("normal aging changes") that are specifically found in virtually every elderly heart* (for example, calcific deposits, vessel tortuosity, myocardial lipofuscin deposits). The sections that follow attempt to separate morphologic changes observed in the very elderly but otherwise normal heart from those morphologic changes that cause clinical cardiac dysfunction, death, or both.

AGING CHANGES IN THE NORMAL ELDERLY HEART

Certain morphologic changes commonly observed at necropsy in the very elderly heart that usually do not produce clinical signs of cardiac dysfunction during life may be divided into seven areas: (1) *myocardium (walls),* (2) *chambers (cavities),* (3) *valves,* (4) *epicardial coronary arteries,* (5) *conduction system,* (6) *pericardium,* and (7) *aorta* (Table 15–1; Figs. 15–1 through 15–24).

Table 15–1. Aging Changes Observed in the Normal Very Elderly Heart

1. *Myocardium (Walls)*
   A. Brown atrophy (lipofuscin deposits)
   B. Basophilic degeneration
   C. Increased subepicardial fat (cardiac adiposity)
   D. Amyloid deposits (focal)
   E. Increased heart weight
2. *Chambers (Cavities)*
   A. Decreased left ventricular cavity
   B. Sigmoid-shaped ventricular septum
   C. Increased left atrial cavity
3. *Valves*
   A. Fibrous thickening at contact points
   B. Fatty alteration of collagen with foci of calcium at base of aortic valve cusps
   C. Fatty alteration of collagen of anterior leaflet of mitral valve
   D. Mitral-valve anular calcium
   E. Protrusion or buckling of mitral leaflets toward the left atrium
4. *Epicardial Coronary Arteries*
   A. Tortuous
   B. Calcific deposits
   C. Increased cross-sectional luminal area (dilated)
   D. Usually mild atherosclerosis
   E. Atherosclerotic plaques composed of fibrosis tissue and calcific deposits ("hard lesions")
5. *Aorta*
   A. Dilated ascending aorta (sinuses of Valsalva) with rightward shift
   B. Related, elongated (tortuous) thoracic aorta
   C. Calcific deposits
   D. Sinotubular junction calcific deposits
   E. Elastic fragmentation and collagen accumulation

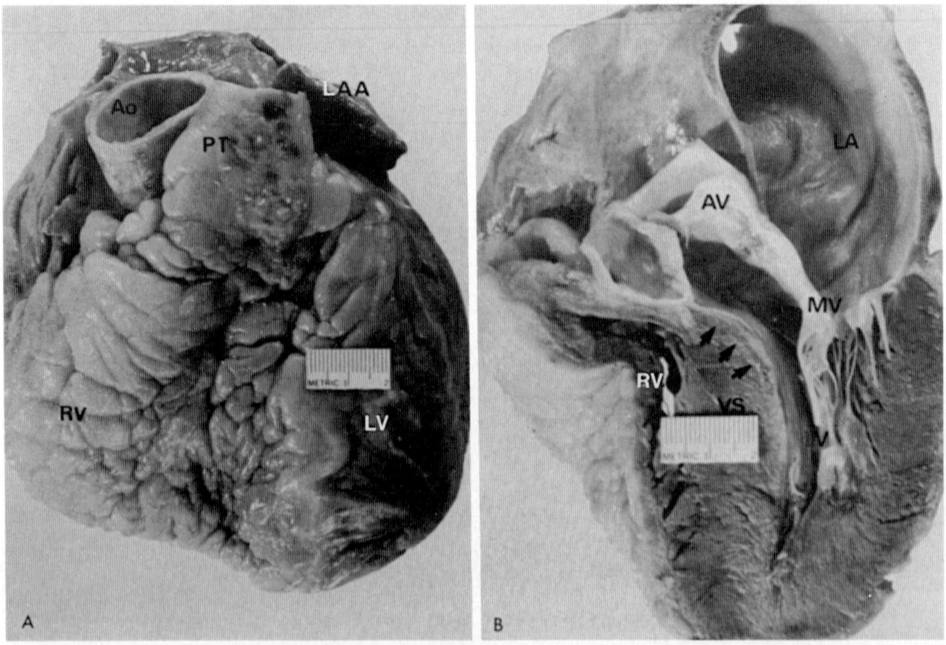

Figure 15–1. *A,* Increased subepicardial fat in the heart of a 92-year-old woman who never had clinical evidence of heart disease and died a noncardiovascular death. *B,* Long-axis cut of heart showing a nondilated left ventricular (LV) cavity, dilated left atrium (LA), and "sigmoid-shaped" ventricular septum (VS) *(arrows).* Ao = aorta, AV = aortic valve, LAA = left atrial appendage, MV = mitral valve, PT = pulmonary trunk, RV = right ventricle.

Myocardium (Walls)

Changes in the myocardium of the very elderly heart related to the aging process include (1) *brown atrophy,* (2) *basophilic degeneration,* (3) *subepicardial fat* (cardiac adiposity) (Figs. 15–1, 15–2), and (4) *focal amyloid deposits.*

Brown Atrophy

Brown atrophy is a term used to describe the browner-than-normal myocardial color observed in the very elderly heart. The histologic basis for the myocardial color is the presence of extensive *lipofuscin deposits* in the paranuclear sarcoplasm. This insoluble inert substance, also referred to as ceroid, lipochrome, wear-and-tear pigment, is generally thought to arise from oxidative polymerization of unsaturated lipids and to exist in combination with components of lysosomes.[33] Lipofuscin accumulates linearly with age (about 0.03 percent per year in humans[34]) and occupies about 6 percent of the intercellular volume of human myocardium.[35] The presence or amount of lipofuscin has not been related to any disease or cause of clinical cardiac dysfunction.

Basophilic Degeneration

Basophilic degeneration of the myocardium is very common, if not universal, in the very elderly heart. The material (basophilic on hematoxylin and eosin staining) is found in the sarcoplasm of the muscle cell. Ultrastructural and biochemical analysis indicates that the material is a glucan, possibly representing a byproduct of glycogen metabolism.[36] Location of the material is variable, with large quantities present in some myocardial cells but absent in others in the same heart. Hutchins[37] suggested that the focal accumulation of this material possibly indicates an acquired disease of individual muscle cells rather than an age-related process.

Subepicardial Fat

The amount of *subepicardial fat* increases with advancing age and is especially prominent over the anterior surface of the right ventricle and atrioventricular groove areas (Figs. 15 – 1, 15 – 2). Frequently, fat cells infiltrate the right ventricular free wall between muscle fibers. A similar fatty accumulation occurs in the cephalad portion of the atrial septum. In its advanced form, the atrial septal fat accumulation is termed "lipomatous hypertrophy of the atrial septum."

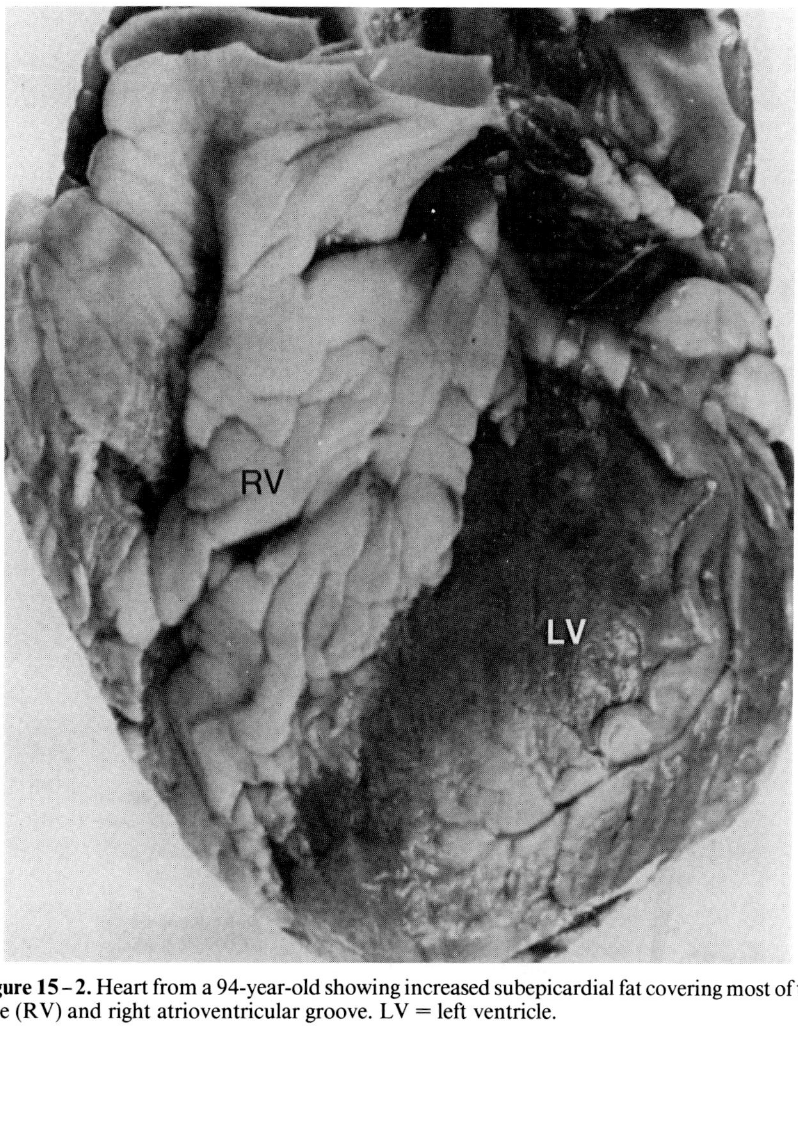

Figure 15 – 2. Heart from a 94-year-old showing increased subepicardial fat covering most of the right ventricle (RV) and right atrioventricular groove. LV = left ventricle.

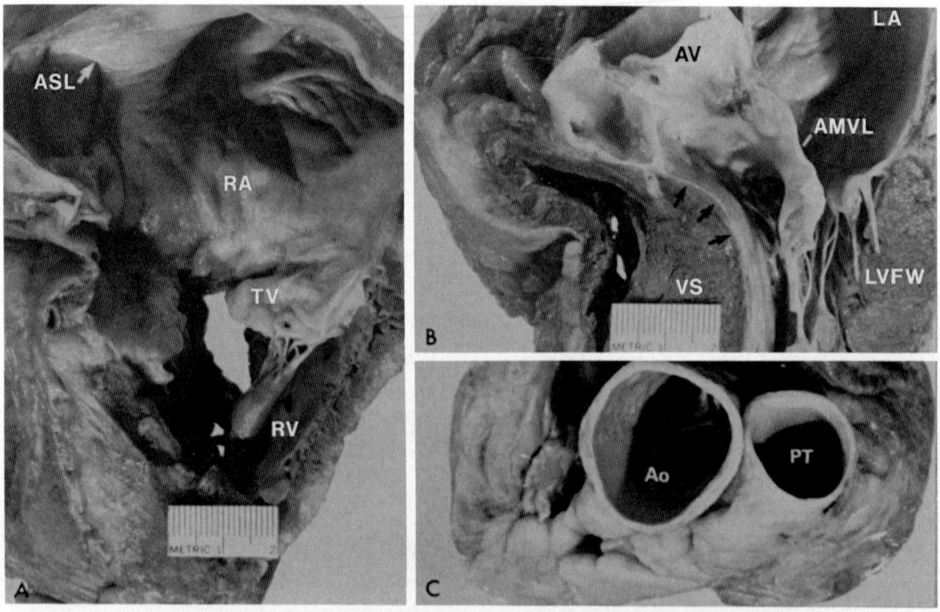

Figure 15–3. Heart from a 92-year-old woman. *A,* View of slightly dilated right atrium (RA), focally thickened tricuspid valve (TV), and normal right ventricle (RV). Note the increased subepicardial fat and atrial septal lipoma (ASL). *B,* Close-up of left ventricular outflow tract showing the "sigmoid" ventricular septum (VS) *(arrows),* and focal calcific deposits on the anterior leaflet of the mitral valve (AMVL). AV = aortic valve, LA = left atrium, LVFW = left ventricular free wall. *C,* View of the ascending aorta (Ao) and pulmonary trunk (PT) showing a dilated Ao and increased basal subepicardial fat.

Amyloid Deposits

Focal cardiac *amyloid deposits* are also a feature of the very elderly myocardium and endocardium. When focal and localized (usually in the left atrium) and observed as an incidental necropsy finding, the condition is termed "senile cardiac amyloidosis." Senile cardiac amyloidosis generally produces no clinically evident cardiac dysfunction, it is uncommon before age 60 years, and its incidence increases dramatically after age 60 years. Pomerance[15] found that the incidence of cardiac amyloid deposits in all subjects over age 60 years was 12.5 percent; in those patients aged over 80 years, it was 23 percent; and in subjects over age 90 years, the incidence increased to 50 percent. Buerger and Braunstein[38] studied 986 autopsies of patients over 55 years of age. The incidence of cardiac amyloid deposits increased with age, occurring in 8 of 33 (24 percent) persons aged 90 to 99 years. The role of age appeared to be in incidence rather than in progressive accumulation in individual hearts. Additional surveys have shown cardiac amyloidosis in 21 percent of patients over 80 years of age,[39] 70 percent in a sampling of 100 hearts from persons aged 60 to 90,[40] and 15 percent in 100 unselected autopsies of men aged 65 to 95 years.[41] Studies thus far have provided information on incidence rather than rates of accumulation in individuals and subpopulations. It remains unclear whether focal amyloid deposition is an aging process that occurs in all members of an elderly population or if it is formed in only some subgroups. Occasionally, extensive amyloid deposits occur in the elderly heart, producing clinical cardiac dysfunction and eventually causing death. Of 54 patients at necropsy with cardiac amyloidosis producing cardiac dysfunction and death reported by Roberts and Waller,[42] only four (7 percent) were aged 90 to 100 years.

Heart Weight

Heart weight in the very elderly patient generally increases.[19] Necropsy data indicate that the human heart "hypertrophies" with advancing age and that its mass increases 1 g to 1.5 g per year between 30 and 90 years of age.[26] In a necropsy study of the very elderly heart, Waller and Roberts[19] found increased heart weight in two thirds of hearts aged 90 to 103 years. The mean heart weight was 0.6 percent of the mean body weight—a 1.3-fold increase over that for younger patients. The increases in mass may be a reflection of the greater content of connective tissue and calcific deposits in the very elderly heart. Reiner[43] concluded that age probably does not markedly influence myocardial weight and that the apparent age-related increase in heart weight is a function of increased subepicardial fat.

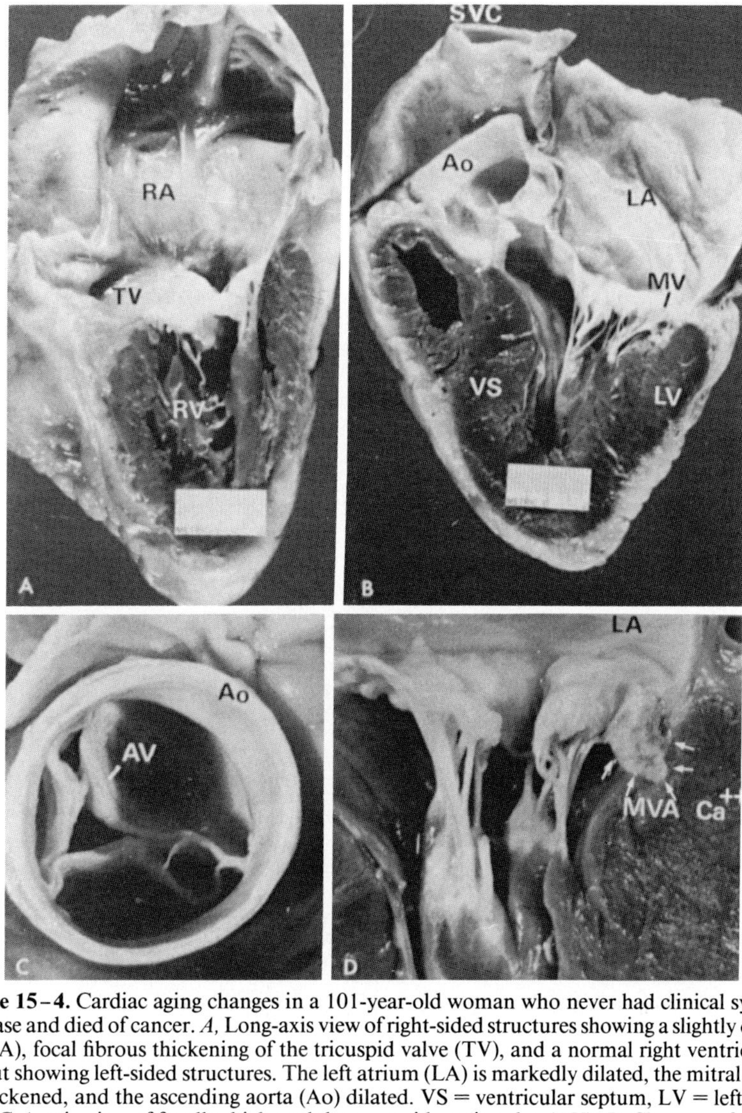

Figure 15–4. Cardiac aging changes in a 101-year-old woman who never had clinical symptoms of heart disease and died of cancer. *A,* Long-axis view of right-sided structures showing a slightly dilated right atrium (RA), focal fibrous thickening of the tricuspid valve (TV), and a normal right ventricle (RV). *B,* Parallel cut showing left-sided structures. The left atrium (LA) is markedly dilated, the mitral valve (MV) focally thickened, and the ascending aorta (Ao) dilated. VS = ventricular septum, LV = left ventricular free wall. *C,* Aortic view of focally thickened three-cuspid aortic valve (AV). *D,* Close-up of mitral valve showing heavy mitral valve anular calcium (MVA Ca^{++}) *(arrows).* LA = left atrium.

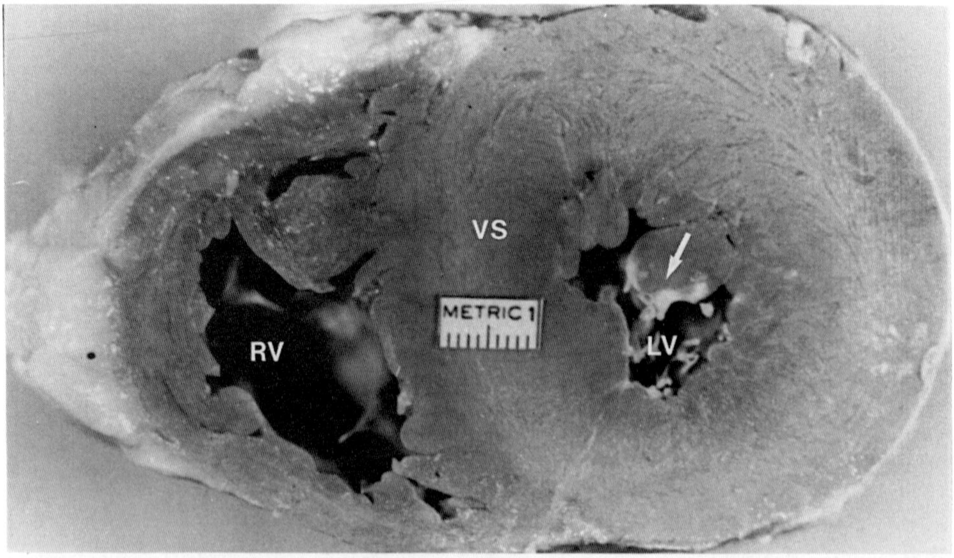

Figure 15–5. Short-axis view of basal half of heart showing small left ventricle (LV), thickened chamber walls, and focal fibrosis of papillary muscle *(arrow)*. VS = ventricular septum; RV = right ventricle.

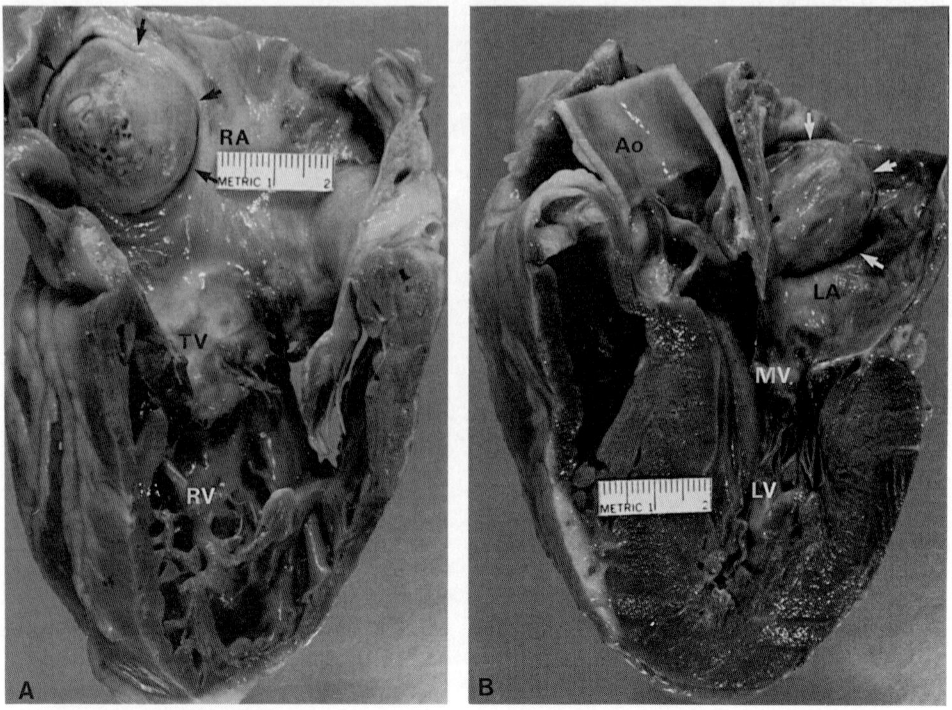

Figure 15–6. Heart from a 90-year-old woman with a "floppy atrial septum" (aneurysm of the foramen ovale) *(arrows)*. Septal aneurysm *(arrows)* moves back and forth between right atrium (RA) *(A)* and left atrium (LA) *(B)*. The foramen ovale is also fenestrated. The ventricular septum has mild sigmoidity and the left ventricle (LV) is small. Ao = aorta, MV = mitral valve, RV = right ventricle, TV = tricuspid valve.

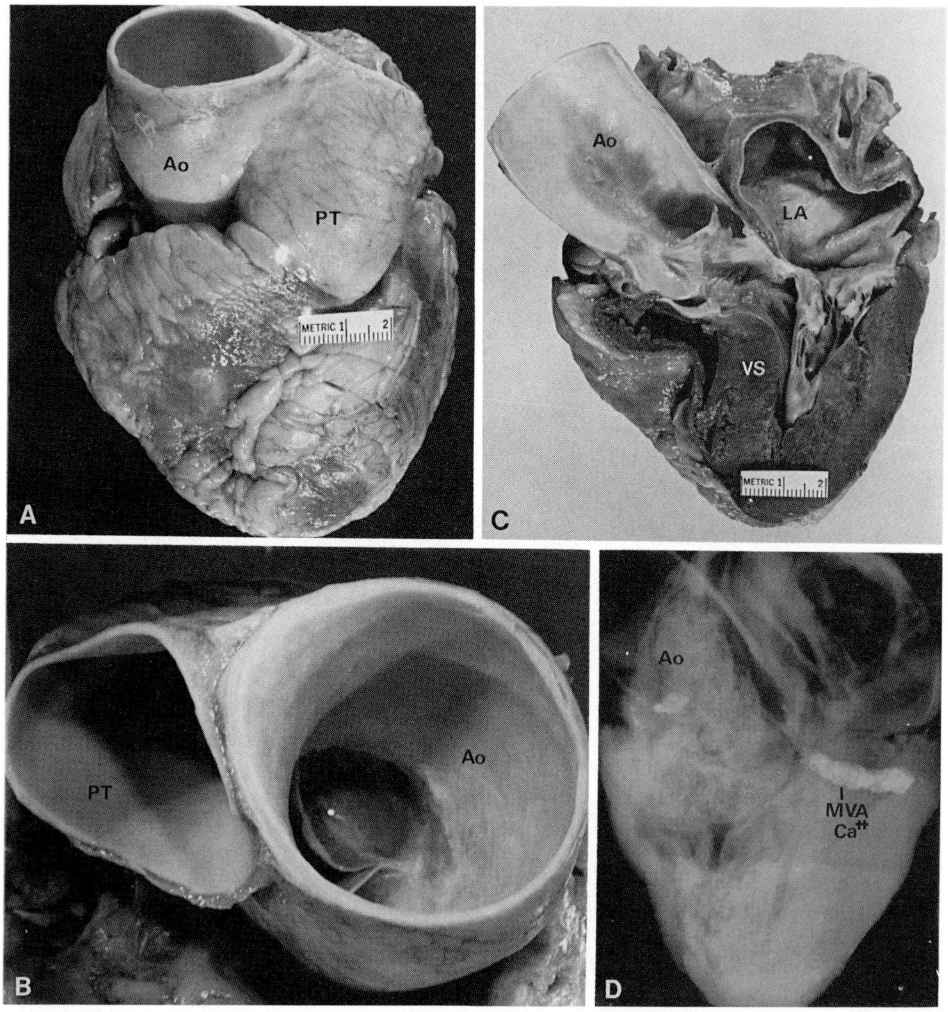

Figure 15-7. *A,* Heart of a 93-year-old patient showing a markedly dilated ascending aorta (Ao) and pulmonary trunk (PT). *B,* Long-axis cut of heart showing markedly dilated Ao, "sigmoid-shaped" ventricular septum (VS), small left ventricular cavity, and dilated left atrium (LA). *C,* Close-up of dilated Ao and PT. *D,* Postmortem radiograph showing mitral valve anular calcium (MVA CA^{++}).

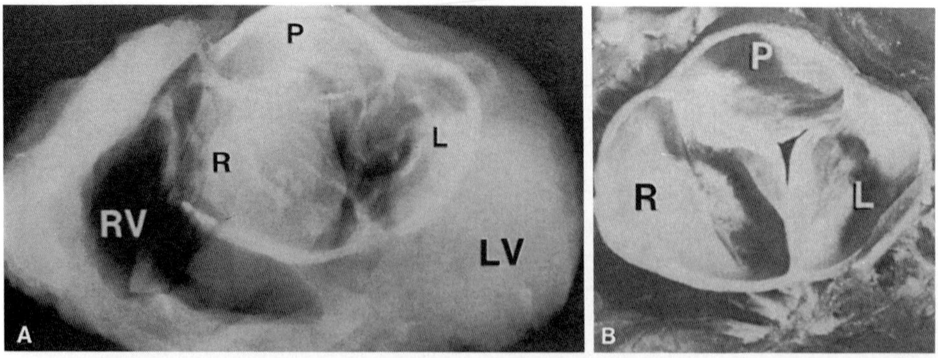

Figure 15–8. A 95-year-old man who never had symptoms of cardiac dysfunction and died of sarcoma. *A,* Radiogram of heart at necropsy showing a dilated aorta. LV, RV = left and right ventricles, respectively; R = right; L = left; P = posterior (noncoronary) sinuses of Valsalva. *B,* Aortic view from above. (From Waller and Roberts,[19] with permission.)

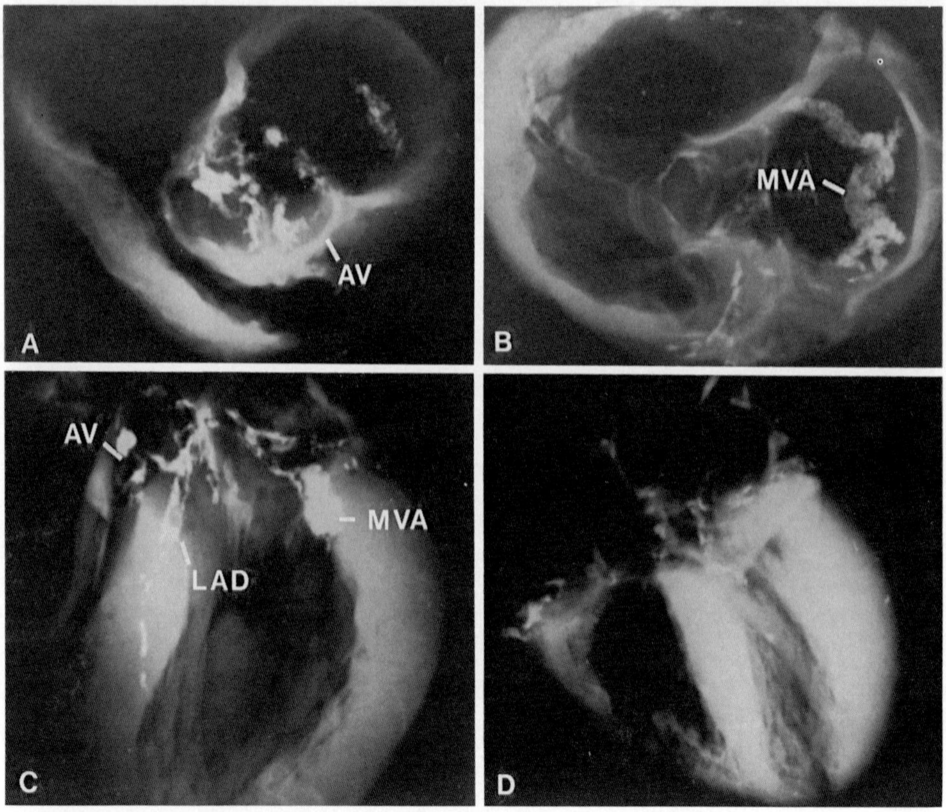

Figure 15–9. Composite radiographs of four old-age hearts showing calcific deposits. *A,* Calcific deposits in aortic valve (AV) and mitral valve anulus (MVA). *B,* Heavy calcific deposits in MVA and focal deposits on AV and coronary arteries. *C,* Heavy calcific deposition MVA, AV, and left anterior descending artery (LAD). *D,* Calcific deposits in AV cusps and coronary tree.

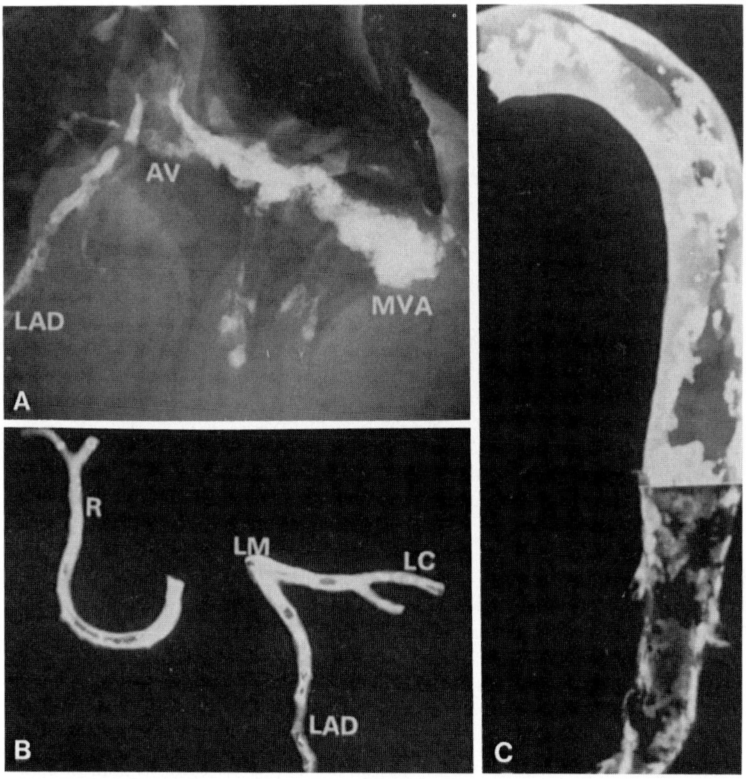

Figure 15–10. Extensive calcific deposits in the cardiovascular system in a 90-year-old woman. *A,* Heavy (4+/4+) mitral valve anular (MVA) calcium and calcific deposits in the aortic valve (AV) and left anterior descending (LAD) coronary artery. *B,* Calcified epicardial coronary arteries. LC = left circumflex, LM = left main, R = right. *C,* Heavy calcific deposits in aorta.

Connective Tissue

The amount and state of *connective tissue* in the heart are of interest because of the role of connective tissue in determining elasticity. An increase in human heart collagen in subendocardial and subepicardial zones with advancing age has been observed.[44] Muscle, as a percentage of heart, decreased from 40 percent in persons less than age 50 years to 27 percent in those older than age 75 years, whereas collagen fibers increased from 17 percent to 36 percent, respectively, in the two groups. It appeared that the muscle loss and fibrosis increase began around 60 years of age. A study of ventricular myocardium free of epicardium and endocardium from 148 previously healthy persons disclosed no significant change in collagen concentration with age.[45]

Chambers (Cavities)

Associated with increasing age is a *reduction in size of the left ventricular cavity.* The reduction in size occurs primarily in the *base-to-apex long-axis dimension* (see Figs. 15–1, 15–3 through 15–6). This decrease in left ventricular cavity size may reflect a generally lower cardiac output observed in elderly patients compared with younger patients. Partly as a result of a decrease in the long-axis dimension of the left

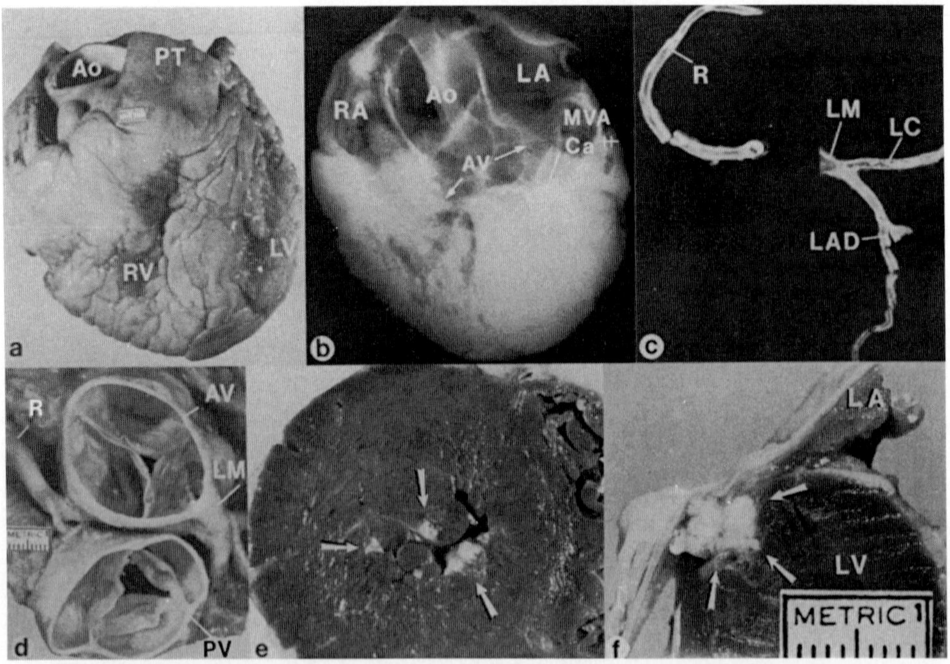

Figure 15-11. Heart from a 97-year-old woman who never had clinical evidence of cardiac dysfunction and who died of cancer. *a,* External view of anterior surface of the heart showing an increased amount of subepicardial fat. Ao = aorta; LV = left ventricle; PT = pulmonary trunk; RV = right ventricle. *b,* Postmortem radiogram showing calcific deposits in the mitral valve anulus (MVA) and aortic valve (AV). LA = left atrium; RA = right atrium. *c,* Radiogram of the excised coronary arteries showing a few calcific deposits. LAD = left anterior descending; LC = left circumflex; LM = left main; R = right. *d,* View of aortic valve (AV) and pulmonic valve (PV) from above. *e,* View of left ventricle showing calcific deposits *(arrows)* in the papillary muscles. *f,* Calcific deposits in mitral anular region. (From Waller and Roberts,[19] with permission.)

ventricle and partly as a result of a rightward shift of a dilated ascending aorta, *the basal ventricular septum bends leftward, bulging into the left ventricular outflow tract* (see Figs. 15-1, 15-3, 15-4, 15-7). This alteration in shape yields a curved ventricular septum, which has been termed the "sigmoid septum."[46] Goor and colleagues[46] also noted that the degree of septal sigmoidality was inversely related to heart weight in the elderly patient: lower heart weights tended to be associated with extremely curved septa and higher heart weights were associated with lesser degrees of curved ventricular septa. This normal aging alteration is important to recognize clinically as well as morphologically because the basal bulging into left ventricular outflow tract may mimic echocardiographically the asymmetric hypertrophy (ASH) of hypertrophic cardiomyopathy.

Although the size of the left ventricular cavity decreases with age, the size of the left atrial cavity typically dilates with advancing age (see Figs. 15-1, 15-4, 15-6). Echocardiographic observations in the elderly heart note increases in left atrial cavity size by as much as 30 percent above normal.[47,48] Occasionally, a floppy atrial septum (aneurysm of the foramen ovale) is encountered in the very elderly heart (Fig. 15-6).

Valves

Morphologic alteration of the *cardiac valves* with increasing age is most prominent on the aortic and mitral valve, presumably related to increased ventricular

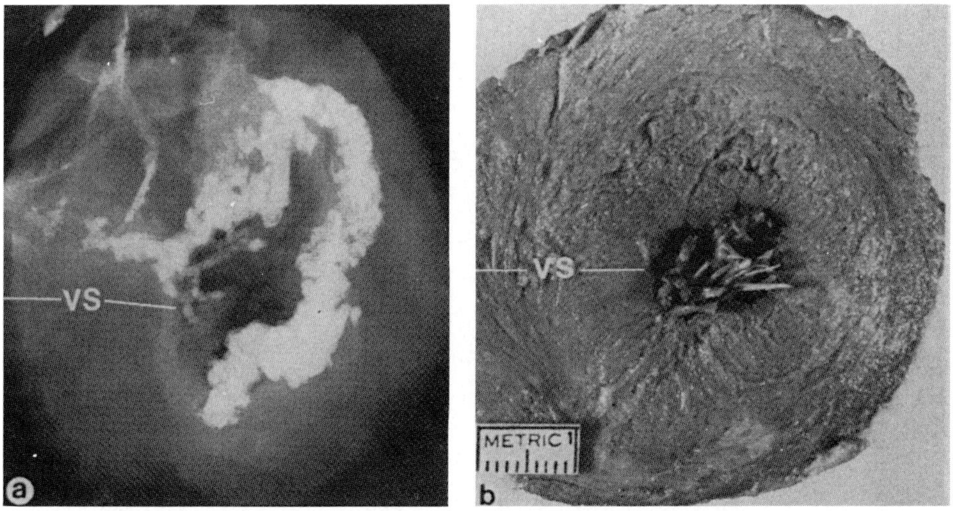

Figure 15-12. A 90-year-old woman with heavy mitral valve anular calcific deposits that reduced the mitral valve orifice to less than 1 cm in diameter. *a,* The unusual feature of the mitral calcium in this patient was that not only was it located behind the posterior mitral leaflet (mitral anular region) but also it extended across the anterior mitral leaflet, nearly producing a letter O. She died from rupture of a descending thoracic aortic aneurysm. VS = ventricular septum. *b,* View of the left ventricle at the level of the tips of the mitral leaflets showing a very small cavity. (From Waller and Roberts,[19] with permission.)

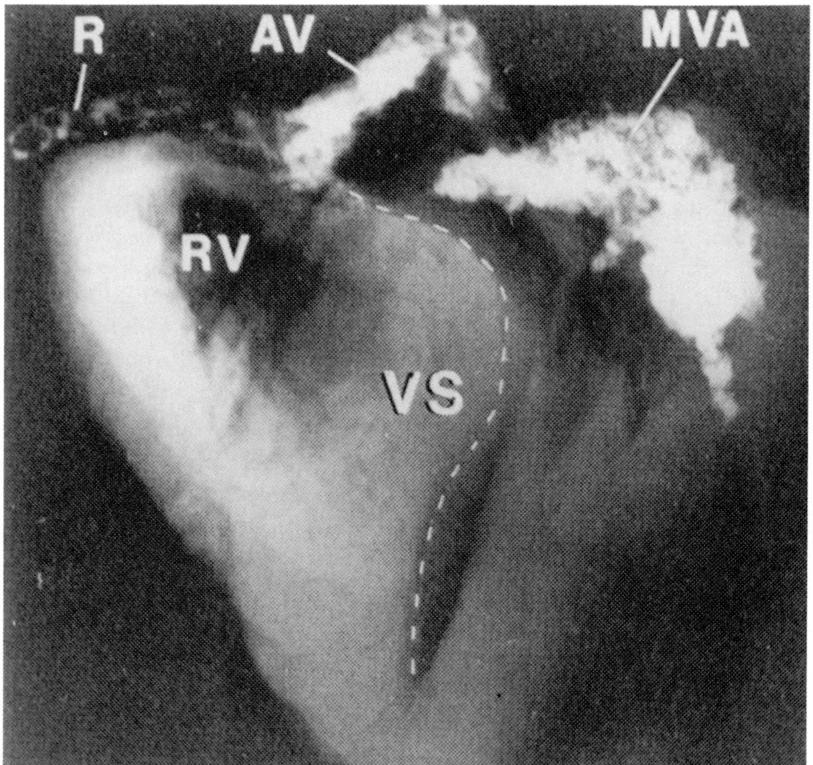

Figure 15-13. Heavy calcific deposits in the heart of a 97-year-old woman located in aortic valve (AV), mitral valve anulus (MVA), and right (R) coronary artery ("senile calcification syndrome"). The ventricular septum (VS) has a sigmoid shape. RV = right ventricle. (From Waller and Roberts,[19] with permission.)

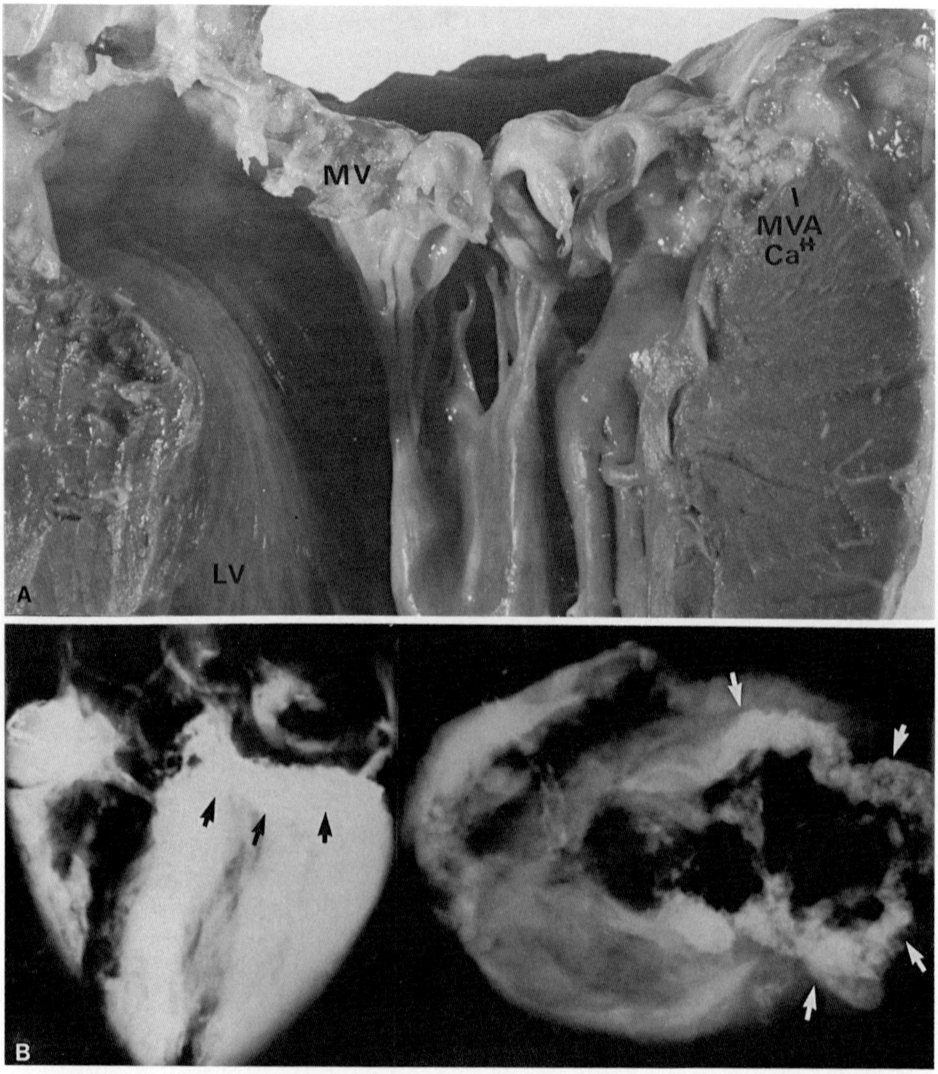

Figure 15–14. Massive mitral valve anular calcium producing mitral valve stenosis. *A,* Close-up of mitral valve (MV) and massive calcific deposits (Ca^{++}) in mitral valve anulus (MVA). *B,* Postmortem radiographs showing massive anular Ca^{++} forming an O shape *(arrows).* LV = left ventricle.

systolic pressure. The valve cusps and leaflets gradually become more rigid and fibrotic from hydrostatic pressures on the heart and from alteration of the properties of collagen (progressive insolubility, stabilization and stiffness). With advancing age the layers of the valves become progressively acellular, with loss of architecture, loosening of the fibrosa and increased elastosis of the spongiosa and fibrosa. At least four changes can be observed in most very elderly hearts:

1. *Focal fibrous thickening at valve contact points* (margins of closure) (see Figs. 15–3, 15–4, 15–6, 15–7, 15–14). The observations of Pomerance[16] are consistent with the interpretation that valve thickening in the elderly patient is largely a function of cumulative injury and repair from continual contact. Assuming an average heart rate of 75 beats per minute for 90 years, the cardiac valve leaflets and cusps make

contact nearly *four trillion times;* it is not surprising that focal to extensive areas of fibrous thickening occur almost universally in normal old-age cardiac valves.

2. *Fatty alteration of valve collagen.* Fatty alteration of valve collagen is characterized by a yellow discoloration of the bases of the aortic valve cusps and the anterior leaflet of the mitral valve. Varying degrees of calcification subsequently occur in these areas of altered collagen. *Calcific deposits are commonly present in the bases of one or more aortic cusps, at the margins of closure on the atrial aspect of the mitral leaflets, and in the mitral valve anulus* (see Figs. 15–3, 15–6, 15–7 through 15–9). Aortic valve calcific deposits ("aortic sclerosis") involve the bases of the sinuses of Valsalva without compromising the three valve commissures (see Figs. 15–8, 15–9). Mounds of calcium build up, producing cuspal rigidity and reduced mobility. Occasionally, these deposits are heavy enough to produce aortic valve stenosis ("senile aortic stenosis") but, more commonly, lesser amounts produce precordial murmurs that may be confused clinically with true aortic valve obstruction.

3. *Anular calcification. The hallmark of the very elderly heart is mitral valve anular calcium* (see Figs. 15–7, 15–9 through 15–14). Mitral anular calcium is the most commonly associated abnormality in the elderly patient with a precordial systolic murmur.[16] Heavy mitral anular calcium is more common in elderly women than in elderly men. Pomerance[15] found an incidence of anular calcium of 43.5 percent in women aged 90 years or older, compared with an incidence of only 17 percent in a similarly aged group of men. Ishii and Sternby,[9] however, noted a

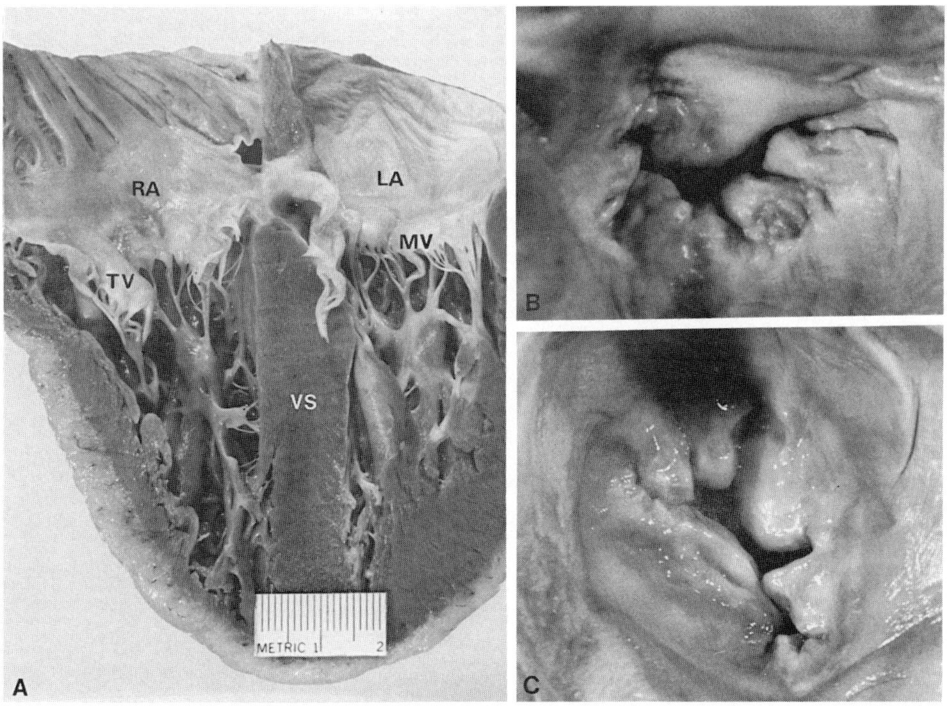

Figure 15–15. "Buckling" mitral valve leaflets in three patients *(A, B, C)* mimicking mitral valve prolapse. *A,* Four-chamber view showing mitral valve leaflets (MV) protruding into left atrium (LA). *B, C,* Atrial views from two patients showing "buckling" MV leaflets. In each patient, the MV leaflet area and anulus were normal.

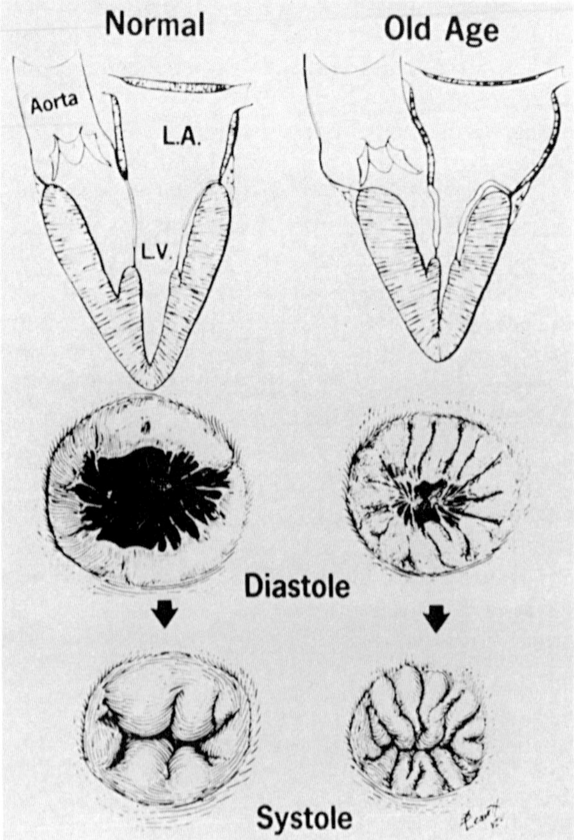

Figure 15–16. Diagram illustrating the protrusion of the mitral leaflets into left atrium (LA) during left ventricular (LV) systole. The amount of space available for the mitral valve leaflets decreases with increasing age, and consequently the leaflets "buckle" into left atrium mimicking a floppy (prolapsed) mitral valve. (From Waller and Roberts,[19] with permission.)

decrease in the incidence of mitral anular calcium in extreme old age. These authors observed anular calcium in only four (1 percent) of 23 centenarians. Calcific deposits can involve a small portion of the mitral anulus or may involve the entire anulus ("C-shaped, J-shaped"), with extension onto the anterior mitral leaflet ("O-shaped") (see Figs. 15–12, 15–14).[49] Extensive calcific deposits in the mitral anulus may produce clinical cardiac dysfunction including heart block, pure mitral regurgitation, and rarely mitral stenosis (see Fig. 15–14).

Many elderly patients have calcific deposits in the aortic valve cusps, mitral valve anulus, and epicardial coronary arteries. This triad of calcific deposits has been termed the "*senile* calcification syndrome" (Figs. 15–9 through 15-11, 15–13).[19] Of 40 necropsy patients studied by Waller and Roberts,[19] 16 (40 percent) had calcific deposits in all three sites.

4. *Leaflet "buckling."* Commonly, the mitral leaflets in the very elderly heart protrude or "buckle" toward the left atrium during ventricular systole, simulating a floppy (prolapsing) mitral valve (see Figs. 15–15, 15–16). Although floppy mitral valves occasionally are observed in the elderly patient,[16] the majority of the valve protrusions observed are not the result of floppy valves but rather the consequence of changes in the size of the left ventricular cavity. With decreasing left ventricular cavity size with advancing age, the area containing the mitral leaflets and chordae tendineae is reduced. Thus, during ventricular systole the leaflets buckle back into the

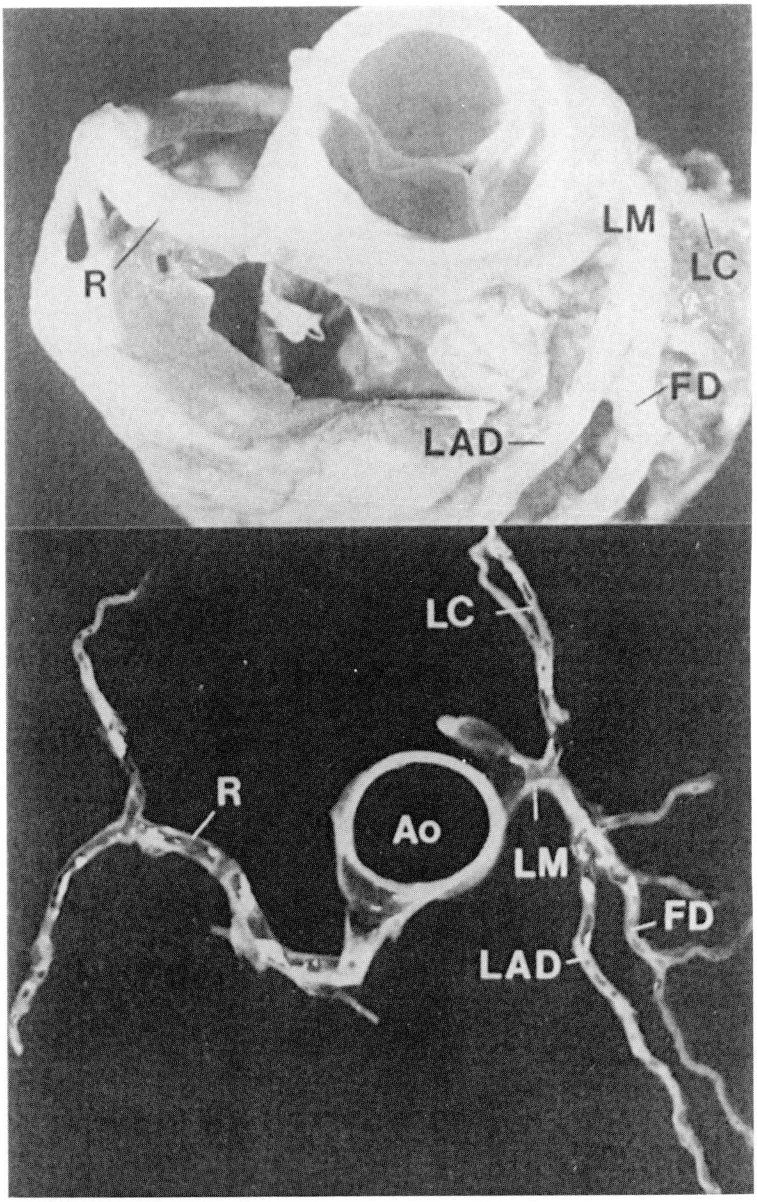

Figure 15–17. Tortuous and calcified epicardial coronary arteries from a 95-year-old man who never had symptoms of cardiac dysfunction. Ao = aorta, FD = first diagonal, LAD = left anterior descending, LC = left circumflex, LM = left main, R = right. (From Waller and Roberts,[19] with permission.)

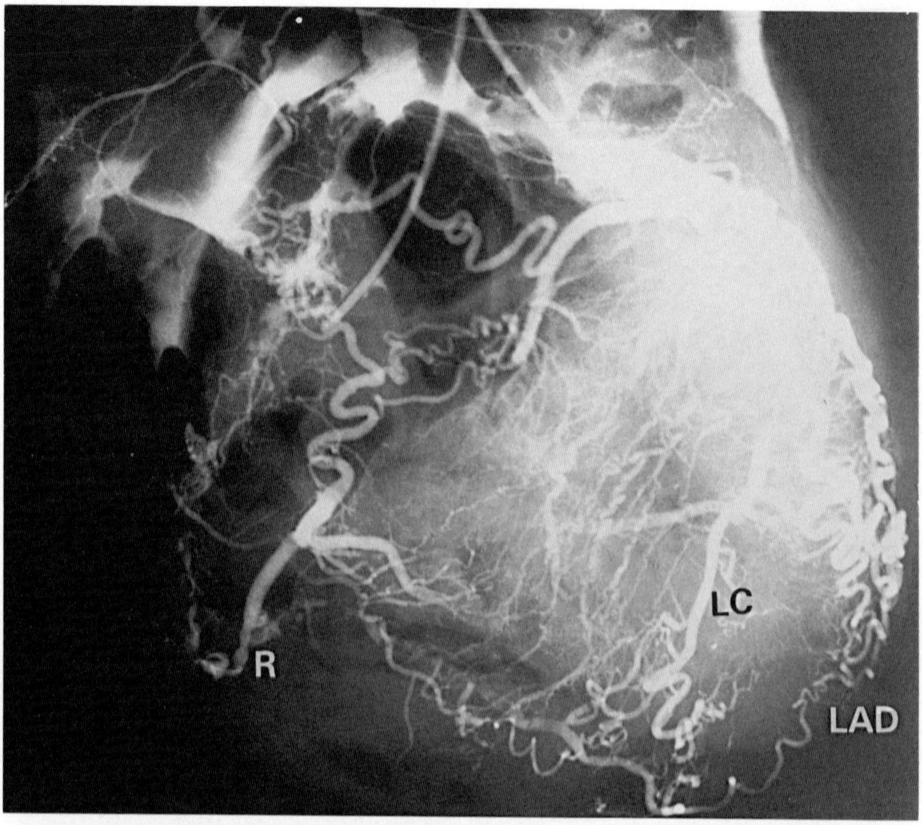

Figure 15-18. Postmortem coronary angiogram in a 92-year-old person showing marked tortuosity of the coronary tree. LAD = left anterior descending, LC = left circumflex, R = right.

left atrium—"leaflet-cavity disproportion." Anatomically, the elderly "buckling valve" has normal leaflet area and normal or reduced anular circumference in distinction to the increased areas and dilated anular circumferences of the floppy mitral valve.[50]

Major Epicardial Coronary Arteries

Several anatomic features characterize the very elderly epicardial coronary arterial tree (see Figs. 15-11, 15-17 through 15-24): (1) *tortuosity,* (2) *increased cross-sectional area (dilated arteries),* (3) *calcific deposits,* (4) usually *minimal atherosclerotic disease,* and (5) atherosclerotic plaques, which when present, consist of dense fibrous tissue and calcific deposits *("hard lesions").* In part, as a result of changes in cardiac size (in particular, a reduction in the long-axis dimension of left ventricle), the major epicardial coronary arteries attempt to "compensate" for this reduction in dimension by becoming "winding" and tortuous (see Figs. 15-17 through 15-20). The caliber of the coronary artery may increase in cross-sectional luminal area with advancing age.[7] As with the aortic valve and mitral valve anulus, epicardial coronary arteries frequently contain varying amounts of calcium (see Figs. 15-11, 15-17, 15-19 through 15-21). Coronary arterial calcification detected by fluoroscopy and at necropsy is usually associated with the presence of atherosclerotic

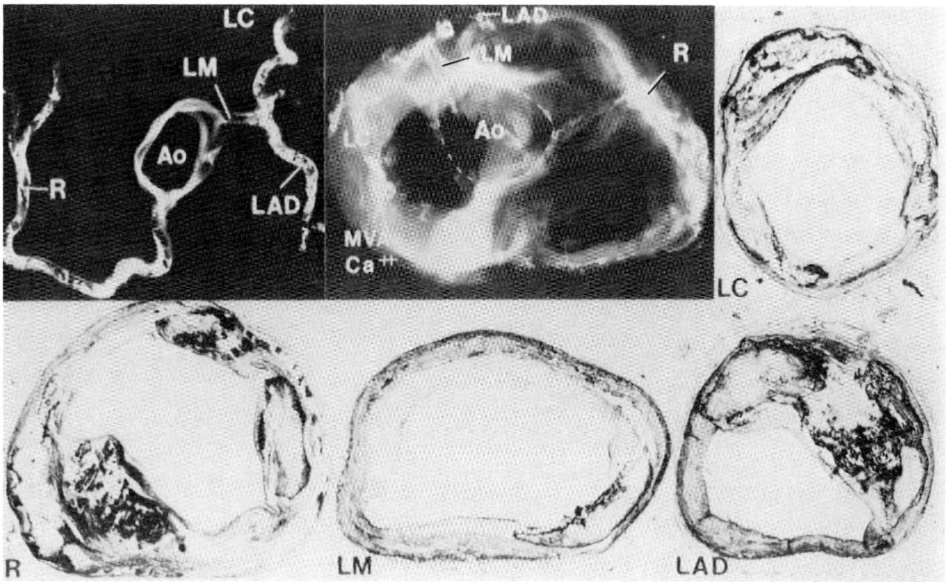

Figure 15–19. Tortuous and heavily calcified coronary arteries in a 95-year-old woman who never had symptoms of cardiac dysfunction and who died of a perforated gastric ulcer. *Top left,* Postmortem radiogram of the excised right (R), left main (LM), left anterior descending (LAD), and left circumflex (LC) coronary arteries. *Top center,* Radiogram of a portion of the heart after removing the walls of the atria and most of the walls of the ventricles. MVA = mitral valve anulus. *Top right and lower panels,* Photomicrographs of coronary arteries at sites of maximal narrowing by calcified atherosclerotic plaques. This case illustrates extensive calcific deposits in the coronary arteries without significant luminal narrowing. (From Waller and Roberts,[19] with permission.)

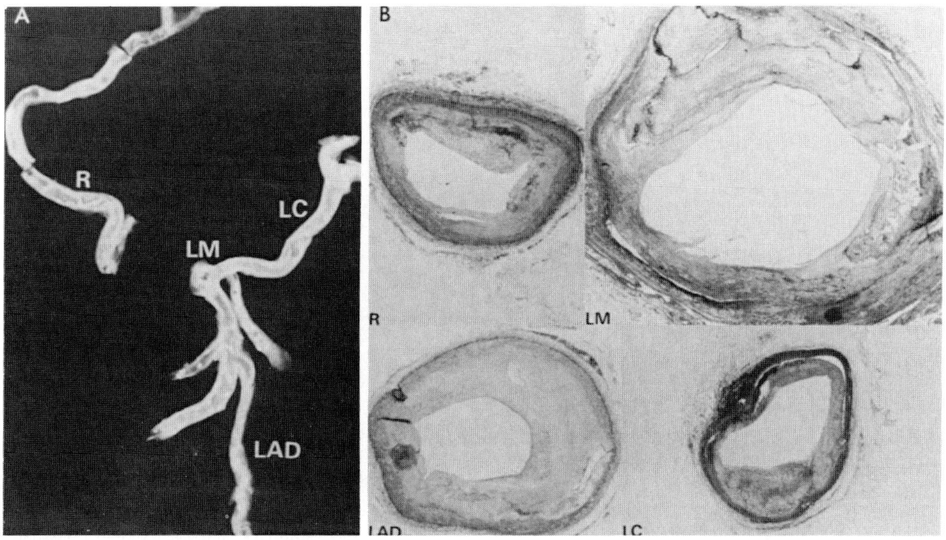

Figure 15–20. *A,* Tortuous epicardial coronary arteries on postmortem radiogram on a 91-year-old man have 2+/4+ calcific deposits. *B,* Sites of maximal narrowing in the four major epicardial coronary arteries: right (R), left main (LM), left anterior descending (LAD), and left circumflex (LC).

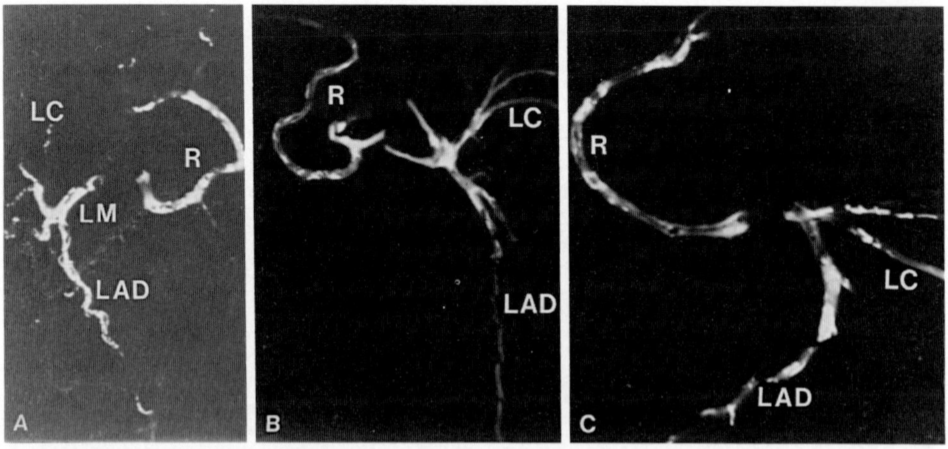

Figure 15–21. Composite of calcific deposits in three coronary arterial trees *(A, B, C)*. LAD = left anterior descending, LC = left circumflex, LM = left main, R = right.

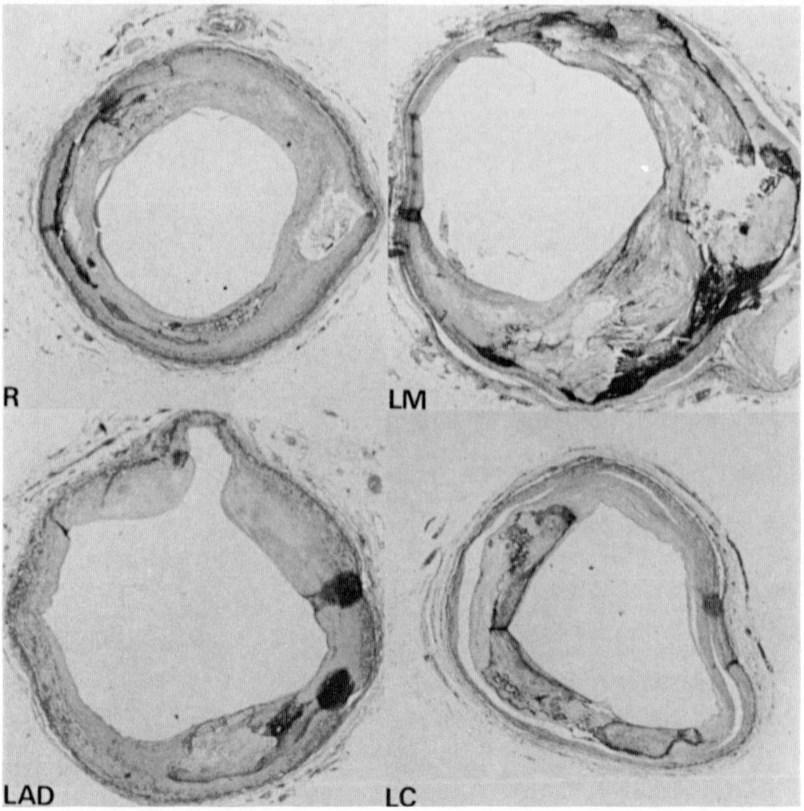

Figure 15–22. Sites of maximal narrowing in the right (R), left main (LM), left anterior descending (LAD), and left circumflex (LC) coronary arteries in a 101-year-old woman who never had symptoms of cardiac dysfunction and died a noncardiovascular death. The coronary arteries have heavy calcific deposits but minimal luminal narrowing by atherosclerotic plaques.

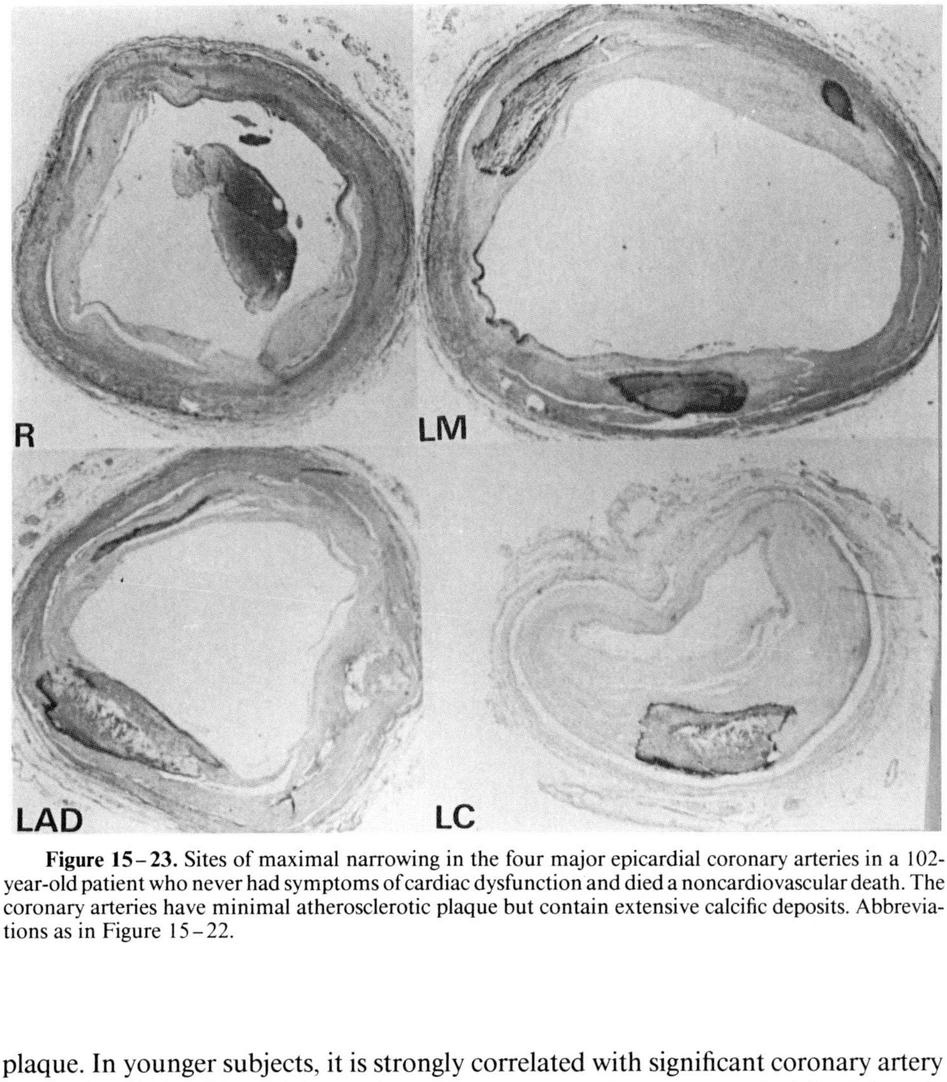

Figure 15–23. Sites of maximal narrowing in the four major epicardial coronary arteries in a 102-year-old patient who never had symptoms of cardiac dysfunction and died a noncardiovascular death. The coronary arteries have minimal atherosclerotic plaque but contain extensive calcific deposits. Abbreviations as in Figure 15–22.

plaque. In younger subjects, it is strongly correlated with significant coronary artery narrowing.[51] In older subjects, the mere presence of coronary arterial calcium is insufficient to predict the presence and severity of atherosclerotic plaque. It is necessary to quantitate the extent of calcific deposits (percent of vessel surface calcified) to observe a difference between atherosclerotic and nonatherosclerotic deaths.[52] Although it is known that the very elderly patient may have severe coronary artery disease, generally the degree of atherosclerosis is less severe than that present in younger necropsy patients.[53–55] Achievement of old age represents escape from the complications of coronary disease (see Figs. 15–22 through 15–24). Edwards[7] has suggested that the person who survives to advanced age has two possibilities with regard to presence or absence of coronary atherosclerosis: (1) the person has harbored this process to significant degree but tolerates it because of well-established collateral channels; or (2) the person does not have significant luminal narrowing by plaque and thus survives. When present in the very elderly heart, atherosclerotic plaque in the coronary tree consists almost exclusively of dense fibrous tissue and extensive calcific deposits.

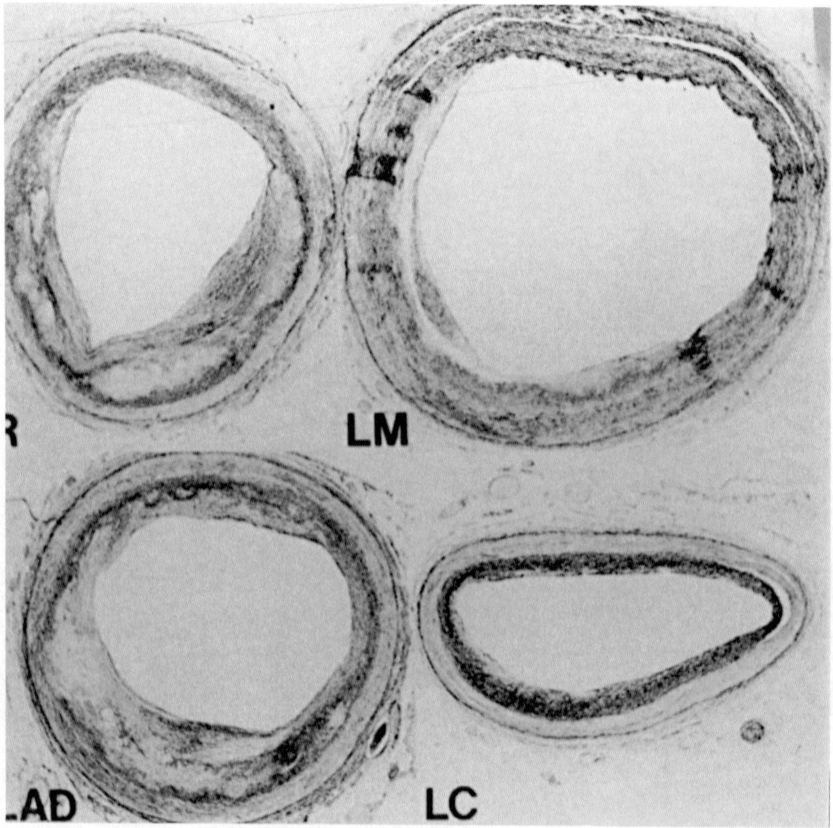

Figure 15–24. Sites of maximal narrowing in the right (R), left main (LM), left anterior descending (LAD), and left circumflex (LC) coronary arteries in a 103-year-old woman who never had symptoms of cardiac dysfunction and died a noncardiovascular death. The coronary arteries are devoid of calcium and significant luminal narrowing. (From Waller and Roberts,[19] with permission.)

Conduction System

Sinus Node

Beginning at age 60, the area of the sinus node shows increased thickening by fibroelastic tissue, whereas the sinus node itself exhibits a decreased number of pacemaker cells. By age 75 years, the heart may have reduced the number of pacemaker cells by 10 percent, compared with the number found in younger adult hearts. In extremely advanced age, fibrous tissue predominates to such a degree that the nodal cells form small areas in an ocean of collagen.[56] Sinus node invasion by fat may also occur with increasing age. The sinoatrial conduction tissue (specialized or non-specialized) of clinically normal old age hearts show loss of muscle fibers and an increased content of collagen.[57,58]

Atrioventricular Node

With increasing age, fine connective tissue extends into the deep surface of the atrioventricular node from the central fibrous body and also concentrates around arteries. The clear sharp margin of the deeper aspect of the atrioventricular node seen in a child is lost with increasing age. Some nodal fibers show minor distortion in old age but is of insufficient magnitude to cause appreciable muscle fiber loss.[59] With advancing age, medial fibrosis and internal thickening of the atrioventricular nodal artery develops, occasionally with luminal obliteration.[59]

Main Bundle and Bundle Branches

With advancing age, the amount of fibrous tissue at the site of the main bundle (bundle of His) (upper ventricular septum) increases and the collagen becomes amorphous and eosinophilic and may calcify.[59] Some degree of this change is universal by age 60 years and occasionally may be grossly visible. Similar changes occur in the central fibrous body, aortic and mitral anuli. The same process was reported by Yater and Cornell,[60] Lenegre,[61] and Lev[62,63] in cases of complete heart block. In these cases, the destruction of the conduction system is far greater than the normal aging process. Excessive stress and strain in a high-pressure left ventricle for many years have been postulated as the underlying etiology.[61–63] Lev[62,63] has named the process "sclerosis of the left side of the cardiac skeleton" and found it accelerated in systemic hypertension. This sclerotic process occurs to some degree *in all hearts* with increasing age and may lead to some loss of conduction fibers, even in patients with normal electrocardiograms.[59] Diffuse fibrosis of the right bundle branch also increases with age but without significant conduction fiber loss.[59]

Pericardium

The parietal layer of pericardium of the elderly heart shows a change in the configuration of collagen fibers compared with that of young adults.[26,64] Collagen fibers are "wavy" at birth and reach their largest wavy amplitude in young adults. In old age the collagen fibers of the parietal pericardium become less wavy and more straight.[65] Waviness of collagen fibers appears to be related to pericardial distensibility. Thus, in the very elderly heart the pericardium would allow only a limited amount of stretch.[26,60] The amount of elastic fibers does not appear to change significantly with increasing age.[26]

Aorta

The aging normal aorta is characterized by *dilation of the ascending portion including all of the sinuses of Valsalva, dilation and elongation of the thoracic aorta, and calcific deposits at the sinotubular junction and in the abdominal aorta* (see Figs. 15–4, 15–7, 15–10). The mechanism for dilation of the ascending aorta and the thoracic aorta is unknown but does not appear to be the result of simple stretching inasmuch as the mass of the elastic media increases as the aorta widens.[66] Generally, "senile aortic dilation" is unassociated with cardiac dysfunction. Rarely, the ascending aorta may widen to such a degree that the aortic valve cusps cannot close completely, and pure aortic regurgitation follows.[7] The sinotubular junction frequently is thickened and calcified in the very elderly aorta. Edwards[7] has noted that the changes occurring at the sinotubular junction are characterized histologically by fatty alteration and calcific deposits that are *distinctive from atherosclerotic plaque.*

Histologic features of aging arteries involve calcium, elastin, and collagen changes. Elastin is a major component of arteries, representing up to 30 percent of dry weight in humans.[67] Thick, discrete, and wavy elastic lamellae seen in younger arteries become thin, fragmented, and diffusely arranged in the elderly arteries. Human arterial elastin has been reported to lose around 30 percent of the cross links and to nearly double the amount of bound or insoluble carbohydrate.[68] The rate of calcification of arteries with increasing age varies with different arteries, being greatest in arteries with the most elastin.[33] It has been suggested that elastin undergoes alterations with age that enable it to bind more calcium.[69] Collagen comprises about 20 percent of normal human aortic interna and most of the adventitia and is focally distributed around smooth muscle cells in the media.[70] Human aortic collagen increases continuously with advancing age in both interna and media.[33] Collagen synthesis is always associated with mucopolysaccharide synthesis, and thus increased amounts of mucopolysaccharides are observed in old-age aortic wall. Aging of collagen is characterized by increased insolubility and stiffness.[45]

The morphologic changes in the heart and aorta just described are frequently (in many instances universally) observed in very elderly patients at necropsy and rarely are associated with or produce clinical cardiac dysfunction. Thus, the "expected" morphologic findings may be considered "age-related changes" of the normal heart and aorta.

CARDIOVASCULAR OBSERVATIONS IN 37 PATIENTS AT NECROPSY, AGED 90 TO 102 YEARS

Between September 1982 and March 1986, 37 hearts from patients aged 90 years or older were entered into the Indiana University Cardiovascular Pathology Registry. Clinical and morphologic observations from these 37 patients (12 of whom have been previously reported[21]) form the basis of this section (Table 15–2; see Figs. 15–1 through 15–9, 15–14, 15–15, 15–18, 15–20 through 15–23; Figs. 15–25 through 15–33).

Clinical Observations

The 37 patients ranged in age from 90 to 102 years (average 92); 27 (73 percent) were women, and 20 (54 percent) were white. Two patients had chest pain described as angina pectoris, one of whom had a fatal acute myocardial infarction and the other had an acute myocardial infarction that healed but produced chronic and eventually fatal congestive heart failure (see Fig. 15–25). Six patients had abnormal dyspnea, including one with aortic stenosis, one with mitral anular calcium producing mitral stenosis, one patient with atherosclerotic coronary disease, and three patients without valvular, coronary, or myocardial heart disease. Three patients had chronic congestive heart failure, two with healed myocardial infarcts and one with massive cardiac amyloidosis. Fourteen patients had a history of systemic hypertension. Of 22 patients with available systemic arterial pressures, two had systolic pressures greater than 140 mmHg and/or diastolic pressures greater than 90 mmHg.

Cause of Death

Cause of death for the 37 very elderly patients was *cardiac* in 11 (30 percent), *vascular* in four (11 percent) and *noncardiovascular* in 22 (59 percent) (see Figs.

Table 15–2. Summary of Clinical and Morphologic Observations in 37 Patients at Necropsy, Aged 90 to 102 Years (Mean 92)

Observation	No. (%) Pts.
1. Gender (Women : Men)	27 (73) : 10 (27)
2. Race (White : Black)	20 (54) : 17 (46)
3. Angina pectoris	2 (5)
4. Hx AMI	3 (8)
5. Abnormal dyspnea	6 (16)
6. Chronic CHF	3 (8)
7. Diabetes mellitus	1 (3)
8. Hx systemic hypertension	14 (39)
9. Systemic arterial pressures (mm Hg) (systolic/diastolic)	$\frac{95-170\ (128)}{50-90\ \ (73)}$ (22 pts)
10. Cause of death	
Cardiac	11 (30)
Vascular	4 (11)
Other	22 (59)
11. Body weight (kg)	42–60 (51)
12. Heart weight (g)	270–565 (mean 404)
13. Heart-body weight ratio	0.005–0.012 (mean 0.008)
14. Calcific deposits	
Coronary arteries	33 (89)
Mitral valve anulus	29 (78)
Aortic valve cusps	21 (57)
Coronary + Mitral + Aortic	18 (49)
15. No. pts with > 75% XSA Narrowing of ≥ 1 LAD, LC, R Coronary arteries (No. arteries)	21 (57) (34/111 [31])
16. No. (%) 5-mm coronary segments > 75% XSA narrowing by plaque	126/1744 (7)
17. Mean coronary score*	2.23
Transmural LV damage	
Necrosis	3 (8)
Fibrosis	3 (8)
Both	0
18. Valve stenosis†	4 (11)
19. Cardiac amyloidosis	
Focal (incidental)	5 (14)
Diffuse	1 (3)

AMI = acute myocardial infarction, CHF = congestive heart failure, g = grams, Hx = history of, Kg = kilograms, LAD = left anterior descending, LC = left circumflex, No. = number, R = right, XSA = cross-sectional area.

* Scoring system utilized by Haider and Roberts.[71]

† Aortic stenosis (3 pts), massive mitral anular calcium (1 pt).

15–14, 15–25 through 15–32). Of the 11 cardiac deaths, six (55 percent) were related to *atherosclerotic coronary heart disease* (see Figs. 15–25 through 15–29), four from *valvular heart disease* (three aortic stenosis and one mitral stenosis from massive anular calcium) (see Figs. 15–14, 15–30, 15–32), and one was from massive *cardiac amyloidosis.* All four vascular deaths resulted from *cerebral vascular accidents.* The 22 noncardiovascular deaths were the result of *neoplasms* (10 patients), complications of *non-neoplastic gastrointestinal problems* (five patients), and *complications of bone fractures* (seven patients).

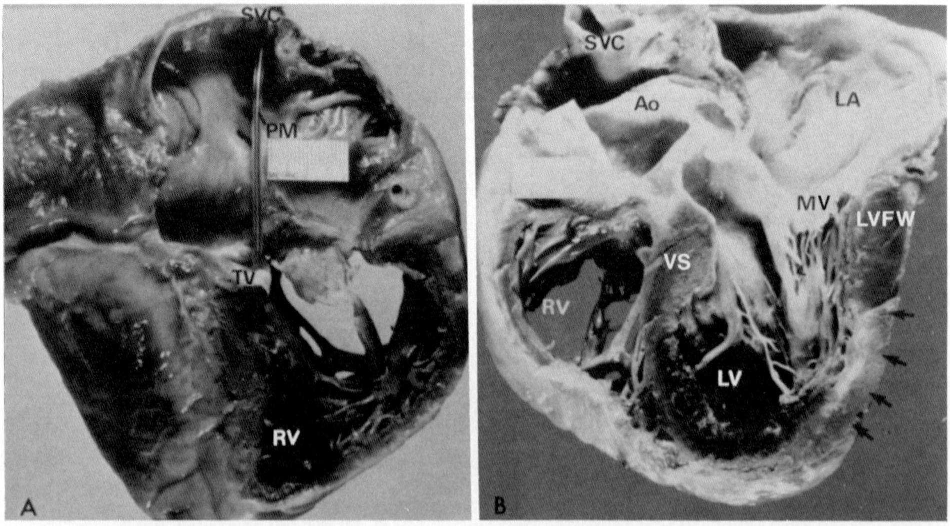

Figure 15–25. Long-axis view of right-sided *(A)* and left-sided *(B)* structures in the heart of a 90-year-old woman who had angina pectoris and an acute myocardial infarction that healed *(arrows, B)*. She had chronic congestive heart failure and required permanent right ventricular (RV) pacing for complete heart block. Ao = aorta, LA = left atrium, LV = left ventricle, LVFW = left ventricular free wall, MV = mitral valve, PM = pacemaker wire, RV = right ventricle, SVC = superior vena cava, TV = tricuspid valve, VS = ventricular septum.

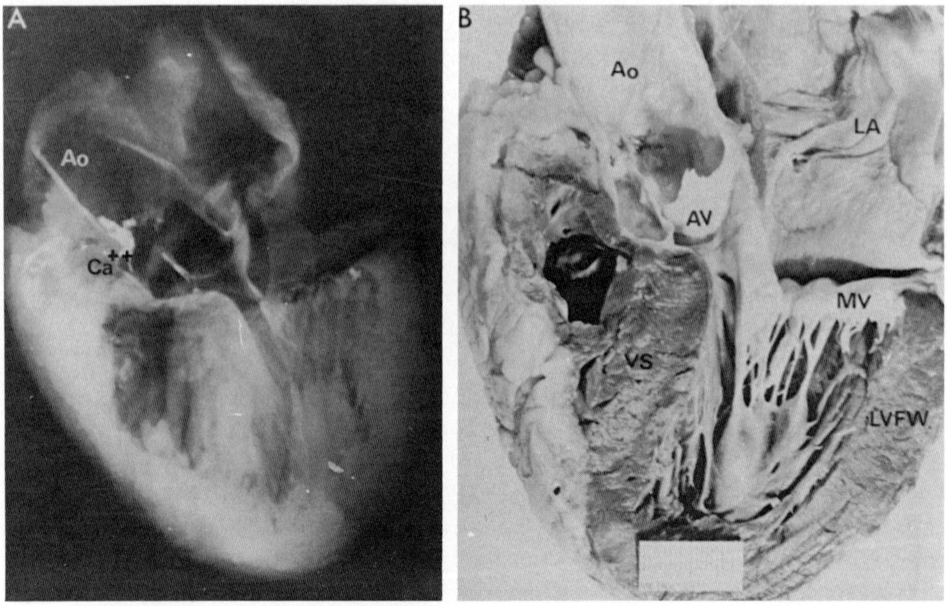

Figure 15–26. Heart of a 96-year-old woman who never had clinical evidence of myocardial ischemia but had severe coronary narrowing at necropsy (see Fig. 15–27). *A,* Postmortem radiogram showing minimal calcific deposits. *B,* Long-axis view of heart showing a dilated left atrium (LA) and basal bulging of ventricular septum (VS) into left ventricular outflow tract. The ventricular myocardium is free of necrosis and fibrosis. Ao = aorta, MV = mitral valve, LVFW = left ventricular free wall.

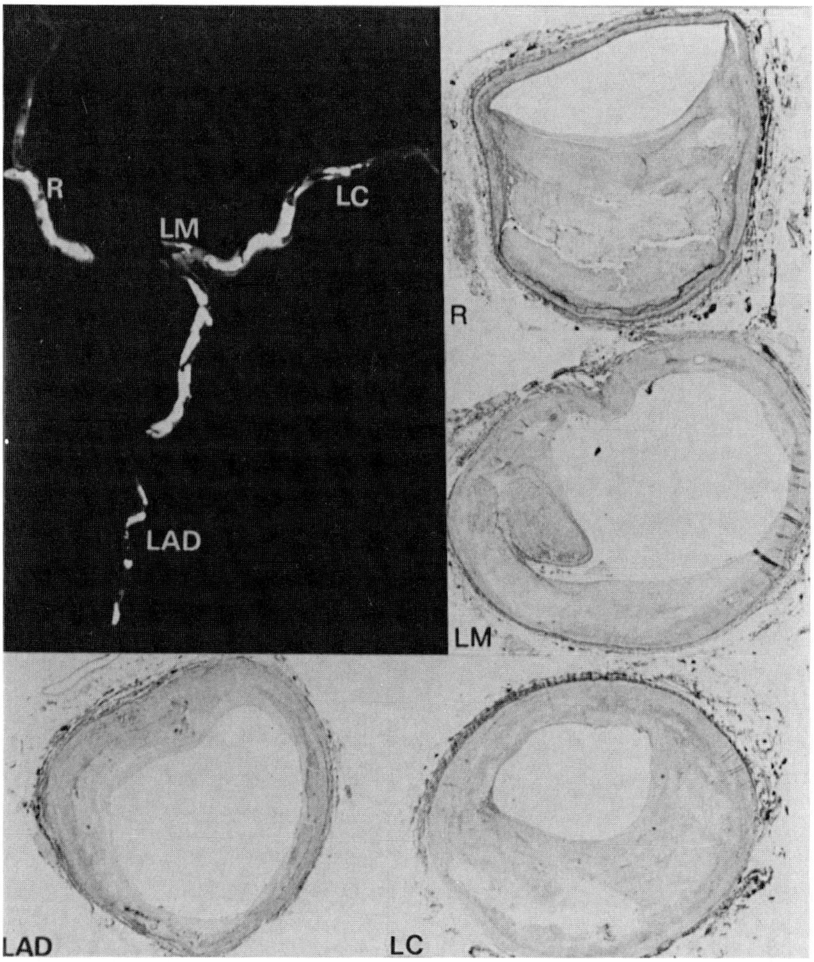

Figure 15–27. Coronary arteries of a 96-year-old patient whose heart is shown in Figure 15–26. Postmortem radiogram shows heavy calcific deposits in each of the major coronary arteries. Sites of maximal coronary narrowing are the right (R), left main (LM), and left anterior descending (LAD) arteries. The R and left circumflex (LC) arteries have severe luminal narrowing by calcified atherosclerotic plaques.

Necropsy Observations

Body weights ranged from 42 to 67 kg, and heart weights ranged from 270 to 565 g (average 404 g) (normal heart weight less than 350 g for women and less than 400 g for men). Only 10 (27 percent) of the 37 hearts had normal weights for the respective subject gender. Of the remaining 27 patients with hearts of increased weight, 15 had a history of systemic hypertension, aortic stenosis, cardiac amyloidosis, or combinations. Heart-body weight ratios were increased, ranging from 0.005 to 0.012 (normal for younger persons 0.004).

Calcific Deposits

Cardiac calcific deposits were found at some site on all 37 hearts (see Figs. 15–7, 15–9, 15–10, 15–14, 15–20, 15–21, 15–26, 15–27, 15–30 through 15–32). Of

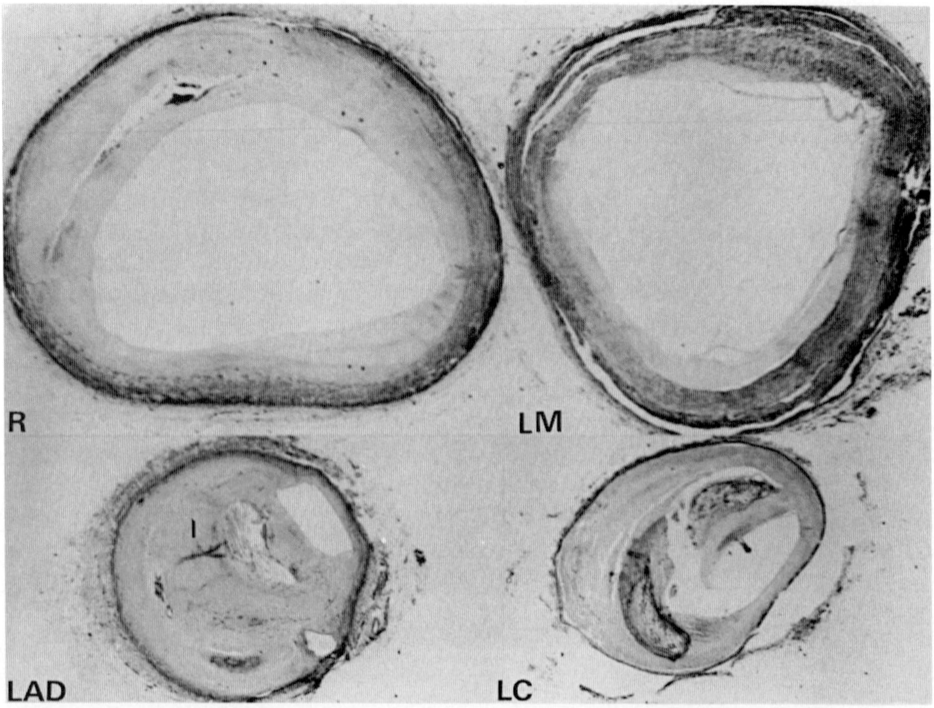

Figure 15–28. Sites of maximal narrowing in the four major epicardial coronary arteries in a 96-year-old patient who died a noncardiac death. Two arteries (LAD, LC) are severely narrowed by atherosclerotic plaque. Abbreviations as in Figure 15–27.

the 37 patients, 33 (89 percent) had calcific deposits on the *coronary arterial tree,* 29 (78 percent) on *mitral valve anulus,* and 21 (57 percent) on *aortic valve cusps.* Eighteen patients (49 percent) had the "senile calcification syndrome," with calcific deposits on all three sites (see Figs. 15–9 through 15–11). Heavy calcific deposits (3–4+/4) were found in 11 mitral anuli, nine coronary arterial trees, and four aortic valves. Of these patients with heavy calcific deposits, 1 of 11 anuli produced mitral valve stenosis, three of four aortic valves were stenotic, and seven of nine coronary arterial trees had at least one artery narrowed greater than 75 percent in cross-sectional area by atherosclerotic plaques.

Epicardial Coronary Arteries and Coronary Atherosclerosis

The epicardial coronary arteries were sectioned into 5-mm segments and the degree of cross-sectional area luminal narrowing graded into four categories: 0 to 25 percent, 26 to 50 percent, 51 to 75 percent, and 76 to 100 percent. Of 1744 5-mm coronary segments, 126 (7 percent) (21 patients) were narrowed more than 75 percent in cross-sectional area by calcified plaques (see Figs. 15–27 through 15–29, 15–32). No segment had occlusive coronary thrombus. Of the 21 patients with at least one of the left anterior descending, left circumflex or right coronary arteries narrowed severely by plaque, six (29 percent) had clinical evidence of myocardial ischemia (angina pectoris, acute myocardial infarction, and/or sudden death) (see Fig. 15-29), and the remaining 15 (71 percent) had no clinical evidence of myocardial ischemia (see Figs. 15-27, 15-28). One of the 15 patients had chest pain not considered to be angina pectoris, and two had abnormal dyspnea unassociated with other cardiac abnormalities.

A scoring system (reported by Harder and Roberts[71]) was used to indicate the severity of the coronary narrowing. Each coronary segment was assigned an arbitrary number (1 to 4), based on the amount of cross-sectional area luminal narrowing by plaques: 1 = 0 to 25 percent; 2 = 26 to 50 percent; 3 = 51 to 75 percent; and 4 = 76 to 100 percent. The total score was calculated for each patient and the average score determined by dividing the total score by the total number of coronary segments examined. Coronary scores ranged from 1.46 to 2.78 (average 2.00). The six patients with *clinical evidence of myocardial ischemia* had scores ranging from 2.04 to 2.78 (average 2.87) (see Fig. 15-29), the 15 patients with severe coronary artery disease *without clinical evidence of myocardial ischemia* had scores ranging from 1.57 to 2.33 (average 2.02) (see Figs. 15-27, 15-28), and the 16 patients *without clinical evidence of myocardial ischemia and no major artery narrowed more than 75 percent in cross-sectional area* had scores ranging from 1.46 to 2.07 (average 1.80) (see Figs. 15-20, 15-22, 15-23, 15-33).

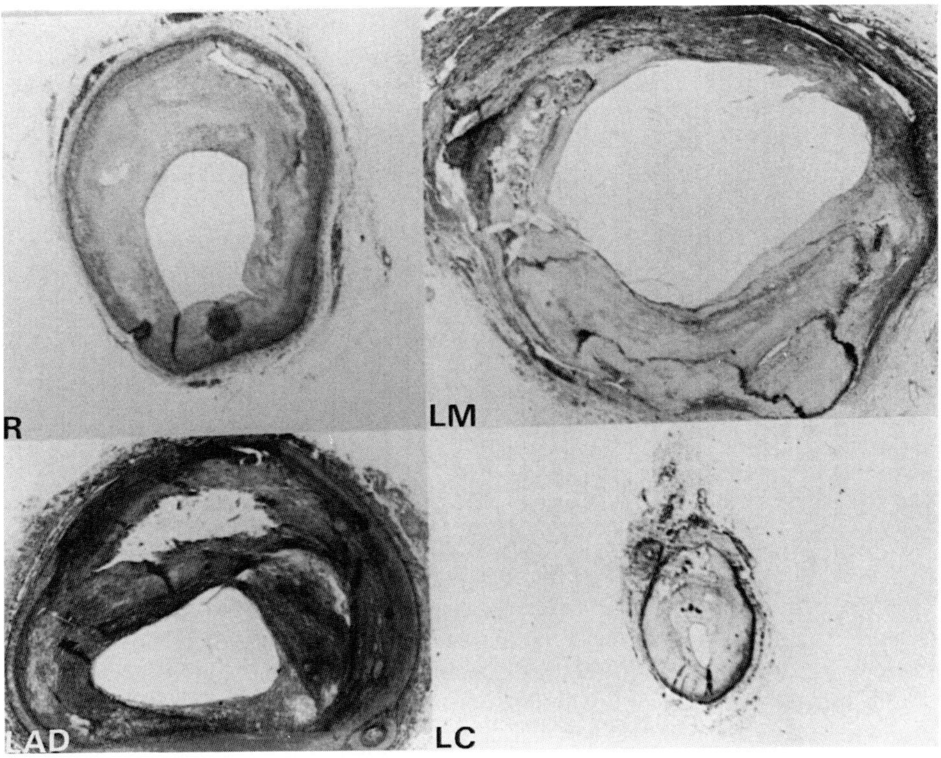

Figure 15-29. Sites of maximal narrowing in the four major epicardial coronary arteries in an elderly patient with fatal coronary atherosclerosis. Abbreviations as in Figure 15-28.

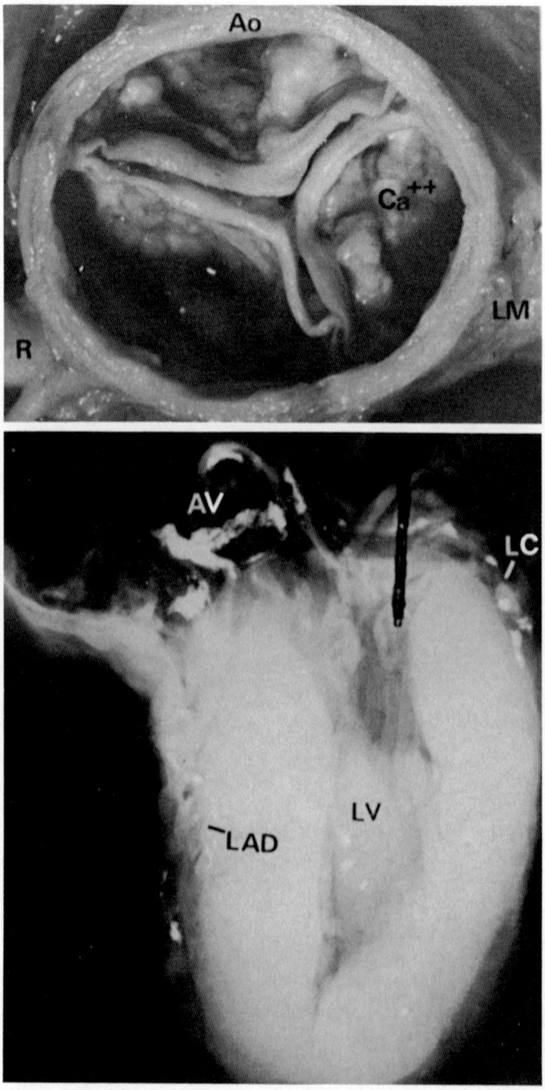

Figure 15–30. Heart of a 91-year-old man with fatal aortic valve (AV) stenosis. *Upper,* Aortic (Ao) view of AV showing all three sinuses of Valsalva filled with calcific deposits (CA^{++}) without commissural fusion. *Lower,* Postmortem radiogram showing calcific deposits in AV and coronary arteries. LAD = left anterior descending, LC = left circumflex, LM = left main, LV = left ventricular cavity.

Left Ventricular Damage

Transmural left ventricular damage (necrosis, fibrosis, or both) was present in nine patients: six *with* clinical evidence of myocardial ischemia and three *without* clinical evidence of myocardial ischemia. Of the nine patients, three had transmural necrosis (acute myocardial infarction) and six had transmural fibrosis (healed myocardial infarction). None of the nine patients had both acute and healed myocardial infarcts. Of the three patients with acute myocardial infarction, two had the clinical diagnosis established, whereas only one of the six patients with healed myocardial infarction had the clinical diagnosis established (see Fig. 15–25).

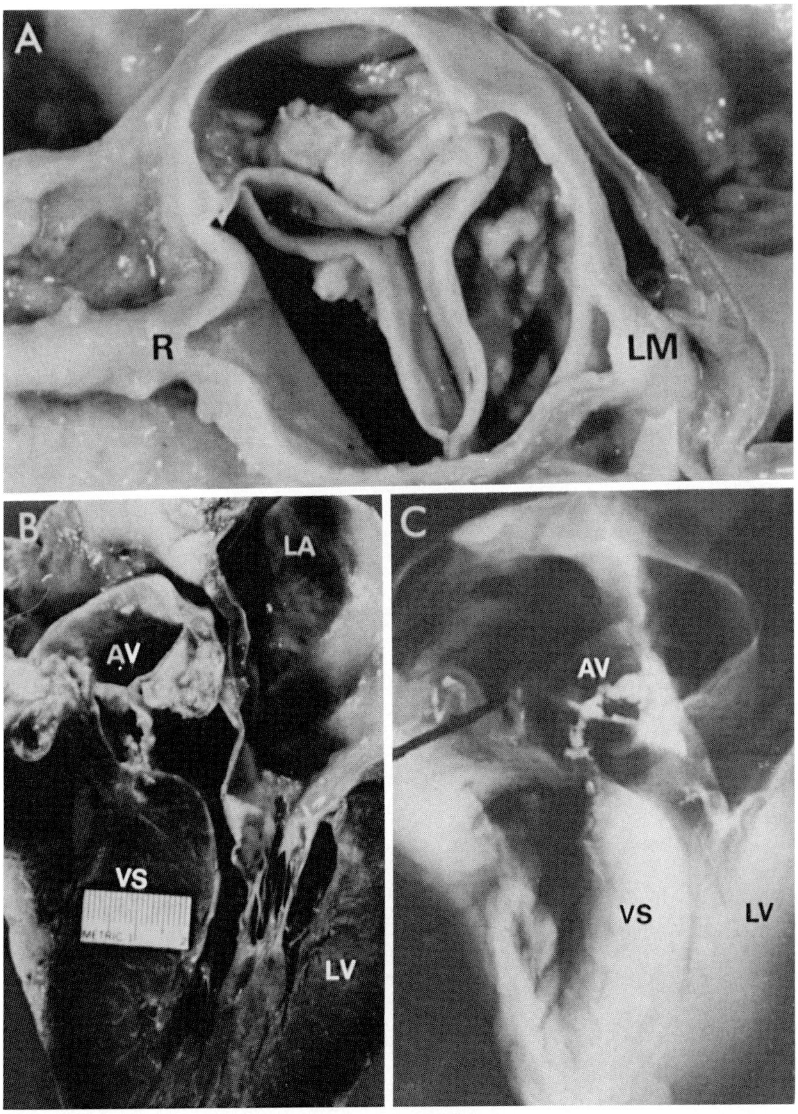

Figure 15–31. Heart of a 98-year-old woman with fatal aortic valve (AV) stenosis. *A,* Aortic view of heavily calcified three-cuspid aortic valve without commissural fusion. LM = left main coronary artery. *B,* Long-axis view through stenotic aortic valve showing a nondilated and hypertrophied left ventricle (LV), dilated left atrium (LA), and sigmoid ventricular septum (VS). *C,* Postmortem radiograph showing AV calcific deposits.

Valvular Heart Disease

Of the 37 patients, four (11 percent) had clinical and/or morphologic evidence of a dysfunctioning cardiac valve. Of the four patients, three had *aortic valve stenosis* with heavy (4+/4+) calcific deposits deposited in the sinuses of Valsalva (see Figs. 15–30, 15–31), and one had massive mitral valve anular calcium producing mitral stenosis (see Fig. 15–14). None of the patients had floppy mitral or tricuspid valves.

Amyloid Deposits

Focal cardiac amyloid deposits were observed histologically in five (14 percent) patients, none of whom had clinical evidence of cardiac dysfunction and all died from noncardiovascular conditions. One patient (3 percent) had massive cardiac amyloid involving all four chambers and clinically had chronic and eventually fatal congestive heart failure.

Thus, of 37 necropsy patients aged 90 to 102 years, 11 (30 percent) had cardiac deaths, 4 (11 percent) had vascular deaths, and 22 (59 percent) had noncardiovascular deaths. In each of 37 hearts, at least one anatomic abnormality was observed.

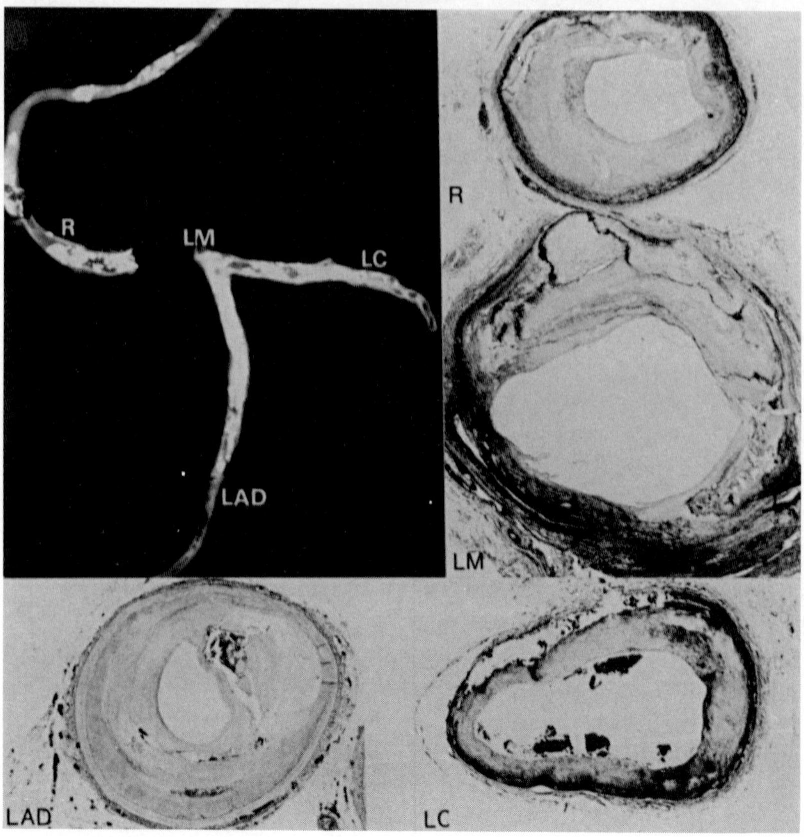

Figure 15–32. Sites of maximal coronary narrowing from a 98-year-old woman whose heart is illustrated in Figure 15–31. All major arteries have heavy calcific deposits, and the left anterior descending (LAD) is severely narrowed by atherosclerotic plaques. LC = left circumflex, LM = left main, R = right.

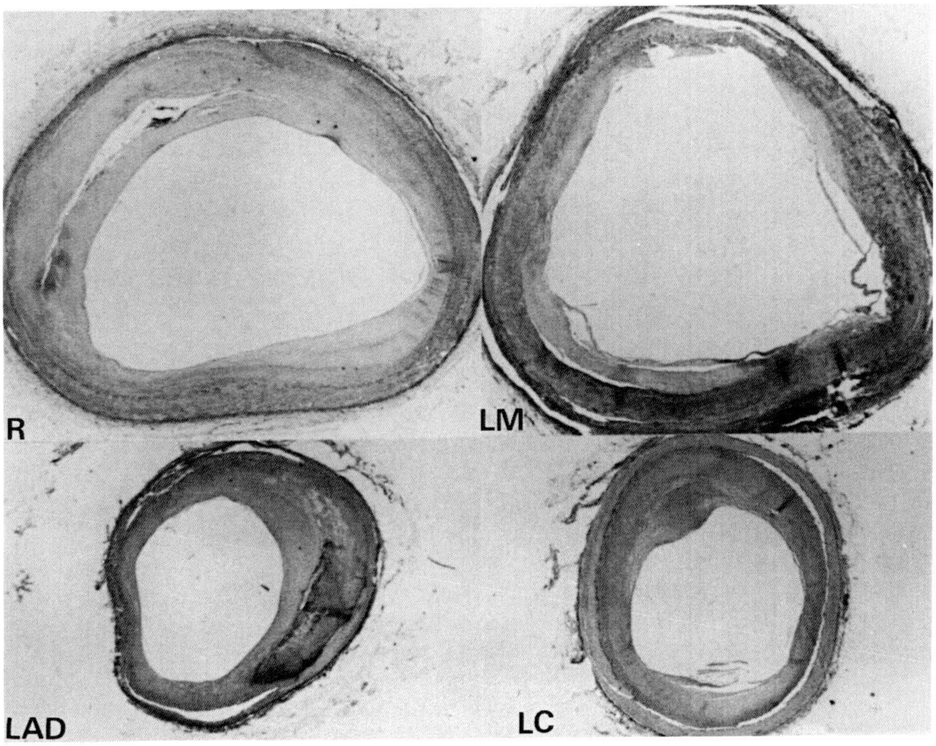

Figure 15–33. Sites of maximal coronary narrowing in a patient who never had symptoms of cardiac disease and died a noncardiac death. Abbreviations as in Figure 15–32.

CARDIOVASCULAR DISEASE IN HEARTS AGED 90 YEARS OR OLDER

Waller and Roberts[19] recently reported clinical and morphologic observations in 40 necropsy patients aged 90 to 103 years. The following discussion is based on analysis of 77 very elderly necropsy patients aged 90 to 103 years (mean = 94): 25 presently described patients, and 52 previously reported patients.[19,21]

General Observations

Certain clinical and morphologic data from the 77 very elderly patients are summarized in Tables 15–3 through 15–11 and Figures 15–1 through 15–49. The month of death was known in 49 of the previously reported 77 patients,[19,21] and in all 25 presently reported patients. Death occurred during *four cold months* (November, December, January, February) in 36 (49 percent), during *four hot months* (June, July, August, September) in 25 (34 percent), and during *four intermediate temperature months* (March, April, May, October) in 13 (17 percent) patients (see Fig. 15–34).

Heart Weight and Body Weight

Heart weight was increased in 53 (69 percent) (Table 15–3). Of the 21 men, 14 (67 percent) had increased heart weights, and of the 56 women, 39 (70 percent) had

Table 15–3. Morphologic Observations in 77 Patients at Necropsy Aged 90 to 103 Years (Mean 94)

Observation	No. (%) Pts.
Heart weight (g)	220–660 (414)
A. Men (n = 21)	320–660 (450)
No. >440 g	14 (67)
HW:BW ratio	0.006–0.13 (0.009)*
B. Women (n = 56)	220–630 (401)
No. >350 g	39 (70)
HW:BW ratio	0.003–0.013 (0.008)†

* Normal for younger men = 0.0045 (Eckner, 1969[72]).

† Normal for younger women = 0.004 (Eckner, 1969[72]).

increased heart weights (normal less than 350 g for women, less than 400 g for men). The average heart-body weight ratio for men was double that predicted for normal younger men,[72] and similarly in the elderly women, the ratio was nearly double that predicted for younger women.[72]

Expected and Unexpected Morphologic Changes

As discussed previously, certain cardiac morphologic changes are "expected" in the very elderly heart ("aging changes of the normal old age heart"). Table 15–4 summarizes the "expected" and "unexpected" morphologic changes in the com-

Table 15–4. Expected and Unexpected Morphologic Findings in 77 Patients at Necropsy Aged 90 to 103 Years (Mean 94)

Expected	No. (%) Pts.
1. Tortuous epicardial coronary arteries	77 (100)
2. Dilated left atrium	77 (100)
3. Dilated ascending aorta	77 (100)
4. Myocardial lipofuscin	77 (100)
5. Calcific deposits	75 (97)
6. Increased subepicardial fat	68 (88)
7. Nondilated left ventricle	67 (87)
8. Amyloid deposits	17 (22)
Unexpected	**No. (%) Pts.**
1. Increased heart weight (>350F, >400M)	53 (69)
2. Narrowing >75% XSA of ≥1 major coronary artery	49 (64)
3. Heavy coronary calcium without >75% XSA narrowing	15 (19)
4. Massive cardiac amyloid	5 (6)
5. Aortic valve stenosis	4 (5)
6. Mitral anular calcium causing stenosis	1(1)

Table 15–5. Coronary Heart Disease (> 75% XSA Narrowing by Atherosclerotic Plaques in ≥ 1 Major Artery) in 49 Patients at Necropsy Aged 90 to 100 Years

Coronary Heart Disease	At Necropsy	Causing Clinical Dysfunction	Causing Death
1. **Clinical Evidence of Myocardial Ischemia**	18	18	18
A. Myocardial infarction	18	15	13
Acute = 7			
Healed = 5			
Both = 6			
B. Angina pectoris	5*	5	0
C. Chronic CHF	3*	3†	3
D. Sudden death	2	2	2
2. **Never Clinical Evidence of Myocardial Ischemia**	31	0	0
A. Myocardial infarction			
Acute = 0			
Healed = 10			
Total Patients	49 (64%)	18 (24%)	18 (24%)

*Each had transmural LV fibrosis or necrosis.

† One patient had excessive dyspnea (while hospitalized with hip fracture) not clinically recognized as AMI.

bined series of 77 very elderly hearts. Each heart had some element of tortuosity of the epicardial coronary vessels, dilated left atrium and ascending aorta, and each heart had myocardial lipofuscin deposits. Calcific deposits (any site) were found in 97 percent of hearts, increased subepicardial fat in 88 percent, nondilated left ventricular cavities in 87 percent, and amyloid deposits in 22 percent (focal in 14 percent). *Unexpected* findings included increased heart weight in 69 percent, severe coronary

Table 15–6. Causes of Death in 77 Patients at Necropsy Aged 90 to 103 Years (Mean 94)

Mode		No. (%) Pts.	
I. **Cardiac**		*29 (38)*	
A. Coronary		18	
Acute MI	13		
Chronic CHF	3		
Sudden	2		
B. Aortic-valve stenosis		4	
C. Mitral-valve stenosis 2-degree anular calcium		1	
D. Myocardial		6	
Dilated cardiomyopathy	1		
Amyloid	5		
II. **Noncardiac**		*48 (62)*	
A. Neoplasm		15	
B. Stroke		8	
C. Bone fracture complications		10	Vascular
D. Ruptured aortic aneurysm		3	
E. Non-neoplastic gastrointestinal problems (obstruction, ulcers)		9	
F. Massive pulmonary embolism		2	
G. Uncertain		1	
Totals		77 (100)	

Table 15–7. Cardiac Calcific Deposits in 77 Patients at Necropsy Aged 90 to 103 Years (Mean 94)

Calcium Location	Amount of CA⁺⁺ Deposits and No. (%) Pts.			
	0	*1–2+*	*3–4+*	*Total*
1. AV cusps	35(46)	37(48)	5(6)	77(100)
A. AV stenosis	0	0	24	
2. MV anulus	29(38)	27(35)	21(27)	77(100)
A. MV stenosis			1	
3. Coronary arteries	7(9)	54(70)	16(21)	77(100)
A. ≥1 artery >75% XSA by plaque	0/6	35/45 (78)	14/16 (88)	
4. AV + anulus + arteries	(1)	⟵ 34(44) ⟶		

calcium without severe coronary luminal narrowing in 19 percent, *massive* cardiac amyloid in 6 percent, severe aortic valve stenosis in 6 percent, and massive mitral anular calcium causing mitral stenosis in 1 percent (Table 15–4).

Clinical Observations

The ages of the 77 patients ranged from 90 to 103 years (mean 94), 56 (73 percent) were women and 50 (65 percent) were black. Of the 77 patients, 20 (26 percent) had some form of chest pain, diagnosed as angina pectoris in 5 (6 percent) of these patients, yet 28 (36 percent) of patients had acute or healed myocardial infarcts at necropsy (Table 15–5). Eleven patients had chronic congestive heart failure (three from coronary disease with healed myocardial infarcts, two with aortic valve stenosis,

Table 15–8. *Morphologic* Observations in 77 Patients at Necropsy Aged 90 to 103 Years (Mean 94)

Observation	No. (%) Pts.
1. Coronary arterial disease	
A. Calcium	71(92)
B. Luminal narrowing 76–100% in XSA by plaques ≥1 major coronary artery	49(64)
C. Acute myocardial infarction	13(17)
D. Healed myocardial infarction	20(26)
2. Aortic valve disease	
A. Calcium	42(55)
B. Stenosis	4 (5)
3. Mitral anular disease	
A. Calcium	48(62)
B. Stenosis	1 (1)
4. Cardiac amyloidosis	
A. Fatal	5 (6)
B. Incidental	12 (16)
5. Dilated cardiomyopathy	1 (1)
6. Obliterative pericardial disease	(3)

Table 15-9. Morphologic Observations in 77 Patients at Necropsy Aged 90 to 103 years (Mean 94)

Observation	No. (%) Pts.
1. No. (%) R, LAD, LC coronary narrowed 76-100% XSA by plaque (avg CA/pt)	80/231 (35) (49 pts) (1.0/3.0)
2. No. coronary arteries (R, LAD, LC) narrowed 76-100% in XSA	
1 artery	26 (53) pts
2 arteries	15 (31) pts
3 arteries	8 (16) pts
3. No. LM coronary arteries narrowed 76-100% in XSA	0
4. No. (%) 5-mm coronary segments narrowed 76-100% in XSA by plaques	279 (8%)
[No. (%) narrowed 96-100%]	6/279 (2%)

Abbreviations: Avg = average, CA = coronary artery; LAD = left anterior descending, LC = left circumflex, LM = left main, R = right, XSA = cross-sectional area.

one with dilated cardiomyopathy, and five with massive cardiac amyloidosis) (Table 15-5). Of the 77 patients, 39 (51 percent) had histories of systemic hypertension. Of 17 patients with available total serum cholesterol levels, the range was 108 to 283 mg/dl (average 220), with 15 of the 17 values greater than 180 mg/dl. Six (8 percent) patients had diabetes mellitus.

Modes of Death

Of the 77 very elderly patients, 29 (38 percent) died from consequences of *cardiac disease* (coronary in 62 percent, myocardial in 21 percent, valvular in 17

Table 15-10. Amount of Narrowing by Atherosclerotic Plaques in Major Coronary Arteries*

	Fatal Coronary Events		Control Subjects	
Item	≥Age 90 (*n* = 18)	<Age 90† (*n* = 98)	≥Age 90 (*n* = 48)	<Age 90 (*n* = 30)
1. Age (years)	90-99 (93)	22-85 (58)	90-103 (94)	21-86 (49)
2. No. (%) men	3 (21) 4 (22)	72 (73)	13 (27)	13 (43)
3. Avg No. R, LAD, LC, CA >75% XSA/pt	2.2/3.0	2.8/3.0	1.0/3.0	1.1/3.0
4. No. LM CA 75% XSA	0	17 (17%)	0	0
5. No. (%) 5-mm CA segments >75% XSA	159 (20)	1836 (37)	103(5)	58(7)

Abbreviations as in Table 15-9.

*In patients with fatal coronary events older and younger than age 90 years and comparison to control subjects.

†Data from Roberts and Jones: Am J Cardiol 44:39, 1979 and Circulation 61:786, 1980; Virmani and Roberts: Am J Med 68:831, 1980 and Br Heart J 45:434, 1981; and Cabin and Roberts: Am J Cardiol 46:754, 1980 and 48:1, 1981.

Table 15–11. Cardiac Disease in 77 Patients at Necropsy Aged 90 to 103 Years (Mean 94)

	No. (%) Pts.		
	At Necropsy	*Causing Clinical Dysfunction*	*Causing Death*
1. Cardiac Abnormality	76 (99%)	29 (38%)	29 (38%)
A. Coronary arterial narrowing (>75% XSA)	49 (64%)	18 (23%)	18 (23%)
B. Cardiomegaly (>350 g F; >400 g M)	54 (69%)	0	0
C. Calcific deposits	75 (97%)	0	0
1. Coronary	71 (92%)	0	0
2. Mitral anulus	48 (62%)	1 (1%)	1 (1%)
3. Aortic valve	42 (55%)	4 (5%)	4 (5%)
4. 1 + 2 + 3	35 (45%)		
D. Amyloid	17 (22%)	5 (6%)	5 (6%)
E. Dilated cardiomyopathy	1 (1%)	1 (1%)	1 (1%)
F. Obliterative pericardial disease	2 (3%)	0	0
2. No Cardiac Abnormality	1 (1%)	0	0
Total Patients	77(100%)	29(38%)	29(38%)

percent); 11 (14 percent) *vascular disease* (stroke in eight patients, ruptured aortic aneurysm in three patients); and *noncardiovascular disease* in 37 (48 percent) (neoplasm in 15 patients, bone fracture complications in 10 patients, gastrointestinal problems in nine patients, massive pulmonary embolism in two patients, uncertain in one patient (Table 15–6, see Fig. 15–35). Two additional studies[10,22] with a total of 1700 necropsy patients also have reported causes of death in patients aged 70 years or older[22] and 85 years or older,[10] respectively (see Figs. 15–36, 15–37). A similarity between these studies is the high frequency of noncardiovascular deaths (43 percent, 48 percent, 75 percent). Cardiovascular causes accounted for 25 percent, 31 percent, and 52 percent of the deaths. Of note, Kohn[10] found no "acceptable cause of death" in 26 percent of 200 patients reported in his study (see Fig. 15–37). This ill-defined category points out the deficiencies in studies relying solely upon autopsy protocols derived from multiple prosectors or studies using death certificate analysis.

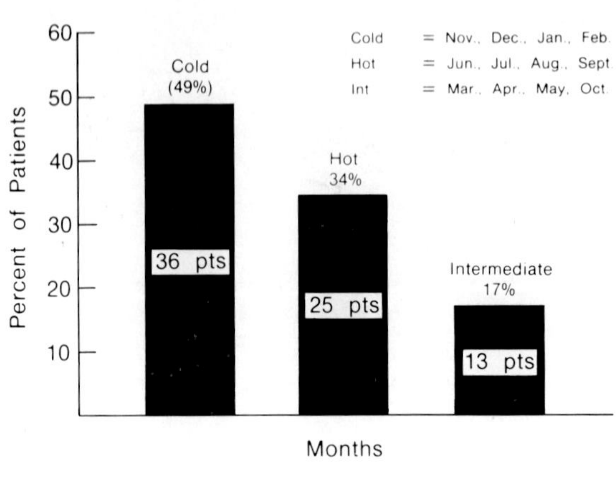

Figure 15–34. Seasonal variation in deaths in 74 necropsy patients aged 90 to 103 years.

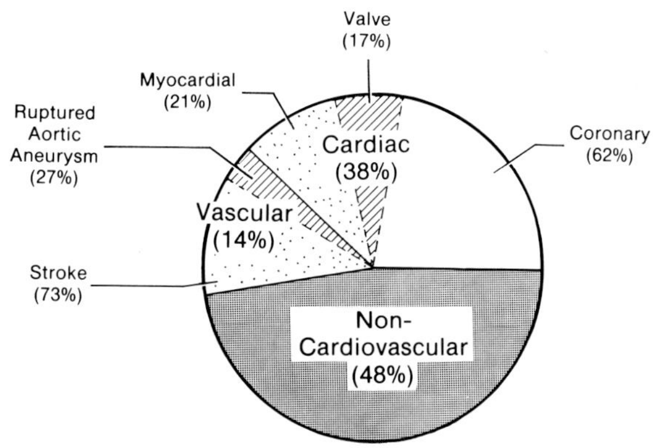

Figure 15-35. Causes of death in 77 necropsy patients aged 90 to 103 years.

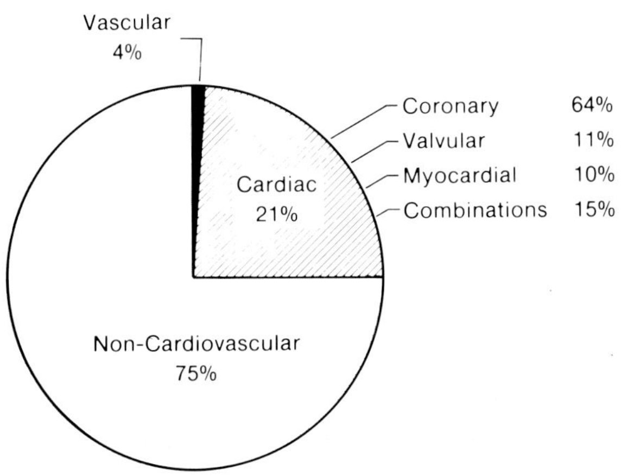

Figure 15-36. Causes of death in 1500 necropsy patients aged 70 years or older. (Modified from McKeown, 1963.[22])

Figure 15-37. Causes of death in 200 necropsy patients aged 85 years or older. (Modified from Kohn, 1982.[23])

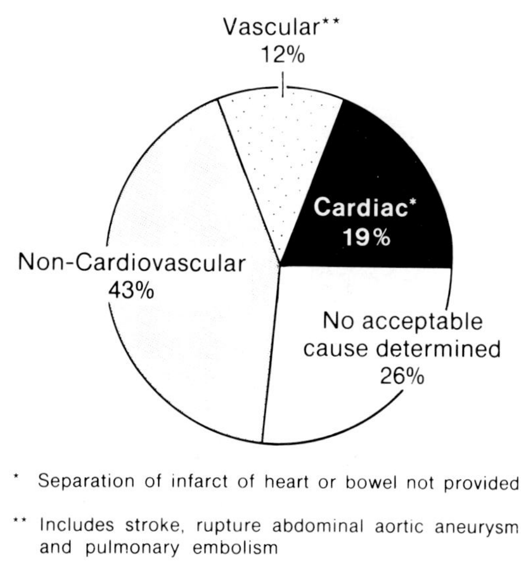

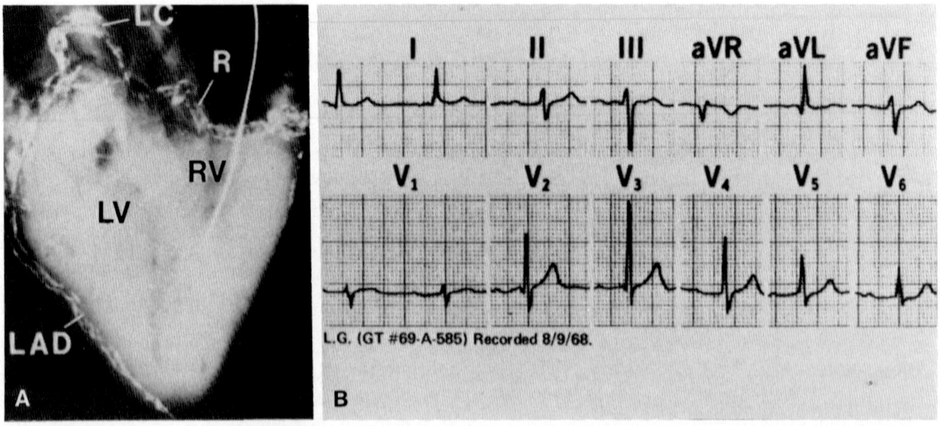

Figure 15–38. This 97-year-old man had complete heart block and had a pacemaker inserted when he was 91 years old. *A,* Radiogram of heart at necropsy showing calcific deposits in the left anterior descending (LAD), left circumflex (LC), and right (R) coronary arteries, and a pacemaker wire in the right ventricle (RV). LV = left ventricle. *B,* Electrocardiogram. (From Waller and Roberts,[19] with permission.)

Necropsy Observations

Calcification

Coronary arterial calcific deposits were observed grossly or on postmortem radiograms in 71 (92 percent) patients (Tables 15–7, 15–8; see Figs. 15–38 through 15–40). In 16 patients the calcific deposits were heavy (3–4+/4+), and in 14 of these patients at least one of the calcified coronary arteries was narrowed more than 75 percent in cross-sectional area by atherosclerotic plaques (see Fig. 15–40). As opposed to younger necropsy patients in whom calcified coronary arteries are sensitive markers for severe luminal narrowing, in the very elderly heart, which commonly has coronary calcific deposits, one in five (20 percent) will have calcific deposits without severe luminal narrowing by atherosclerotic plaques.

Correlation of coronary luminal narrowing with the presence of calcific deposits improves when analyzing those patients with heavy calcific deposits. Of 16 patients with heavy (3–4+/4+) coronary calcific deposits, 14 (88 percent) had at least one major artery narrowed more than 75 percent in cross-sectional area by atherosclerotic plaques (Table 15–7).

Mitral valve anular calcific deposits were found in 48 (62 percent) patients (see Tables 15–7, 15–8). In 21 (27 percent) patients, the anular calcific deposits had secondary mitral valve stenosis. Calcific deposits extended onto the mitral valve leaflets, considerably reducing their mobility.

Aortic valve cusps had calcific deposits in 42 (55 percent) patients (see Tables 15–7, 15–8; see Fig. 15–41). In four (5 percent) patients, aortic valve calcific deposits in the cuspal bases filled the sinuses of Valsalva causing severe aortic valve obstruction ("senile aortic stenosis"). In each of these aortic valves, the commissures were open.

Senile calcification syndrome (calcific deposits in coronary arteries, mitral valve anuli, and aortic valve cusps) was found in 34 (44 percent) of the patients. Only one patient (1 percent) had *no* cardiac deposits (see Table 15–7).

Coronary Arterial Atherosclerosis

At necropsy, one or more of the three major epicardial coronary arteries (left anterior descending, left circumflex, right) was narrowed more than 75 percent in cross-sectional area by atherosclerotic plaques in 49 (64 percent) patients (Tables 15–8, 15–9; see Figs. 15–27 through 15–29, 15–32, 15–40, 15–42), averaging one artery per patient. In 53 percent of patients, one artery was severely narrowed (single-vessel disease), in 31 percent of patients, two arteries (double-vessel disease), and in 16 percent all three major arteries were severely narrowed by plaques (triple-vessel disease) (see Fig. 15–42). The distribution of arteries severely narrowed was as follows: left anterior descending 59 percent, right 27 percent, left circumflex 14 percent. *No patient older than age 90 years had severe narrowing of the main left coronary artery.* The amount of coronary arterial atherosclerosis was quantitated in 73 patients (Table 15–9). Of 5-mm coronary segments from these 73 patients, 279 (8 percent) segments were narrowed more than 75 percent in cross-sectional area by atherosclerotic plaques. Of these 279 segments, only six (2 percent) were narrowed 96 to 100 percent (nearly totally occluded) in cross-sectional area.

Clinical Myocardial Ischemia

Of the 49 necropsy patients with at least one major coronary artery severely narrowed, 18 (37 percent) patients had *clinical evidence of myocardial ischemia*

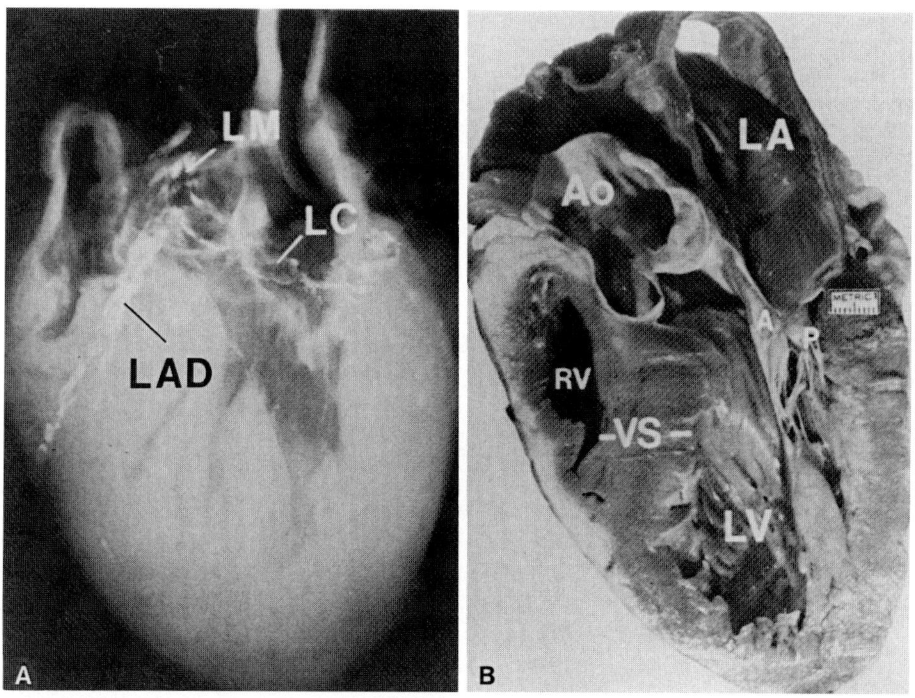

Figure 15–39. This 90-year-old woman had no symptoms of cardiac dysfunction and died of a ruptured fusiform abnormal aortic aneurysm. *A,* Postmortem radiogram of the entire heart showing calcific deposits in the left anterior descending (LAD), left circumflex (LC), and left main (LM) coronary arteries. *B,* View of heart cut in an anteroposterior fashion (M-mode or long-axis two-dimensional echocardiographic view) showing a dilated left atrium (LA) and left ventricle (LV). A and P = anterior and posterior mitral valve leaflets; Ao = aorta; RV = right ventricle; VS = ventricular septum. (From Waller and Roberts,[19] with permission.)

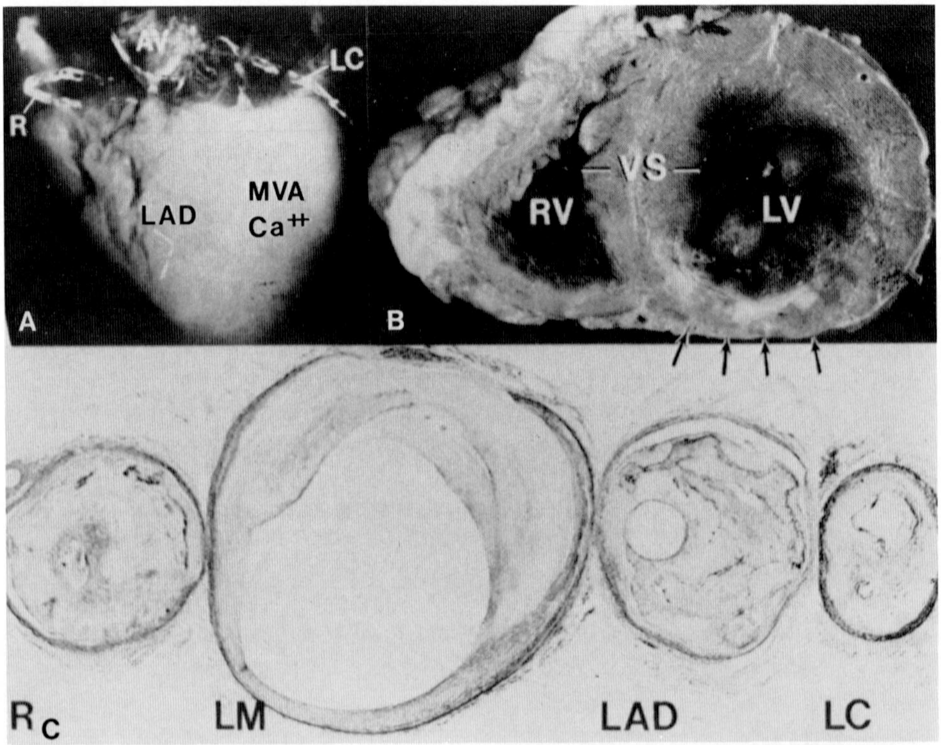

Figure 15-40. Heart and coronary arteries in a 93-year-old woman who was hospitalized with worsening chronic congestive heart failure. *A,* Postmortem radiogram showing calcific deposits in the right (R), left anterior descending (LAD), and left circumflex (LC) coronary arteries and in the mitral valve anulus (MVA) and aortic valve. *B,* View of right (RV) and left ventricles (LV) and ventricular septum (VS) showing a transmural scar *(arrows). C,* Coronary arteries at sites of maximal narrowing. LM = left main. (From Waller and Roberts,[19] with permission.)

(angina pectoris, acute myocardial infarction, sudden death) (see Tables 15-6, 15-8; see Figs. 15-25, 15-29, 15-40, 15-43). Of these 18 patients, 13 had transmural myocardial necrosis (clinically recognized events in five [28 percent]), and 11 had transmural healed myocardial infarcts (clinically recognized events in 2 [18 percent]). The number of coronary segments narrowed more than 75 percent in cross-sectional area by calcified atherosclerotic plaques ranged from 11 to 33 percent (average 20 percent). The mean coronary score for this group of patients was 2.51. The average percent luminal narrowing in the 18 patients was 63 percent (see Fig. 15-44). Breakdown of average percent luminal narrowing according to type of fatal coronary event indicates a similar amount of narrowing in 13 patients with acute myocardial infarction (64 percent), healed myocardial infarction with chronic congestive heart failure (59 percent), and sudden coronary death (with or without previous healed myocardial infarction) (62 percent) (see Fig. 15-45). None of the patients with fatal coronary events had occlusive coronary arterial thrombi.

"Silent" Coronary Atherosclerosis

Of the 49 necropsy patients with at least one major coronary artery severely narrowed by atherosclerotic plaques, 31 (63 percent) *did not have clinical evidence of*

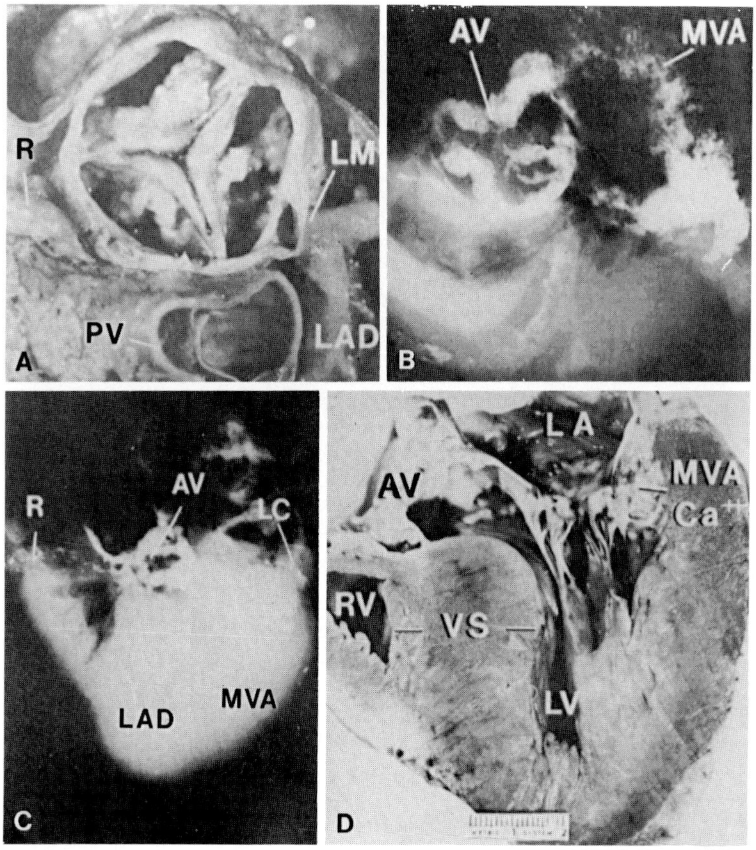

Figure 15–41. Heart from a 92-year-old woman with clinically recognized and eventually fatal aortic valve (AV) stenosis. *A,* Aortic view of stenotic AV. *B,* Radiograph showing heavy calcific deposits in AV and mitral valve anulus (MVA). *C,* Radiograph at necropsy showing calcium in coronary arteries, MVA, and AV. *D,* Long-axis view of heart showing "sigmoid-shaped" ventricular septum (VS) and nondilated and hypertrophied left ventricle (LV). LA = left atrium, LAD = left anterior descending, LC = left circumflex, LM = left main, RV = right ventricle. (From Waller and Roberts,[19] with permission.)

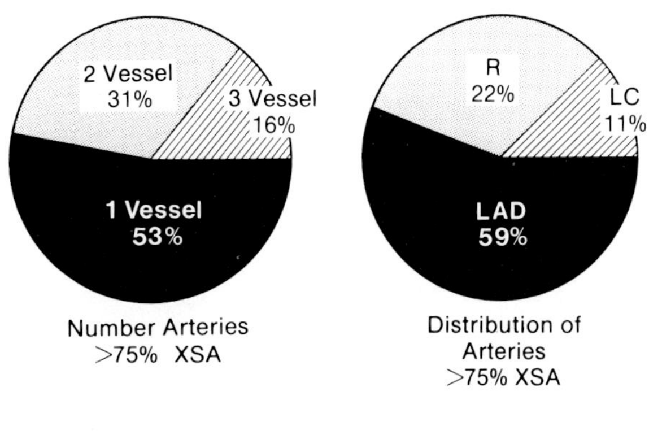

Figure 15–42. Number *(left)* and distribution *(right)* of severely narrowed epicardial coronary arteries in 49 necropsy patients aged 90 to 100 years.

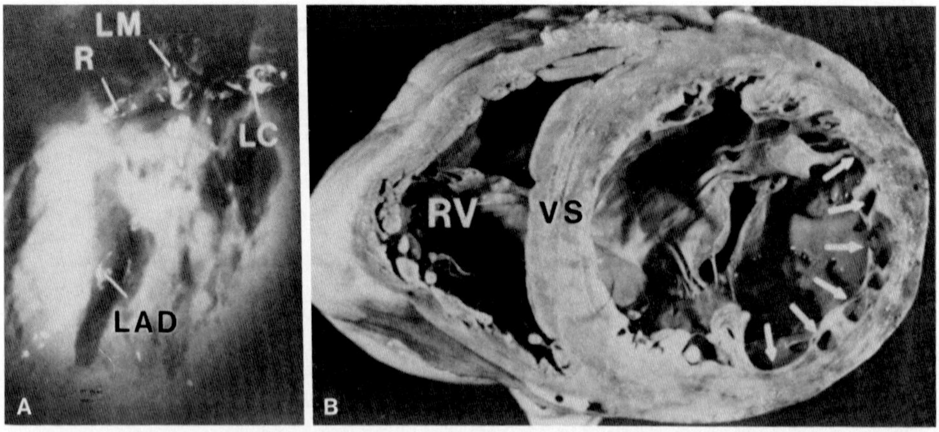

Figure 15–43. This 91-year-old woman had a "typical" clinical acute myocardial infarct, which was fatal. *A,* Postmortem radiogram showing calcific deposits in the right (R), left main (LM), left anterior descending (LAD), and left circumflex (LC) coronary arteries. *B,* View of left and right (RV) ventricles showing transmural necrosis and fibrosis *(arrows)* and dilated ventricles. VS = ventricular septum. (From Waller and Roberts,[19] with permission.)

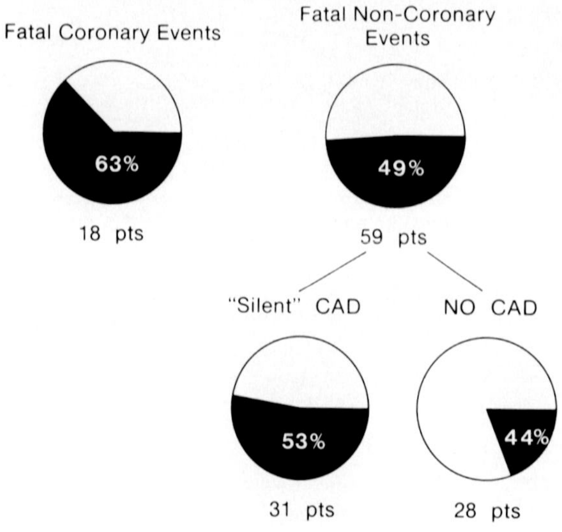

Figure 15–44. Average percent luminal cross-sectional area narrowing by atherosclerotic plaque in necropsy patients aged 90 to 103 years. CAD = coronary atherosclerotic disease.

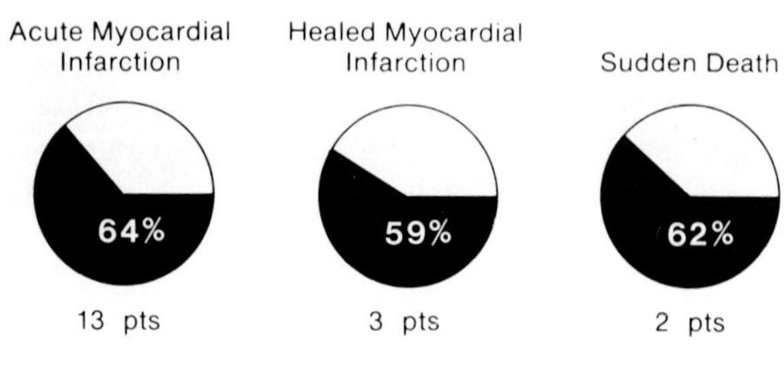

Figure 15–45. Average percent luminal narrowing in 18 patients with fatal coronary events aged 90 to 100 years.

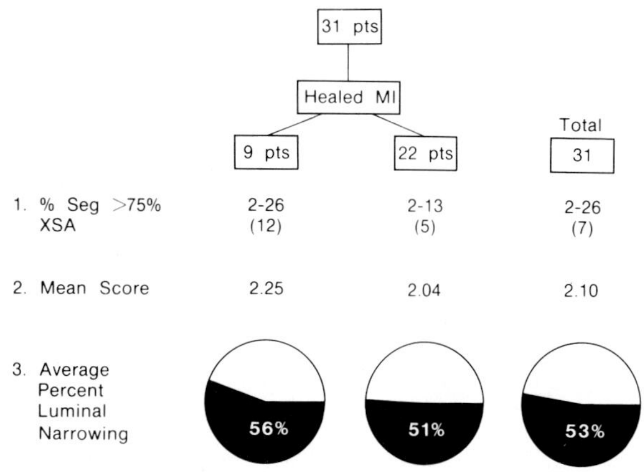

Figure 15–46. "Silent" coronary artery disease in patients with noncoronary deaths. MI = myocardial infarction, XSA = cross-sectional area.

myocardial ischemia, i.e., clinically "silent" coronary atherosclerosis (see Figs. 15–27, 15–28, 15–46). Of these 31 patients, nine (29 percent) had transmural healed myocardial infarcts *(all clinically silent events).* The number of coronary segments narrowed 76 to 100 percent in cross-sectional area ranged from 2 to 26 percent (average 7 percent). The mean coronary score for this group of patients was 2.10 (see Figs. 15–44, 15–46). The average percent luminal narrowing in patients with clinically "silent" coronary atherosclerosis was 53 percent, compared with 63 percent in patients with clinical evidence of myocardial ischemia and fatal coronary events (see Fig. 15–44). Breakdown of the 31 patients with "silent" coronary artery disease with noncoronary deaths disclosed the nine patients with healed myocardial infarcts ("silent" infarcts) had a similar average percent luminal narrowing as did the remaining 22 patients without healed infarcts (see Fig. 15–44).

Absent Myocardial Ischemia, Myocardial Damage and Severe Coronary Artery Disease

The remaining 28 (36 percent) patients had none of the major coronary arteries narrowed more than 75 percent in cross-sectional area by plaques. The mean coronary score was 1.76. None of these patients had transmural left ventricular myocardial damage. The average percent luminal narrowing by atherosclerotic plaque was 44 percent (see Fig. 15–44).

Comparison of Younger Versus Very Elderly Patients With Fatal Coronary Events

Table 15–10 compares the amounts of coronary narrowing in patients at necropsy *with* and *without fatal coronary events* (acute myocardial infarction, sudden coronary death, chronic congestive heart failure after healing of a myocardial infarct) in two age categories: *older and younger than 90 years.* Striking differences between these two groups occurred in three areas: the frequency of *men,* the frequency of *left main coronary* arteries severely narrowed by plaques, and the frequency of coronary segments of the *three major coronary arteries narrowed more than 75 percent* in cross-sectional area by plaques. In each of these areas, the very elderly patients with fatal coronary events had significantly *lower* percentages. In patients without fatal coronary events ("control subjects") in the same age categories, the average number of right, left anterior descending, and left circumflex arteries per patient narrowed

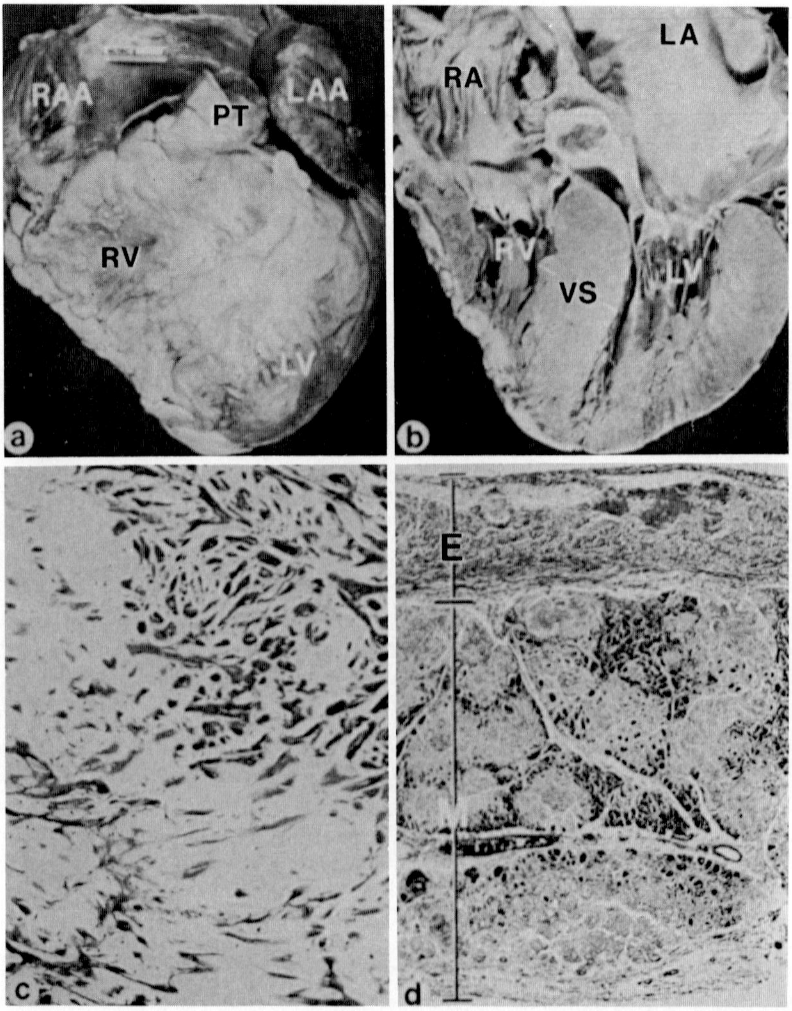

Figure 15–47. Massive cardiac amyloidosis in a 90-year-old man with chronic and eventually fatal congestive heart failure. *A,* External view of heart showing prominent left ventricle (LV). LAA = left atrial appendage, RAA = right atrial appendage. *B,* Four-chamber view of heart showing thickened LV walls. *C,* Photomicrograph of LV showing extensive amyloid deposits. *D,* Photomicrograph of left atrial wall showing amyloid deposits in endocardium (E) and myocardium (M). (From Waller and Roberts,[19] with permission.)

more than 75 percent in cross-sectional area was similar at 1.1 of 3.0 on patients aged less than 90 years and 1.0 of 3.0 in patients aged 90 years or older. The number of 5-mm coronary segments narrowed more than 75 percent in cross-sectional area was also similar at 7 percent and 5 percent, respectively (Table 15–10).

Valvular Heart Disease

Four patients (5 percent) had fatal aortic valve stenosis, clinically recognized in two patients (see Tables 15–6, 15–8; see Figs. 15–30, 15–31, 15–41). In each patient the valve was three-cuspid, the commissures were not fused, and heavy calcific deposits within the sinuses of Valsalva immobilized the aortic valve cusps. No patient had rheumatic mitral stenosis. One patient (1 percent) had massive anular calcium, producing mitral valve stenosis (see Fig. 15–14). No patient had floppy mitral or tricuspid valves, although many had leaflet "buckling" simulating mitral valve prolapse.

Myocardial (Nonatherosclerotic) Disease

One of the 37 currently reported patients had fatal amyloidosis (see Tables 15–6, 15–8). In the series by Waller and Roberts,[19] a total of five patients had either fatal cardiac amyloidosis (four patients) (Fig. 15–47) or dilated cardiomyopathy (one patient) (see Fig. 15–48). In each of the five patients, the myocardial abnormality produced chronic congestive heart failure.

Cardiac Diseases in the Very Elderly Heart

Of 77 very elderly necropsy patients, 76 (99 percent) *had at least one cardiac abnormality at necropsy, and only one patient (1 percent) was free of any recognizable cardiac abnormality* (see Table 15–11; see Fig. 15–49). Of the 76 patients with at least one anatomic cardiac abnormality, 29 (38 percent) had clinical evidence of cardiac dysfunction and death resulting from the abnormality. Of the 29 patients with symptoms of cardiac disease, 64 percent had severe *coronary atherosclerosis,* 21 percent had *myocardial disease,* and 17 percent had *valvular disease.* Of the 48 (62

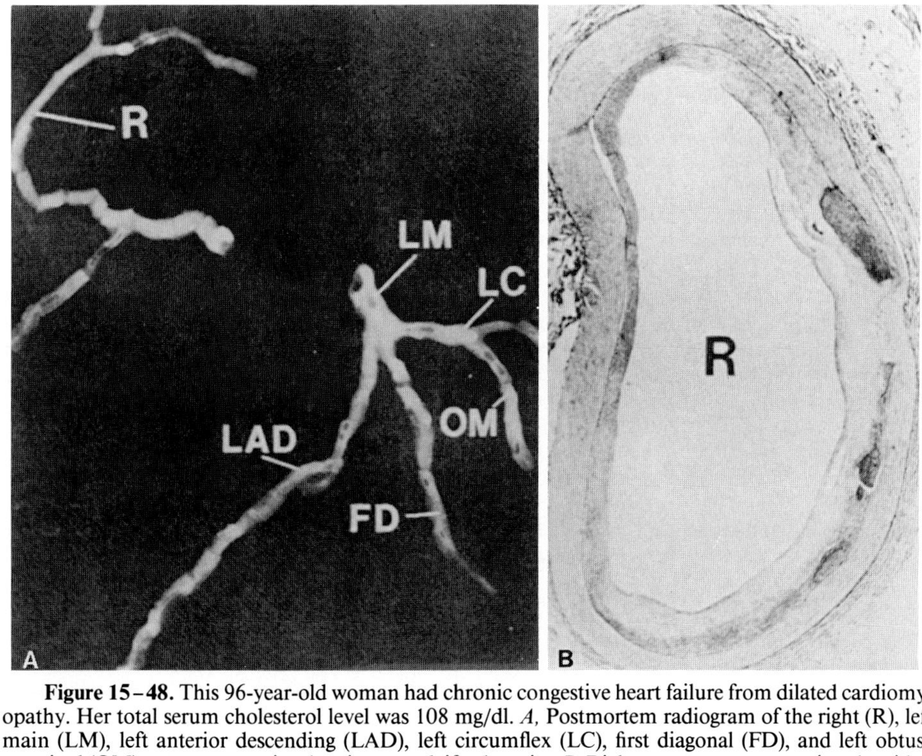

Figure 15–48. This 96-year-old woman had chronic congestive heart failure from dilated cardiomyopathy. Her total serum cholesterol level was 108 mg/dl. *A,* Postmortem radiogram of the right (R), left main (LM), left anterior descending (LAD), left circumflex (LC), first diagonal (FD), and left obtuse marginal (OM) coronary arteries showing no calcific deposits. *B,* Right coronary artery section devoid of calcium or narrowing. (From Waller and Roberts,[19] with permission.)

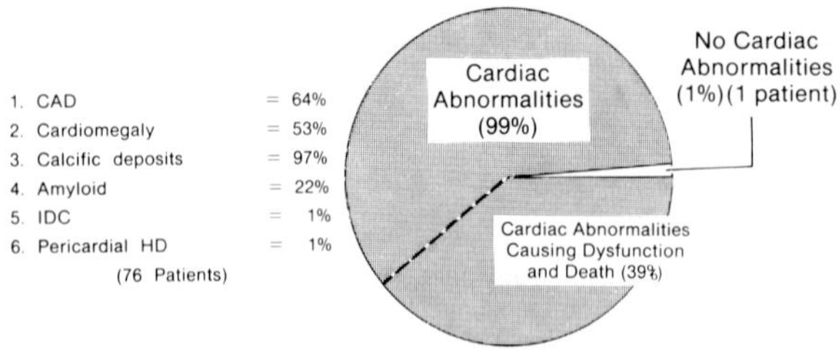

Figure 15-49. Cardiac disease in 77 necropsy patients aged 90 to 103 years. CAD = coronary atherosclerotic disease, HD = heart disease, IDC = idiopathic dilated cardiomyopathy.

percent) patients without clinical evidence of cardiac disease, 23 (48 percent) had "silent" coronary disease, 25 (32 percent) had morphologic abnormalities considered under age-related changes, and 1 (1 percent) patient had none of the morphologic cardiac changes usually observed in the very elderly heart.

ACKNOWLEDGMENTS

We wish to thank Marcy Culp for her expert typing of this manuscript and George Buckley and Ken Wilhite for their graphic and photographic assistance.

REFERENCES

1. Fries, JF: Aging, natural history, and the compression of morbidity. N Engl J Med 303:130, 1980.
2. McWhirter, N: Guinness Book of World Records. Bantam Books, New York, 1986, p 14.
3. Leaf, A: Search for the oldest people: Every day is a gift when you are over 100. National Geographic, January:93, 1973.
4. Mazess, RB and Forman, SH: Longevity and age exaggeration in Vilcabamba, Ecuador. J Gerontol 34:94, 1979.
5. Coe, RM: Social epidemiology of diseases of aging. In Blumenthal, HT (ed): Handbook of Diseases of Aging. Van Nostrand Reinhold, New York, 1983, p 45.
6. Siegel, JS: Recent and prospective demographic trends for the elderly population and some implications in health care. I. In Haynes, SG and Feinleib, M (eds): Second Conference on the Epidemiology of Aging. US Department of Health and Human Services, Washington, DC, NIH Pub No 80-969, 1980, p 293.
7. Edwards, JE: Pathology of the aging heart. In Liebow, LS (ed): Cardiovascular Aspects of Geriatric Medicine, Vol 2. Hoffman-LaRoche, Inc, Nutley, NJ, 1981, p 29.
8. Hutchins, GM: Structure of the aging heart. In Weisfeldt, ML (ed): Aging: The Aging Heart. Vol 12, Raven Press, New York, 1980, p 7.
9. Ishii, T and Sternby, NH: The pathology of centenarians. I. The cardiovascular system and lungs. J Am Geriatr Soc 26:108, 1978.
10. Kohn, RR: Cause of death in very old people. JAMA 247:2793, 1982.
11. McMillan, JB and Lev, M: The aging heart. I. Endocardium. J Gerontol 14:268, 1959.
12. McMillan, JB and Lev, M: The aging heart. II. The valves. J Gerontol 19:1, 1964.
13. Pomerance, A: Cardiac pathology in the elderly. In Noble, RJ and Rothbaum, DA (eds): Geriatric Cardiology. FA Davis, Philadelphia, 1981, p 9.
14. Pomerance, A: Pathology of the heart with and without cardiac failure in the aged. Br Heart J 27:697, 1965.
15. Pomerance, A: The pathology of senile cardiac amyloidosis. Br J Pathol Bacteriol 91:357, 1966.
16. Pomerance, A: Cardiac pathology and systolic murmurs in the elderly. Br Heart J 30:687, 1968.
17. Surgiura, M, Hiraoka, K, Ohkawa, S, et al: A clinicopathologic study on the heart disease in the aged: The morphologic classification of 1000 consecutive autopsy cases. Jpn Heart J 16:526, 1975.
18. Sell, S and Scully, RE: Aging changes in the aortic and mitral valves. Am J Pathol 46:345, 1965.
19. Waller, BF and Roberts, WC: Cardiovascular disease in the very elderly: Analysis of 40 necropsy patients aged 90 years or older. Am J Cardiol 51:403, 1983.

20. Jonsson, A, Agnarsson, BA, and Hallgrimsson, J: Coronary atherosclerosis and myocardial infarction in nonagenarians: A retrospective autopsy study. Age Ageing 14:109, 1985.
21. Waller, BF, Bloch, T, Barker, BG, et al: The old age heart: Aging changes of the normal elderly heart and cardiovascular disease in 12 necrospy patients aged 90 to 101 years. Cardiology Clinics 2(4):753, 1984.
22. McKeown, F: Heart disease in old age. J Clin Pathol 16:532, 1963.
23. Kohn, RR: Heart and cardiovascular system. In Finch, CE and Hayflick, L (eds): Handbook of the Biology of Aging. Van Nostrand Reinhold, New York, 1977, p 281.
24. Strehler, BL and Mildvan, AS: General theory of mortality and aging. Science 132:14, 1960.
25. Belt, E: Leonardo da Vinci's study of the aging process. Geriatrics 7:205, 1952.
26. Harris, R: Clinical Geriatric Cardiology: Management of the Elderly Patient. JB Lippincott, Philadelphia, 1986, p 3.
27. Sobel, H: Aging and age—associated disease. Lancet 2:1191, 1970.
28. Bernard, C: An Introduction to the Study of Experimental Medicine. (Trans HE Greene.) Henry Ackerman, New York (Originally published in 1865), 1978.
29. Charcot, JM: Clinical Lectures on the Diseases of Old Age. 1881. (Trans LH Hunt.) Wood, New York (cited by Freeman, JT: Of aging and illness. Geriatric Psychiatry 1:263, 1968).
30. Kleemeier, RW: Infinitely eliminable. Contemporary Psychology 10:53, 1965.
31. McKeown, T: De Senectute. F.E. Williams' lecture. J Roy Coll Phys (Lond) 10:79, 1975.
32. Hayflick, L: Perspectives on human longevity. In Havighurst, R and Neugarten, BL (eds): Extending the Human Lifespan: Social Policy and Social Ethics. Washington, DC, US Government Printing Office, NSF/RA 770123, 1976, p 53.
33. Kohn, RR: Heart and Cardiovascular System. In Finch, CE and Hayflick, L (eds): Handbook of the Biology of Aging. Van Nostrand Reinhold, New York, 1977, p 281.
34. Strehler, BL, Mark, D, Mildran, AS, et al: Rate and magnitude of age pigment accumulation in the human myocardium. J Gerontol 14:430, 1959.
35. Koobs, DH, Schultz, RL, and Jutzy, RV: The origin of lipofuscin and possible consequences to the myocardium. Arch Pathol Lab Med 102:66, 1978.
36. Rosai, J and Lascano, EF: Basophilic (mucoid) degeneration of myocardium. A disorder of glycogen metabolism. Am J Pathol 61:99, 1970.
37. Hutchins, GM: Structure of the Aging Heart. In Weisfeldt, ML (ed): Aging: The Aging Heart, Vol 12, New York, Raven Press, 1980, p 9.
38. Buerger, L and Braunstein, H: Senile cardiac amyloidosis. Am J Med 28:357, 1960.
39. Wright, JR, Calkins, E, Breen, WJ, et al: Relationship of amyloid to aging. Medicine 48:39, 1969.
40. Katenkamp, D and Stiller, D: Histotopographische untersuchungen zur senilen herzamyloidose. Pathol Eur 6:109, 1971.
41. Cohen, AS: The constitution and genesis of amyloid. Intern Rev Exp Pathol 4:159, 1965.
42. Roberts, WC and Waller, BF: Cardiac amyloidosis causing cardiac dysfunction. Analysis of 54 necropsy patients. Am J Cardiol 52:137, 1983.
43. Reiner, L: Gross examination of the heart, ed 3. Charles C Thomas, Springfield, IL, 1968, p 1111.
44. Lenkiewicz, JE, Davies, MJ, and Rosen, D: Collagen in human myocardium as a function of age. Cardiovasc Res 6:549, 1972.
45. Kohn, RR and Rollerson, ER: Age changes in swelling properties of human myocardium. Proc Soc Exp Biol Med 100:253, 1959.
46. Goor, D, Lillehei, CW, and Edwards, JE: The "sigmoid septum": Variation in the contour of the left ventricular outlet. Am J Roentgenol 107:366, 1969.
47. Gardin, JM, Henry, WL, Savage, DD, et al: Echocardiographic measurements in normal subjects: Evaluation of an adult population without clinically apparent heart diseases. JCU 7:439, 1979.
48. Gerstenblith, G, Frederiksen, JW, Yin, FC, et al: Echocardiographic assessment of a normal adult aging population. Circulation 56:273, 1978.
49. Roberts, WC and Waller, BF: Mitral valve "anular" calcium forming a complete circle or "O" configuration: Clinical and necropsy observations. Am Heart J 101:619, 1981.
50. Waller, BF, Morrow, AG, Maron, BJ, et al: Etiology of clinically isolated, severe, chronic, pure mitral regurgitation. Analysis of 97 patients over 30 years of age with mitral valve replacement. Am Heart J 104:276, 1982.
51. Rifkin, RD, Porisi, AF, and Folland, E: Coronary calcification in the diagnosis of coronary artery disease. Am J Cardiol 44:141, 1979.
52. Eggen, DA, Strong, JP, and McGill, HC: Coronary calcification: Relationship to clinically significant coronary lesions and race, sex and topographic distribution. Circulation 32:948, 1965.

53. Waller, BF and Roberts, WC: Comparison of luminal narrowing by atherosclerotic plaques in young and very old necropsy patients with fatal coronary events. In Roskamn, H (ed): Myocardial Infarction at Young Age. Springer-Verlag, Berlin, 1981, p 104.
54. White, NK, Edwards, JE, and Dry, TJ: The relationship of the degree of coronary atherosclerosis with age in men. Circulation 1:645, 1950.
55. Ackerman, RF, Dry, TJ, and Edwards, JE: Relationship of various factors to the degree of coronary atherosclerosis in women. Circulation 1:1345, 1950.
56. Davies, MJ, Anderson, RH, and Becker, AE: The Conduction System of the Heart. Butterworths, London, 1983, p 18.
57. Davies, MJ and Pomerance, A: Quantitative study of aging changes in the human sinoatrial node and internodal tracts. Br Heart J 34:150, 1972.
58. Lev, M: Aging changes in the human sinoatrial node. J Gerontol 9:1, 1954.
59. Davies, MJ: Pathology of Conducting Tissue of the Heart. Appleton-Century-Crofts, New York, 1971, p 38.
60. Yater, WM and Cornell, VH: Heart block due to calcarious lesions of the bundle of His: Review and report of a case with detailed histopathologic study. Ann Intern Med 8:777, 1935.
61. Lenegre, J: Etiology and pathology of bilateral branch block in relation to complete heart block. Prog Cardiovasc Dis 6:409, 1962.
62. Lev, M: The pathology of complete atrio-ventricular block. Prog Cardiovasc Dis 6:317, 1964.
63. Lev, M: Anatomic basis for atrioventricular block. Am J Med 37:740, 1964.
64. Ishihara, T, Ferrans, VJ, Jones, M, et al: Histologic and ultrastructural features of normal human parietal pericardium. Am J Cardiol 46:744. 1980.
65. Hort, W and Braeun, H: Studies on normal and pathologically changed pericardium. Verh Dtsch Ges Pathol 45:271, 1961.
66. Wellman, WE and Edwards, JE: Thickness of the media of the thoracic aorta in relation to age. Arch Pathol 50:183, 1950.
67. Linder, J and Johannes, G: Contribution on the aging of arterial connective tissue. In Vogel, HG (ed): Connective Tissue and Aging. Excerpta Medica, Amsterdam, 1973, p 68.
68. John, R and Thomas, J: Chemical composition of elastins isolated from aortas and pulmonary tissues of humans of different ages. Biochem J 127:261, 1972.
69. Eisenstein, R, Ayer, J, Papajiannis, S, et al: Mineral binding by human arterial elastic tissue. Lab Invest 13:1198, 1964.
70. Levene, CI and Poole, JCF: The collagen content of the normal and atherosclerotic human aortic intima. Br J Exp Pathol 43:469, 1962.
71. Haider, YS and Roberts, WC: Coronary arterial disease in systemic lupus erythematosus. Quantification of degrees of narrowing in 22 necropsy patients (21 women) aged 16 to 37 years. Am J Med 70:775, 1981.
72. Eckner, FAD, Brown, BW, Davidson, DL, et al: Dimensions of normal hearts: After standard fixation by controlled pressure coronary perfusion. Arch Pathol Lab Med 88:497, 1969.

Index

Page numbers followed by F indicate figures; page numbers followed by T indicate tables.